Medical Insurance
A Guide to Coding and Reimbursement
Second Edition

Joanne Valerius, MPH, RHIA

Health Information Program Director, College of Saint Catherine

Nenna Bayes

Associate Professor, Ashland Community and Technical College

Cynthia Newby, CPC

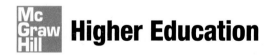 **Higher Education**

Boston   Burr Ridge, IL   Dubuque, IA   Madison, WI   New York   San Francisco   St. Louis
Bangkok   Bogotá   Caracas   Kuala Lumpur   Lisbon   London   Madrid   Mexico City
Milan   Montreal   New Delhi   Santiago   Seoul   Singapore   Sydney   Taipei   Toronto

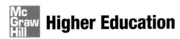

Higher Education

MEDICAL INSURANCE: A GUIDE TO CODING AND REIMBURSEMENT, SECOND EDITION

 This book is printed on recycled, acid-free paper containing 10% postconsumer waste.

2 3 4 5 6 7 8 9 0 QPD/QPD 0 9 8 7 6

ISBN-13: 978-0-07-295023-6
ISBN-10: 0-07-295023-4

Publisher: *David T. Culverwell*
Senior Sponsoring Editor: *Roxan Kinsey*
Developmental Editor: *Patricia Forrest*
Senior Project Manager: *Kay J. Brimeyer*
Senior Production Supervisor: *Sherry L. Kane*
Senior Media Project Manager: *Sandra M. Schnee*
Media Technology Producer: *Janna Martin*
Senior Coordinator of Freelance Design: *Michelle D. Whitaker*
Cover/Interior Designer: *Studio Montage*
(USE) Cover Image: Computer monitor: © *Photodisc/Vol. OS52*
Supplement Producer: *Brenda A. Ernzen*
Compositor: *Shepherd, Inc.*
Typeface: *11/13 Berkeley*
Printer: *Quebecor World Dubuque, IA*

Codeveloped by McGraw-Hill Higher Education and Chestnut Hill Enterprises, Inc.
chestnuthl@aol.com

Between the time that Web site information is gathered and published, some sites may have closed or changed their addresses. Also, the transcription of URLs can result in typographic errors. The publisher would appreciate notification where these occur so that they may be corrected in subsequent editions.

CPT codes are based on CPT 2004.
ICD-9-CM codes are based on ICD-9-CM 2004.

www.mhhe.com

Brief Contents

Contents

PART 2   PHYSICIAN PRACTICE CODING AND COMPLIANCE   107

Chapter 4   Diagnostic Coding: Introduction to ICD-9-CM 108

Chapter 5   Procedural Coding: Introduction to CPT and HCPCS 143

PART 4   HEALTH CARE PAYERS   329

Preface

The second edition of *Medical Insurance: A Guide to Coding and Reimbursement* is designed for medical insurance courses. This text/workbook provides medical assisting, medical insurance, and health information technology students with the knowledge and skills needed to successfully perform insurance-related duties. It focuses on three components required to handle the billing and reimbursement cycle:

- **Knowledge of procedures**—including the administrative duties important in medical practices and an understanding of how to work with payers.
- **Communications skills**—effectively working with physicians, patients, other members of the health care team, and payers using written and oral communications.
- **Health information management skills**—using information technology (IT) to manage patients' records and the billing/collections process, electronically transmit claims, conduct research, and for communications.

Medical insurance specialists must also understand medical coding guidelines and principles in order to verify diagnosis and procedure codes and use them to report patients' conditions on health care claims and encounter forms. For this reason, the text/workbook provides a fundamental understanding of current diagnostic and procedural coding, preparing students to effectively and efficiently submit claims in accordance with payers' requirements.

Of special importance is the coverage of HIPAA (Health Information Portability and Accountability Act). In today's health care environment, claims cannot be simply correct. Claims, as well as the process used to create them, must also comply with the rules imposed by federal and state law and by government and private payer health care program requirements. Medical insurance specialists help ensure that physician practices receive maximum appropriate reimbursement for reported services by submitting correct and complaint claims, reducing the chance of an investigation of the practice and the risk of liability if an audit occurs. *Medical Insurance 2e* provides students with the concepts and facts needed to understand applicable rules and to stay current with the changing regulatory environment.

Organization of the Text

The second edition of *Medical Insurance* introduces a ten-step billing and reimbursement cycle that is used to organize the topical presentation.

Billing and Reimbursement Cycle

1. Collection of patient information
2. Insurance verification
3. Encounter form preparation
4. Coding
5. Linkage and compliance review
6. Physician charge calculation
7. Claims preparation
8. Claims transmission
9. Payer adjudication
10. Reimbursement follow-up and record retention

The four parts of the text/workbook follow this sequence:

- **Part 1**, *The Health Care Environment*, introduces the major types of medical insurance, payers, and regulators; the medical insurance specialist's functions, ethical responsibilities, and certification; the claims and reimbursement process; and HIPAA Privacy, Security, and Electronic Health Care Transactions/Code Sets rules.
- **Part 2**, *Physician Practice Coding and Compliance*, builds skills in correct coding procedures, use of coding references, and compliance with proper linkage guidelines.
- **Part 3**, *Claims Processing*, covers the general procedures for calculating reimbursement, preparing and transmitting claims, verifying reimbursement, handling collections, and record retention.
- **Part 4**, *Health Care Payers*, provides descriptions of the major third-party private and government-sponsored payers' procedures and regulations. Each chapter contains specific filing guidelines. The final chapter discusses hospital billing and reimbursement.

Chapter Structure

Each chapter provides background information and current procedures in a clear, comprehensive presentation. Many figures and tables are included to enhance the learning process. The chapters also contain the following elements to ensure that students grasp the key points:

- **Chapter Outline:** A list of the major headings in the chapter and the pages on which they appear.
- **Objectives:** A description of the most important concepts and abilities that can be acquired by studying the chapter.
- **Thinking It Through:** Thought-provoking questions that require students to think about major sections' important concepts.
- **Chapter Summary:** A list of the chapter's key concepts.
- **Key Terms:** An alphabetic list of important vocabulary words and the page on which they first appear in the chapter. Key terms are highlighted and defined when introduced in the text.
- **Review Questions:** Questions in matching, true-false, completion, and short answer format that cover the facts and points made in the chapter.
- **Applying Your Knowledge:** Cases that require the student to apply the knowledge gained by studying the chapter for correct answers.

Special Features

Additional features are included in *Medical Insurance 2e* to provide more information, practice new skills, or permit students to extend their knowledge through Internet research and computer applications:

HIPAA, Billing, and Compliance Tips

These tips on HIPAA rules, billing points, and ensuring compliance with correct coding practices are located in the margins near the related chapter topics.

Focus on Careers

In each chapter, a feature box describes the tasks and educational/employment background required for a particular job in the medical insurance, billing, and coding fields.

Internet Activity

The first part of each chapter's optional Computer Exploration section describes relevant Web sites and directs students to use the Internet to research and report their findings. The goal of the activities is to extend the students' knowledge of the selected topics and use of the Internet as a research tool.

NDC*Medisoft Activity*

The second part of the Computer Exploration permits students to explore the functions of a patient billing software program, NDC*Medisoft Advanced*, which is free to adopters of *Medical Insurance 2e*. The Student Data Disk that accompanies the text/workbook contains a sample medical practice with which students work. Basic instruction in using NDCMedisoft, which must be studied before students work through the activities, is contained in the Quick Guide to NDCMedisoft on pages 521–526.

Information on ordering and installing NDC*Medisoft* is contained in the Instructor's Manual that accompanies the program. To use the software and the NDCMedisoft activities, the following equipment and supplies are needed:

—IBM or IBM-compatible computer with Pentium III or faster processor, 64 MB RAM, and 1 gig hard drive (500 MB available hard drive space)

—Microsoft Windows 98 (with current updates), Windows ME, Windows NT (Version 4.0 with current updates), Windows 2000, or Windows ME, 2000, or XP operating system

—NDCMedisoft Advanced, Version 9 (*free to adopters*)

—*Medical Insurance* Student Data Disk

—A blank, formatted 3.5" floppy diskette

—mouse or compatible pointing device

—CD ROM 2X or faster

—Printer

Health Care Claim Simulations

Chapters 11–14 contain case studies to test the student's ability to process various types of insurance claims. The claims can be prepared using NDCMedisoft Advanced or by completing a paper CMS-1500 form. Details are supplied in the Instructor's Manual.

Related Materials

Instructor's Manual for Medical Insurance, 2e

An *Instructor's Manual* provides the instructor with a course overview, answers to the review questions and case studies in the text, teaching suggestions, SCANS, AAMA, and AMT correlations, resources for insurance information, and information on ordering and installing NDC*MediSoft: Advanced*. The Instructor's CD ROM packaged with the manual contains a testbank for each chapter and a chapter-by-chapter PowerPoint presentation that can be used for lecture, review, or make-up work.

Medical Insurance Coding Workbook for Physician Practices, 2004–2005 Edition

The *Medical Insurance Coding Workbook* provides practice and instruction in coding and compliance skills. Since medical insurance specialists verify diagnosis and procedure codes and use them to report physicians' services, a fundamental understanding of coding principles and guidelines is the baseline for correct claims. The workbook reinforces and enhances skill development by applying the coding principles introduced in *Medical Insurance 2e* and extending knowledge through additional coding guidelines, examples, and compliance tips. The workbook, updated annually, is also accompanied by an Instructor's Manual.

Acknowledgments

A number of people made significant contributions to the second edition of *Medical Insurance*. For insightful reviews, criticisms, helpful suggestions, and information, we would like to acknowledge the following:

Lisa Ann Cook, B.S.H.S.

Mercedes A. Fisher
Indian River Community College

Linda Iavarone B.X., R.T. (R)
National Institute of Technology

Dr. Linda F. Samson
Governors State University

Anne Marti-Segrini, RHIA
Santa Fe Community College,
Gainesville, FL

Kristi Sopp
MTI College

Valeria D. Truitt
Craven Community College

For technical review of coding instruction in Chapters 4, 5, and 6:
Daphne Balacos, CPC, approved AAPC PMCC isntructor

All these reviewers offered invaluable assistance in reviewing the text for accuracy. Any errors, however, are the authors' responsibility. You are encouaged to report them, and to send other comments, to Cynthia Newby at CHESTNUTHL@aol.com

Part 1 The Health Care Environment

Chapter 1

Introduction to Medical Insurance

Objectives

After studying this chapter, you should be able to:

1. Explain why employment opportunities for medical insurance specialists are increasing.

2. Describe the basic types of medical insurance policies.

3. Define the two main methods of payment for medical services.

4. Compare indemnity and managed care plans.

5. Identify the chief differences between health maintenance organizations, point-of-service plans, and preferred provider organizations.

6. List the major types of private-sector payers and government-sponsored health care programs.

7. Discuss the regulation of health plans.

8. Identify seven important skills of medical insurance specialists.

9. Describe the employment and professional credentialing opportunities for medical insurance specialists.

10. Compare medical ethics and etiquette.

The Health Care Industry

The trillion-dollar health care industry—including pharmaceutical companies, hospitals, doctors, medical equipment makers, nursing homes, assisted-living centers, and insurers—is a fast-growing and dynamic sector of the American economy. Spending for health care is projected to rise to over $3 trillion by 2012, as shown in Figure 1.1. Professional services—the work of physicians and other clinical professionals—and hospital care make up the largest increases. Two factors have caused this growth in health care spending: (1) advances in medical technology and (2) an aging American population that is living longer and requiring more health care services.

Advances in Medical Technology

Continual technological improvements add costs in every area of medicine. For example, an X-ray machine that cost $175,000 ten years ago is being replaced by a more powerful CT scan device that costs over $1 million. The latest PET (positron emission tomography) scanner—a device used to better diagnose cancer—costs $2 million. A new type of pacemaker that coordinates the action of both sides of the heart for patients with congestive heart failure sold units totaling more than $470 million in its first year on the medical device market. Many other types of medical costs have increased steadily. For example, the amount spent on prescription drugs continues to rise. Drug companies advertise new, more expensive drugs, such as cholesterol and arthritis treatments, directly to consumers, who ask their doctors to prescribe them. More people buy alternative medical treatments, such as herbal medicines and massage therapy, along with conventional therapies.

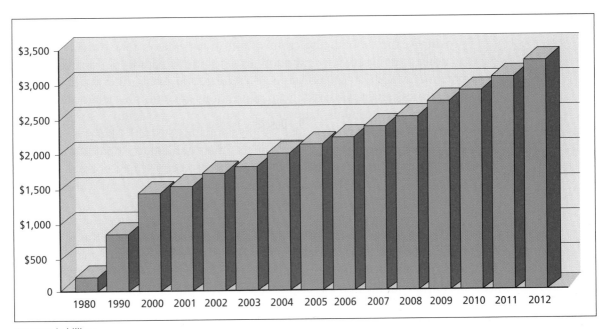

Amounts in billions.
Source: Centers for Medicare & Medicaid Services, Office of the Actuary

Figure 1.1 Spending on Health Care in the United States (Projected from 2002 to 2012)

Health Care Needs of the Aging U.S. Population

The average age of the population—and the need for health care—are both increasing in the United States. In 1950, the over-sixty-five population totaled 7 percent, or 9 million people. By 2000, more than 34 million Americans, or 12.6 percent of the population, were over sixty-five. The baby boom generation (people born between 1946 and 1964) will reach retirement age between 2010 and 2030, and by 2030 people over sixty-five will likely make up 20 percent of the population. The number of people over eighty-five is growing at a much faster rate than the overall population. In 2000, 1.6 percent of the population—more than 4 million people—was over eighty-five years of age. In 2050, the over-eighty-five population is projected to be 4.6 percent, or more than 18 million people.

The elderly need more health care services than do the young. About 60 percent of all medical dollars are spent on managing chronic diseases, such as diabetes, hypertension, osteoporosis, and arthritis, which are more common among those age sixty-five and older. Many older individuals have at least one chronic condition, and some have multiple conditions. Because of medical advances, people are living longer even when they have chronic conditions. For example, hypertension is associated with heart disease, which has been the leading cause of death since the 1920s. The average age of heart patients is sixty-seven, about ten years older than it was in 1980.

Increasing Employment Opportunities

Higher health care costs and an aging population together create pressure on the health care industry to control costs and regulate services. Employers have paid larger and larger amounts for their employees' medical insurance and are searching for ways to reduce these costs. In response, **health plans**—those plans, programs, or organizations that provide some form of medical insurance, such as an insurance policy or a government program—adopt methods intended to manage medical care and costs. In particular, these payers continually scrutinize the need for—and at times deny reimbursement for—various medical procedures. They negotiate lower prices for the services of health care **providers**, the individuals, groups, and organizations that provide medical or other health services and supplies. Providers include physicians, nurse-practitioners, physician assistants, therapists, and many other types of health care professionals. Groups and organizations include physician and practitioner groups, hospitals, laboratories, long-term care facilities, and suppliers such as pharmacies and medical supply companies. Health plans also examine each bill they pay to make sure it meets their guidelines. In addition, federal and state governments have enacted laws to protect private information about patients and to curtail fraud and abuse in the delivery of heath care. Compliance with government regulations is essential for providers.

Because of this competitive, complex situation, knowledgeable medical office employees are in demand (see Figure 1.2). Service is the defining factor in health care today. As cost and quality are presumed to be equal in doctors' offices, the only remaining competitive force is service excellence. The potential for improving the operational success of most physician practices is based on the expectations of their staff and patients. Medical insurance specialists, in particular, are increasingly important. They help ensure both top-quality service and increased revenue for practices in the following ways:

Occupational Outlook Handbook

Health Information Technicians

- Health Information technicians are projected to be one of the 20 fastest growing occupations.
- Job prospects for formally trained technicians should be very good. Employment of health information technicians is expected to grow much faster than the average for all occupations through 2010, due to rapid growth in the number of medical tests, treatments, and procedures which will be increasingly scrutinized by third-party payers, regulators, courts, and consumers.
- Most technicians will be employed in hospitals, but job growth will be faster in offices and clinics of physicians, nursing homes, and home health agencies.

Medical Assistants

- Employment of medical assistants is expected to grow much faster than the average for all occupations through 2010 as the health services industry expands due to technological advances in medicine and a growing and aging population. It is one of the fastest growing occupations.
- Employment growth will be driven by the increase in the number of group practices, clinics, and other health care facilities that need a high proportion of support personnel, particularly the flexible medical assistant who can handle both administrative and clinical duties. Medical assistants work primarily in outpatient settings, where much faster than average growth is expected.
- Job prospects should be best for medical assistants with formal training or experience, particularly those with certification.

Medical Secretaries

- Growth in the health services industry will spur faster than average employment growth for medical secretaries.
- Medical secretaries are a type of specialized secretary. They transcribe dictation, prepare correspondence, and assist physicians or medical scientists with reports, speeches, articles, and conference proceedings. They also record simple medical histories, arrange for patients to be hospitalized, and order supplies. Most medical secretaries need to be familiar with insurance rules, billing practices, and hospital or laboratory procedures.

Figure 1.2 Employment Opportunities

- By keeping up to date on changes in the health care field, and verifying compliance with the guidelines of patients' medical insurance coverage and with governmental regulations, medical insurance specialists make sure that payment for medical services will not be withheld.
- By completing health care claims with technical accuracy and clarity, they correctly communicate which services providers performed to the health plans that pay for the services.
- By understanding the billing regulations and filing procedures involved with claims processing, medical insurance specialists help ensure that payments are prompt and at the maximum level for the services provided.

- By using interpersonal skills in dealing with a diversity of people every day—those who work for health plans as well as patients and their families, all with different backgrounds and communication styles—, they establish professional and courteous relationships that enhance the billing and reimbursement process.

Medical insurance specialists' effective and efficient work is critical for the satisfaction of the patients—the physician's customers—and for the financial success of the practice.

Thinking It Through—1.1

Based on the history of health care expenditures and the statistics about the population of the United States, what is your projection for the direction of health care costs? Will they increase, decrease, or stay the same over the next ten years? How do you think the direction of health care costs affects employment opportunities for medical insurance specialists?

Insurance Basics

Medical insurance, which is also known as health insurance, is a written contract in the form of a policy or a certificate of coverage between a **policyholder** and a health plan. Under this contract, the policyholder, who may also be referred to as the insured or the member, pays a **premium**. In exchange, the health plan provides **benefits**—defined by the HIAA (Health Insurance Association of America) as payments for medical services—for a specified time period.

There are actually three participants in the relationship. The patient (policyholder) is the *first party*, and the physician is the *second party*. Under the laws governing contracts, a patient–physician contract is created when a physician agrees to treat a patient who seeks medical services. Through this unwritten contract, the patient is legally responsible for paying for services. The patient may have a policy with a health plan, the *third party*, which agrees to carry the risk of paying for those services and therefore is called a **third-party payer**.

Health Care Benefits

The insurance policy contains a **schedule of benefits**, which is a list of covered medical expenses. Benefits commonly include payment of medically necessary medical services incurred by policyholders and their dependents. Typical medical services include surgical, primary care, emergency care, and specialists' services. Other medically related expenses, such as hospital-based services, are usually included. However, if a new policyholder has a medical condition that was diagnosed before the policy was written—known as a **pre-existing condition**—a health plan may not cover medical services for the treatment of that condition.

Many health plans also cover **preventive medical services**, such as annual physical examinations, pediatric and adolescent immunizations, prenatal care, and routine cancer screening procedures such as mammograms. Policies also list treatments that are covered at different rates and noncovered services. For example, plans usually do not cover routine dental procedures, and many pay

Medical insurance specialists, also called medical billers, are employed by single-specialty and multispecialty medical group practices. They also work in clinics, for insurance companies and managed care organizations, for hospitals or nursing homes, and in other health care settings. Medical insurance specialists analyze patients' medical records and collect payment for the physicians' services from health plans and from patients.

Medical insurance specialists also handle the administrative work that is part of the payment process. These activities include preparing and sending insurance claims, communicating with health plans to follow up on claims, entering charges and payments in a patient billing computer system, and collecting bills. They may also gather information from patients and answer written or oral questions from both patients and payers, while maintaining the confidentiality of patients' data. Medical insurance specialists may also be responsible for assigning codes to patients' diagnoses and services.

Completion of a medical insurance specialist or medical assisting program at a postsecondary institution is an excellent background for an entry-level position. Professional certification, additional study, and work experience contribute to advancement to positions such as medical billing manager and medical office manager. Billers may also advance through specialization in a field, such as radiology billing management.

a smaller percentage of the charges for mental health services than they do for physically related treatments.

Types of Medical Insurance Policies

Health plans create a variety of insurance products that offer different levels of coverage for various prices. In each product, they must manage the risk that some individuals they insure will require extremely expensive medical services by spreading that risk among many policyholders. Either groups or individuals may be insured. In general, policies that are written for groups cost policyholders less than those written for individuals.

Group plans are usually offered to employers or organizations The employer or the organization agrees to the contract and offers the coverage to its group members (also called subscribers or enrollees). People who are not eligible for group insurance—for example, independent contractors or unemployed people—may purchase individual policies directly from a health plan. The policyholder's dependents, customarily the spouse and children, may also be covered under a group or an individual policy.

Disability, Workers' Compensation, and Liability Insurance

Other types of health-related insurance are available. A patient may have disability insurance that provides reimbursement for income lost because of the person's inability to work. Disability insurance is discussed in Chapter 14.

Workers' compensation insurance is also offered by insurance companies. It is purchased by employers to pay benefits and provide medical care for employees who are injured in job-related accidents and to pay benefits to employees' dependents in the event of a work-related death. State laws determine the coverage that is required. Chapter 14 also covers workers' compensation insurance.

Physicians and other professional employees usually also have liability insurance, which covers situations in which an individual causes a loss or injury to another party. When liability insurance is involved in a patient's injury, the patient's medical insurance usually does not provide benefits until the liability case is resolved. Liability insurance is discussed in Chapter 6.

Medical Insurance Payment Methods and Plans

Before medical insurance was available, patients usually paid the fees their physicians set. During the 1940s, companies began to offer medical insurance to attract workers from the small work pool that was not serving in the military, and the federal government enacted legislation that permitted employers to deduct this cost as a business expense. By the 1960s, nearly 75 percent of the U.S. population had medical insurance. At that point, health plans began to develop lists of standard fees that they would pay for specified physicians' services. As costs for medical services increased in the 1970s, health plans felt that changes were needed in the way they paid providers. To curtail cost increases, these payers analyzed standard fees and reduced some by accounting for factors such as the locale of the provider and the relative difficulty of a procedure (see Chapter 7).

Currently, two main payment methods, fee-for-service and capitation, are used by health plans.

Fee-for-Service

The **fee-for-service** payment method is referred to as a **retroactive payment**. Payment is made *after* the patient receives services from the physician (see Figure 1.3). Payers reimburse policyholders for medical expenses they have paid or, if so instructed by the policyholder, make payments to providers on behalf of patients.

Capitation

Capitation (from *capit-*, Latin for *head*) is a fixed prepayment to a medical provider for all necessary, contracted services provided to a patient who is a plan member (see Figure 1.4). The capitated rate is referred to as a **prospective payment** because it is paid in advance. The health plan makes this payment whether the provider provides no medical services or performs multiple services to the enrolled patient during a given period.

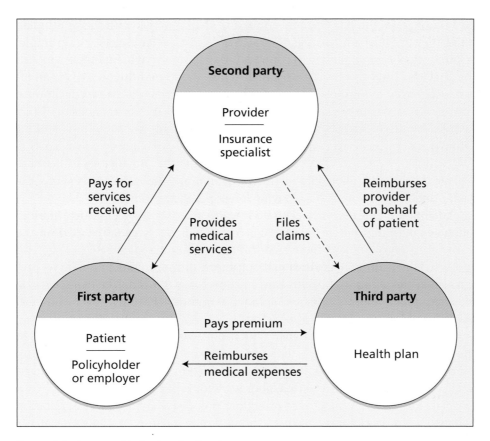

Figure 1.3 Payment Under Fee-for-Service

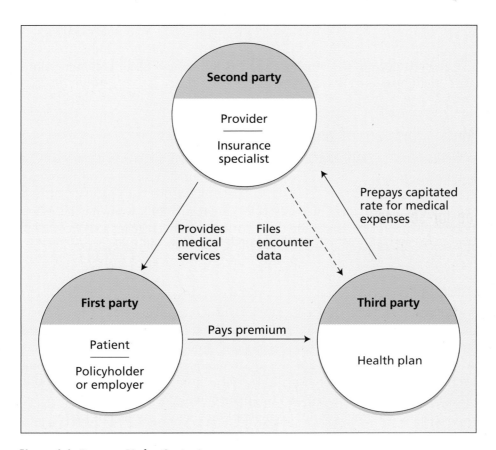

Figure 1.4 Payment Under Capitation

In capitation, the physician is required to share the risk with the health plan that an insured person will use more services than the fee covers. For example, a family physician might have a contract for a capitated payment of $30 a month for each of a hundred patients in a plan. This $3,000 monthly fee covers all office visits from all of those patients. If half the patients see the physician once during a given month, the provider in effect receives $60 for each visit ($3,000 divided by fifty visits). If, however, half of the patients see the physician four times in a month, the average fee is $3,000 divided by two hundred visits, or $15 for each visit. In fee-for-service, the more patients the provider sees, the more charges the health plan reimburses. In capitation, the payment remains the same, and the provider risks receiving lower per-visit revenue.

Patients are enrolled in a capitated health plan for a specific time period, such as a month, quarter, or year. The capitated rate is usually based on the number of enrollees and their health-related characteristics, such as age and gender. The health plan analyzes these factors and sets a rate based on its prediction of the amount of health care each person will need. The capitated rate of prepayment, referred to as **per member per month (PMPM)**, covers only services listed on the schedule of benefits.

Health plans usually establish capitation-based contracts with groups of physicians who provide the listed services. In some cases, the physician group hires other providers to handle certain services. For example, a group of physicians may have a contract with a laboratory for clinical laboratory work. Or a specialist, such as an oncologist or endocrinologist, may have a subcapitation agreement from a group of general practitioners. These specialists receive a PMPM from the physician group for the enrollees who use their services.

Another payment variation is an **episode of care (EOC) option**. The EOC option is a flat fee that is negotiated with a specialist for all services for a particular treatment. For example, a set fee is established for coronary bypass surgery or hip replacement surgery; the fixed rate per patient includes preoperative and postoperative treatment as well as the surgery itself. If complications arise, additional fees are usually paid.

Medical Insurance Plans

A wide array of health care plan options are offered by payers. Each plan has somewhat different policies and options (see Table 1.1). Medical insurance specialists must keep track of each plan held by the practice's patients, including its particular payment methods, rules, and regulations. Knowing these facts is essential in order to be certain that a patient has coverage for a service and to process health care claims and other billing documents for patients.

Indemnity Plans

Indemnity, the basis of fee-for-service insurance plans, refers to security against loss. Under an indemnity plan, the health plan indemnifies the policyholder against costs of medical services and procedures as listed on the benefits schedule. Indemnity plans usually reimburse medical costs on a fee-for-service basis. Patients receive medical services from the providers they choose, who usually file the required claims for payment on behalf of patients.

For each claim, four conditions must be met before payment is made:

1. The medical service must be covered by the insured's health plan.
2. The policy's premium payment must be up to date.

TABLE 1.1	Comparison of Health Plan Options		
Plan Type	**Provider Options**	**Cost Containment**	**Features**
Indemnity	Any provider	• Little or none • Preauthorization required for some procedures	• Higher costs • Deductibles • Coinsurance • Preventive care not usually covered
Preferred Provider Organization (PPO)	Network or out-of-network providers	• Referral not required for specialists • Fees are discounted • Preauthorization for some procedures	• Higher cost for out-of-network providers • Preventive care coverage varies
Point-of-Service (POS)	Network providers or out-of-network providers	• Within network, primary care physician manages care	• Lower copayments for network providers • Higher costs for out-of-network providers • Covers preventive care
Health Maintenance Organization (HMO)	Only HMO network providers	• Primary care physician manages care; referral required • No payment for out-of-network nonemergency services • Preauthorization required	• Low copayment • Limited provider network • Covers preventive care

3. A **deductible**—the amount that the insured pays on covered services before benefits begin—must be paid. Deductibles usually range from $200 to $500 annually. Higher deductibles usually mean lower premiums.

4. Any **coinsurance**—the percentage of each claim that the insured pays—must be taken into account. The coinsurance rate presents the health plan's percentage of the charge followed by the insured's percentage, such as 80/20.

For example, a typical high-deductible plan might specify that the first $1,000 in covered annual medical fees are **out-of-pocket** (paid by the patient) expenses for the insured, and the coinsurance rate is 80/20 for the next $6,000 of fees. In this case, the patient with a first medical bill of $8,000 would owe the $1,000 deductible plus 20 percent of the remaining $7,000, or $1,400, for a total of $2,400. In this instance, the health plan payment is $5,600.

Managed Care Plans

Managed care plans, first introduced in California in 1929, are the predominant type of insurance (see Figure 1.5 on page 13). Over 90 percent of all insured workers are enrolled in some type of managed care plan, and thousands of different plans are offered. The term **managed care** describes the goals of these plans: to manage care by establishing effective and efficient health care delivery systems that ensure quality and at the same time control health care costs.

To accomplish managed care goals, the financing and management of health care are combined with the delivery of services. **Managed care organizations (MCOs)** establish links between provider, patient, and payer. Instead of only the patient having a policy with the health plan, under managed care both the patient and the provider have agreements with the MCO. This arrangement gives the managed care plan more control over what services the provider performs and the fees that are charged for the services.

Health Maintenance Organizations

One type of MCO is the **health maintenance organization (HMO)**, which combines coverage of medical costs and delivery of health care for a prepaid premium. About 23 percent of insured workers are enrolled in HMOs.

The HMO creates a network of physicians, hospitals, and other providers by employing or negotiating contracts with them, and then enrolls members in a health plan under which they use those providers' services. In most states, HMOs are licensed and are legally required to provide certain services to members and their dependents. For example, preventive care may be required as appropriate for each age group, such as immunizations and well-baby checkups for infants and screening mammograms for women.

Medical Management Practices in HMOs

Health maintenance organizations seek to control rising medical costs and at the same time improve health care.

Cost control   An HMO uses the following methods to control costs:

- *Restricting patients' choice of providers:* After enrollment in an HMO, members must receive services from the network of physicians, hospitals, and other providers who are employed by or under contract to the HMO. This provision of the HMO's contract with members is referred to as a lock-in. Visits to out-of-network providers are not covered, except for emergency care or urgent health problems that arise when the member is temporarily away from the service area.

- *Controlling access to services:* Patients are required to select a **primary care physician (PCP)**—also called a "gatekeeper" from the HMO's list of general or family practitioners, internists, and pediatricians. A PCP coordinates patients' overall care to ensure that all services provided are, in the PCP's judgment, necessary. In gatekeeper plans, HMO members need a medical **referral** from the PCP before seeing a specialist or a consultant and for hospital admission. Members in those plans who visit providers without a referral are directly responsible for the total cost of the service.

- *Requiring preauthorization for services:* HMOs often require **preauthorization** (also called precertification or prior authorization) before the physician delivers many types of services. The HMO may require a second opinion—the judgment of another physician that a planned procedure is necessary—before authorizing it. If the preauthorization requirement is not met, the services are not covered.

  Preauthorization controls unnecessary tests and treatments. It is intended to match the level of care to the patient's level of need. For example, preauthorization is almost always needed for nonemergency hospital admission, and it is usually required within a certain number of days after an emergency admission.

- *Controlling use of services:* HMOs develop standard **utilization** guidelines that regulate what is considered appropriate and necessary medical care. For example, the HMO may set a number of times each year that a patient can have a particular service, such as once a year for a physical examination. The HMO holds the provider accountable for any questionable service and may deny a patient's or provider's request for preauthorization.

  For example, a patient who has a rotator cuff shoulder injury can receive a specific number of physical therapy sessions; more sessions will not be

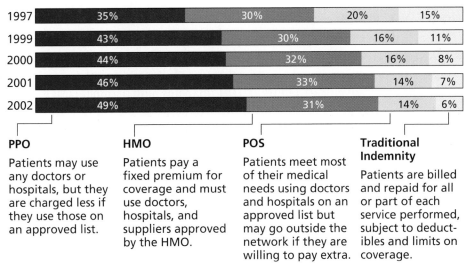

1997	35%	30%	20%	15%
1999	43%	30%	16%	11%
2000	44%	32%	16%	8%
2001	46%	33%	14%	7%
2002	49%	31%	14%	6%

PPO

Patients may use any doctors or hospitals, but they are charged less if they use those on an approved list.

HMO

Patients pay a fixed premium for coverage and must use doctors, hospitals, and suppliers approved by the HMO.

POS

Patients meet most of their medical needs using doctors and hospitals on an approved list but may go outside the network if they are willing to pay extra.

Traditional Indemnity

Patients are billed and repaid for all or part of each service performed, subject to deductibles and limits on coverage.

Source: Mercer's National Survey of Employer-Sponsored Health Plans, 2003.

Figure 1.5 Health Plan Coverage Choices in Employer-Sponsored Plans

covered without additional approval. Experimental treatments are typically not covered. Emergency care is particularly tightly controlled because it is generally the most costly way to deliver services. For example, if a patient suspects he or she is having a heart attack and seeks emergency service, but the cause of chest pain is found to be indigestion, some plans will not cover that emergency-room visit. These guidelines are also applied to hospitals in the network, which, for instance, limit the number of days patients can spend in the hospital following particular surgeries.

• *Controlling drug costs:* Providers are usually required to prescribe drugs for patients only from the HMO's **formulary**, a list of selected pharmaceuticals and their appropriate dosages as determined by the HMO. Drugs that are not on the formulary require preauthorization.

• *Cost-sharing:* At the time HMO members see a provider, they pay a specified charge called a **copayment** (or copay). A lower copayment is usually charged for an office visit to the primary care physician, and a higher copayment is required for a visit to the office of a specialist or for the use of emergency-department services.

• *Using nonphysician practitioners:* HMOs encourage the use of nonphysician practitioners, such as physician's assistants, because the costs are lower when they provide services.

The first HMOs emphasized cost-containment methods and were effective in reducing costs. However, cost-containment policies also created widespread dissatisfaction among both physicians and patients. Physicians working under managed-care contracts omplained that they were not allowed to order needed treatments and tests. Patients often reported that needed referrals were denied. In response, the medical management practices of HMOs have changed, increasingly emphasizing the quality of health care as well as the cost of its delivery. Just as providers must demonstrate that their services are both effective and efficient, HMOs must demonstrate to their customers that they can offer these services at competitive prices while improving the quality of health care. Most HMOs have switched from "gatekeeper" plans that required referrals to all specialists to **open-access plans**, in which members can visit any specialists in the network without a referral.

Health care quality improvements The quality improvements made by HMOs are illustrated by these features, which most plans contain:

- *Disease management practices:* Some patients face difficult treatments, such as for high-risk pregnancies, and others need chronic care for conditions such as congestive heart failure (CHF), diabetes, and asthma. HMOs often assign case managers to work with these patients. Some conditions require case managers who are health care professionals. Other types of cases are assigned to someone familiar with the health care system, such as a social worker. The goal of case managers is to make sure that patients have access to all needed treatments. For example, physician case managers coordinate appropriate referrals to consultants, specialists, hospitals, and other services. Other types of case managers provide patient education, special equipment like a blood glucose meter for a diabetic, and ongoing contact to monitor a patient's condition.
- *Preventive care:* Preventive care, which seeks to prevent the occurrence of conditions through early detection of disease, is emphasized through provisions for annual checkups, screening procedures, and inoculations.
- *Best practices:* HMOs collect and analyze large amounts of data about patients' clinical treatment and their responses to it. In this way, the most effective protocols—detailed, precise treatment regimens—are established. HMOs use these protocols to advise their providers about the best course of treatment for patients with particular conditions.

Business Models for Health Maintenance Organizations

An HMO is organized around one of three business models. Each model is based on how the terms of the agreement connect the provider and the plan.

1. Staff Model

   In a staff HMO, physicians are employed by the organization. All the premiums and other revenues come to the HMO, which in turn pays the physicians salaries. For medical care, patients visit the clinics and health centers owned by the HMO.

2. Group or Network Model

   In a group or network managed care organization, the HMO contracts with more than one physician group, creating a network of physicians. The medical practices under contract are usually paid a capitated rate for the HMO members. In some plans, HMO members receive medical services in HMO-owned facilities from providers who work only for that HMO. In other group or network HMOs, members visit the providers' facilities, and the providers also have nonmember patients.

3. Independent Practice Association Model

   An independent practice association (IPA) type of HMO is physician-led. The HMO contracts with a central administrative group of providers that has its own contracts with individual physicians or practices. Under the terms of the contract, the HMO pays negotiated fees for medical services to the IPA. The IPA, in turn, pays its physician members, either by a capitated rate or according to an agreed-on fee. Providers may join more than one IPA and usually also have nonmember patients.

Point-of-Service Plans

Many patients dislike HMO rules that restrict their access to physicians. In order to better compete for membership, a **point-of-service (POS) plan**, also called an open HMO, reduces restrictions and allows members to choose providers who are not in the HMO's network. About 22 percent of workers covered by employers' health care plans are enrolled in this type of plan.

Members must pay additional fees that are set by the plan when they use out-of-network providers. Typically, 20 to 30 percent of the charge for service must be paid by the patient, and the deductible can be very high. The HMO pays out-of-network providers on a fee-for-service basis.

Preferred Provider Organizations

A **preferred provider organization (PPO)** is another health care delivery system that manages care. PPOs usually create a network of physicians, hospitals, and other providers with whom they have negotiated **discounted fee-for-service** payment schedules. For example, a practice might charge $80 for a brief appointment under a fee-for-service health plan, but charge $60 under the discounted schedule of a PPO. In exchange for accepting lower fees, providers—in theory, at least—see more patients, thus making up the revenue that is lost through the reduced fees. Almost 50 percent of American workers insured through their employers are members of PPOs.

PPOs do not generally require a primary care physician to oversee patients' care. Referrals to specialists are not required, so patients have an *open access* or an *open panel* plan under a PPO. Premiums and copayments, however, are higher than in HMO or POS plans. Members choose from many in-network generalists and specialists, usually for a copayment. Members also can use out-of-network providers, usually for a higher copayment or deductible. For example, for using an in-network provider, the patient might pay a copayment or be reimbursed at the 80 to 100 percent level, compared with 60 to 70 percent for treatment from out-of-network providers.

PPOs also:

- *Direct patients' choice of providers:* PPO members are encouraged to receive services from the PPO's network of physicians, hospitals, and other providers.
- *Control utilization of services:* PPOs also establish utilization guidelines for appropriate and necessary medical care.
- *Require preauthorization for services:* PPOs usually require preauthorization for nonemergency hospital admission and for some outpatient procedures.
- *Require cost-sharing:* PPO members are also required to pay a copayment for general or specialist services.

Table 1.2 on page 17 summarizes the types of managed care health plan structures.

Consumer-Driven Health Plans/Health Savings Accounts

Many employers that offer health plans to their employees have increased the managed care plan options to control costs. They have also asked employees to pay for a greater share of these costs, through increasing the employees' annual premiums as well as copayments. A number of new plan structures are aimed at increasing employee awareness of and contribution to these costs. One example is a **consumer-driven health plan.** This option combines a low-cost high-deductible health plan (it may be a PPO or an indemnity plan) with a health savings plan that covers some out-of-pocket expenses. Employers put an amount of money in individual cash accounts for employees. Patients with

Health maintenance organizations often require different payments for different services. Figure 1.7 shows the copayments for one HMO health plan. Study this schedule and respond to these questions:

- Does this health plan cover diabetic supplies? Dental exams? Emergency services?

- Is the copayment amount for a PCP visit higher or lower than the charge for specialty care?

	Copayments
Primary Care Physician Visits	
Office Hours	$20 copay
After Hours/Home Visits	$20 copay
Specialty Care	
Office Visits	$30 copay
Diagnostic Outpatient Testing	$20 copay
Phys, Occ, Speech Therapy	$20 copay
SPU Surgery	$20 copay
Hospitalization	$250 copay
Emergency Room (copay waived if admitted)	$35 copay
Maternity	
First OB Visit	$30 copay
Hospital	$250 copay
Mental Health	
Inpatient	$250 copay, 60 days
Outpatient	30% copay
Substance Abuse	
Detoxification	$250 copay
Inpatient Rehab (combined w/MH)	$250 copay
Outpatient Rehabilitation	30% copay
Preventive Care	
Routine Eye Exam	Not covered
Routine GYN Exam	$30 copay
Pediatric Preventive Dental Exam	Not covered
Chiropractic Care (20 visits/condition)	$20 copay
Prescriptions	$15/$20/$20 copay $150 deductible/calendar year
Contraceptives	Covered
Diabetic Supplies	Covered
31–90 Day Supply (Retail & Mod)	$30/40/60 copay
Durable Medical Equipment	No copay

Figure 1.6 Example of Benefits Under an HMO

TABLE 1.2	Comparison of Managed Care Health Plan Structures		
Plan Type	Patient Base	Provider Payment Method	Plan Employment of Physicians
Health Maintenance Organization (HMO): Staff HMO	Only HMO patients	By Employment Contract	Yes
Group HMO	HMO or nonHMO	By Employment Contract or Capitation	Yes or No
Independent Practice Association (IPA)	HMO or nonHMO	PCP—Capitation Specialist—Fee-for-Service	No
Point-of-Service (POS)	HMO or nonHMO	By Contract, but Specialist Is Fee-for-Service	No
Preferred Provider Organization (PPO)	Managed Care and Non-Managed Care	By Contract	No

these plans are responsible for all costs until the deductible is met. They can use the cash account to cover medical spending, and roll over remaining money from year to year.

Medical Insurance Payers

More than 240 million people in the United States have medical coverage through either private insurance or government-sponsored programs (see Figure 1.7 on page 18). Most private health insurance is employer-sponsored. Insurance companies in the private sector may be either for-profit or nonprofit organizations. About 70 million people are covered by government-sponsored programs. More than 43 million people—about 15 percent of the population—have no medical insurance.

Insurance Companies

A small number of large firms dominate the national market: Aetna, Cigna, United Healthcare Group, Health Net, Humana, Pacificare Health Systems, and Wellpoint Health Networks. Small companies compete for regional business. Increasingly, private-sector payers are national companies that offer all the leading types of health plans. There are also a number of nonprofit organizations, such as Kaiser Permanente, which is the largest nonprofit HMO. Some organizations, such as the Blue Cross and Blue Shield Association, have both for-profit and nonprofit components.

Self-Insured Health Plans and Third-Party Administrators

Some 50 million employees have health insurance through their employers that have established themselves as **self-insured health plans.** Rather than paying a premium to an insurance carrier, the organization "insures itself." It assumes the risk of paying directly for medical services, establishes contracts with local physician practices, and sets up a fund with which it pays for claims. The organization itself establishes the benefit levels and the plan types it will offer. Most self-insured health plans are set up as fee-for-service or PPOs; fewer than 10 percent are set up as HMOs. Some firms hire a **third-party administrator (TPA)** to operate their health plans.

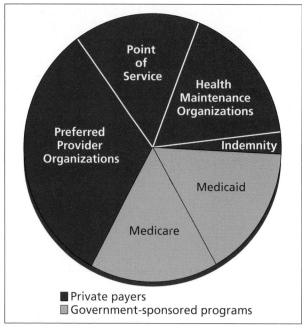

Source: Centers for Medicare & Medicaid Services, 2001 data

Figure 1.7 Types of Insurance Held

Government-Sponsored Health Care Programs

A number of government-sponsored health care programs offer benefits for which various groups in the population are eligible:

- Medicare is a 100 percent federally funded health plan that covers people who are sixty-five and over, are disabled, or have permanent kidney failure (end-stage renal disease, or ESRD).
- Medicaid, a federal program that is jointly funded by federal and state governments, covers low-income people who cannot afford medical care. Medicaid is administered by each state, which determines the program's qualifications and benefits under broad federal guidelines.
- TRICARE, a Department of Defense program, covers medical expenses for spouses, children, and other dependents of active-duty members of the uniformed services, retired military personnel and their dependents, and family members of deceased active-duty personnel. (This program replaced CHAMPUS, the Civilian Health and Medical Program of the Uniformed Services, in 1998.)
- CHAMPVA, the Civilian Health and Medical Program of the Department of Veterans Affairs, covers veterans with permanent service-related disabilities and their dependents. It also covers surviving spouses and dependent children of veterans who died from service-related disabilities.

Regulations and Accreditation in Medical Insurance

Health care is a highly regulated industry. To protect consumers' health, both federal and state governments pass laws that affect the types of services all patients are offered. In addition, to protect the privacy of patients' health information, federal laws address how health care plans and providers exchange this information in the conduct of business.

Federal Regulation

The main federal government agency responsible for health care is the **Centers for Medicare and Medicaid Services**, known as **CMS** (formerly the Health Care Financing Administration, or HCFA). An agency of the Department of Health and Human Services (HHS), CMS administers the Medicare and Medicaid programs to more than 70 million Americans. CMS implements annual federal budget acts and laws such as the Medicare Prescription Drug, Improvement, and Modernization Act of 2003 that create additional benefits—help in paying for drugs and an annual physical examination—for Medicare beneficiaries.

CMS also performs activities to ensure the quality of health care, such as

- Regulating all laboratory testing, except research performed on humans
- Preventing discrimination based on health status for people buying health insurance
- Conducting research on the effectiveness of various methods of health care management, treatment, and financing
- Assessing the quality of health care facilities and services

Because of these activities, CMS policy is often the health care industry leader. When government regulations change the way Medicare reimbursement is calculated, for example, insurance companies often adopt the same formulas for paying practitioners.

HIPAA

When federal laws regarding Americans' rights to health care are enacted, CMS often has a key role in developing and implementing them. For example, major legislation entitled the **Health Insurance Portability and Accountability Act (HIPAA) of 1996** is designed to protect peoples' private health information (see Chapter 2), to ensure health insurance coverage for workers and their families when they change or lose their jobs, and to uncover fraud and abuse against the government (see Chapter 6). This act includes administrative simplification provisions that require the adoption of standards for electronic transactions involving health plans, providers, individuals, and employers (see Chapter 8). CMS must ensure that all medical practices comply with these regulations.

Fraud and Abuse Regulation

Another major activity of CMS is to combat fraud and abuse in government-sponsored programs. In conjunction with HHS's Office of the Inspector General (OIG), the agency is charged with enforcing fraud and abuse rules and regulations. The number of lawsuits that the federal government has filed against health care providers has increased greatly in the last ten years. Compliance plans to avoid illegal actions, such as billing for Medicare services that were not performed, are a very important part of every medical practice (see Chapter 6).

State Regulation

States are a major regulator of the health care industry. Operating an insurance company without a license is illegal in all states. State commissioners of insurance investigate consumer complaints about the quality and financial aspects of health care. State laws ensure the solvency of insurance companies and

Compliance Guideline

Emergency Services
Under federal law, hospital emergency departments must provide care for all patients in need of medical services, regardless of their ability to pay.
The law is the Emergency Medical Treatment and Active Labor Act, or EMTALA. It requires hospital emergency departments to provide any individual coming to their premises with a medical screening exam (MSE) to determine if an emergency condition or active pregnancy labor is present. If so, the hospital must supply either stabilization prior to transferring the patient or a certification (signed by the physician) that the transfer is appropriate and meets certain conditions.

managed care organizations, so that they will be able to pay enrollees' claims. States may also restrict price increases on premiums and other charges to patients.

Many states have laws requiring managed care organizations to accept any qualified physician who wants to be a participating provider in their plan. This regulation helps reduce the number of patients who have to switch physicians if they change from one plan to another.

Accrediting Organizations

Several organizations accredit health plans:

- *NCQA:* The National Committee for Quality Assurance (NCQA), an independent nonprofit organization, is the leader in accrediting HMOs. Working with the health care industry, NCQA developed a standardized set of sixty performance measures called HEDIS (Health Plan Employer Data and Information Set). HEDIS provides employers and consumers with information about each plan's effectiveness in preventing and treating disease, access to care, and members' satisfaction with their care. NCQA's guidelines on the process by which HMOs select physicians and hospitals to join their networks, called **credentialing**, include performance measures. NCQA requires HMOs to review the credentials of all providers in their plan every two years to ensure that they continue to meet appropriate standards of professional competence. The organization also sets precise standards for the way physicians document and update patients' medical records.
- *URAC:* The Utilization Review Accreditation Commission (URAC), also known as the American Accreditation Healthcare Commission, is another leading accrediting group. Like NCQA, it is a nonprofit organization that establishes accreditation standards for managed health care plans. URAC has accreditation programs addressing both the security and privacy of health information as required by HIPAA.
- *JCAHO:* Standards for many types of patient care are set and monitored by the Joint Commission on Accreditation of Healthcare Organizations (JCAHO), often referred to as the Joint Commission. JCAHO is made up of members from the American College of Surgeons, the American College of Physicians, the American Medical Association, the American Hospital Association, and the American Dental Association. JCAHO verifies compliance with accreditation standards for hospitals, long-term care facilities, psychiatric facilities, home health agencies, ambulatory care facilities, and pathology and clinical laboratory services. JCAHO works with NCQA and the American Medical Accreditation Program to coordinate the measurement of the quality of health care across the entire health care system.
- *AMAP:* The American Medical Accreditation Program is designed to help alleviate the pressures facing physicians, health plans, and hospitals by reducing cost and administrative effort while simultaneously documenting quality. As a comprehensive program, AMAP measures and evaluates individual physicians against national standards, criteria, and peer performance in five areas: credentials, personal qualifications, environment of care, clinical performance, and patient care.

Employment as a Medical Insurance Specialist

The health care industry offers many rewarding career paths for employees who are well qualified. Providers must compete in a complex environment of various health plans, managed care contracts, and federal and state regulations. Employment in positions that help providers handle these demands is growing, as are opportunities for career development.

Characteristics for Success

The following skills are required for successful mastery of the tasks of a medical insurance specialist:

- *Knowledge of medical terminology, anatomy, and physiology:* Medical insurance specialists must analyze physicians' descriptions of patients' conditions and treatments and relate these descriptions to the systems of codes used in the health care industry. The codes are required by federal law in order to standardize reporting of health data and also by third-party payers for processing health care claims.
- *Communication skills:* The job of a medical insurance specialist requires excellent communication skills, both oral and written. For example, patients often need explanations of insurance benefits or clarification of instructions such as referrals. Courteous, helpful answers to questions strongly influence patients' desire to continue to use the practice's services. Memos, letters, the telephone, and e-mail are used to research and follow up on changes in health plans' rules and governmental regulations, to accompany claims as documentation of special conditions or treatments to obtain maximum reimbursement from payers, and to solve billing problems.
- *Attention to detail:* Many aspects of the job involve paying close attention to detail, such as correctly completing health care claims, filing patients' medical records, recording preauthorization numbers, calculating the correct payments, and posting third-party and patients' payments for services.
- *Flexibility:* Working in a changing environment requires the ability to adapt to new procedures, handle varying kinds of problems and interactions during a busy day, and work successfully with different types of people.
- *Computer skills:* Most medical practices use computers to handle billing and to process claims. General computer literacy, including a working knowledge of (1) the Microsoft Windows operating system, (2) a word-processing program, (3) a medical office billing program, and (4) Internet-based research, is essential. Data entry skills are also necessary.
- *Honesty and integrity:* Medical insurance specialists work with patients' medical records and with finances. It is essential to maintain the confidentiality of patient information and communications, as well as to act with integrity when handling these tasks.
- *Ability to work as a team member:* Patient service is a team effort. To do their part, medical insurance specialists are cooperative and focus on the best interests of patients and the practice.

Billing Tip

Keeping Up to Date: The Internet
The Internet, along with other tools, is frequently used for research about government regulations, payer updates on reimbursement and other procedural changes, and information on changes in coding systems. Ignorance of new instructions or rules is not an excuse for incorrect billing. Experienced medical insurance specialists make it a habit to check the most important Web sites for their billing environment regularly.

Thinking It Through—1.4

Which of the skills of medical insurance specialists do you think are most important in avoiding incomplete or inaccurate claims?

Roles and Responsibilities

Duties of employees in the medical insurance field differ, depending on the size of the institution. Medical insurance specialists may work in small practices or clinics or in large hospitals or long-term care facilities. In smaller practices, medical insurance specialists or employees trained as medical assistants usually handle most insurance billing and coding tasks. To do so, they must be familiar with the provider contracts that are in effect, be knowledgeable about patients' *insurance* coverage, and have coding skills.

Most positions, however, are found in larger medical practices, which have advantages over physicians who practice alone or in small groups. They can negotiate better contracts with managed care plans and hire trained staff, such as medical insurance specialists, to keep up with changing rules and regulations. For this reason, employment opportunities in larger practices are growing rapidly. Jobs in large practices or for networks of providers are usually found in insurance departments, and the duties are more specialized. For example, billing and coding duties may be separated—medical insurance specialists handle insurance and reimbursement, and medical coders relate patients' conditions and treatments to the health care coding systems. In a specialized structure, a medical insurance specialist may work exclusively with claims sent to just one of many third-party payers. The administrative functions in larger groups or networks are usually headed by a practice manager, office manager, or administrator to whom the administrative staff, such as medical transcriptionists, receptionists, accounting personnel, and medical insurance specialists, report.

In most practice-based employment, medical insurance specialists are likely to *be responsible for*:

- Verifying patient insurance information, eligibility, and authorization requirements before medical services are provided
- Maintaining up-to-date information about patients, third-party payers' reimbursement guidelines, and government programs' regulations
- Following federal, state, and local legal guidelines and regulations on the confidentiality of all information about patients and their illnesses
- Analyzing the information in patients' medical records to provide accurate codes and billing information
- Calculating provider reimbursement, billing the appropriate payer—health plan, patient, or government program—and maintaining effective communication to avoid problems or delays
- Assisting patients with insurance information and required documents
- Processing payments and requests for further information about claims and bills
- Maintaining financial records
- Maintaining current coding systems and updating the forms the practice uses for patient information and claims processing

There are also employment opportunities in many other areas. For example, payers and service companies such as billing agencies hire medical assistants. Employment may also be found in other areas, such as consulting and teaching.

Education, Certification, and Continuing Education Opportunities

Completion of a medical insurance specialist program, coding specialist program, or medical assisting or health information technology program at a postsecondary institution provides an excellent background for many types of positions in the medical insurance field. Another possibility is to earn an associate degree or a certificate of proficiency by completing a program in a curriculum area such as health care business services. Further baccalaureate and graduate study enable advancement to managerial positions.

Career advancement is often aided by membership in professional organizations that offer certification in various areas. Certification by a professional organization provides evidence to prospective employers that the applicant has demonstrated a superior level of skill on a nationally developed test.

Medical Assisting Certification

Two organizations offer tests in the professional area of medical assisting. After earning a diploma in medical assisting from an accredited school (or having a year's work experience), medical assistants may sit for certification from the American Association of Medical Assistants or the registration designation from the American Medical Technologists.

Health Information Technician Certification

Students who are interested in the professional area of health information (also known as medical records) may complete an associate's degree from an accredited college program and pass a credentialing test from the American Health Information Management Association (AHIMA) to be certified as a Registered Health Information Technician, or RHIT. An RHIT examines medical records for accuracy, reports patient data for reimbursement, and helps with information for medical research and statistical data.

Coding Certification

Medical coders are expert in classifying medical data. They assign codes to physicians' descriptions of patients' conditions and treatments. For employment as a medical coder, employers typically prefer—or may require—certification. The AHIMA offers three coding certifications: the Certified Coding Associate (CCA), intended as a starting point for entering a new career as a coder; the Certified Coding Specialist (CCS); and the Certified Coding Specialist-Physician-based (CCS-P). The American Academy of Professional Coders grants the Certified Professional Coder (CPC) and the Certified Professional Coder-Hospital (CPC-H) certifications, as well as an associate-level certification.

Continuing Education

Most professional organizations require certified members to keep up to date by taking annual training courses to refresh or extend their knowledge. Continuing education sessions are assigned course credits by the credentialing organizations, and satisfactory completion of a test on the material is often required for credit. Employers often approve attendance at seminars that apply to the practice's goals and ask the person who attends to update other staff members.

Obtaining a Position

In each chapter of this book, a *Career Focus* feature highlights a different type of job related to medical insurance and coding. These features describe the tasks that are done; the working environment; the background, skills, and credentials needed; and the possibilities for advancement. For example, the

Certified Medical Assistant (CMA)

American Association of Medical Assistants (AAMA)
20 N. Wacker Drive, Suite 1575
Chicago, IL 60606-2903
800-228-2262
http://www.aama-ntl.org

Registered Medical Assistant (RMA)

American Medical Technologists (AMT)
710 Higgins Road
Park Ridge, IL 60068-5765
847-823-5169
http://www.amt1.com

Registered Health Information Technician (RHIT); Coding Certification (CCA, CCS, CCS-P)

American Health Information Management Association (AHIMA)
919 North Michigan Avenue, Suite 1400
Chicago, IL 60611-1683
312-787-2672
http://www.ahima.org

Certified Professional Coder (CPC, CPC-H)

American Academy of Professional Coders
309 West 700 South
Salt Lake City, UT 84101
800-626-2633
http://www.aapc.com

Focus on Careers at the top of page 7 describes the job of the medical insurance specialist. In the text, these other opportunities are described:

Chapter	Focus on Careers
2	Privacy Official/Security Official
3	Administrative Medical Assistant
4	Medical Coder Physician Practice
5	Medical Coding Manager
6	Coding Compliance Auditor
7	Billing Manager
8	Consulting and Educational Career Opportunities
9	Collection Specialist
10	Payer Customer Service Representative, Claims Examiner, and Provider Relations Representative
11	Medicare Compliance Specialist
12	Physician Practice Manager
13	Billing Manager
14	Workers' Compensation Specialist
15	Medical Coder—Hospital

Jobs for well-trained medical insurance and coding specialists are available in all regions of the United States. According to *The Physician's Advisory,* a health care journal, "good, experienced billing/coding specialists are in short supply; to retain good workers in these very important positions, going up in salary is a bargain compared to risking their going to another employer . . . the work of insurance specialists is an increasingly complex job."

In addition to employment in medical practices, insurance specialists may work in hospitals and outpatient settings, nursing homes, and mental health care facilities. Many positions are available with managed care organizations, insurance companies, and third-party administrators as claims examiners, provider relations representatives, or benefits analysts. Positions are also available in government and public health agencies. Employment with companies that offer billing or consulting services to health care providers is an option, as is self-employment as a claims assistance professional who helps consumers with medical insurance problems or as a billing service.

Many excellent publications offer advice on conducting an effective job hunt. Critical skills include:

- Having a well-prepared resume and securing personal references. The key words employers look for should be highlighted in the resume.
- Being able to discuss professional objectives, strengths, and potential contributions with interviewers.
- Locating job leads on the Internet. For example, states usually have Web sites that list jobs as well as advice on interviewing and resume preparation. Use other types of research, review printed advertisements for jobs, and use employment services or the school's placement program as well.
- Networking to establish and maintain contacts with friends, relatives, and others who may know of opportunities, especially through membership in professional organizations.

- Following up every interview with a letter thanking the employer for conducting the interview.

Medical Ethics and Etiquette in the Practice

Licensed medical staff and other employees working in physicians' practices share responsibility for observing a code of ethics and for following correct etiquette.

Ethics

Medical **ethics** are standards of behavior requiring truthfulness, honesty, and integrity. Ethics guide the behavior of physicians, who have the training, the primary responsibility, and the legal right to diagnose and treat human illness and injury. All medical office employees and those working in health-related professions share responsibility for observing the ethical code.

Each professional organization has a code of ethics that is to be followed by its membership. In general, this code states that information about patients, other employees, and confidential business matters should not be discussed with anyone not directly concerned with them. Behavior should be consistent with the values of the profession. For example, it is unethical for an employee to take money or gifts from a company in exchange for giving them business.

Figures 1.8 and 1.9 illustrate two codes of ethics. Figure 1.8 on page 26 shows the code of ethics of the American Health Information Management Association (AHIMA), which applies to workers in the health information field. Figure 1.9 on page 27 shows the code of ethics of the American Academy of Professional Coders (AAPC), which applies to the job of medical coder.

Etiquette

Professional **etiquette** is also important for medical insurance specialists. Correct behavior in a medical practice is generally covered in the practice's employee policy and procedure manual. For example, guidelines establish which types of incoming calls must go immediately to a physician or to a nurse or assistant, and which require a message to be taken. Of particular importance are guidelines about the respectful and courteous treatment of patients and all others who interact with the practice's staff.

Thinking It Through—1.5

- Dorita McCallister, the office manager of Clark Clinic, ordered medical office supplies from her cousin, Gregory Hand. When the supplies arrived, Gregory came to the office to check on them and to take Dorita out to lunch. Is Dorita's purchase of supplies from her cousin ethical? Why?

- George McGrew is working as a medical insurance specialist for Dr. Sylvia Grets. Dr. Grets consistently writes down codes that stand for one-hour appointments, but George knows that these visits were all very short, no longer than fifteen minutes each. This overcoding of the office visits has been happening for the last few weeks. Is it ethical for George to report these codes on insurance claims?

AHIMA Code of Ethics

Preamble

This Code of Ethics sets forth ethical principles for the health information management profession. Members of this profession are responsible for maintaining and promoting ethical practices. This Code of Ethics, adopted by the American Health Information Management Association, shall be binding on health information management professionals who are members of the Association and all individuals who hold an AHIMA credential.

I. Health information management professionals respect the rights and dignity of all individuals.

II. Health information management professionals comply with all laws, regulations, and standards governing the practice of health information management.

III. Health information management professionals strive for professional excellence through self-assessment and continuing education.

IV. Health information management professionals truthfully and accurately represent their professional credentials, education, and experience.

V. Health information management professionals adhere to the vision, mission, and values of the Association.

VI. Health information management professionals promote and protect the confidentiality and security of health records and health information.

VII. Health information management professionals strive to provide accurate and timely information.

VIII. Health information management professionals promote high standards for health information management practice, education, and research.

IX. Health information management professionals act with integrity and avoid conflicts of interest in the performance of their professional and AHIMA responsibilities.

Source: Copyright © 2003, American Health Information Management Association. Reprinted by permission.

Figure 1.8 AHIMA Code of Ethics

American Academy of Professional Coders

Code of Ethical Standards

- Members of the American Academy of Professional Coders shall be dedicated to providing the highest standard of professional coding and billing services to employers, clients and patients. Behavior of AAPC members must be exemplary.

- AAPC members shall maintain the highest standard of personal and professional conduct. Members shall respect the rights of patients, clients, employers and all other colleagues.

- Members shall use only legal and ethical means in all professional dealings, and shall refuse to cooperate with or condone by silence, the actions of those who engage in fraudulent, deceptive or illegal acts.

- Members shall respect the laws and regulations of the land, and uphold the mission statement of the AAPC.

AAPC Mission Statement

Establish and maintain ethical and educational standards for professional coders.

Provide a national certification and credentialing process.

Support the national and local membership by providing educational products and opportunities to network.

Increase and promote national recognition and awareness of procedural and diagnostic coding.

- Members shall pursue excellence through continuing education in all areas applicable to their profession.

- Members shall strive to maintain and enhance the dignity, status, competence and standards of coding for professional services.

- Members shall not exploit professional relationships with patients, employees, clients or employers for personal gain.

- Above all else, we will commit to recognizing the intrinsic worth of each member.

This code of Ethical Standards for members of the American Academy of Professional Coders strives to promote and maintain the highest standard of professional service and conduct among its members. Adherence to these standards assures public confidence in the integrity and service of professional coders who are members of the American Academy of Professional Coders.

Source: © Copyright American Academy of Professional Coders. Published by permission.

Figure 1.9 Code of Ethical Standards, American Academy of Professional Coders

Review

Chapter Summary

1. Higher health care costs and an aging population mean that medical providers are experiencing financial pressures and have an increasing need for knowledgeable medical insurance specialists on their staffs.

2. Group and individual policies provide medical insurance coverage; disability insurance, covers loss of income due to a person's inability to work; workers' compensation provides benefits for job-related claims; and liability insurance covers loss or injury inflicted on another party by the policyholder.

3. Fee-for-service reimbursement is a retroactive payment method in which payment is made after services are provided. In capitation, a fixed prospective payment is made for services to be provided during a specified period of time.

4. Indemnity health plans reimburse beneficiaries according to the contract's schedule of benefits in exchange for payment of a specified premium, deductibles, and coinsurance. Patients receive care from the providers of their choice. Managed care plans, in contrast, have agreements with both beneficiaries and providers that control the delivery and cost of health care services. In exchange for lower premiums and other cost reductions, plan members agree to a reduced choice of health care providers and tighter regulation of access to services.

5. An HMO locks patients into receiving services from providers with whom it has contracts; usually a primary care physician coordinates care and makes required referrals to specialists. A

POS offers more flexibility to choose providers, but at an increased cost. A PPO offers patients lower fees in exchange for receiving services from plan providers, but does not usually require care coordination or referrals.

6. Private-sector payers of health benefits are either insurance companies or self-insured employers. Most private health insurance is employer-sponsored. Government-sponsored health care programs include Medicare, Medicaid, TRICARE, and CHAMPVA.

7. The medical insurance industry is regulated by the federal government and by state law. Several organizations also accredit health plans.

8. Medical insurance specialists must know medical terminology, anatomy, and physiology, have communication and computer skills, pay attention to detail, be flexible and honest, and be able to work as team members.

9. Medical insurance specialists work in a variety of environments ranging from small to very large medical practices and for insurance companies, government-sponsored programs, and billing services. Certification includes designation as a Certified Medical Assistant, Registered Medical Assistant, and Registered Health Information Technician.

10. Ethical conduct in medical practices means following standards of behavior to ensure that medical employees are honest, truthful, and act with integrity. Professional etiquette sets the standards for good manners in dealing with others.

Key Terms

benefits *page 6*
capitation *page 8*
Centers for Medicare and Medicaid
   Services (CMS) *page 19*
coinsurance *page 11*
consumer-driven health plan *page 15*
copayment *page 13*

credentialing *page 20*
deductible *page 10*
discounted fee-for-service *page 15*
episode-of-care (EOC) option *page 10*
ethics *page 25*
etiquette *page 25*
fee-for-service *page 8*

formulary *page 13*
Health Insurance Portability and Accountability Act (HIPAA) of 1996 *page 19*
health maintenance organization (HMO)
   page 12
health plan *page 4*
indemnity *page 10*

Review Questions

Match the key terms in the left column with the definitions in the right column.

A. health maintenance organization (HMO)

B. capitation

C. schedule of benefits

D. fee-for-service

E. coinsurance

F. deductible

G. copayment

H. premium

I. preferred provider organization (PPO)

J. indemnity

_____ 1. A list of the medical services covered by an insurance policy

_____ 2. The amount of money paid to an health plan to buy an insurance policy

_____ 3. A managed care network of providers under contract to provide services at discounted fees

_____ 4. An amount that an insured person pays at the time of a visit to a provider

_____ 5. The percentage of each claim that an insured person must pay

_____ 6. A prospective payment to a provider made for each plan member

_____ 7. A health plan that reimburses policyholders based on the fees charged

_____ 8. An organization that contracts with a network of providers for the delivery of health care for a prepaid premium

_____ 9. The amount that an insured person must pay before reimbursement for medical expenses begins

_____ 10. A retroactive reimbursement method based on providers' charges

Decide whether each statement is true or false, and write T for true or F for false.

_____ 1. Employment opportunities for medical insurance specialists are increasing because providers need trained, knowledgeable staff to maximize revenue and ensure patient satisfaction.

_____ 2. The third party to a medical insurance contract is the policyholder.

_____ 3. A discounted fee-for-service schedule provides for prospective payment.

_____ 4. In order to receive PMPM payments for enrollees in a capitated managed care plan, a provider must have given medical services to each member at least once a month.

_____ 5. Under an indemnity plan, the premium, deductible, and coinsurance are taken into account before the insured is reimbursed.

_____ 6. In a POS plan, members must use network providers to be covered by the plan.

_____ 7. Both HMOs and PPOs use capitation as their main reimbursement method.

_____ 8. About two-thirds of medical coverage is employer-sponsored and one-third is government-sponsored.

_____ 9. CMS stands for the Centers for Medicare and Medicaid Services.

_____ 10. Everyone who works in a medical practice, whether a physician, nonphysician practitioner, or administrative staff member, has ethical responsibilities.

Write the letter of the choice that best completes the statement or answers the question.

_____ 1. In an HMO, a _____ coordinates the patient's care and provides referrals.
A. PPO C. PCP
B. EPO D. NPP

_____ 2. Which of the following permits members to see out-of-network providers?
A. POS C. URO
B. PCP D. EOC

_____ 3. The _____ sets a fee that covers all routine services for a treatment.
A. POS C. EPO
B. EOC D. PCP

_____ 4. In an HMO, securing a _____ is often required before services are provided.
A. preauthorization C. gatekeeper
B. utilization D. formulary

_____ 5. A self-insured employer may use a _____ to operate its health plan.
A. third-party payer C. third-party administrator
B. referral D. gatekeeper

_____ 6. Unlike an HMO, a PPO permits its members to use _____ providers, but at a higher cost.
A. subcapitated C. nonphysician practitioner
B. out-of-network D. primary care

_____ 7. The Centers for Medicare and Medicaid Services administers
A. TRICARE and CHAMPVA C. Medicare and Medicaid
B. HEDIS D. Medicare and TRICARE

_____ 8. An HMO is generally licensed as a business by
A. the federal government C. the state banking administration
B. the state insurance department D. a local government

_____ 9. The _____ regulations govern patients' private health information.
A. formulary C. PMPM
B. HEDIS D. HIPAA

_____ 10. In a medical practice, professional _____ provides guidelines on how to treat patients and visitors.
A. credentialing C. utilization
B. etiquette D. subcapitation

Provide answers to the following questions in the spaces provided.

1. Describe three features of HMOs that are designed to ensure high-quality patient care.

A. _____

B. _____

C. _____

2. List four government-sponsored health care programs.

A. _____

B. _____

C. _____

D. _____

3. List at least four important skills of medical insurance specialists.

A. _____

B. _____

C. _____

D. _____

4. Define the following abbreviations:

A. CCS _____

B. CCS-P _____

C. RHIT _____

D. CPC _____

Applying Your Knowledge

Case 1.1

A patient shows the following insurance identification card to the medical insurance specialist:

Connecticut HealthPlan

I.D.#:	1002.9713
Employee:	DANIEL ANTHONY
Group #:	A0000323
Eff. date:	03/01/2004
Status:	Dependent Coverage? F
In-network:	$10 Co-Pay
Out-of-network:	$250 Ded; 80%/20%

Front of card

IMPORTANT INFORMATION
Notice to Members and Providers of Care
To avoid a reduction in your hospital benefits, you are responsible for obtaining certification for hospitalization and emergency admissions. The review is required regardless of the reason for hospital admission. For specified procedures, Second Surgical Opinions may be mandatory.
For certification, call Utilization Management Services at 800-837-8808:
• At least 7 days in advance of Scheduled Surgery of Hospital Admissions.
• Within 48 hours after Emergency Admissions or on the first business day following weekend or holiday Emergency Admissions.

CONNECTICUT HEALTHPLAN C/O
WEISS   Robert S. Weiss
& Company
Silver Hill Business Center
500 S. Broad Street
P.O. Box 1034
Meriden, CT 06450
(800) 466-7900

THIS CARD IS FOR IDENTIFICATION ONLY AND DOES NOT ESTABLISH ELIGIBILITY FOR COVERAGE BY CONNECTICUT HEALTH PLAN. Please refer to your insurance booklet for further details.

Back of card

1. What copayment is due when the patient sees a network physician?

2. What payment rules apply when the patient sees an out-of-network physician?

3. What rules apply when the patient needs to be admitted to the hospital?

Computer Exploration

1. The World Wide Web is a valuable source of information about many topics of interest to medical insurance specialists, such as career opportunities. To explore the job statistics gathered by the *Occupational Outlook Handbook* of the Bureau of Labor Statistics, visit

   http://stats.bls.gov/oco

   Using the site map at that home page, choose Keyword Search of BLS Web Pages, and enter a job title of interest to you. Two possible choices are (1) medical assistants and (2) health information technicians. In particular, review the job outlook information.

2. Investigate the following organizations' Web sites, studying their membership, career ladders, and certification or credentials offered.

   ACA International (formerly American Collectors Association)
   http://www.collector.com

   American Academy of Professional Coders
   http://www.aapc.com

   American Association of Healthcare Administrative Management
   http://www.aaham.org

   American Health Information Management Association
   http://www.ahima.org

   Association of Medical Billers
   http://www.billers.com

   Healthcare Billing and Management Association
   http://www.hbma.com

   Healthcare Financial Management Association
   http://www.hfma.org

   Medical Group Management Association
   http://www.mgma.org

   Professional Association of Health Care Office Management
   http://www.pahcom.com

3. State insurance commissions protect consumers in the area of health insurance. For example, many states set up an ombudsman office to provide information on managed care. Locate your state's organization that provides health insurance help, or visit

   http://www.omc.state.ct.us

   to explore this state's information.

Computer Exploration

Many excellent medical billing programs are available, such as those from American Medical Software, MEDIC Computer Systems, NDCMediSoft, and Medical Manager Corporation. In this text, NDCMediSoft is used to illustrate a typical billing program's data entry screens and printed reports. NDCMediSoft is available free to adopters of *Medical Insurance*, 2e; instructions appear in the program, *Instructors Manual*. Quick-start instructions are on page 521 of the text. Detailed instructions on installing and using NDCMediSoft are on the student media that accompanies the text. This media, a student data disk, and a CD ROM, both contain all necessary introductory material as well as the Valley Associates, P.C., datasave which serves as an example of practice management software in use.

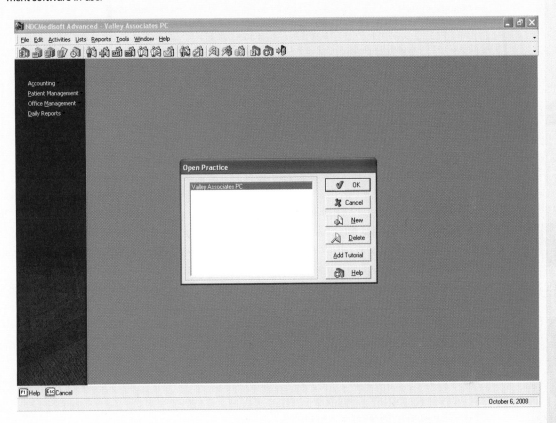

Computer Exploration

1.1 Review Patients' Copayment Requirements

The patients' insurance plans in the Valley Associates, P.C., database represent a variety of types, such as HMOs, PPOs, and traditional fee-for-service plans. This activity views the plans of selected patients and compares their copayment requirements.

1. Open the Lists menu, and select Patients/Guarantors and Cases. The Patient List dialog box appears.

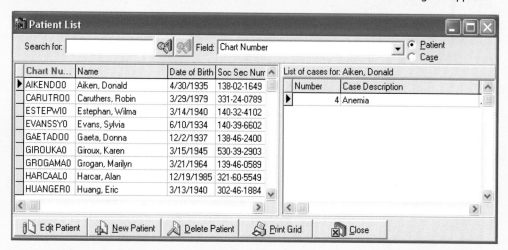

The Patient List dialog box is divided into two sections: patient information and case information. The left side of the dialog box lists basic information about patients. The right side of the dialog box lists cases for the patient who is selected in the left section of the window. Depending on which pane is active, the Patient or Case radio button in the upper right corner of the dialog box will be selected.

The patient's insurance plan information is attached to the case information. Therefore, to look up a patient's insurance coverage, the patient's Case dialog box must be opened.

2. The Search For box located at the top left of the dialog box can be used to search for a specific patient. Once the patient's information is selected in the Patient List dialog box, his or her case information can be accessed.

Patients can be searched for based on several criteria, for example chart number, assigned provider, or name. The Field box to the right of the Search For box contains the list of seach critieria. Click the triangle button in the Field box to display the list.

3. The drop-down list is displayed. By default, MediSoft searches for patients based on their chart numbers, the first item in the list. For the purposes of these exercises, we will also search for patients using their chart numbers. Click Chart Number in the drop-down list now to make sure this option is displayed in the Field box. Then Key "EV" to select information for Sylvia Evans.

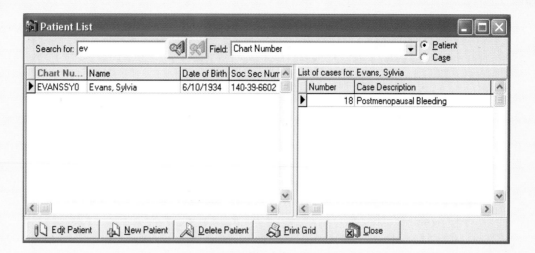

4. When Sylvia Evans' chart number is selected, her case description, "Postmenopausal Bleeding," is displayed in the right pane. If she had more than one case, additional cases would be listed. Click the case name to select it, and then click the Edit Case button at the bottom of the dialog box.

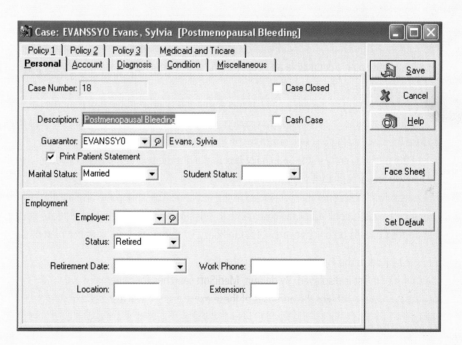

5. Sylvia Evans' Case dialog box for postmenopausal bleeding is displayed. It contains nine tabs. To view insurance information for this case, click the Policy 1 tab.

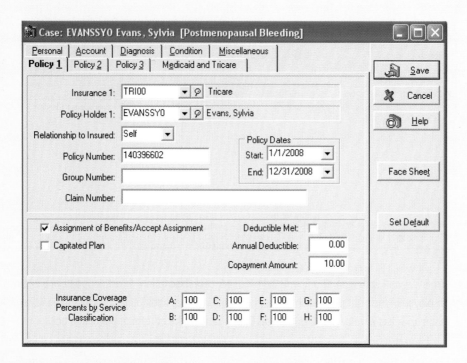

6. The Insurance 1 box indicates that Evans' primary insurance plan is Tricare. The middle section of the dialog box displays the plan's deductible and copayment requirements. The plan has no deductible and requires a $10 copayment for each visit.

7. In the bottom section of the dialog box, boxes A through H indicate the different rates at which the payer covers different types of services. Tricare covers 100 percent of all covered services. Click the Cancel button to close the Case dialog box and return to the Patient List dialog box.

8. Delete the previous entry in the Search For box (highlight the text and press the Delete key) and key "RUFFJ" to locate Jean Ruff's information.

9. When Jean Ruff's chart number is selected in the left pane, the right pane displays the name of the case "Ventricular Fibrillation." Click the case name to select it, and then click the Edit Case button.

10. Jean Ruff's Case dialog box appears. Click the Policy 1 tab to view her insurance plan data.

Computer Exploration

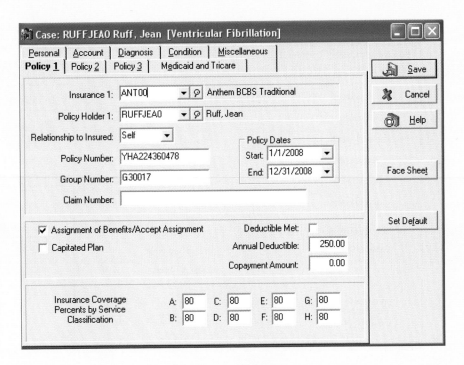

11. Jean Ruff's insurance plan is Anthem BCBS Traditional. Because this plan is a traditional fee-for-service plan, no copayments are required. The plan has a $250 deductible.

12. In addition, as indicated by the Insurance Coverage Percents by Service Classification boxes, the plan covers 80 percent of covered services. The patient pays the remaining 20 percent. Click the Cancel button to exit the Case dialog box and return to the Patient List dialog box.

13. Delete the previous entry in the Search For box, and key "V" to display information for Jose Velaquez.

14. Click his case description, "Mitral Valve Stenosis," to select it, and then click the Edit Case button.

15. Click the Policy 1 tab to display insurance information for this case.

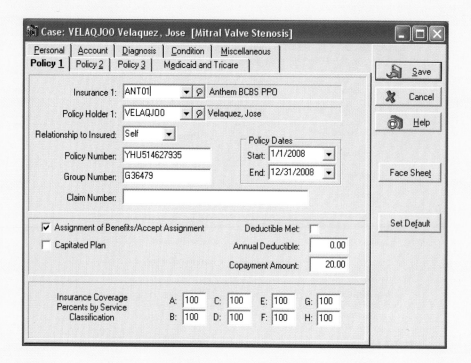

16. Jose Velaquez's insurance plan is Anthem BCBS PPO. PPOs generally have higher copayment requirements than other types of managed care programs. Jose Velaquez's copayment requirement is $20.

17. The Insurance Coverage Percents by Service Classification for this PPO indicate that Anthem BCBS PPO pays for covered services at the rate of 100 percent. Click the Cancel button to close the Case dialog box.

18. Click the Close button to close the Patient List dialog box and return to the main MediSoft window.

HIPAA and the Legal Medical Record

Objectives

After studying this chapter, you should be able to:

1. Discuss the importance of medical records.
2. List eight standards for medical documentation.
3. Describe the elements that are documented in patients' initial examinations and assessments, and discuss the documentation of patients' termination records.
4. Explain the purpose of the HIPAA Privacy Rule.
5. Distinguish between a covered entity and a business associate under HIPAA.
6. Define protected health information (PHI).
7. Describe the Notice of Privacy Practices.
8. Discuss patients' authorizations to use or disclose their health information.
9. Briefly describe the purpose of the HIPAA Security Rule.
10. Describe the HIPAA Electronic Health Care Transactions and Code Sets standards and the four National Identifiers.

Medical Records

Patients' **medical records** contain all facts, findings, and observations about their health history. They also contain all communications with and about each patient. In physicians' practices, the medical record begins with a patient's first contact with the practice and continues through all treatments and services. These records provide continuity and communication among physicians and other health care professionals who are involved in a patient's care. Patient medical records are also used in research and for education.

Patient medical records are kept by medical practices, hospitals, surgery centers, clinics, and other health care facilities. General practitioners and specialists use them to help make accurate diagnoses of patients' conditions and to trace the course of therapeutic care. For example, a patient's medical record contains the results of all tests a primary care physician (PCP) ordered during a comprehensive physical examination. By studying this medical record, a specialist treating a referred patient learns the outcome of those tests and avoids repeating them unnecessarily.

General practitioners often have medical records for patients that extend for many years. Other providers may have comparatively briefer encounters to record, after which patients are discharged. For example, a surgeon's file on a patient's cholecystectomy (surgical removal of the gallbladder) might include notes on the initial patient meeting for preoperative examination and discussion of the planned surgery, the operation itself, the postoperative review, and the instructions given to the patient at discharge from the surgeon's care.

Electronic Versus Paper Records

Patient medical records are created with the use of computers, as written notes on paper, or as some combination of both. **Electronic medical records (EMR)** offer both patients and providers significant advantages over paper records. For example, a patient who is away from home or in an accident can authorize a local physician to access the record to locate needed history. These records also improve inpatient care. Large amounts of information gathered over many years about a patient's chronic condition can be organized for quick review. Such records for thousands of patients with similar diagnoses can be analyzed to determine which treatment plans have given the best results. This protocol can then be provided to physicians who have patients with similar problems.

Electronic medical records are typically created on computers, rather than being written. The patient information is entered or checked off on a screen-based form (see Figure 2.1). Not just electronic versions of physicians' notes, electronic medical records include digital files of X-ray images, lab test results, medical history, and perhaps other images, such as a picture of the patient. An EMR system in a large health care center such as a hospital often includes a computerized physician order-entry system (CPOE) and a medication administration record (MAR) system. These electronic systems improve patient care by helping reduce medical errors. Physicians use desktop, laptop or handheld computers to access patient information on the hospital's EMR network.

Although electronic medical records are the preferred way to store, access, and process patient information, implementing an EMR system requires money and time. Many physician practices and other providers are gradually changing to electronic systems, so medical insurance specialists work with paper records as well. These records may be written and then stored on paper, or they may be

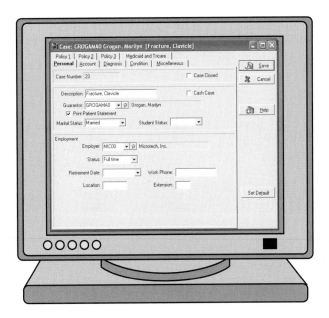

Figure 2.1 Example of an Electronic Record

written and then converted to electronic media such as computer disks. When a manual system is used, providers' notes are usually written on the patients' records or transcribed from dictation and placed in the record, where they are signed and dated by the responsible provider. Lab test results are printed; Xrays, ECGs, and other routine test results are included.

Documentation

In medical record **documentation**, a patient's health status is recorded in chronological order using a systematic, logical, and consistent method. One system is SOAP notes, reviewed on page 44. A patient's health history, examinations, tests, and results of treatments are all documented.

Medical Standards of Care

Complete and comprehensive records are important in providing evidence that physicians have followed states' medical standards of care. In legal terms, a standard of care is the degree of attention called for in a particular situation— what any reasonable party would do in the same circumstance. Medical **standards of care** are defined as using the care and expertise that under the circumstances could be reasonably expected of a professional with similar experience and training.

Health care providers are liable (that is, legally responsible) for providing the state-required standard of care to their patients. The term *medical professional liability* describes this responsibility, which extends to all licensed health care professionals, such as nurses and physician's assistants, as well as physicians.

Negligence

Health care professionals can be charged with **negligence** when they fail to perform their medical duties properly. A medical professional may be negligent in a number of ways. Here are examples:

- A physician assistant may perform a wrongful act, such as acting beyond the authority of the license and dispensing medications.

- Care may be provided in an improper way, such as a physician overlooking a test that is customarily done for a patient with a given condition, causing the physician to misdiagnose the illness.
- A registered nurse may not act when the situation and the law demand it, such as by failing to treat an AIDS patient because of fear of transmission of the disease.

Ensuring Proper Documentation

Patient medical records are legal documents. Properly documented patient medical records become part of the physician's defense against accusations that patients were not treated correctly. They clearly state who performed what service and describe why, where, when, and how it was done. Physicians document the rationale behind their treatment decisions. This rationale is the basis for the concept of medical necessity—a clinically logical link between a patient's condition and the treatment or procedure provided. For example, when a test or drug is ordered for a patient, the physician documents the diagnosis or condition that is being confirmed or ruled out.

Although they do not make entries in patient medical records, medical insurance specialists work with the records in the billing and reimbursement process. The documentation of diagnoses and procedures is used as proof of the services that they report to payers for reimbursement. An unwritten law of medical insurance is that if it was not documented, it was not done, and if it was not done, it cannot be billed. Payers also use documentation to decide whether the reported services should be reimbursed. The record must clearly document where, why, when, and how each service occurred.

Standards

Because of the importance of patient medical records, the leading health care industry groups, including the American Medical Association and the American Hospital Association, have set standards for documentation. Standardization helps make medical records more efficient and improves the quality of patient care. Although not responsible for documentation, medical insurance specialists help organize and maintain patient medical records. They must be aware of the following standards and encourage their use to ensure that the practice maintains complete and proper documentation of all patient-related issues:

- *Records must be clear:* Medical records should be complete and accurate. If the records are handwritten, the entries should be legible to others, made in black ink (not pencil), and dated.
- *Entries must be signed and dated:* Whether digitally entered by the provider, handwritten, or transcribed, each entry must have the signature or initials and title of the responsible provider and the date.
- *Changes must be clearly made:* An incorrect entry is marked with a single line through the words to be changed; the correct information is entered after it, so that the previous copy can be read. Corrections are also dated and signed by the person making the change. No part of a record should be otherwise altered or removed, deleted, or destroyed.

Example

Correct	Incorrect	Guideline
85 5/7/2007 this 80-year old *jrb* ^	85 this 85-year old	Corrections should be clear, signed, and dated

- *No blank spaces may be left between entries:* Entries are made chronologically, without spaces between them, to prevent out-of-order entries.
- *Each patient should have a single record:* Each patient should have one medical record, often called a unit record. (Note, however, that practices should be sure to have a separate file in a patient's medical record when workers' compensation claims are involved; see Chapter 14.)
- *Records should use consistent vocabulary and format:* All entries should reflect standard, accepted medical vocabulary and abbreviations. All medical records in a practice should be consistently labeled and have logical sections.
- *Diagnostic information must be easy to locate:* Past and present diagnoses should be placed so that they are easy to locate by each physician who uses the medical record.
- *Practitioners' entries must be made promptly:* Entries should be made in a timely manner and filed in a consistent chronological order, either ascending or descending.

Billing Tip

Documentation and Billing
The connection between documentation and billing bears repeating: If a service is not documented, it was not done, and if it was not done, it cannot be billed.

Documenting Encounters

Every patient **encounter**—face-to-face meeting with a patient—should be documented with the following information:

- The patient's name
- The encounter date and reason
- Appropriate history and physical examination
- Review of all tests that were ordered
- The diagnosis
- The plan of care, or notes on treatments that were given
- The instructions or recommendations that were given to the patient
- The signature of the provider who saw the patient.

In addition to this encounter information, a patient's medical record must contain:

- Biographical and personal information, including the patient's full name, Social Security number, date of birth, full address, marital status, home and work telephone numbers, and employer information as applicable
- Duplicates of all documents that communicate with the patient, including letters, telephone calls, faxes, and e-mail messages; the patient's responses; and a note of the time, date, topic, and physician's response to each communication from the patient
- Duplicates of prescriptions and instructions given to the patient, including refills
- Any original documents that the patient has signed, such as an authorization to release information (see page 56) and an advance directive
- Medical allergies and reactions, or the lack of them
- Up-to-date immunization record and history if appropriate, such as for a child
- Previous and current diagnoses, test results, health risks, and progress
- Copies of referral or consultation letters
- Hospital admissions and release documents
- A record of any missed or canceled appointments
- Any requests for information about the patient (from a health plan or an attorney, for example), and a detailed log of to whom information was released

The patient medical record also includes the identification number assigned by the practice to the patient. Billing and insurance information is usually stored separately from the medical record.

SOAP Format

Medical insurance specialists work with a number of methods that are used to organize patient medical records. The most common format used in general medical practices is called a *problem-oriented medical record* (POMR). The problem-oriented medical record contains a general section with data from the initial patient examination and assessment. When the patient makes subsequent visits, the reasons for those encounters are listed separately and have their own notes. For example, the patient's record might have a general section followed by sections labeled "skin disorder" and "right eye scleral abrasion" with notes about these conditions.

A problem-oriented medical record contains SOAP notes. In the SOAP format, a patient's encounter documentation is grouped into four parts: Subjective, Objective, Assessment, and Plan:

S: The *subjective* information is based on the patient's descriptions of symptoms along with other comments.

O: The *objective* information includes the physician's descriptions of the presenting problem and data from examinations and tests.

A: The *assessment,* also called the impression or conclusion, is the physician's diagnosis, or interpretation of the subjective and objective information.

P: The *plan,* also called treatment, advice, or recommendations, includes the necessary patient monitoring, follow-up, procedures, and instructions to the patient.

The Initial Examination: The History and Physical

Providers follow generally recognized guidelines to document encounters during which they evaluate a patient's condition and select the treatment that will be used to manage it.

These initial examinations and assessments are often called history and physical. The order of documentation is (1) the chief complaint, (2) the history and physical examination, (3) the diagnosis, and (4) the treatment plan (see Figure 2.2).

The physician first documents the patient's **chief complaint (CC)**, a concise statement that describes the symptom, problem, condition, diagnosis, or other factor the patient gives as the reason for the encounter. It is usually stated in the patient's words. For clarity, the physician may restate it as a "presenting problem," using medical terminology.

The physician then takes the patient's history and conducts the examination. The extent of the history and of the examination is determined by what the physician considers appropriate. Following the history and examination, the physician documents the diagnosis—the interpretation of the information that has been gathered. The treatment plan, or plan of care, includes the treatments and medications, specifying dosage and frequency of use.

To document the process of **informed consent** for a procedure or anesthesia, physicians discuss the assessment and recommendations with patients, including the risks and benefits of the recommended course of treatment and other treatment options. Immediately after, physicians document in the medical record that the activity occurred, and include a brief summary of the content that was discussed. Often, patients are asked to sign their chart entry describing the informed consent or a form to show they consent to the procedure.

James E. Ribielli
5/19/2006

CHIEF COMPLAINT: This 79-year-old male presents with sudden and extreme weakness. He got up from a seated position and became light-headed.

PAST MEDICAL HISTORY: History of congestive heart failure. On multiple medications, including Cardizem, Enalapril 5 mg qd, and Lasix 40 mg qd.

PHYSICAL EXAMINATION: No postural change in blood pressure. BP, 114/61 with a pulse of 49, sitting; BP, 111/56 with a pulse 50, standing. Patient denies being light-headed at this time.

HEENT: Unremarkable.

NECK: Supple without jugular or venous distension.

LUNGS: Clear to auscultation and percussion.

HEART: S1 and S2 normal; no systolic or diastolic murmurs; no S3, S4. No dysrhythmia.

ABDOMEN: Soft without organomegaly, mass, or bruit.

EXTREMITIES: Unremarkable. Pulses strong and equal.

LABORATORY DATA: Hemoglobin, 12.3. White count, 10.800. Normal electrolytes. ECG shows sinus bradycardia.

DIAGNOSIS: Weakness on the basis of sinus bradycardia, probably Cardizem induced.

TREATMENT: Patient told to change positions slowly when moving from sitting to standing, and from lying to standing.

John R. Ramirez, MD

Figure 2.2 Example of Examination Documentation

Progress Reports and Discharge Summaries

Progress reports document the patient's progress and response to the treatment plan (see Figure 2.3 on page 46). They explain whether the plan should be continued or changed. Progress reports include:

- Comparisons of objective data with the patient's statements
- Goals and progress toward the goals
- The patient's current condition and prognosis
- Type of treatment still needed and for how long

Jennifer Delgado
8/14/2006

SUBJECTIVE: The patient has had epilepsy since she was 10. She takes her medication as prescribed; denies side effects. She reports no convulsions or new symptoms. She is a full-time student at Riverside Community College.

OBJECTIVE: Phenobarbital 90 mg twice a day as prescribed since 1994. The motor and sensory examination results are normal.

ASSESSMENT: Well-controlled epilepsy.

PLAN: Patient advised to continue medication regimen. Schedule for follow-up in 6 months.

Jared R. Wandaowsky, MD

Figure 2.3 Example of a Progress Report

Myrna W. Pearl
8/20/2006

SUBJECTIVE: Myrna came in for suture removal from a right-knee wound. She reports that she is healing well.
OBJECTIVE: The wound appears dry and clean, with no signs of infection.
ASSESSMENT: Uncomplicated suture removal.
PLAN: All six sutures were removed and a bandage applied. Patient was advised to continue to keep the wound clean. No further treatment is required.

Grady Lonquier, MD

Figure 2.4 Example of a Discharge Summary

Discharge summaries are prepared during the patient's final visit for a particular treatment plan (see Figure 2.4). Discharge summaries include:

- The final diagnosis
- Comparisons of objective data with the patient's statements
- Whether goals were achieved
- Reason for and date of discharge

Dear _____:

I find it necessary to inform you that I am discharging you as a patient for the reason that you have continually refused to follow my medical advice and treatment. Because your condition requires medical attention, I suggest that you find another physician to provide you with care promptly. If you wish, I will provide care for a period of up to five days after you receive this letter. This should give you enough time to select a physician from the many competent providers in this area. With your authorization, I will make your medical record available to the physician you select.

Sincerely,

_____, MD

Figure 2.5 Example of a Termination Letter

- The patient's current condition, status, and final prognosis
- Instructions given to the patient at discharge, noting any special needs such as restrictions on activities and medications

Termination of the Provider–Patient Relationship

At times, either the patient or the provider terminates the relationship. In these cases, the provider must still maintain the patient's medical record. The provider also sends the patient a letter that documents the situation and provides for continuity of care with the next provider. For example, if a patient wishes to be released from a physician's care, the provider documents this fact and any part of the treatment plan that was still underway at the time of termination. On the other hand, the patient's actions, such as refusing to observe a treatment plan, take required medication, or keep appointments, may cause the provider to decide to terminate the relationship. In this event, the patient is informed in writing (see Figure 2.5). A copy of this letter becomes part of the patient's medical record.

Health maintenance organizations have specific regulations concerning a primary care physician's decision to terminate a relationship with a patient. The PCP must first request approval to do so from the HMO, and then send the patient a certified letter. A receipt must be signed by the patient and returned. The PCP must provide emergency care until the transfer takes place.

HIPAA

Patients' medical records—the actual progress notes, reports, and other materials—are legal documents that belong to the provider that created them. Although the provider owns the actual records, the provider cannot use or withhold the information in them according to its own wishes. This information—the nature of the patient's diagnosis, for example, rather than the actual progress note where it is written—belongs to the patient.

Nicholas J. Kramer, MD
2200 Carriage Lane
Currituck, CT 07886

Consultation Report
on John W. Wu
(Birth date 12/06/1933)

Dear Dr. Kramer:

At your request, I saw Mr. Wu today. This is a sixty-five-year-old male who stopped smoking cigarettes twenty years ago, but continues to be a heavy pipe smoker. He has had several episodes of hemoptysis; a small amount of blood was produced along with some white phlegm. He denies any upper respiratory tract infection or symptoms on those occasions. He does not present with chronic cough, chest pain, or shortness of breath. I reviewed the chest X-ray done by you, which exhibits no acute process. His examination was normal.

A bronchoscopy was performed, which produced some evidence of laryngitis, tracheitis, and bronchitis, but no tumor was noted. Bronchial washings were negative.

I find that his bleeding is caused by chronic inflammation of his hypopharynx and bronchial tree, which is related to pipe smoking. There is no present evidence of malignancy.

Thank you for requesting this consultation.

Sincerely,

Mary Lakeland Georges, MD

This letter is in the patient medical record of John W. Wu.

What is the purpose of the letter?

How does it demonstrate the use of a patient medical record for continuity of care?

Patients have rights to the information their records contain. Patients control the amount and type of information that is released, except for the use of the data to treat them or conduct the normal business transactions of the practice. Only patients, or their legally appointed representatives, have the authority to authorize the release of information to anyone not directly involved in their care.

Medical insurance specialists handle issues such as requests for information from patients' medical records, and they need to know what information can be released about patients' conditions and treatments. The information in this section explains the rules concerning information that can be legally shared with other providers and health plans, and what information the patient must specifically authorize to be released.

Administrative Simplification: Three Rules

The rules about answering this type of question are based on the HIPAA Administrative Simplification provisions, which affect providers' responsibilities and patients' rights related to their private health information. Congress passed the Administrative Simplification provisions partly because of concern over rising health care costs (see Chapter 1). A significant portion of every health care dollar is spent on administrative and financial transactions. These costs can be controlled if the business transactions of health care are standardized and handled electronically, just like ATM transactions for the banking industry. The Administrative Simplification provisions are also intended to protect the privacy of people's health information once transactions are handled electronically.

There are three parts to HIPAA's Administrative Simplification provisions:

- *HIPAA privacy requirements:* The privacy requirements cover patients' health information.
- *HIPAA security requirements:* The security requirements state the administrative, technical, and physical safeguards that are required to protect patients' health information.
- *HIPAA electronic transaction and code sets standards:* These standards require every provider who does business electronically to use the same health care transactions, code sets, and identifiers.

Complying with HIPAA

Health care organizations that are required by law to obey the HIPAA regulations are referred to as **covered entities.** A covered entity is an organization that electronically transmits any information that is protected under HIPAA. Other organizations that work for the covered entities must also agree to follow the HIPAA rules when they are using information that is protected under the regulations.

Covered Entities

Under HIPAA, three types of covered entities must follow the regulations:

- Health plans—the individual or group plan that provides or pays for the cost of medical care
- Health care **clearinghouses**—companies that help providers handle electronic transactions such as submitting claims
- Health care providers—people or organizations that furnish, bill, or are paid for health care in the normal course of business

Almost all physician practices are included under HIPAA. A practice is *not a* covered entity only if it does not send any claims (or other HIPAA transactions) electronically *and* does not employ any other firm to send electronic claims for it. Since CMS requires Medicare claims to be sent electronically from all but the smallest groups—those with fewer than ten employees—noncompliance is both impractical and potentially costly for physician practices.

Business Associates

HIPAA also affects many others in the health care field. For instance, software billing vendors are not covered entities—they are not themselves required to comply with the law. However, they may need to make changes in order to do business with a covered entity. In HIPAA terms, they are called **business associates**, a category that includes law firms, accountants, information technology (IT) contractors, compliance consultants, and collection agencies. Through agreements with their business associates, covered entities make sure that they will perform their work as required by HIPAA.

HIPAA Privacy Rule

The HIPAA Standards for Privacy of Individually Identifiable Health Information (known as the **HIPAA Privacy Rule**) is the first comprehensive federal protection for the privacy of health information. These national standards protect individuals' medical records and other personal health information. Before the HIPAA Privacy Rule became law, the personal information stored in hospitals, physicians' practices, and health plans fell under a patchwork of federal and state laws. Some state laws were strict, but others were not. The privacy rule is a baseline of safeguards to protect the confidentiality of medical information. State laws that provide stronger privacy protections apply over and above the federal privacy standards. For example, states may have special privacy requirements for patients tested, diagnosed, or treated for alcohol and drug abuse, sexually transmitted diseases, or mental health disorders.

The privacy rule must be followed by all covered entities—health plans, health care clearinghouses, and health care providers—and their business associates. The rules mandate that a covered entity must

- Adopt a set of privacy practices that are appropriate for its health care services
- Notify patients about their privacy rights and how their information can be used or disclosed
- Train employees so that they understand the privacy practices
- Appoint a staff member to be the privacy official responsible for seeing that the privacy practices are adopted and followed
- Secure patient records containing individually identifiable health information so that they are not readily available to those who do not need them

Protected Health Information

The HIPAA privacy rule covers the use and disclosure of patients' **protected health information (PHI)**. PHI is defined as individually identifiable health information that is transmitted or maintained by electronic media, such as over the Internet or by computer modem, or on magnetic tape or compact disks. This information includes a person's

- Name
- Address (including street address, city, county, ZIP code)
- Names of relatives and employers
- Birth date
- Telephone numbers
- Fax number
- E-mail address
- Social Security number

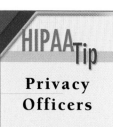

HIPAA Tip

Privacy Officers

The privacy official at a small physician practice may be the office manager who has other duties. At a large health plan, the position of privacy official may be full time.

The HIPAA Privacy Rule and the HIPAA Security Rule both require providers to appoint a staff person to take responsibility for compliance. In large facilities, the Privacy Officer and the Security Officer each lead a team of people focused on planning and implementing the necessary steps. In smaller practices, where the responsibilities may overlap, the two roles may be combined.

Because the Privacy Rule requires release of just the minimum necessary information, the Privacy Officer's job includes analyzing what information employees need in order to do their jobs. Often, the officer oversees the work of experts in clinical areas who determine the minimum necessary information for various jobs. Another common practice is to ask managers to tell the privacy officer which computer applications their workers need ready access to. When this analysis is complete, the secu-

rity officer sets up each person's controlled access to the computer files. For example, a person-authentication system is designed to verify that people seeking access to PHI are who they claim to be.

Professional certification in the area of privacy is offered by the American Health Information Management Association (AHIMA) with the credential of Certified in Healthcare Privacy (CHP). The Health Information Management Systems Society (HIMSS), through AHIMA, offers the credential of Certified in Healthcare Security (CHS). Jointly, the organizations offer the credential of Certified in Healthcare Privacy and Security (CHPS). Applicants for the examinations must have an RHIT or RHIA credential, a baccalaureate degree, and a minimum of two year's on-the-job experience in the health care management field.

- Medical record number
- Health plan beneficiary number
- Account number
- Certificate or license number
- Serial number of any vehicle or other device
- Web site address
- Fingerprints or voiceprints
- Photographic images

Disclosure for Treatment, Payment, and Health Care Operations

Patients' PHI under HIPAA can be shared for treatment, payment, and health care operations. *Use of PHI* means sharing or analysis *within* the entity that holds the information, while *disclosure* means the release, transfer, provision of access to, or divulging of PHI *outside* the entity holding the information.

Both use and disclosure of PHI are necessary and permitted for patients' treatment, payment, and health care operations (TPO). *Treatment* means providing and coordinating the patient's medical care; *payment* refers to the exchange of information with health plans; and health care *operations* are the general business management functions.

Minimum necessary standard   When using or disclosing protected health information, a covered entity must try to limit the information shared to the minimum amount of PHI necessary to accomplish the intended purpose. The **minimum necessary standard** means taking reasonable safeguards to protect PHI from incidental disclosure. For example, a medical insurance specialist would

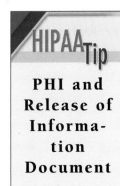

HIPAATip

PHI and Release of Information Document

No patient release of information document is needed when PHI is shared for treatment, payment, or health care operations (TPO) under HIPAA.

not disclose a patient's history of cancer on a workers' compensation claim for a sprained ankle. Only the information the recipient needs to know is given.

Designated record set　A covered entity must disclose individuals' PHI to them (or their personal representatives) when they request access to, or an accounting of disclosures of, their protected health information. According to the "AHIMA Practice Brief: Defining the Designated Record Set," patients' rights apply to a **designated record set (DRS)**. For a provider, the designated record set means the medical and billing records the provider maintains. It does not include appointment and surgery schedules, requests for lab tests, and birth and death records. It also does not include mental health information, psychotherapy notes, and genetic information. For a health plan, the designated record set includes enrollment, payment, claims decisions, and medical management systems of the plan.

Within the designated record set, patients have the right to

- Access, copy, and inspect their PHI
- Request an amendment to their health information
- Obtain an accounting of most disclosures of their health information
- Receive communications from providers via other means, such as in Braille or in foreign languages
- Complain about alleged violations of the regulations and the provider's own information policies

Notice of privacy practices　Covered entities must give each patient a notice of privacy practice at their first contact or encounter. To satisfy this requirement, physician practices give patients a copy of their **Notice of Privacy Practices** (see Figure 2.6) and ask them to sign an acknowledgment that they have received it. The notice explains how their PHI may be used and describes their rights. Practices may choose to use a layered approach to giving patients the notice. A short notice that briefly describes the uses and disclosures of PHI and the person's rights is on top of the information packet. The longer notice is placed next in the packet.

Authorizations

For use or disclosure other than for treatment, payment, or operations, the covered entity must have the patient sign an **authorization** to release the information. For example, information about alcohol and drug abuse may not be released without a specific authorization from the patient. The authorization document must be in plain language and include the following:

- A description of the information to be used or disclosed
- The name or other specific identification of the person(s) authorized to use or disclose the information
- The name of the person(s) or group of people to whom the covered entity may make the use or disclosure
- A description of each purpose of the requested use or disclosure
- An expiration date
- Signature of the individual (or authorized representative) and date

In addition, the rule states that a valid authorization must include:

- A statement of the individual's right to revoke the authorization in writing
- A statement about whether the covered entity is able to base treatment, payment, enrollment, or eligibility for benefits on the authorization

Valley Associates, P.C.

NOTICE OF PRIVACY PRACTICES

THIS NOTICE DESCRIBES HOW MEDICAL INFORMATION ABOUT YOU MAY BE USED AND DISCLOSED AND HOW YOU CAN GET ACCESS TO THIS INFORMATION. PLEASE REVIEW IT CAREFULLY.

WHY ARE YOU GETTING THIS NOTICE?

Valley Associates, P.C. is required by federal and state law to maintain the privacy of your health information. The use and disclosure of your health information is governed by regulations under the Health Insurance Portability and Accountability Act of 1996 (HIPAA) and the requirements of applicable state law. For health information covered by HIPAA, we are required to provide you with this Notice and will abide by this Notice with respect to such health information. If you have questions about this Notice, please contact our Privacy Officer at 877-555-1313. We will ask you to sign an "acknowledgment" indicating that you have been provided with this notice.

WHAT HEALTH INFORMATION IS PROTECTED?

We are committed to protecting the privacy of information we gather about you while providing health-related services. Some examples of protected health information are:

- Information indicating that you are a patient receiving treatment or other health-related services from our physicians or staff;
- Information about your health condition (such as a disease you may have);
- Information about health care products or services you have received or may receive in the future (such as an operation); or
- Information about your health care benefits under an insurance plan (such as whether a prescription is covered);

when combined with:

- Demographic information (such as your name, address, or insurance status);
- Unique numbers that may identify you (such as your Social Security number, your phone number, or your driver's license number); and
- Other types of information that may identify who you are.

SUMMARY OF THIS NOTICE

This summary includes references to paragraphs throughout this notice that you may read for additional information.

1. Written Authorization Requirement

We may use your health information or share it with others in order to treat your condition, obtain payment for that treatment, and run our business operations. We generally need your written authorization for other uses and disclosures of your health information, unless an exception described in this Notice applies.

2. Authorizing Transfer of Your Records

You may request that we transfer your records to another person or organization by completing a written authorization form. This form will specify what information is being released, to whom, and for what purpose. The authorization will have an expiration date.

3. Canceling Your Written Authorization

If you provide us with written authorization, you may revoke, or cancel, it at any time, except to the extent that we have already relied upon it. To revoke a written authorization, please write to the doctor's office where you initially gave your authorization.

4. Exceptions to Written Authorization Requirement

There are some situations in which we do not need your written authorization before using your health information or sharing it with others. They include:

Treatment, Payment and Operations
As mentioned above, we may use your health information or share it with others in order to treat your condition, obtain payment for that treatment, and run our business operations.

Family and Friends
If you do not object, we will share information about your health with family and friends involved in your care.

(a)

Figure 2.6 Example of a Summary of Privacy Practices

Research
Although we will generally try to obtain your written authorization before using your health information for research purposes, there may be certain situations in which we are not required to obtain your written authorization.

De-Identified Information
We may use or disclose your health information if we have removed any information that might identify you. When all identifying information is removed, we say that the health information is "completely de-identified." We may also use and disclose "partially de-identified" information if the person who will receive it agrees in writing to protect your privacy when using the information.

Incidental Disclosures
We may inadvertently use or disclose your health information despite having taken all reasonable precautions to protect the privacy and confidentiality of your health information.

Emergencies or Public Need
We may use or disclose your health information in an emergency or for important public health needs. For example, we may share your information with public health officials at the State or city health departments who are authorized to investigate and control the spread of diseases.

5. How to Access Your Health Information

You generally have the right to inspect and get copies of your health information.

6. How to Correct Your Health Information

You have the right to request that we amend your health information if you believe it is inaccurate or incomplete.

7. How to Identify Others Who Have Received Your Health Information

You have the right to receive an "accounting of disclosures." This is a report that identifies certain persons or organizations to which we have disclosed your health information. All disclosures are made according to the protections described in this Notice of Privacy Practices. Many routine disclosures we make (for treatment, payment, or business operations, among others) will not be included in this report. However, it will identify any non-routine disclosures of your information.

8. How to Request Additional Privacy Protections

You have the right to request further restrictions on the way we use your health information or share it with others. However, we are not required to agree to the restriction you request. If we do agree with your request, we will be bound by our agreement.

9. How to Request Alternative Communications

You have the right to request that we contact you in a way that is more confidential for you, such as at home instead of at work. We will try to accommodate all reasonable requests.

10. How Someone May Act On Your Behalf

You have the right to name a personal representative who may act on your behalf to control the privacy of your health information. Parents and guardians will generally have the right to control the privacy of health information about minors unless the minors are permitted by law to act on their own behalf.

11. How to Learn about Special Protections for HIV, Alcohol and Substance Abuse, Mental Health and Genetic Information

Special privacy protections apply to HIV-related information, alcohol and substance abuse treatment information, mental health information, psychotherapy notes and genetic information.

12. How to Obtain A Copy of This Notice

If you have not already received one, you have the right to a paper copy of this notice. You may request a paper copy at any time, even if you have previously agreed to receive this notice electronically. You can request a copy of the privacy notice directly from your doctor's office. You may also obtain a copy of this notice from our website or by requesting a copy at your next visit.

13. How to Obtain A Copy of Revised Notice

We may change our privacy practices from time to time. If we do, we will revise this notice so you will have an accurate summary of our practices. You will be able to obtain your own copy of the revised notice by accessing our website or by calling your doctor's office. You may also ask for one at the time of your next visit. The effective date of the notice is noted in the top right corner of each page. We are required to abide by the terms of the notice that is currently in effect.

14. How To File A Complaint

If you believe your privacy rights have been violated, you may file a complaint with us or with the federal Office of Civil Rights. To file a complaint with us, please contact our Privacy Officer.

No one will retaliate or take action against you for filing a complaint.

(b)

Figure 2.6 (*Continued*)

Based on the information in Figure 2.6,

1. What document is required when a patient asks Valley Associates to transfer a record to another person or organization?

2. Is written authorization from a patient needed to use or disclose health information in an emergency?

3. What is the purpose of an "accounting of disclosures"?

- A statement that information used or disclosed after the authorization may be disclosed again by the recipient and may no longer be protected by the rule

A sample authorization form is shown in Figure 2.7.

Uses or disclosures for which the covered entity has received specific authorization from the patient do not have to follow the minimum necessary standard. Incidental use and disclosure are also allowed. For example, the practice may use reception-area sign-in sheets.

Exceptions

There are a number of exceptions to the privacy rule:

- Court orders
- Workers' compensation cases
- Statutory reports
- Research

All these types of disclosures must be logged, and the release information must be available to the patient who requests it.

Release under court order   If the patient's PHI is required as evidence by a court of law, the provider may release it without the patient's approval upon judicial order. In the case of a lawsuit, a court sometimes decides that a physician or medical practice staff member must provide testimony. The court issues a **subpoena**, an order of the court directing a party to appear and testify. If the court requires the witness to bring certain evidence, such as a patient medical record, it issues a **subpoena** *duces tecum,* which directs the party to appear, to testify, and to bring specified documents or items.

Workers' compensation cases   State law may provide for release of records to employers in workers' compensation cases (see Chapter 14). The law may also authorize release to the state Workers' Compensation Administration board and to the insurance company that handles these claims for the state.

Statutory reports   Some specific types of information are required by state law to be released to state health or social services departments. For example, physicians must make such statutory reports for patients' births and deaths and for cases of abuse. Because of the danger of harm to patients or others, communicable diseases such as tuberculosis, hepatitis, and rabies must usually be reported.

A special category of communicable disease control is applied to patients with diagnoses of human immunodeficiency virus (HIV) infection and acquired immunodeficiency syndrome (AIDS). Every state requires AIDS cases to be

HIPAA Tip

PHI and Practice Policy

The release of protected health information must follow the practice's policies and procedures. The practice's privacy official trains medical insurance specialists on how to verify the identity and authority of a person requesting PHI.

Patient Name: _____

Health Record Number: _____

Date of Birth: _____

1. I authorize the use or disclosure of the above named individual's health information as described below.

2. The following individual(s) or organization(s) are authorized to make the disclosure: _____

3. The type of information to be used or disclosed is as follows (check the appropriate boxes and include other information where indicated)

What specific information can be released

❑ problem list

❑ medication list

❑ list of allergies

❑ immunization records

❑ most recent history

❑ most recent discharge summary

❑ lab results (please describe the dates or types of lab tests you would like disclosed): _____

❑ x-ray and imaging reports (please describe the dates or types of x-rays or images you would like disclosed): _____

❑ consultation reports from (please supply doctors' names): _____

❑ entire record

❑ other (please describe): _____

4. I understand that the information in my health record may include information relating to sexually transmitted disease, acquired immunodeficiency syndrome (AIDS), or human immunodeficiency virus (HIV). It may also include information about behavioral or mental health services, and treatment for alcohol and drug abuse.

5. The information identified above may be used by or disclosed to the following individuals or organization(s):

Name: _____

To whom

Address: _____

Name: _____

Address: _____

6. This information for which I'm authorizing disclosure will be used for the following purpose:

For what purpose

❑ my personal records

❑ sharing with other health care providers as needed/other (please describe): _____

7. I understand that I have a right to revoke this authorization at any time. I understand that if I revoke this authorization, I must do so in writing and present my written revocation to the health information management department. I understand that the revocation will not apply to information that has already been released in response to this authorization. I understand that the revocation will not apply to my insurance company when the law provides my insurer with the right to contest a claim under my policy.

8. This authorization will expire (insert date or event): _____

If I fail to specify an expiration date or event, this authorization will expire six months from the date on which it was signed.

9. I understand that once the above information is disclosed, it may be redisclosed by the recipient and the information may not be protected by federal privacy laws or regulations.

10. I understand authorizing the use or disclosure of the information identified above is voluntary. I need not sign this form to ensure health care treatment.

Signature of patient or legal representative: _____ Date: _____

If signed by legal representative, relationship to patient

Signature of witness: _____ Date: _____

Distribution of copies: Original to provider; copy to patient; copy to accompany use or disclosure

Note: This sample form was developed by the American Health Information Management Association for discussion purposes. It should not be used without review by the issuing organization's legal counsel to ensure compliance with other federal and state laws and regulations.

Figure 2.7 Example of an Authorization to Use or Disclose Health Information

reported. Most states also require reporting of the HIV infection that causes the syndrome. However, state law varies concerning whether just the fact of a case is to be reported, or if the patient's name must also be reported. The practice guidelines reflect the state laws and must be strictly observed, as all these regulations should be, to protect patients' privacy and to comply with the regulations.

Research data   PHI may be made available to researchers approved by the practice. For example, if a physician is conducting clinical research on a type of diabetes, the practice may share information from appropriate records for analysis. When the researcher issues reports or studies based on the information, specific patients' names may not be identified.

De-identified health information   There are no restrictions on the use or disclosure of **de-identified health information** that neither identifies nor provides a reasonable basis to identify an individual. For example, these identifiers must be removed: names, medical record numbers, health plan beneficiary numbers, device identifiers (such as pacemakers), and biometric identifiers, such as fingerprints and voiceprints.

Enforcement and Penalties

Patients who observe privacy problems in their providers' offices can complain either to the practice or to the Department of Health and Human Services (HHS). Complaints must be put in writing, either on paper or electronically, and sent to the **Office of Civil Rights (OCR)**, which is part of HHS, usually within 180 days. A covered entity must cooperate with an HHS investigation and give HHS access to its facilities, books, records, and systems, including relevant protected health information.

There are civil and criminal penalties for violating the rule. Civil penalties for HIPAA privacy violations—which can be imposed only on covered entities, not on business associates—can be up to $100 for each offense, with an annual cap of $25,000 for repeated violations of the same requirement. Criminal penalties are as follows:

- For knowing misuse of individually identifiable health information: up to $50,000 and/or one year in prison
- For misuse under false pretenses: up to $100,000 and/or five years in prison
- For offenses to sell for profit or malicious harm: up to $250,000 and/or ten years in prison

HIPAA Security Rule

The **HIPAA Security Rule** requires covered entities to establish administrative, physical, and technical safeguards to protect the confidentiality, integrity, and availability of PHI. The security rule specifies how to secure such protected health information on computer networks, the Internet, disks and magnetic tape, and over other networks.

Security Requirements

The security rule also mandates the following:

- A security official must be assigned responsibility for the entity's security.
- All staff members must receive security awareness training.

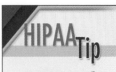

PHI and the Security Rule

The security regulations require controlling access to PHI. For example, in a practice, receptionists may view the names of patients coming to the office on one day, but they should not see those patients' medical records. However, the nurse or physician in charge of X-rays needs to view the patient records. To build two types of access, receptionists are given an individual computer password that lets them view the day's schedule, but denies entry to patient records. The physicians and nurses possess computer passwords that allow them to see all patient records.

- Organizations must control and monitor staff access to patients' records.
- Organizations must limit physical access to facilities that contain electronic PHI.
- Organizations must determine where they have information security risks and vulnerabilities to illegal access.

Enforcement and Penalties

The regulations are enforceable for most covered entities on April 21, 2005. Small health plans (those with less than $5 million in annual revenue) will have an additional year to comply.

HIPAA Electronic Health Care Transactions and Code Sets

The **HIPAA Electronic Health Care Transactions and Code Sets (TCS)** standards eliminate the huge variety of e-commerce methods used in the health care industry. Following these standards, a physician can submit electronic claims in the same format, using standard codes, regardless of the payer. Every health plan must accept the standard format and standard codes and send electronic messages back to the provider, also in standard formats, advising the provider of claim status, payment, and other key information.

Standard Transactions

The HIPAA transactions standards apply to the financial and administrative information that is regularly exchanged between providers and health plans. Each standard is labeled with both the transaction number and the name. Either the number or the name may be used to refer to the particular electronic document.

Number	Name
X12 837	(1) Health care claims or equivalent encounter information/coordination of benefits
	(2) Coordination of benefits (COB)—an exchange of information between payers when a patient is covered by more than one medical insurance plan
X12 276/277	Health care claim status inquiry/response
X12 270/271	Eligibility for a health plan inquiry/response
X12 278	Referral authorization inquiry/response
X12 835	Health care payment and remittance advice
X12 820	Health plan premium payments
X12 834	Health plan enrollment and disenrollment

Medical insurance specialists use the first six transactions in performing their jobs. This topic is covered in detail in Chapters 3 and 8.

TABLE 2.1	HIPAA Standard Code Sets
Purpose	**Standard**
Codes for diseases, injuries, impairments, and other health-related problems	*International Classification of Diseases,* Ninth Edition, *Clinical Modification* (ICD-9-CM), Volumes 1 and 2
Codes for procedures or other actions taken to prevent, diagnose, treat, or manage diseases, injuries, and impairments	*Physicians' Services: Current Procedural Terminology,* Fourth Edition (CPT) *Inpatient Hospital Services: International Classification of Diseases,* Ninth Revision, *Clinical Modification,* Volume 3: *Procedures*
Codes for dental services	*Current Dental Terminology* (CDT-4)
Codes for other hospital-related services	Healthcare Common Procedures Coding System (HCPCS)

Standard Code Sets

Under HIPAA, a **code set** is any group of codes used for encoding data elements, such as tables of terms, medical concepts, medical diagnosis codes, or medical procedure codes. Medical code sets used in the health care industry include coding systems for diseases; treatments and procedures; and supplies or other items used to perform these actions. These standards, listed in Table 2.1, are covered in Chapters 4, 5, and 15.

HIPAA National Identifiers

The Administrative Simplification provisions mandate the creation of **HIPAA National Identifiers** for

- Employers
- Health care providers
- Health plans
- Patients

Identifiers are numbers of predetermined length and structure, such as a person's Social Security number. They are important because the unique numbers can be used in electronic transactions as a standard system. Two have been established.

Employer Identification Number (EIN)

The employer identifier is used to identify the patient's employer on claims to a plan. In addition, employers must identify themselves in transactions when they enroll or disenroll employees in a health plan, or make premium payments to plans on behalf of their employees. The final regulation establishes the Employer Identification Number (EIN) issued by the Internal Revenue Service as the HIPAA standard.

National Provider Identifier (NPI)

The National Provider Identifier (NPI) is the standard unique health identifier for health care providers to use in filing and processing health care claims and other transactions. The effective date of this final rule is 2005. NPIs will be issued through the National Provider System (NPS), which is being developed by CMS. The NPI will replace all identifiers that are currently being used.

PHI and Electronic Transmission

Medical insurance specialists receive training in handling electronically transmitted information using the practice's computer system and the Internet. E-mail systems and fax machines should be designed for secure transmission of confidential information.

All health care providers are eligible to be assigned NPIs. The NPI is 10 positions in length, with 9 numbers plus a check digit in the last position. The numbers will be assigned to individuals, such as doctors, nurses, and hygienists; numbers will also be assigned to organizations, such as hospitals, pharmacies, and clinics. For example, if a physician is in a group practice, both the individual and the practice will have NPIs.

Enforcement and Penalties

CMS enforces the transaction and code set standards. Failure to comply with the transaction and code set rule may result in monetary penalties. CMS may impose a penalty of not more than $100 per violation on the entity failing to comply, with a cap of $25,000 for violations of a single standard in a calendar year.

Thinking It Through—2.3

Gloria Traylor, an employee of National Bank, called Marilyn Rennagel, a medical insurance specialist who works for Dr. Judy Fisk. The bank is considering hiring one of Dr. Fisk's patients, Juan Ramirez, and Ms. Traylor would like to know if he has any known medical problems. Marilyn, in a hurry to complete the call and get back to work on this week's claims, quickly explains that she remembers that Mr. Ramirez was treated for depression some years ago, but that he has been fine since that time. She adds that she thinks he would make an excellent employee.

In your opinion, did Marilyn handle this call correctly?
What problems might result from her answers?

Review

Chapter Summary

1. Patients' medical records, which contain the complete, chronological, and comprehensive documentation of patients' health history and status, are used by providers to communicate and coordinate patients' health care. The records are used by medical insurance specialists to prepare and support insurance claims.

2. The standards for documentation are that (a) records must be clear; (b) entries must be signed and dated by the responsible provider; (c) changes must be clearly marked, and the record must not be otherwise altered; (d) no blank spaces are to appear between entries; (e) each patient should have a single record; (f) consistent vocabulary and format should be used; (g) diagnostic information must be easy to locate; and (h) practitioners' entries should be made promptly.

3. Documentation of an examination includes the chief complaint (CC), the history, the examination, the diagnosis, and the treatment plan. The process leading to the patient's informed consent for procedures is also documented. A progress report documents a patient's response to a treatment plan and provides justification for continued treatment. At the end of a treatment plan, a discharge summary documents the patient's final status and prognosis. If the provider–patient relationship is terminated, the reasons for termination and the status of the patient's treatment plan are documented, and the patient is informed in writing.

4. The HIPAA Privacy Rule, a part of the Administrative Simplification provisions, regulates the use and disclosure of patients' protected health information (PHI), individually identifiable health information that is transmitted or maintained by electronic media.

5. Under HIPAA, a covered entity is a health plan, health care clearinghouse, or health care provider that transmits any health information in electronic form in connection with a HIPAA transaction. A business associate, such as a law firm or billing service that performs work for a covered entity, must agree to follow applicable HIPAA regulations to safeguard protected health information.

6. Protected health information (PHI) is individually identifiable health information that is transmitted or maintained by electronic media, including data such as a patient's name, Social Security number, address, and phone number.

7. A Notice of Privacy Practices is a HIPAA-mandated document that presents a covered entity's principles and procedures related to the protection of patients' PHI. Covered entities must give patients copies of their notices.

8. For use or disclosure for treatment, payment, or operations (TPO), no release is required from the patient. To release PHI for other than TPO, a covered entity must have the patient sign an authorization. The authorization document must be in plain language and have a description of the information to be used, who can disclose it and for what purpose, who will receive it, an expiration date, and the patient's signature.

9. The HIPAA Security Rule, a part of the Administrative Simplification provisions, requires covered entities to establish administrative, physical, and technical safeguards to protect the confidentiality, integrity, and availability of health information.

10. The HIPAA Electronic Health Care Transactions and Code Sets establishes standards for the exchange of financial and administrative data among covered entities that require them to use common electronic transaction methods and code sets. The four National Identifiers are for employers, health care providers, health plans, and patients.

Key Terms

authorization *page 52*
business associate *page 50*
chief complaint (CC) *page 44*
clearinghouse *page 48*
code set *page 59*
covered entity *page 48*
de-identified health information *page 57*
designated record set (DRS) *page 52*
documentation *page 41*

electronic medical record (EMR) *page 40*
encounter *page 43*
HIPAA Electronic Health Care Transactions
   and Code Sets (TCS) *page 58*
HIPAA National Identifier *page 59*
HIPAA Privacy Rule *page 50*
HIPAA Security Rule *page 57*
informed consent *page 44*
medical records *page 40*

minimum necessary standard *page 51*
negligence *page 41*
Notice of Privacy Practices *page 52*
Office of Civil Rights (OCR) *page 57*
protected health information (PHI)
   page 50
standards of care *page 41*
subpoena *page 55*
subpoena *duces tecum page 55*

Review Questions

Match the key terms in the left column with the definitions in the right column.

A. HIPAA Privacy Rule

B. authorization

C. minimum necessary
   standard

D. business associate

E. clearinghouse

F. Notice of Privacy
   Practices

G. code set

H. HIPAA Security Rule

I. covered entity

J. documentation

_____ 1. Law under the Administrative Simplification provisions of HIPAA requiring covered entities to establish administrative, physical, and technical safeguards to protect the confidentiality, integrity, and availability of health information

_____ 2. The systematic, logical, and consistent recording of a patient's health status—history, examinations, tests, results of treatments, and observations—in chronological order in a patient's medical record

_____ 3. A person or organization that performs a function or activity for a covered entity but is not part of its workforce

_____ 4. The principle that individually identifiable health information should be disclosed only to the extent needed to support the purpose of the disclosure

_____ 5. Under HIPAA, a health plan, health care clearinghouse, or health care provider that transmits any health information in electronic form in connection with a HIPAA transaction

_____ 6. Law under the Administrative Simplification provisions of HIPAA regulating the use and disclosure of patients' protected health information, individually identifiable health information that is transmitted or maintained by electronic media

_____ 7. A HIPAA-mandated document that presents a covered entity's principles and procedures related to the protection of patients' protected health information

_____ 8. A coding system used to encode elements of data

_____ 9. A company that offers providers, for a fee, the service of receiving electronic or paper claims, checking and preparing them for processing, and transmitting them in proper data format to the correct carriers

_____ 10. Document signed by a patient that permits release of medical information under the specific stated conditions

Decide whether each statement is true or false, and write T for true or F for false.

_____ 1. Electronic medical records offer advantages over paper records.

_____ 2. Medical standards of care are based on the expertise that any reasonable layperson would follow in the situation.

_____ 3. The chief complaint is usually documented using clinical terminology.

_____ 4. The three major parts of the Administrative Simplification provisions are the privacy requirements, the security requirements, and the electronic transactions and code sets.

_____ 5. When federal and state privacy laws disagree, the federal rule is always followed.

_____ 6. Under HIPAA regulations, each physicians' practice must appoint a privacy official.

_____ 7. Protected health information includes the various numbers assigned to patients, such as their medical record numbers and their health plan beneficiary numbers.

_____ 8. The minimum necessary standard does not refer to the patient's health history.

_____ 9. Patients have the right to access, copy, inspect, and request an amendment of their medical and billing records.

_____ 10. A patient's authorization is needed to disclose protected information for payment purposes.

Write the letter of the choice that best completes the statement or answers the question.

_____ 1. Under the HIPAA Privacy Rule, physician practices must
   A. train employees about the practice's privacy policy
   B. appoint a staff member as the privacy officer
   C. both A and B
   D. neither A nor B

_____ 2. A Notice of Privacy Practices is given to
   A. a practice's patients
   B. a practice's business associates
   C. the health plans a practice contracts with
   D. none of the above

_____ 3. Patients' PHI may be released without authorization to
   A. local newspapers
   B. employers in workers' compensation cases
   C. social workers
   D. family and friends

_____ 4. Which government group has the authority to enforce the HIPAA Privacy Rule?
   A. CIA   C. OCR
   B. OIG   D. Medicaid

_____ 5. Patients always have the right to
   A. withdraw their authorization to release information
   B. alter the information in their medical record
   C. block release of information about their communicable disease to the state health department
   D. none of the above

_____ 6. The authorization to release information must specify
   A. the number of pages to be released
   B. the Social Security number of the patient
   C. to whom the information is to be released
   D. the name of the treating physician

_____ 7. Health information that does not identify an individual is referred to as
   A. protected health information
   B. authorized health release
   C. statutory data
   D. de-identified health information

_____ 8. Violating the HIPAA Privacy Rule can result in
   A. civil penalties
   B. criminal penalties
   C. both civil and criminal penalties
   D. neither civil nor criminal penalties

_____ 9. The main purpose of the HIPAA Security Rule is to
   A. regulate electronic transactions
   B. protect research data
   C. control the confidentiality and integrity of and access to protected health information
   D. protect medical facilities from criminal acts such as robbery

_____ 10. Under HIPAA, National Identifiers will be created for
   A. health plans, employers, health care providers, and patients
   B. physicians, nurses, aides, and medical office staff
   C. health plans, employees, dependents, and spouses
   D. all of the above

Provide answers to the following questions in the spaces provided.

1. List eight standards for documentation.

2. Define the following abbreviations:

   A. OCR _____

   B. PHI _____

   C. TCS _____

   D. DRS _____

   E. EMR _____

   F. CC _____

   G. NPI _____

Applying Your Knowledge

Case 2.1

The X-ray report shown on the next page contains four documentation errors. Identify each, and indicate the guideline that has not been followed.

X-RAY REPORT

Patient name
Salvia, Leonard X.

Examination
Esophagus

Report

jdl
7-20-2005

1

① The patient experiences no difficulty in swallowing barium. A 2 cm. tablet was given and

② passes readily down to the distal esophagus. After considerable swallowing, the barium

③ tablet remained in place, indicating a significant area of narrowing, less than 1 cm in

④ diameter, located between this distal esophagus that probably represents a stricture related

⑤ to a small hiatus hernia and possible esophagitis. There are no shelf-like defects or masses

Jane

portion
⑥ to correspond to neoplasm. The mid and upper ~~position~~ of the esophagus is unremarkable.

⑦ Conclusion: Small hiatus hernia with an area of stenosis, probably on the basis of

major
⑧ esophagitis, appears to represent a ~~significant~~ lesion.

jdl

Case 2.2

Rosalyn Ramirez is a medical insurance specialist employed by Valley Associates, P.C., a midsized multispecialty practice with an excellent record of complying with HIPAA rules. Rosalyn answered the telephone and heard this question:

"This is Jane Mazloum, I'm a patient of Dr. Olgivy. I just listened to a phone message from your office about coming in for a checkup. My husband and I were talking about this. Since this is my first pregnancy and I am working, we really don't want anyone else to know about it yet. Has this information been given to anybody outside the clinic?"

How do you recommend that she respond?

Case 2.3

Angelo Diaz signed the authorization form on the next page. When his insurance company called for an explanation of a reported procedure that Dr. Handlesman performed to treat a stomach ulcer, George Welofar, the clinic's registered nurse, released copies of his complete file. On reviewing Mr. Diaz's history of treatment for alcohol abuse, the insurance company refused to pay the claim, stating that Mr. Diaz's alcoholism had caused the condition. Mr. Diaz complained to the practice manager about the situation.

Should the information have been released?

Patient Name: _Angelo Diaz_

Health Record Number: _ADI00_

Date of Birth: _10-12-1945_

1. I authorize the use or disclosure of the above named individual's health information as described below.

2. The following individual(s) or organization(s) are authorized to make the disclosure: _Dr. L. Handlesman_

3. The type of information to be used or disclosed is as follows (check the appropriate boxes and include other information where indicated)

❑ problem list

❑ medication list

❑ list of allergies

❑ immunization records

☑ most recent history

❑ most recent discharge summary

❑ lab results (please describe the dates or types of lab tests you would like disclosed): _____

☑ x-ray and imaging reports (please describe the dates or types of x-rays or images you would like disclosed): _____

❑ consultation reports from (please supply doctors' names): _____

❑ entire record

☑ other (please describe): _Progress notes_

4. I understand that the information in my health record may include information relating to sexually transmitted disease, acquired immunodeficiency syndrome (AIDS), or human immunodeficiency virus (HIV). It may also include information about behavioral or mental health services, and treatment for alcohol and drug abuse.

5. The information identified above may be used by or disclosed to the following individuals or organization(s):

Name: _Blue Cross & Blue Shield_

Address: _____

Name: _____

Address: _____

6. This information for which I'm authorizing disclosure will be used for the following purpose:

❑ my personal records

❑ sharing with other health care providers as needed/other (please describe): _____

7. I understand that I have a right to revoke this authorization at any time. I understand that if I revoke this authorization, I must do so in writing and present my written revocation to the health information management department. I understand that the revocation will not apply to information that has already been released in response to this authorization. I understand that the revocation will not apply to my insurance company when the law provides my insurer with the right to contest a claim under my policy.

8. This authorization will expire (insert date or event): _____

If I fail to specify an expiration date or event, this authorization will expire six months from the date on which it was signed.

9. I understand that once the above information is disclosed, it may be redisclosed by the recipient and the information may not be protected by federal privacy laws or regulations.

10. I understand authorizing the use or disclosure of the information identified above is voluntary. I need not sign this form to ensure healthcare treatment.

Signature of patient or legal representative: _Angelo Diaz_ Date: _3-1-2006_

If signed by legal representative, relationship to patient

Signature of witness: _____ Date: _____

Distribution of copies: Original to provider; copy to patient; copy to accompany use or disclosure

Note: This sample form was developed by the American Health Information Management Association for discussion purposes. It should not be used without review by the issuing organization's legal counsel to ensure compliance with other federal and state laws and regulations.

Computer Exploration

1. The Computer-based Patient Record Institute (CPRI) promotes the development of the electronic (computer-based) medical record. Go to

    http://www.aafp.org/x518.xml

    and research the present status of electronic medical records in the United States. In the opinion of this group, how can electronic records improve patient care?
2. Visit the Web site of the American Medical Association:

    http://www.ama-assn.org

    Do a site search for *medical records,* and report on the summary findings of a recent study on this subject.
3. Visit the Web site of the Centers for Medicare and Medicaid Services (CMS) to research the current status of HIPAA National Identifiers. Determine whether standards have been adopted for health plan or patient identifiers.

NDCMedisoft Activity

2.1 Review Security Features in MediSoft

The HIPAA security rule is designed to enforce the HIPAA privacy standards by securing protected health information (PHI). Patient information containing individually identifiable health information must not be readily available to those who do not need the information. In compliance with the HIPAA standards, MediSoft provides security features to protect the practice's data from unauthorized access. The program can be set up to limit the access of users to certain areas of MediSoft. In addition, security procedures can deny specific users the ability to edit or change data in the program.

The security features in MediSoft are set up as follows.

1. Select Security Setup on the File menu. The Security Setup dialog box appears. (On your screen, the dialog box is blank because no security features have been activated. The illustration below is an example of a Security Setup dialog box with data.) The names, login names, and access levels are shown for all existing users. Names are added to the list using the New button.

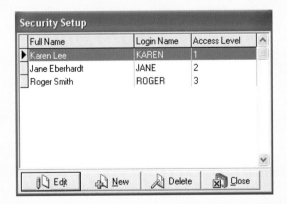

Each person who will be using the MediSoft program is assigned a login name and password, as well as an access level. There are five access levels, Level 1 through Level 5. Level 1 permits unlimited access and should be assigned to a supervisor or office manager. Level 1 allows the designated person to set up and modify security levels for all other users. Level 1 users have unrestricted access to all of MediSoft's features.

Level 5 is assigned to individuals whose task is limited to data entry. Level 5 users can record transactions, enter new patient information, and generate day sheet reports. However, they cannot generate most of the other reports available in MediSoft, such as practice analysis or aging reports. Nor can they create claims, delete entries, or perform general billing tasks.

The levels between Levels 1 and 5 represent a range of access levels. Levels 2 and 3 are generally assigned to individuals in charge of billing. Users with Level 2 and 3 access can create and edit claims, print practice analysis and aging reports, create new reports, and perform other tasks related to billing.

Once a Level 1 access person is assigned in the Security Setup dialog box, a new option, Permissions, appears on the File menu. When the Permissions option is clicked by a Level 1 access person, the MediSoft Security Permissions dialog box appears.

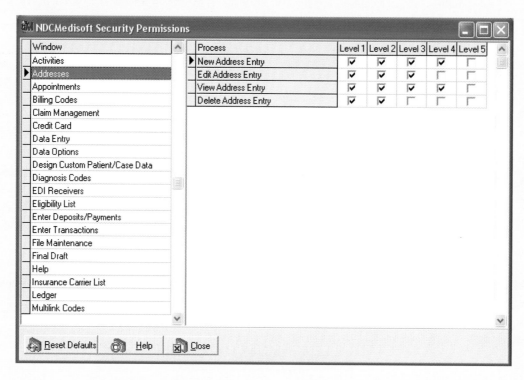

The MediSoft Security Permissions dialog box defines the different levels of access permitted for each level. All available MediSoft functions are listed on the left, and the grid on the right indicates whether a user with a given access level has permission to use the dialog box connected with that function. All the default settings displayed in the MediSoft Security Permissions dialog box can be modified by a Level 1 access person, with the exception that Level 1 access can not be changed—Level 1 must have access to all functions.

Once users are assigned a security access level, they must log in and enter a password every time they enter MediSoft. If they try to perform a task that is not allowed for their access level, the following Security Warning dialog box is displayed:

Computer Exploration

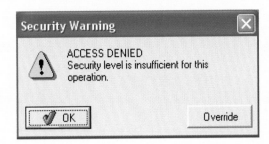

The Override button is available in the event a person with a higher level of access temporarily wants to log in and give the current user a higher level of access to the program. Otherwise, access is denied to the current user for that task.

2. Click the Close button to exit the Security Setup dialog box.

The HIPAA security rule also mandates that organizations have records of workers who have logged into information systems that contain PHI. The MediSoft Data Audit Report is designed to produce this information. Once the MediSoft security setup has been completed (users have been assigned login names, passwords, and access levels), MediSoft tracks changes made to the data by each user. At any time, the individual with Level 1 access can print a report, the Data Audit Report, that displays these changes.

The report is accessed via the Reports menu. It can be created for any date or period of dates and for any user or users. For example, a billing supervisor might print a weekly list of all changes made to the data, or see changes made by a certain user.

Chapter 3

Introduction to the Billing and Reimbursement Cycle

Objectives

After studying this chapter, you should be able to:

1. List the ten steps in the health care billing and reimbursement cycle.

2. Identify the information that is collected from new and established patients.

3. Explain the purpose of the HIPAA Acknowledgment of Receipt of Notice of Privacy Practices.

4. Discuss the procedures and transactions that are used to verify patients' insurance benefits.

5. Describe the basic billing and reimbursement procedures and transactions that medical insurance specialists perform following patients' encounters.

6. Explain the importance of communications skills in working with patients, health plans, and providers.

7. Discuss the use of information technology in billing and reimbursement.

Overview of the Billing and Reimbursement Cycle

The billing and reimbursement cycle follows a set of steps that lead to maximum appropriate, timely payment for patients' medical services.

Basic Billing and Reimbursement Steps

These basic steps (see Figure 3.1) are followed:

1. *Collection of patient information:* Personal and demographic information about patients is recorded.
2. *Insurance verification:* Patients' insurance coverage is checked, and documents are scanned or copied, current benefits are verified, and payers' conditions for payment, such as preauthorization, are met.
3. *Encounter form preparation:* Encounter forms (the forms providers use to summarize patients' visits) are prepared for scheduled appointments.
4. *Coding:* Following patient encounters, patients' diagnoses, as well as the providers' procedures and services, are assigned codes.
5. *Linkage and compliance review:* A review is performed to check that the diagnosis and the medical services received are logically connected and that all applicable regulations on adequate documentation in the patient medical record have been followed.
6. *Physician charge calculation:* The fees for medical services are calculated, based on the payer's conditions for payment, and the patients' portions or copayments are collected.
7. *Claims preparation:* Health care claims for reimbursement from payers are promptly prepared and checked.
8. *Claims transmission:* Claims are sent to patients' health plans.
9. *Payer adjudication:* Payers process claims, request missing or more detailed information if needed, and decide whether they will pay or deny claims.
10. *Reimbursement follow-up and record retention:* Payments are received and recorded. Patients are billed for the amounts they owe. Patients' medical records are updated and filed according to practice guidelines.

Billing and Reimbursement Cycle

1. Collect Patient Information
2. Verify Insurance
3. Prepare Encounter Form
4. Code Diagnoses and Procedures
5. Review Linkage and Compliance
6. Calculate Physician Charges
7. Prepare Claims
8. Transmit Claims
9. Payer Adjudication
10. Follow Up Reimbursement/Record Retention

Figure 3.1 **Billing and Reimbursement Steps**

Procedures, Communication, and Information Technology

The billing and reimbursement cycle involves three components: (1) procedures, (2) communications, and (3) information technology.

Procedures

Each step in billing and reimbursement involves following medical office procedures. Some procedures involve administrative duties, such as scanning an insurance card. Others are performed to comply with HIPAA and other regulations, such as protecting PHI in computer files from unauthorized viewing. Some procedures, such as medical coding, are based on technical skills. Most of the procedures are handled by medical insurance specialists working as a team with providers and other professional health care staff, such as physician assistants (PA), nurse-practitioners (NP), clinical social workers, physical therapists, occupational therapists, audiologists, and clinical psychologists.

This chapter discusses general procedures. In physician practices, the procedures are usually established by the practice manager and described in the practice's policy and procedures manual.

Communications

Communication skills are as important as knowing about specific forms, codes, and regulations. For instance, when a medical insurance specialist gathers information from patients, a pleasant tone and a helpful manner increase patient satisfaction with the services they are receiving. The ability to communicate with a diverse audience is very important. The basic guidelines of courtesy and consideration also apply to communications with the staff members of health plans.

Equally important are effective communications with busy physicians and other professional staff. These conversations must be brief and to the point, showing that the speaker values the physician's time. Remember that people are more likely to listen when the speaker is smiling and has an interested expression. In addition, nonverbal cues such as good listening skills are important. Speakers should be aware of their facial expressions and maintain moderate eye contact.

Information Technology

Medical insurance specialists use **information technology (IT)**—the development of computer hardware and software information systems—to handle administrative tasks electronically in almost all physician practices.

Electronic data interchange An important information technology application involves **electronic data interchange**, known as **EDI**. EDI is the computer-to-computer exchange of routine business information using publicly available standards. Administrative staff use EDI to exchange health information about their practices' patients with payers and clearinghouses. Each electronic exchange is a **transaction**, which is the electronic equivalent of a business document. An example of a nonmedical transaction is the process of getting cash from an ATM.

Note that EDI transactions are not visible in the way an exchange of paperwork such as letters is. In the example of an ATM transaction, the computer-to-computer exchange is made up of computer language that is sent and answered between the machines. This exchange happens "behind the scenes." It is documented on the customer's end with the transaction receipt that is printed; the bank also has a record at its location.

HIPAA Tip

Electronic Information Exchange

When information is exchanged electronically between providers, health plans, and clearinghouses, the HIPAA electronic transaction standards must be followed.

on Careers Administrative Medical Assistant

Administrative medical assistants are employed by medical group practices and clinics. Possible duties include preparing and maintaining medical records, handling the office-staff payroll, ordering equipment and supplies, performing medical transcription, greeting patients and scheduling appointments, arranging for patients' hospital admissions, and billing, bookkeeping, and insurance-processing tasks. In large practices, duties may be specialized; in small practices, medical assistants perform a wide range of tasks.

Administrative medical assistants must understand the use of office equipment and computer software programs—word processing, database management, and accounting and billing—as well as banking, billing, collections, and accounts payable procedures. Equally important are the skills needed for effective interactions with the practice's patients. Administrative medical assistants maintain a safe and welcoming patient reception area, help educate patients about the practice's policies or preparation for a medical procedure, and ensure patient data confidentiality.

A postsecondary medical assisting program is an excellent background for an entry-level position. Fulfilling the requirements for certification from either the American Association of Medical Assistants (for a Certified Medical Assistant, or CMA, designation) or the American Medical Technologists (for a Registered Medical Assistant, or RMA, designation) and successful job performance contribute to advancement to positions such as medical office manager and medical records manager.

Many exchanges of billing and reimbursement information use the Internet. For example, many health plans offer an online "platform"—a Web site where providers who are part of their network can exchange information with the plan about patients' insurance coverage, the plan's benefits, and the status of claims that have been sent.

Medical billing programs   Information technology is critical in managing prospective payments from managed care organizations (MCOs) as well as reimbursements from health plans. Medical billing programs are typically used for this administrative work. Billing programs streamline the important process of creating and following up on health care claims sent to payers and bills sent to patients. For example, a large medical practice with a group of providers and thousands of patients receives a phone call from a patient who wants to know the amount owed on an account. With a computerized billing program, the medical insurance specialist enters the first few letters of the patient's last name, and the patient's account data appear on the monitor. The outstanding balance is communicated to the patient.

Before use by a practice, the medical billing program is set up with data about the practice's income and expense accounting. The provider database, or collection of related facts, is then entered. It contains data about all physicians in the practice, such as their medical license numbers, tax identification numbers, and office hours, as well as facts about referring physicians and lab services. The practice's most common diagnoses and services, with associated fees, are also entered in the medical billing program's databases.

Medical insurance specialists enter information about patients' visits as appointments are made and encounters occur. They use the billing program to

• Organize patient and payer information

- Collect data on patients' diagnoses and services
- Generate, transmit, and report on the status of health care claims
- Record payments from payers
- Provide information on patients' payments and accounts
- Generate financial and productivity reports

A note of caution: What information technology cannot do   Although computers increase efficiency and reduce errors, they are not more accurate than the individual who is entering the data. If humans make mistakes while entering data, the information the computer produces will be incorrect. Computers are very precise and also very unforgiving. While the human brain knows that *flu* is short for *influenza,* the computer regards them as two distinct conditions. If a computer user accidentally enters a name as *ORourke* instead of *O'Rourke,* a human might know what is meant; the computer does not. It would probably respond with a message such as "No such patient exists in the database."

Many human errors occur during data entry, such as pressing the wrong key on the keyboard. Other errors are a result of a lack of computer literacy—not knowing how to use a program to accomplish tasks. For this reason, proper training in data-entry techniques so that errors are caught, as well as knowing how to use computer programs, are both essential for medical insurance specialists.

Collection of Patient Information

The first step in billing and reimbursement is gathering and verifying information about patients. This is perhaps the most important step, because if it is not done correctly, the provider may be unable to collect payment for services. Missing or invalid birth dates, mismatches between a patient's name in the medical record and in the health plan record, and other incorrect information cause payers to return claims unpaid.

To gather accurate patient information, medical insurance specialists follow one procedure for patients who are new to the medical practice and another procedure for existing patients. A **new patient** has not received any services from the provider (or another provider of the same specialty who is a member of the same practice) within the past three years. An **established patient**, on the other hand, has seen the provider (or another provider in the practice who has the same specialty) within the past three years.

New Patient Information

When a new patient calls or is referred for an appointment, the collection of patient information begins. Most medical practices gather facts about patients before their first appointments. This information is used to ensure that patients' health care requirements are appropriate for the medical practice, to schedule appointments of appropriate length, and to establish responsibility for payment. The facts about a patient typically include:

- Full name
- Telephone number
- Address
- Date of birth
- Gender
- Social Security number
- Reason for call or nature of complaint

- If insured, the name of the health care plan (uninsured patients are often referred to as self-pay patients)
- If referred, the name of the primary care physician (PCP)

Provider Participation

New patients, too, may need information before deciding to make an appointment. For example, a patient who is a member of a preferred provider organization (PPO) must use network physicians to avoid paying higher charges. For this reason, the patient needs to know whether the provider is a **participating provider**, or **PAR**, in the PPO plan. A PAR provider follows the plan's rules regarding fees. For instance, often a participating provider has signed a contract with the PPO to charge the plan's members lower fees. **Nonparticipating**, or **nonPAR, providers** can charge their usual fees for services, so the patient may choose not to make an appointment because of the additional expense. (The calculation of provider charges under various plans is discussed in Chapter 7.) Patients may check with their health plan or the provider's office to find out whether the provider is a PAR or a nonPAR provider in their plan.

Patient Information Form

When new patients arrive at the office for appointments, they are asked to fill out a **patient information form** (see Figure 3.2 on page 76). This form is used to collect and verify the following information about the patient:

- First name, middle initial, and last name.
- Gender (*F* for female or *M* for male).
- Martial status (*S* for single, *M* for married, *D* for divorced, *W* for widowed).
- Birth date, using four digits for the year
- Home address and telephone number.
- Social Security number.
- Employer's name, address, and telephone number.
- Spouse's name and employer.
- A contact for the patient in case of a medical emergency.
- If the patient is a minor (under the age of majority according to state law), the minor's personal representative's name, gender, marital status, birth date, address, Social Security number, telephone number, and employer information, and the child's status if a full-time or part-time student. In most cases, the personal representative is a parent, guardian, or other person acting with legal authority to make health care decisions on behalf of the minor.
- The patient's health plan.
- The health plan's policyholder's (insured's or guarantor's) name (the policyholder may be a spouse, divorced spouse, guardian, or other relation), birth date, plan type, Social Security number, policy number, group number, telephone number, and employer.
- Policyholder information about other insurance coverage.
- Other related information, such as allergies.

Assignment of Benefits

Physicians who submit claims for patients are usually authorized to receive payments for medical services directly from third-party payers. This saves patients paperwork and benefits the provider, since payments are faster. The policyholder must also authorize this procedure by signing and dating an **assignment of benefits** statement (see Figure 3.3 on page 77). It is usually worded

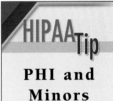

HIPAA Tip

PHI and Minors

A covered entity may choose to provide or deny a parent access to a minor's personal health information (PHI) if doing so is consistent with state or other applicable law, and provided that the decision is made by a licensed health care professional. These options apply whether or not the parent is the minor's personal representative.

VALLEY ASSOCIATES, P.C.
1400 West Center Street
Toledo, OH 43601-0123
614-321-0987

PATIENT INFORMATION FORM

Patient

Last Name	First Name	MI	Sex __ M __ F	Date of Birth / /

Address	City	State	Zip

Home Ph # ( )	Marital Status	Student Status

SS#	Allergies:

Employment Status	Employer Name	Work Ph # ( )	Primary Insurance ID#

Employer Address	City	State	Zip

Referred By	Ph # of Referral ( )

Responsible Party (Complete this section if the person responsible for the bill is not the patient)

Last Name	First Name	MI	Sex __ M __ F	Date of Birth / /

Address	City	State	Zip	SS#

Relation to Patient __ Spouse __ Parent __ Other	Employer Name	Work Phone # ( )

Spouse, or Parent (if minor):	Home Phone # ( )

Insurance (If you have multiple coverage, supply information from both carriers)

Primary Carrier Name	Secondary Carrier Name
Name of the Insured (Name on ID Card)	Name of the Insured (Name on ID Card)
Patient's relationship to the insured __ Self __ Spouse __ Child __Other (Specify)_____	Patient's relationship to the insured __ Self __ Spouse __ Child __Other (Specify)_____
Insured ID #	Insured ID #
Group # or Company Name	Group # or Company Name
Insurance Address	Insurance Address
Phone #	Copay $	Phone #	Copay $

Other Information

Is patient's condition related to: Reason for visit:
__ Employment   __ Auto Accident (if yes, state in which accident occurred: ___)   __ Other Accident
Date of Accident: /   /   Date of First Symptom of Illness: /   /

Authorization

I hereby authorize release of information necessary for my insurance company to process my claim. The above information is correct to the best of my knowledge.	I hereby authorize payment directly to VALLEY ASSOCIATES, P.C. insurance benefits otherwise payable to me. I understand that I am financially responsible for charges not paid in a timely manner by my insurance.
Signed: _____Date: _____	Signed: _____Date: _____

Figure 3.2 Patient Information Form

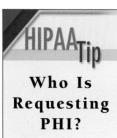
something like "I authorize payment of medical benefits to the undersigned physician or supplier for services described below." The assignment of benefits statement is also filed in the patient medical record.

Acknowledgment of Receipt of Notice of Privacy Practices

Under the HIPAA Privacy Rule (see Chapter 2), providers may use patients' PHI without specific authorization for treatment, payment, and operations (TPO) purposes:

Assignment of Benefits

I hereby assign to Valley Associates, PC, any insurance or other third-party benefits available for health care services provided to me. I understand that Valley Associates has the right to refuse or accept assignment of such benefits. If these benefits are not assigned to Valley Associates, I agree to forward to Valley Associates all health insurance and other third-party payments that I receive for services rendered to me immediately upon receipt.

Signature of Patient/Legal Guardian: _____

Date: _____

Figure 3.3 **Assignment of Benefits Form**

1. *Treatment:* This purpose primarily consists of discussion of the patient's case with other providers. For example, the physician may document what each member of the health care team is expected to do in providing care. Each team member then records actions and observations, so that the ordering physician knows how the patient is responding to treatment.
2. *Payment:* In most instances, providers submit claims on the behalf of patients. Providers are required by Centers for Medicare and Medicaid Services (CMS) to do so for Medicare patients. Other patients appreciate this service, since they often find the paperwork unfamiliar and difficult to handle. It also benefits the practice by expediting payments.
3. *Operations:* This purpose includes activities such as staff training and quality improvement.

Providers must have patients' authorization to use or disclose information that is not for TPO purposes. For example, a patient who wishes a provider to disclose PHI to an insurance company for an application for life insurance must authorize this release in writing.

Providers must inform each patient about their privacy practices once. The most common method is to give the patient a copy of the medical office's privacy practices to read, and then a separate form called an **Acknowledgment of Receipt of Notice of Privacy Practices** to sign (see Figure 3.4 on page 78). Providers must make a good-faith effort to have patients sign this document, which states that the patient has read the privacy practices and understands how the provider intends to protect the patient's rights to privacy under HIPAA. The provider must also document in the medical record whether the patient signed the form. The format for the acknowledgment is up to the practice.

HIPAA does not require that the parent or guardian of a minor must sign. If a child is accompanied by a parent or guardian who is completing other paperwork on behalf of the minor, then it is reasonable to ask that adult to sign the acknowledgement of receipt. On the other hand, if the child or teen is unaccompanied, the minor patient may be asked to sign.

Established Patient Information

When established patients schedule appointments, they are asked whether any pertinent personal information has changed, and whether they have the same

Prescription Refills

If a patient who has not received a privacy notice or signed an acknowledgement calls for a prescription refill, the recommended procedure is to mail the patient a copy of the privacy notice, along with an acknowledgment of receipt form, and document the mailing to show a good faith effort that meets the office's HIPAA obligation, even if the patient does not return the signed form.

Acknowledgment of Receipt of Notice of Privacy Practices

I understand that the providers of Valley Associates, PC, may share my health information for treatment, billing and healthcare operations. I have been given a copy of the organization's notice of privacy practices that describes how my health information is used and shared. I understand that Valley Associates has the right to change this notice at any time. I may obtain a current copy by contacting the practice's office or by visiting the Web site at www.xxx.com.

My signature below constitutes my acknowledgment that I have been provided with a copy of the notice of privacy practices.

_____

Signature of Patient or Legal Representative   Date

If signed by legal representative,
relationship to patient:_____

Figure 3.4 Acknowledgment of Receipt of Notice of Privacy Practices

---

insurance plan. Different employment, marital status, or dependent status, for instance, may affect patients' insurance coverage. Changes, such as new addresses or employers, may also be phoned in by patients. To double-check that information is current, most practices periodically ask established patients to review their patient information when they come in. This review should be done at least once a year; some practices do this twice annually. Practices often ask for the updated document when established patients have their first appointment in a new year The file is also checked to be sure that the patient has been given a current Notice of Privacy Practices.

Communications with Patients

Service to patients, who are the customers of medical practices, is critically important. Satisfied customers are essential to the financial health of every business, including medical practices. Medical practice staff must be dedicated to retaining patients by providing excellent service.

The following are examples of good communication practices:

- Established and new patients who call or arrive for appointments are always given a friendly greeting and referred to by name.
- Patients' questions about forms they are completing and insurance matters are answered with courtesy.
- When possible, patients in the reception area are told the approximate waiting time until they will see the provider.
- Fees for providers' procedures and services are explained to patients.
- The medical practice's guidelines about patients' responsibilities, such as when payments are due from patients and the need to have referrals from primary care physicians, are prominently posted in the office.
- Patients are called a day or two before their appointments to remind them of the appointment time.

Like all businesses, medical practices, even though very well managed, have problems and complaints to deal with. Patients sometimes become upset over scheduling or bills, or have problems understanding a lab report or instructions they have been given. Medical insurance specialists often handle patients' questions about benefits and charges. They must become good problem solvers, willing to listen to and empathize with the patient while sorting out emotions from facts to get accurate information. Phrases such as these reduce patients' anger and frustration:

"I'm glad you brought this to our attention. I will look into it further."

"I can appreciate how you would feel this way."

"It sounds like we have caused some inconvenience, and I apologize."

"I'm sorry you are angry. Let me try to help."

"Thank you for taking the time to tell us about this. Because you have, we can resolve issues like the one you raised."

Medical insurance specialists need to use the available resources and investigate solutions to problems. Following through on promised information is also critical. A medical insurance specialist who says to a patient, "I will call you by the end of next week with that information," must do exactly that. Even if the problem is not solved, the patient needs an update on the situation within the stated time frame.

Information Technology: The Patient Database and the Scheduling Program

To use the medical billing program, the database of patients must be created and maintained by the medical insurance specialist, who enters the data that are gathered or updated on the patient information forms. A new record must be created for a new patient, and established patients' information may need to be updated. Usually, a new *case* or record for the patient is set up in the program when the patient's chief complaint for an encounter is different. For example, a patient might have an initial appointment for a comprehensive physical examination. Subsequently, this patient sees the provider because of stomach pain. Each visit is set up as a separate case in the medical billing program.

Many medical practices also use computer-based patient-appointment scheduling systems. The appointment system may be a separate program or part of the medical billing program. It is used to send patient reminders automatically, to trace follow-up appointments, and to schedule recall appointments according to the provider's instructions. Such programs make providers' schedules more efficient. Scheduling techniques are used to ensure a continuous flow of patients through the practice and minimize waiting time. Scheduling programs also make it easier to change patients' appointments. When a patient calls to reschedule an appointment, the system can locate the next available time slot with the patient's physician.

Billing Tip

MCOs and Appointments
Many managed care contracts require participating physicians to see enrolled patients within a short time of their calling for appointments. Some also require PCPs to handle emergencies in the office, rather than sending patients to an emergency department. Juggling schedules is often a reality because of these requirements, and scheduling systems may help.

Insurance Verification

To be paid for services provided, medical practices need to verify patients' insurance coverage. Medical insurance specialists verify patients' eligibility for benefits before services are provided, except in the case of medical emergencies, which are handled immediately. The medical insurance specialist checks patients' eligibility by contacting the payer. An electronic transaction or a telephone or fax may be used to communicate with health plans.

The payer's provider representative (also called the provider consultant or customer representative) checks to confirm that the patient is currently enrolled, has paid all required premiums or other charges, and how much of the plan deductible for the current period (if there is one) has been met. The medical insurance specialist also finds out if there is a copayment for the visit.

In a general or family practice, for patients in plans that require the use of network PCPs, three facts are checked:

1. The provider must be a plan participant.
2. The patient must be listed on the plan's enrollment master.
3. The patient must be assigned to the PCP as of the date of service.

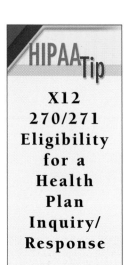

Insurance Cards

When a new patient arrives for an appointment, the medical insurance specialist scans or photocopies the front and back of the insurance card, and verifies the member and/or group numbers that the patient has written on the patient information form. If the insurance of an established patient has changed, both sides of the new card are scanned or photocopied, and the member and group numbers are checked.

Most insurance cards contain the following information (see Figure 3.5):

- Group identification number
- Date on which the member's coverage became effective
- Member name
- Member identification number
- The health plan's name, type of coverage, copayment requirements, frequency limits or annual maximums for services, and annual deductible
- Optional items, such as prescription drugs that are covered, with the copayment requirements

HIPAA Eligibility for a Health Plan Transaction

The **HIPAA Eligibility for a Health Plan** transaction (the inquiry from the provider and the response from the payer) is the electronic format used to verify benefits. An advantage of using the electronic format is that the medical insurance specialist does not have to wait on the telephone for the health plan representative to check and answer or call back.

Inquiries

The provider transmits this information electronically to the health plan:

- The insured's name, plan ID number, date of birth, and gender
- The patient's name (exactly as it appears on the insurance card), plan ID number, insurance group ID number, date of birth, gender, and relationship to the insured
- A code that indicates a query for Health Benefit Plan Coverage, if the provider wants to know only whether the patient is covered
- Another type of service code if the provider also wants to know if a particular service is covered for the patient

When an eligibility benefits transaction is sent by the medical insurance specialist, the computer program assigns a unique **trace number** to the inquiry. Often, eligibility transactions are sent the day before patients arrive for appointments. The office's scheduling system may have a program that automates this job.

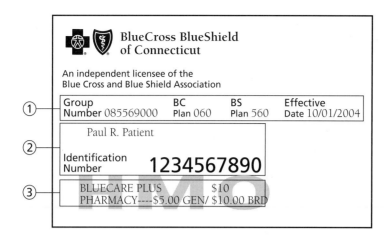

1. **Group identification number**
   The 9-digit number used to identify the member's employer.

   Blue Cross Blue Shield plan codes
   The numbers used to identify the codes assigned to each plan by the Blue Cross Blue Shield Association; used for claims submissions when medical services are rendered out-of-state.

   Effective date
   The date on which the member's coverage became effective.

2. **Member name**
   The full name of the cardholder.

   Identification number
   The 10-digit number used to identify each Anthem Blue Cross and Blue Shield of Connecticut or BlueCare Health Plan member.

3. **Health plan**
   The name of the health plan and the type of coverage; usually lists any copayment amounts, frequency limits or annual maximums for home and office visits; may also list the member's annual deductible amount.

   Riders
   The type(s) of riders that are included in the member's benefits (DME, Visions).

   Pharmacy
   The type of prescription drug coverage; lists copayment amounts

Figure 3.5 A Sample Insurance Card

Responses

The health plan responds to an eligibility inquiry with this information:

- The trace number, as a double-check on the inquiry
- Benefit information, such as whether the insurance coverage is active
- Service type, to answer the question on coverage for the particular service
- Covered period—the period of dates that the coverage is active
- Benefit units, such as how many physical therapy visits
- Coverage level—that is, who is covered, such as spouse and family or individual

Often, this information, as applicable, is also transmitted:

- The copay amount

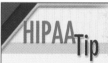

Double-Checking Patients' Information

Medical insurance specialists review the health plan's spelling of the insured's and the patient's first and last names, as well as the dates of birth and identification numbers. Any mistakes in the record are corrected, so that when a health care claim is later transmitted for the patient's encounter, it will be accepted by the plan for processing.

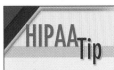
- The yearly deductible amount and amount paid to date
- The coinsurance amount
- The out-of-pocket expenses
- The health plan's information on the insured's/patient's first and last names, dates of birth, and identification numbers
- Primary care provider

HIPAA Referral Certification and Authorization Transaction

Payers may require prior approval before the patient sees a specialist, is admitted to the hospital, or has a particular procedure. The **HIPAA Referral Certification and Authorization** electronic transaction is used for this purpose. It is similar to the HIPAA Eligibility for a Health Plan transaction. The physician transmits information with a trace number to the health plan, which reviews the request for approval. If the health plan approves the service, the electronic response contains a **certification number.**

When an authorization is needed, the patient with a managed care plan receives a referral document from the PCP and is usually responsible for bringing it to the encounter with the specialist or to the hospital. In some cases, this approval may be communicated electronically. A referral document (see Figure 3.6) describes the services the patient is certified to receive.

The specialist's office handling a referred patient must

- Check that the patient has a certification number
- Verify patient enrollment in the plan

Referral Form

> **Label with Patient's Demographic & Insurance Information**

Physician referred to _____

Referred for:
❑ Consult only
❑ Follow-up
❑ Lab
❑ X-Ray
❑ Procedure
❑ Other

Reason for visit _____

Number of visits _____

Appointment Requested: Please contact patient; phone: _____

Primary care physician

Name _____

Signature _____

Phone _____

Figure 3.6 Referral

- Understand restrictions to services, such as regulations that require the patient to visit a specialist in a specific period of time after receiving the referral or that limit the number of times the patient can receive services from the specialist
- Ask patients who "self-refer" (managed care plan members who come for specialty care without a referral) to sign a form stating that they acknowledge that they must pay for the services (see Figure 3.7a)

If a patient is required to present a referral document but does not have one, the medical insurance specialist asks the patient to sign a document such as that shown in Figure 3.7 b. This referral waiver ensures that the patient will pay for services received if in fact a referral is not documented in the time specified.

Primary and Secondary Insurance

The medical insurance specialist also determines each patient's **primary insurance** coverage. A patient may have coverage under more than one group plan, such as a person who has both employer-sponsored insurance and a policy from union membership. A person may have primary insurance coverage from

---

Member Self-Referral Acknowledgment

I, _____, understand that I am seeking the care
of this specialty physician or health care provider, _____,
without a referral from my primary care physician. I understand that
the terms of my Plan coverage require that I obtain that referral, and
that if I fail to do so, my Plan will not cover any part of the charges,

costs or expenses related to this specialist's services to me.

Signed,

_____   _____
(member's name)   (date)

****
Specialty physician or other health care provider:

Please keep a copy of this form in your patient's file

(a)

Referral Waiver

I did not bring a referral for the medical services I will receive today.
If my primary care physician does not provide a referral within two
days, I understand that I am responsible for paying for the services I
am requesting.

Signature: _____

Date: _____

(b)

Figure 3.7 (a) Self-Referral Document, (b) Referral Waiver

an employer, but also be covered as a dependent under a spouse's insurance, making the spouse's plan the person's **secondary insurance.**

Insurance carriers' policies cover situations when more than one plan applies. For example, when an active employee has a plan with the present employer and is still covered by a former employer's plan as a retiree or a laid-off employee, the plan covering that person as an active employee is primary.

A child's parents may each have primary insurance. If both parents cover dependents on their plans, the child's primary insurance is usually determined by the **birthday rule.** This rule states that the parent whose date of birth is earlier in the calendar year is primary. For example, Rachel Foster's mother and father both work and have employer-sponsored insurance policies. Her father, George Foster, was born on October 7, 1971, and her mother, Myrna, was born on May 15, 1972. Since the mother's date of birth is earlier in the calendar year (although the father is older), her plan is Rachel's primary insurance. The father's plan is secondary for Rachel. Note that if a dependent child's primary insurance does not provide for the complete reimbursement of a bill, the balance may usually be submitted to the other parent's plan for consideration.

Another way to determine a child's primary coverage is the **gender rule.** When this rule applies, if the child is covered by two health plans, the father's plan is primary. In some states, insurance regulations require a plan that uses the gender rule to be primary to a plan that follows the birthday rule.

The insurance policy also covers which parent's plan is primary for dependent children of separated or divorced parents. If the parents have joint custody, usually the birthday rule applies. If the parents do not have joint custody of the child, unless otherwise directed by a court order, usually the primary benefits are determined in this order:

- The plan of the custodial parent
- The plan of the spouse of the custodial parent, if the parent has remarried
- The plan of the parent without custody

HIPAA Coordination of Benefits Transaction

Finding out which policy is primary is important because under state and/or federal law, insurance policies contain a provision called **coordination of benefits (COB).** The coordination of benefits guidelines ensure that when a patient is covered under more than one policy, maximum appropriate benefits are paid, but without duplication.

If the patient has signed an assignment of benefits statement, it is the provider's responsibility to supply the information about the secondary insurance coverage to the primary payer. Based on the information about their insurance coverage that patients supply to the provider, medical insurance specialists use the **HIPAA Coordination of Benefits** transaction to transmit the necessary data to payers.

Coordination of benefits in government-sponsored programs follows specific guidelines. Primary and secondary coverage under Medicare, Medicaid, and other programs is discussed in Chapters 11 through 14. Note that COB information can also be exchanged between provider and health plan, or between a health plan and another payer, such as an auto insurance plan.

Communications with Payers

Communications with payers' representatives—whether to check on eligibility, receive referral certification, or resolve billing disputes—are frequent and vitally important to the medical practice. Getting answers quickly means quicker payment for services. Medical insurance specialists follow these guidelines for effective communications:

- Learn the name and telephone extension of the appropriate representative at each payer. If possible, invite the representative to visit the office and meet the staff.
- Use a professional, courteous telephone manner or writing style to help build good relationships.
- Keep current with changing reimbursement policies and utilization guidelines by regularly reviewing information from payers. Usually, the medical practice receives Internet or printed bulletins or newsletters from health plans and government-sponsored programs that contain up-to-date information.

All communications with payer representatives should be documented in the patient's financial record. The representative's name, the date of the communication, and the outcome should be described. This information is sometimes needed later to explain or defend a charge on a patient's insurance claim.

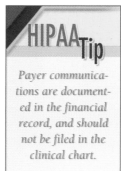

HIPAA Tip

Payer communications are documented in the financial record, and should not be filed in the clinical chart.

Information Technology: The Insurance Database

A medical billing program used by medical insurance specialists contains a database of the payers from whom the medical practice receives payments. The database contains each payer's name and the contact's name; the plan type, such as HMO, PPO, Medicare, Medicaid, or other; and telephone and fax numbers. This database must be updated to reflect changes. Because of corporate mergers in the insurance field (as noted in Chapter 1), company addresses change frequently. Also, a new representative may be assigned to the practice, or the terms of a contract may be altered, as described in Chapter 10.

When patient information is entered in the program, the medical insurance specialist indicates which payer is the patient's primary insurance coverage. Secondary coverage is also selected for the patient as applicable. Other related facts, such as policy numbers and effective dates, are entered for each patient.

Encounter Form Preparation

An **encounter form** is a document that is completed during an office visit with a provider. It is used to record the services provided to a patient as the basis for billing (see Figure 3.8 on page 87). The encounter form, which is called a **superbill**, charge slip, or routing slip in some medical practices, lists the medical practice's most frequently performed services. It also often lists the diagnoses that are most frequently made by the practice's physicians. (Some forms have a blank where diagnostic information will be entered rather than a checklist.) Other information is often included:

- A checklist of managed care plans under contract, and their utilization guidelines
- The patient's prior balance due, if any
- Check-off boxes to indicate the timing and need for a follow-up appointment to be scheduled for the patient

Encounter forms may be electronic or paper. An electronic encounter form is designed to appear on a computer screen or a handheld device. Using the electronic form, providers enter the services provided and patients' diagnoses. If a paper form is used, it is usually a full page or longer.

PATIENT INFORMATION FORM

THIS SECTION REFERS TO PATIENT ONLY				
Name: Mary Anne C. Kopelman		Sex: F	Marital status: ☐ S ☒ M ☐ D ☐ W	Birth date: 9/7/73
Address: 45 Mason Street		SS#: 465-99-0022		
City: Hopewell	State: OH	Zip: 43800	Employer:	
Home phone: 999-555-6877		Employer's address:		
Work phone:		City:	State:	Zip:
Spouse's name: Arnold B. Kopelman		Spouse's employer: U.S. Army, Fort Tyrone		
Emergency contact: Arnold B. Kopelman		Relationship: husband	Phone #: 999-555-0018	

INSURANCE INFORMATION	
Primary insurance company: TriCare	Secondary insurance company:
Policyholder's name: Birth date: Arnold B. Kopelman 4/10/73	Policyholder's name: Birth date:
Plan: SS#: TriCare 230-56-9874	Plan:
Policy #: Group #: 230-56-9874 USA9947	Policy #: Group #:

According to the information supplied by the patient, who is the policyholder? What is the patient's relationship to the policyholder?

Billing Tip

Signing and Dating Encounter Forms
Encounter forms may be completed by the physicians who provided the care, or medical office staff may complete encounter forms based on physicians' documentation. In either case, physicians should sign and date the completed encounter forms for their patients.

- The paper form may be designed by the practice manager and/or physicians based on analysis of the practice's medical services. It is then printed, usually with carbonless copies available for distribution according to the practice's policy. For example, the top copy may be filed in the medical record, the second copy filed in the financial record, and the third copy given to the patient.
- The form may be printed for each patient's appointment using the billing program. A customized encounter form lists the date of the appointment, the patient's name, and the identification number assigned by the medical practice. It can also be designed to show the patient's previous balance, the day's fees, payments made, and amount due.

Medical practitioners use encounter forms to summarize the patient's diagnoses and the services received for use in billing; the medical record contains the full documentation of the physician's findings. The practitioner gives completed encounter forms to the medical insurance specialist, who uses the information to prepare the patient's billing information. The encounter form is

VALLEY ASSOCIATES, P.C.
Christopher M. Connolly, M.D. - Internal Medicine
555-967-0303
FED I.D. #16-1234567

PATIENT NAME	APPT. DATE/TIME	
Deysenrothe, Mae J.	10/06/2008	9:30am

PATIENT NO.	DX
DEYSEMA0	**1.** V70.0 Exam, Adult **2.** **3.** **4.**

DESCRIPTION	✓	CPT	FEE	DESCRIPTION	✓	CPT	FEE
EXAMINATION				**PROCEDURES**			
New Patient				Diagnostic Anoscopy		46600	
Problem Focused		99201		ECG Complete	✓	93000	70
Expanded Problem Focused		99202		I&D, Abscess		10060	
Detailed		99203		Pap Smear		88150	
Comprehensive		99204		Removal of Cerumen		69210	
Comprehensive/Complex		99205		Removal 1 Lesion		17000	
Established Patient				Removal 2-14 Lesions		17003	
Minimum		99211		Removal 15+ Lesions		17004	
Problem Focused		99212		Rhythm ECG w/Report		93040	
Expanded Problem Focused		99213		Rhythm ECG w/Tracing		93041	
Detailed		99214		Sigmoidoscopy, diag.		45330	
Comprehensive/Complex		99215					
				LABORATORY			
PREVENTIVE VISIT				Bacteria Culture		87081	
New Patient				Fungal Culture		87101	
Age 12-17		99384		Glucose Finger Stick		82948	
Age 18-39		99385		Lipid Panel		80061	
Age 40-64	✓	99386	180	Specimen Handling		99000	
Age 65+		99387		Stool/Occult Blood		82270	
Established Patient				Tine Test		85008	
Age 12-17		99394		Tuberculin PPD		85590	
Age 18-39		99395		Urinalysis	✓	81000	17
Age 40-64		99396		Venipuncture		36415	
Age 65+		99397					
				INJECTION/IMMUN.			
CONSULTATION: OFFICE/ER				DT Immun		90702	
Requested By:				Hepatitis A Immun		90632	
Problem Focused		99241		Hepatitis B Immun		90746	
Expanded Problem Focused		99242		Influenza Immun	✓	90659	68
Detailed		99243		Pneumovax		90732	
Comprehensive		99244					
Comprehensive/Complex		99245		**TOTAL FEES**			335.00

Figure 3.8 Sample of a Completed Encounter Form

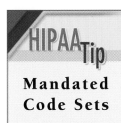
also used to update the patient's account information by recording payments made by the patient during the visit.

Coding

Patients' diagnoses and procedures are documented in their medical records by the physicians providing their care. To report these diagnoses and procedures for payment, the medical terminology is converted to codes. In some medical practices, the physicians assign these codes; in others, a medical coder or a medical insurance specialist handles this task. The codes that are selected are shown on the encounter form (see Figure 3.8) that is completed after the patient encounter.

Diagnoses and Procedures

The description of the patient's primary illness is assigned a **diagnosis code**. The code is a standardized number located in the *International Classification of Diseases,* Ninth Revision, *Clinical Modification* (ICD-9-CM), an internationally recognized set of diagnosis codes (see Chapter 4). For example, the code for Alzheimer's disease is 331.0, and the code for influenza with bronchitis or with a cold is 487.1.

Similarly, each procedure the physician performs is converted to a **procedure code** representing the particular service, treatment, or test. The code is selected from the *Current Procedural Terminology* (CPT) (see Chapter 5). A large group of codes cover the physician's evaluation and management of a patient's condition during office visits or visits at other locations, such as nursing homes. Other codes cover groups of specific procedures, such as surgery, pathology, and radiology. For example, 99431 is the CPT code for the physician's examination of a newborn infant, and the code for magnetic resonance imaging of the temporomandibular joints is 70336.

Information Technology: Encounter Forms and the Databases of Codes

Encounter forms and billing programs both contain diagnosis and procedure codes. Medical insurance specialists must be sure that these databases are up-

---

Thinking It Through—3.2

Review the completed encounter form shown in Figure 3.8 on page 87.

What is the age range of the patient?

_____

Is this a new or an established patient?

_____

What procedures were performed during the encounter?

_____

What laboratory test was ordered?

_____

dated annually when new codes are issued and old codes are modified or dropped. For example, if a new surgical method of implanting a pacemaker in a patient is developed, a new procedure code is issued in the annual CPT update to distinguish this method from older approaches. Likewise, diagnosis codes are changed to reflect the needs of those who report and analyze patients' conditions. Usually, codes are added to make the coding system more specific. For example, in the 2003 edition, ten codes were added under 765 (disorders relating to short gestation and low birth weight) in order to allow the coder to specify the weeks of gestation, from less than twenty-four weeks to thirty-seven or more weeks. Some codes may be added to report new diseases or conditions, such as SARS or West Nile virus.

Linkage and Compliance Review

The medical insurance specialist and medical coder work with the patient's encounter form and medical record in order to analyze the services that should be billed. The codes and the documentation are also reviewed to make sure that errors have not been made. (Chapter 6 covers these topics in depth.) The review checks these key points:

- *The appropriateness of the codes:* For example, some procedure codes are related to the age of the patient. The CPT code 99381, for instance, covers the initial examination of an infant under twelve months old. If this code appears on the encounter form of an adult patient, a mistake would be suspected and the physician queried.
- *The link between the diagnosis and the procedure:* For example, a simple, obvious error may be identified, such as a patient with a diagnosis of a concussion (ICD 850.9) and a procedure for dislocation of a radiocarpal joint, such as CPT 25660.
- *The payer's rules about the diagnosis and the procedure:* Medicare beneficiaries, for example, are covered for a periodic bone mass measurement if they meet certain diagnostic criteria. The medical insurance specialist might review the file to see if an eligibility inquiry was correctly processed for this treatment to be accepted for payment.
- *The documentation of the procedure:* All procedures to be billed must be documented in the patient's medical record as well as checked or written on the encounter form.
- *Compliance with regulations:* The use of the procedure code must comply with regulations. For example, Medicare does not pay separate charges for some procedures if they are all done on the same date of service.

Physician Charge Calculations

The next task in the billing and reimbursement cycle is to calculate the charges for services (see Chapter 7). Each charge, or fee, is related to a specific procedure code. The provider's fees for services are listed on the medical practice's fee schedule. Most medical practices have a standard fee schedule listing their usual fees. Many also have additional fee schedules for contractual arrangements on fees. For example, PPOs negotiate discounted fees with practices.

Some medical practices collect coinsurance or other payments at the time of service, rather than sending bills to patients later. Any copayment required under a managed care plan is also collected before patients leave the office.

In medical practices that do not file health care claims on the behalf of patients, the medical insurance specialist informs patients that they need to file their own claims and attach the encounter forms they receive. The majority of practices, however, do file claims for their patients. Some practices file claims for the patients' primary insurance, but ask the patients to handle claims with secondary plans.

Communications with Providers

Medical practices are extremely busy. Providers often have crowded schedules, especially if they see many patients, and have little time to go over billing and coding issues. Changes that relate only to the administrative staff, such as a new telephone number for an HMO or a changed address for an insurance carrier, do not need to be communicated to the providers. However, when new diagnosis or procedure codes are issued, or coverage of procedures is added or deleted by a health plan, physicians need to know. Medical insurance specialists need to be sure that key changes are brought to providers' attention. Usually the practice manager arranges a time to discuss such matters with the physicians.

At times, a medical insurance specialist must be able to explain insurance changes to patients on the physician's behalf. When they are given their bills, patients may have questions or find discrepancies that must be clarified before they leave the office. In a large practice, the medical insurance specialist usually asks the practice manager for clarification, and the practice manager will consult with the provider if necessary. In a small medical practice, the medical insurance specialist may work directly with the physician or nurse to resolve billing questions.

Information Technology: Patient Charges, Payments and Receipts, and Accounts

The medical practice's billing program is used to process the financial transactions that result from patients' appointments. The medical insurance specialist enters information from the encounter form, and the program calculates charges. The program also records patients' payments, provides receipts, and computes patients' outstanding account balances.

Patient Charges

Using the encounter form, the medical insurance specialist posts (that is, enters in the computer program) the patient's case information and diagnosis. Then the day's procedures are posted, and the program calculates the charges.

Patient Payments and Receipts

Next, payments made by patients are posted. The billing program can print a receipt for the payment, called a **walkout receipt**, which is given to the patient who has made the payment. The walkout receipt is dated and summarizes the diagnosis, procedures, charges, payment made, and account balance (amount due). For example, if a plan requires a copayment, the medical insurance specialist collects this payment, posts it to the patient's account, and prints out a walkout receipt for the patient. Some health plans accept a walkout receipt instead of an encounter form when the patient submits an insurance claim.

Patient Accounts

When patients' charges and payments are posted, the billing program also updates the **patient ledger,** or patient account record, which collects all the financial activity in each patient's account. Later, when insurance payments are received by the medical practice for patients with reimbursement plans, those payments are also posted to the patient's account, reducing the balance that the patient owes.

Claim Preparation

A health care claim communicates information about a patient's diagnosis, procedures, and charges to a payer. A claim contains both clinical and financial information. It is not part of the patient medical record, but it is based on the data located there. The claim may be for reimbursement for services rendered or to report an encounter to an MCO.

The HIPAA transaction for electronic claims is the **HIPAA Health Care Claims or Equivalent Encounter Information.** There are also versions for dental claims, hospital claims, and pharmacy claims.

Another claim form that is sometimes used is the **CMS-1500** paper claim. (It was called the HCFA-1500 until the Health Care Financing Administration was renamed the Centers for Medicare and Medicaid Services.) This paper form is mailed or faxed to payers.

The data needed to complete a health care claim are ready as soon as the medical insurance specialist enters the billing transactions—the charges and payments—for the patient's visit. After these are entered, the program is instructed to prepare the corresponding claims for transmission.

Claim Transmission

Health care claims must next be transmitted to payers. This step can be done by the billing program, if it is programmed for this task. Many practices, though, prefer to use a clearinghouse to transmit their health care claims to payers. In this case, the practice's billing program transmits claim data to the clearinghouse's computer system (see Figure 3.9 on page 92). The clearinghouse, for a fee, reformats the claim so that it is HIPAA-compliant and transmits it to the payer. Most practices also have a schedule that the medical insurance specialist follows for claim transmission, such as every day or every other day. The billing program maintains a log of transmitted claims.

Claim Attachments

At times supporting documents or reports, such as X-rays or referral paperwork, must be attached to claims. In these situations, the electronic claim carries a code that indicates that a separate paper attachment is coming to the payer or is on file in the provider's records for the payer to examine if necessary

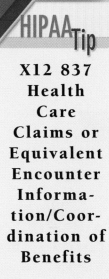

HIPAATip

X12 837 Health Care Claims or Equivalent Encounter Information/Coordination of Benefits

The HIPAA Health Care Claims or Equivalent Encounter Information/Coordination of Benefits transaction is also called the X12 837. It is used both to send a claim to the primary payer and to a secondary payer.

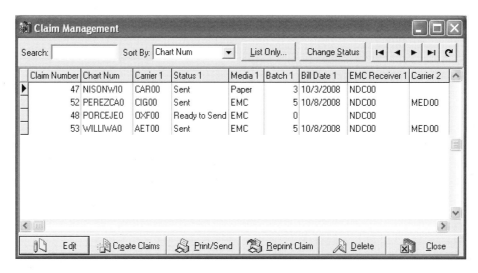

Figure 3.9 Health Care Claim Transmittal Screen (NDCMediSoft)

(see Chapter 8). Copies of paper claims and attachments are filed in patients' financial records.

HIPAA Claim Status Transaction

The **HIPAA Claim Status** transaction is the electronic format used by practices to ask payers about the status of claims (see Chapters 8 and 9). Like the HIPAA Eligibility for a Health Plan, it has two parts: an inquiry and a response.

Payer Adjudication

Health care claims received by payers undergo a process known as **adjudication**. This term means that the claim goes through a series of steps designed to judge whether it should be paid (see Chapter 9). The basic steps in claim adjudication are

1. *Initial processing:* A preadjudication review of electronic claims rejects any with mistakes—such as invalid patient numbers or missing information—and instructs the medical practice that sent the claims to fix and resubmit them. Paper attachments are date-stamped and entered into the payer's computer system, either by data-entry personnel or by the use of a scanning system.

2. *Automated review:* Claims go through an automated review, which checks for eligibility, status of deductible or other required payments, coverage of billed procedures, provider certification, authorization, effective dates of coverage, preexisting conditions, and other facts. If problems result from the automated review, the claim is set aside for *development*—the term used by payers to indicate that more information is needed before processing can be continued.

3. *Medical necessity review:* The **medical necessity** of the procedures is reviewed by the payer's claims examiner. *Medically necessary* is defined by the HIAA (Health Insurance Association of America) as a "term that is used by insurers to describe medical treatment that is appropriate and rendered in accordance with generally accepted standards of medical

practice." As a general measure, the procedure must meet these conditions to be considered medically necessary:

- Procedure codes match diagnosis codes.
- Procedures are not elective (not required to treat a condition, but elected to be done by the patient).
- Procedures are not experimental. The procedures must be approved by the appropriate federal regulatory agency, such as the Food and Drug Administration.
- Procedures are furnished at an appropriate level. Simple diagnoses need simple procedures; complex or time-consuming procedures are reserved for complex conditions.

4. *Determination:* The payer determines whether to pay the fee, deny the claim, or pay less for some or all procedures. If benefits have been assigned, the amount of the patient's responsibility for charges under a required deductible, copayment, or coinsurance is calculated and subtracted from the payer's reimbursement to the provider. If the benefit is paid to the patient, the patient is responsible for paying the provider.

5. *Payment:* The **HIPAA Health Care Payment and Remittance Advice** is the electronic transaction that the payer uses to send the claim payment to the provider. (For paper claims, this document is called an explanation of benefits, or EOB.) This claim payment transaction, often called the **remittance advice (RA)**, provides detailed payment information. One claim payment transaction provides payment for more than one health care claim (see Figure 3.10 on page 94). Codes are used to represent the adjustments the payer made. For example, the code 110 stands for the payer's subtraction of a charge because the billing date predated the date of service.

   If there are questions about a claim that extend beyond the normal review, the third-party payer may want to check documentation to confirm
   - Where the service took place
   - Whether the treatments were appropriate and a logical outcome of the facts and conditions shown in the medical record
   - That services were accurately reported

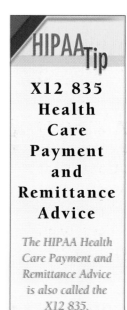

Reimbursement Follow-up and Record Retention

All payment transactions are checked by the medical insurance specialist, who compares the payments and claims to check that

- All procedures that were listed on the claim also appear on the payment transaction
- Any unpaid charges are explained
- The codes on the payment transactions match those on the claim
- The payment listed for each procedure is correct

If discrepancies are found, an appeal process may be started (see Chapter 9). The payments are posted to the appropriate patients' accounts. The total paid by the patient and all third-party payers (the primary insurance and any other insurance) should equal the expected charge. Occasionally, an overpayment may be received, and a refund check is issued by the medical practice. More often, a patient is to be billed for charges that were not fully reimbursed by third-party payers. The patient account ledger can be printed from the billing program (see Figure 3.11 on page 95). Statements show the dates and services

Anthem Blue Cross Blue Shield
900 West Market Street
Cleveland, OH 44101-3456

Date prepared: 6/22/2008

Patient's name	Dates of service from - thru	POS	Proc	Qty	Charge amount	Eligible amount	Patient liability	Amt paid provider
Claim number 0347914								
Daiute, Angelo X	06/17/08 - 06/17/08	11	36415	1	$11.00	$11.00	$00.00	$11.00
Daiute, Angelo X	06/17/08 - 06/17/08	11	80050	1	$98.00	$98.00	$00.00	$98.00
Daiute, Angelo X	06/17/08 - 06/17/08	11	81000	1	$12.00	$12.00	$00.00	$12.00
Daiute, Angelo X	06/17/08 - 06/17/08	11	93000	1	$51.00	$51.00	$00.00	$51.00
Daiute, Angelo X	06/17/08 - 06/17/08	11	99386	1	$123.00	$123.00	$00.00	$123.00
Claim number 0347915								
Daiute, Brian G	06/17/08 - 06/17/08	11	99383	1	$98.00	$98.00	$00.00	$98.00
Daiute, Brian G	06/17/08 - 06/17/08	11	90711	1	$74.00	$74.00	$00.00	$74.00
Claim number 0347916								
Daiute, Mary F	06/17/08 - 06/17/08	11	36415	1	$11.00	$11.00	$00.00	$11.00
Daiute, Mary F	06/17/08 - 06/17/08	11	80050	1	$98.00	$98.00	$00.00	$98.00
Daiute, Mary F	06/17/08 - 06/17/08	11	81000	1	$12.00	$12.00	$00.00	$12.00
Daiute, Mary F	06/17/08 - 06/17/08	11	93000	1	$51.00	$51.00	$00.00	$51.00
Daiute, Mary F	06/17/08 - 06/17/08	11	99386	1	$123.00	$123.00	$00.00	$123.00
Daiute, Mary F	06/17/08 - 06/17/08	11	88150	1	$24.00	$24.00	$19.00	**A
Claim number 0347917								
Daiute, Rosemary B	06/17/08 - 06/17/08	11	99384	1	$122.00	$122.00	$00.00	$122.00
Daiute, Rosemary B	06/17/08 - 06/17/08	11	90707	1	$82.00	$82.00	$00.00	$82.00
Daiute, Rosemary B	06/17/08 - 06/17/08	11	90702	1	$30.00	$30.00	$00.00	$30.00

**A Total for patient exceeds $300 annual maximum for preventive care.

* * * * * * * * Check #109876 is attached in the amount of $1001.00 * * * * * * * *

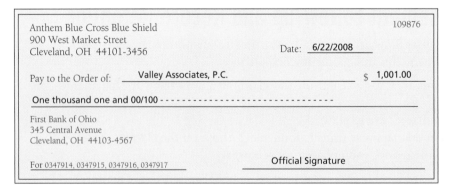

Anthem Blue Cross Blue Shield   109876
900 West Market Street
Cleveland, OH 44101-3456   Date: 6/22/2008

Pay to the Order of: ___Valley Associates, P.C._____ $ 1,001.00

One thousand one and 00/100 -

First Bank of Ohio
345 Central Avenue
Cleveland, OH 44103-4567

For 0347914, 0347915, 0347916, 0347917   Official Signature

Figure 3.10 Claim Payment Transaction

provided, payments made by the patient and the third-party payer, and the balances due. Bills based on the account ledger are mailed periodically—usually monthly—to patients with balances due.

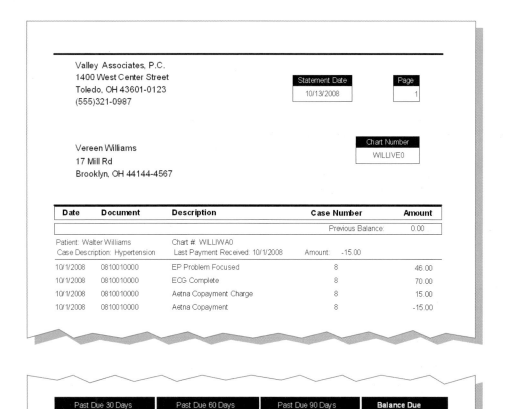

Valley Associates, P.C.
1400 West Center Street
Toledo, OH 43601-0123
(555)321-0987

Statement Date
10/13/2008

Page
1

Vereen Williams
17 Mill Rd
Brooklyn, OH 44144-4567

Chart Number
WILLIVE0

Date	Document	Description	Case Number	Amount
			Previous Balance:	0.00

Patient: Walter Williams   Chart #: WILLIWA0
Case Description: Hypertension   Last Payment Received: 10/1/2008   Amount: -15.00

Date	Document	Description	Case Number	Amount
10/1/2008	0810010000	EP Problem Focused	8	46.00
10/1/2008	0810010000	ECG Complete	8	70.00
10/1/2008	0810010000	Aetna Copayment Charge	8	15.00
10/1/2008	0810010000	Aetna Copayment	8	-15.00

Past Due 30 Days	Past Due 60 Days	Past Due 90 Days	Balance Due
0.00	0.00	0.00	**116.00**

Figure 3.11 Patient Ledger (NDCMediSoft)

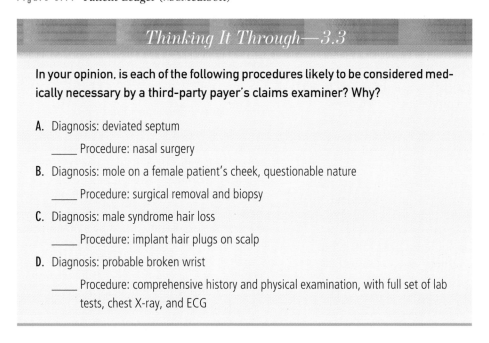

Thinking It Through—3.3

In your opinion, is each of the following procedures likely to be considered medically necessary by a third-party payer's claims examiner? Why?

A. Diagnosis: deviated septum

_____ Procedure: nasal surgery

B. Diagnosis: mole on a female patient's cheek, questionable nature

_____ Procedure: surgical removal and biopsy

C. Diagnosis: male syndrome hair loss

_____ Procedure: implant hair plugs on scalp

D. Diagnosis: probable broken wrist

_____ Procedure: comprehensive history and physical examination, with full set of lab tests, chest X-ray, and ECG

Patient medical records and financial records are filed and retained according to the medical practice's policy (see Chapter 9). Federal and state regulations often affect what materials are retained and for how long.

Review

Chapter Summary

1. The ten steps in the billing and reimbursement cycle are (a) collection of patient information, (b) insurance verification, (c) encounter form preparation, (d) coding, (e) linkage and compliance review, (f) physician charge calculations, (g) claims preparation, (h) claims transmission, (i) payer adjudication, and (j) reimbursement follow-up and record retention.

2. The patient information form is used to record new patient information, including personal, demographic, and employment information; insurance coverage; and emergency contact and related information. This form is reviewed at each visit by established patients to confirm the information. An assignment of benefits statement may also be signed by a patient.

3. All patients must be given the office's Notice of Privacy Practices once, and asked to sign an Acknowledgment of Receipt of Notice of Privacy Practices. This process is followed and documented to show that the office has made a good-faith effort to inform patients of the privacy practices.

4. Medical insurance specialists contact payers to verify patients' plan enrollment and eligibility for benefits. If done electronically, the HIPAA Eligibility for a Health Plan transaction is used. Patients' insurance cards are scanned or photocopied, and the patient information or update form is checked against the cards. Restrictions to benefits, various copayment requirements, and/or deductible status may also be checked. Referrals and authorizations for services are handled electronically with the HIPAA Referral Certification and Authorization transaction. Primary insurance coverage is also determined when more than one policy is in effect. The HIPAA Coordination of Benefits transaction may be used to transmit data to payers.

5. After patient encounters, the completed encounter form and the patient medical record are used by the medical insurance specialist to code or verify assigned codes and to analyze the billable services. The charges for these services are calculated, based on the applicable fee schedule. Copayments are collected from patients according to practice policy, and patients' accounts are updated. Health care claims are prepared and transmitted to payers using either the electronic HIPAA Health Care Claims or Equivalent Encounter Information transaction or the paper method. Remittance advices that are returned by payers are checked to verify that all billed services have been appropriately reimbursed. Patients are billed for the part of charges not covered by their health care plans.

6. Throughout the billing and reimbursement cycle, communication skills are critical to keeping patients satisfied. Equally important are good relationships with third-party payer representatives who can help smooth the payment process. Medical insurance specialists also communicate important changes in payers' policies to providers and work with the health care team to answer patients' billing questions.

7. In most medical practices, information technology is used throughout the claims-processing sequence. Electronic data interchange (EDI) is the basis for the computer-to-computer exchange of routine business information. Medical billing programs store patient and insurance information and can be used to schedule appointments and create encounter forms for patient encounters. After the medical insurance specialist enters diagnosis and procedure codes from encounter forms, the billing program is instructed to generate and transmit health care claims. Patient payments and payer payments are posted to the program to update patients' accounts.

Key Terms

Acknowledgment of Receipt of Notice of
   Privacy Practices *page 77*
adjudication *page 92*
assignment of benefits *page 75*
birthday rule *page 84*
certification number *page 82*
coordination of benefits (COB) *page 84*
CMS-1500 *page 91*
diagnosis code *page 88*
direct provider *page 77*
electronic data interchange (EDI) *page 72*
encounter form *page 85*
established patient *page 74*
gender rule *page 84*

HIPAA Claim Status *page 92*
HIPAA Coordination of Benefits *page 85*
HIPAA Eligibility for a Health Plan
   page 80
HIPAA Health Care Claims or Equivalent
   Encounter Information *page 91*
HIPAA Health Care Payment and Remittance Advice *page 93*
HIPAA Referral Certification and Authorization *page 82*
indirect provider *page 77*
information technology (IT) *page 72*
medical necessity *page 93*
new patient *page 74*

nonparticipating provider (nonPAR)
   page 75
participating provider (PAR) *page 75*
patient information form *page 75*
patient ledger *page 91*
primary insurance *page 83*
procedure code *page 88*
remittance advice (RA) *page 93*
secondary insurance *page 83*
superbill *page 85*
trace number *page 80*
transaction *page 72*
walkout receipt *page 91*

Review Questions

Match the key terms in the left column with the definitions in the right column.

A. direct provider

B. assignment of benefits

C. new patient

D. secondary insurance

E. electronic data
   interchange

F. adjudication

G. remittance advice

H. coordination of benefits

I. walkout receipt

J. medical necessity

_____ 1. The computer-to-computer exchange of routine business
   information

_____ 2. A document from a payer that shows how the benefit amount was
   determined

_____ 3. Authorization by a policyholder that allows a payer to pay benefits
   directly to a provider

_____ 4. The insurance plan that pays benefits after payment by the primary
   payer when a patient is covered by more than one medical
   insurance plan

_____ 5. The provider who treats the patient

_____ 6. A clause in an insurance policy that explains how the policy will
   pay if more than one insurance policy applies to the claim

_____ 7. The process followed by payers to examine claims and determine
   payments

_____ 8. A term describing a payer's judgment that a reported procedure or
   service matches the diagnosis, is not elective, is not experimental,
   has not been performed at the convenience of the patient, and has
   been provided at an appropriate level

_____ 9. A patient who has not received professional services from a
   provider, or another provider in the same practice with the same
   specialty, in the past three years

_____ 10. Document given to a patient who makes a payment

Decide whether each statement is true or false, and write T for true or F for false.

_____ 1. The HIPAA Health Care Claims or Equivalent Encounter Information/Coordination of Benefits transaction is
   the electronic format for the health care claim.

_____ 2. If Gary's parents each have primary medical insurance, his father's date of birth is February 13, 1969, and his mother's date of birth is March 4, 1968, his mother's plan is Gary's primary insurance under the birthday rule.

_____ 3. The patient ledger contains a record of all the patient's financial charges and payments.

_____ 4. A provider may not treat a patient unless the patient has first signed an Acknowledgment of Receipt of Notice of Privacy Practices.

_____ 5. The provider does not need authorization to release a patient's PHI for treatment, payment, or operations purposes.

_____ 6. The HIPAA Eligibility for a Health Plan transaction may be used to determine a patient's insurance coverage.

_____ 7. Patients' dates of birth should be recorded using all four digits of the year of birth.

_____ 8. Patients' insurance benefits are usually verified after provider encounters.

_____ 9. The policyholder and the patient are always the same individual.

_____ 10. Most providers have fee schedules listing the fees that they charge most patients in most instances.

Write the letter of the choice that best completes the statement or answers the question.

_____ 1. A patient's group insurance number written on the patient information or update form must match
   A. the patient's Social Security number
   B. the number on the patient's insurance card
   C. the practice's identification number for the patient
   D. the diagnosis codes

_____ 2. If a health plan member receives medical services from a provider who does not participate in the plan, the cost to the member is
   A. lower   C. the same
   B. higher   D. negotiable

_____ 3. The patient information form gathers the following information:
   A. the patient's personal and demographic information, employment data, and insurance information
   B. the patient's history of present illness, past medical history, and examination results
   C. the patient's chief complaint
   D. the patient's insurance plan deductible and/or copayment requirements

_____ 4. If a husband has an insurance policy but is also eligible for benefits as a dependent under his wife's insurance policy, the wife's policy is considered _____ for him.
   A. primary   C. secondary
   B. participating   D. coordinated

_____ 5. A certification number for a procedure is the result of which transaction?
   A. claim status
   B. health care payment and remittance advice
   C. coordination of benefits
   D. referral and authorization

_____ 6. A completed encounter form contains
   A. information about the patient's diagnosis
   B. information on the procedures performed during the encounter
   C. both A and B
   D. neither A nor B

_____ 7. The encounter form is a source of _____ information for the medical insurance specialist.
   A. billing   C. third-party payment
   B. treatment plan   D. credit card

____ 8. Under HIPAA, what must be verified about a person who requests PHI?
   A. identity
   B. authorization to access the information
   C. either A or B
   D. both A and B

____ 9. Health care claims for patients contain
   A. clinical information only
   B. clinical and financial information
   C. X-ray reports, primarily
   D. medical histories

____ 10. The remittance advice is issued by
   A. a payer   C. a patient
   B. a provider   D. none of the above

Provide answers to the following questions in the spaces provided.

1. List the ten steps in the billing and reimbursement cycle.

   _____

   _____

   _____

   _____

2. Define the following abbreviations:

   A. RA _____

   B. COB _____

   C. PAR_____

   D. EDI _____

Applying Your Knowledge

Case 3.1

Carol Viragras saw Dr. Alex Roderer, a gynecologist with the Alper Group, a multispecialty practice of 235 physicians, on October 24, 2003. On December 3, 2005, she made an appointment to see Dr. Judy Fisk, a gastroenterologist also with the Alper Group. Did the medical insurance specialist handling Dr. Fisk's patients classify Carol as a new or an established patient?

Case 3.2

Harry Cornprost, a patient of Dr. Connelley, calls on October 25, 2005, to cancel his appointment for October 31 because he will be out of town. The appointment is rescheduled for December 4. How would you document this call?

Case 3.3

Based on the following RA:

1. What is the total amount paid? (Fill in the "amount paid provider" column before calculating the total.)

2. Were any procedures paid at a rate less than the claim indicated? If so, which?

3. Why do you think there is no third-party payment for services for Gloria Vanderhilt?

4. Were any claims rejected? For what reason?

Date prepared: 6/22/2004   **Claim number: 0347914**

Patient's name	Dates of service from - thru	POS	Proc	Qty	Charge amount	Eligible amount	Patient liability	Amt paid provider
Kavan, Gregory	04/15/04 - 04/15/04	11	99213	1	$48.00	$48.00	$4.80	_____
Ferrara, Grace	05/11/04 - 05/11/04	11	99212	1	$35.00	$35.00	$3.50	_____
Cornprost, Harry	05/12/04 - 05/12/04	11	99214	1	$64.00	$54.00	-0-	_____
Vanderhilt, Gloria	05/12/04 - 05/12/04	11	99212	1	$35.00	$35.00	$35.00	-0-
Dallez, Juan	05/13/04 - 05/13/04	11	99212	1	$35.00	*	*	-0-

* * * * * * * *   Check #1039242 is attached in the amount of _____   * * * * * * * *

* Procedure not covered under Medicaid

Computer Exploration

Internet Activity

1. Research commonly asked questions and their answers on the HIPAA Privacy Rule at the Office of Civil Rights (OCR):
   http://www.hhs.gov/ocr/hipaa/assist.html
2. Visit the Website of the Centers for Medicare and Medicaid Services (CMS) and research patients' privacy rights. Locate and read the Notice of Privacy Practices for the Original Medicare Plan.

NDCMediSoft Activity

3.1 Review Patient Information

In NDCMediSoft, general information about a patient is located in the Patient/Guarantor dialog box. This activity provides an overview of this information.

1. Open the Lists menu, and select Patients/Guarantors and Cases. The Patient List dialog box appears.

Computer Exploration

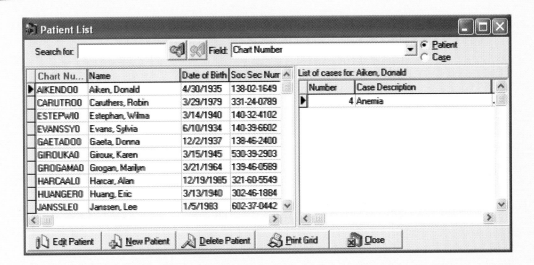

2. The Patient List dialog box contains basic information on each patient/guarantor in the database. It is divided into two sections: patient information and case information. The patient information, on the left side of the dialog box, lists basic information, such as chart number, name, and date of birth, for each patient in the database. To obtain detailed information for a specific patient, the patient's chart number and name is first selected.

3. The Field box to the right of the Search For box should already be set to Chart Number. (If it is not, click the triangle button to display the drop-down list of search criteria and then click Chart Number from the list.) Key "GI" in the Search For box to select Karen Giroux's chart number and name.

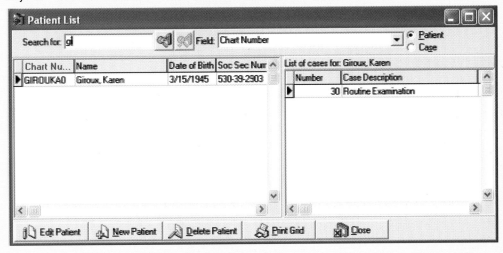

4. Click the Edit Patient button to display detailed information on Karen Giroux in the Patient/Guarantor dialog box.

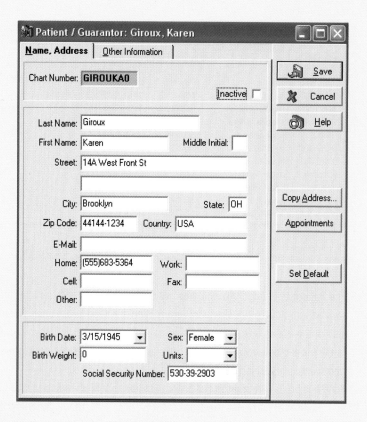

5. The Name, Address tab of the Patient/Guarantor dialog box is displayed. The Patient/Guarantor dialog box contains two tabs: Name, Address and Other Information. The Name, Address tab contains the individual's name, address, e-mail address, various phone numbers, date of birth, gender, birth weight and unit (for newborns), and Social Security Number. Notice that the date of birth is entered in century format (MMDDCCYY).

6. Click the Other Information tab to display its contents.

Computer Exploration

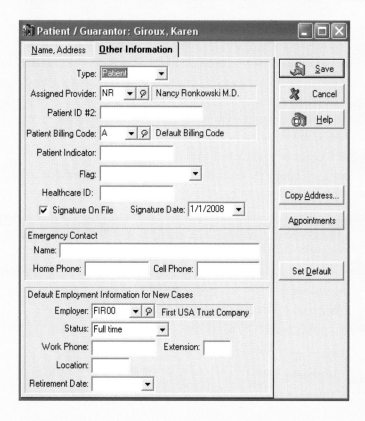

This Other Information tab, which is divided into three parts, contains a variety of information about the patient. The Type box in the top portion indicates whether the individual is a patient or a guarantor. A guarantor is someone who is responsible for an account but who is not a patient of the practice. For example, suppose a woman is a patient of the practice, but has insurance coverage through a group plan offered by her husband's employer. He is not a patient of the practice. She would be entered in MediSoft as a patient. Even though he is not a patient, information about him, such as his employer and insurance coverage, would need to be entered because he is the guarantor. Otherwise, no insurance claims could be created for his wife's office visits.

The other information listed in the top section of the tab includes items such as the patient's assigned provider, billing code, and whether the patient has signed a release form permitting the practice to share information about medical treatment and diagnoses with the insurance carrier.

7. The middle section of the tab contains emergency contact information, including name and phone number(s).

8. The bottom section lists information about the patient or guarantor's employment, including the name of the employer, employment status (full-time, part-time, retired, unemployed, and so on), work phone number, work location, and retirement date (if applicable).

9. Click the Cancel button to exit the Patient/Guarantor dialog box for Karen Giroux and return to the Patient List dialog box.

Computer Exploration

3.2 Review Patient Insurance Information

In MediSoft, information about a patient's insurance coverage is located in the Case dialog box. As with patient information, case information is accessed through the Patient List dialog box. This activity provides an overview of the kind of information that is stored in MediSoft about a patient's insurance coverage.

1. With Karen Giroux's name and case description ("Routine Examination") still selected in the Patient List dialog box, click the case description in the right pane to select it. (Notice the radio button in the upper right corner of the dialog box automatically changes from Patient to Case.)
2. Click the Edit Case button at the bottom of the dialog box.
3. Giroux's Case dialog box for the selected case appears. To view information about the patient's primary insurance plan, click the Policy 1 tab.

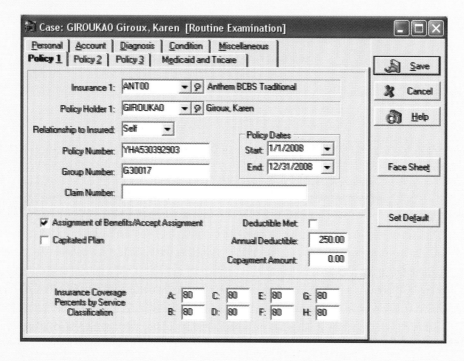

4. In addition to the name of the insurance carrier, notice that the upper section of the Policy 1 tab lists the policyholder's name, the patient's relationship to the policyholder, the policy number, the group number, the claim number (if applicable), and the policy start and end dates. This information is required when creating claims in MediSoft.
5. The middle section of the tab lists specific information about the coverage, including:
   • Whether the provider accepts assignment
   • Whether the plan is capitated
   • The annual deductible
   • The copayment amount
6. The Insurance Coverage Percents by Service Classification boxes in the bottom of the tab list the percentage the insurance will pay for different types of procedures. For example, field A could be for office visits, which are paid at 80 percent. Field B could be for lab work, which is paid at 100 percent, and so on. The amount not covered by the insurance carrier is the patient's coinsurance percentage. For example, in this case, the patient coinsurance for an office visit is 20 percent.

Computer Exploration

7. If a patient has more than one insurance carrier, the Policy 2 and Policy 3 tabs in the Case dialog box are used to record information on the additional carriers. With a few exceptions, the Policy 2 and Policy 3 tabs contain the same fields as the Policy 1 tab. Click the Policy 2 and Policy 3 tabs to view the fields in each.

8. As Karen Giroux has only one insurance carrier, the Policy 2 and Policy 3 tabs do not contain any information at this time. Click the Cancel button to exit the Case dialog box.

9. Click the Close button to close the Patient List dialog box and return to the main MediSoft window.

Part 2 Physician Practice Coding and Compliance

Diagnostic Coding: Introduction to ICD-9-CM

Objectives

After studying this chapter, you should be able to:

1. Discuss the purpose of the ICD-9-CM and the importance of its annual updates.
2. Describe the structure and content of the Alphabetic Index and the Tabular List.
3. Interpret the conventions that are followed in the Alphabetic Index and the Tabular List.
4. Identify the purpose and correct use of V codes and E codes.
5. List the three steps in the diagnostic coding process.
6. Describe and provide examples of key coding guidelines.
7. Discuss the coding process for circulatory diseases, neoplasms, burns, and fractures.
8. Given diagnostic statements, apply coding guidelines to determine correct ICD-9-CM diagnosis codes.

Introduction to Diagnostic Coding

For more than a hundred years, scientists and researchers have gathered information from hospitals about illnesses and causes of death. Their goal has been to better understand the disease process. In the United States, data about morbidity (illness) and mortality (cause of death) are reported to government agencies. For example, the National Center for Health Statistics (NCHS) tracks infant mortality rates, which are an important measure of the quality of health care in a country.

Until the 1950s, physicians used written descriptions of conditions, and different terms were used for similar illnesses. As the amount of information gathered increased, however, researchers needed a better way to analyze and store data. For this purpose, systems were developed that replace written diagnoses with codes. In a coding system, a code number is assigned to each type of disease, and the codes are grouped by disease or by the area of the body that is involved.

Medical practices and hospitals now work with coded diagnostic information. Over time, more-detailed information has been captured. For example, in the predominant diagnostic system, a single code was used for diabetes mellitus at first. Currently, multiple codes are used for the various types and complications of diabetes. As detailed diagnostic information is analyzed, new information about the outcomes of the procedures used to treat diseases becomes available. The goal is to use the statistical information to identify better ways to keep people healthy and to plan for needed resources, as well as to record morbidity and mortality data.

Medical insurance specialists verify diagnosis codes and use them to report patients' conditions on insurance claims and encounter forms. In a medical practice, physicians, medical coding specialists, or medical insurance specialists may be responsible for code selection. Expertise in diagnostic coding requires knowledge of medical terminology, anatomy and physiology, and pathophysiology, as well as experience in correctly applying the rules of the coding system. This chapter provides a fundamental understanding of current diagnostic coding principles and guidelines so that medical insurance specialists can work effectively with encounter forms and health care claims.

The ICD-9-CM

The diagnosis codes used in the United States are based on the *International Classification of Diseases* (ICD). The ICD lists diseases and their three-digit codes according to a system created by the World Health Organization of the United Nations. It has been revised a number of times since the coding system was first developed more than a hundred years ago. The ICD is the classification used by the federal government to categorize mortality data from death certificates.

History

A U.S. version of the ninth revision of the ICD (ICD-9) was published in 1979. A committee of physicians from various organizations and specialties prepared this version, which is called the ICD-9's *Clinical Modification,* or **ICD-9-CM.** It is used to code and classify morbidity data from patient medical records, physician offices, and surveys conducted by the National Center for Health Statistics. Codes in the ICD-9-CM describe conditions and illnesses more precisely than does the World Health Organization's ICD-9 because the codes are intended to provide a more complete picture of patients' conditions. The Medicare Catastrophic Coverage Act of 1988 mandated the change from written diagnoses to ICD-9-CM diagnosis codes for Medicare claims. After the Medicare ruling, private payers also began to require physicians to report diagnoses with ICD-9-CM codes. The use of these diagnosis codes in the health care industry is now standard.

ICD-9-CM diagnosis codes are made up of three, four, or five digits, and a description. The system uses three-digit categories for diseases, injuries, and symptoms. Many of these categories are subcategorized into four-digit codes. Some codes are further subdivided into five-digit codes. For example:

> **Category 415: Acute pulmonary heart disease (three digits)**
> *Subcategory 415.1: Pulmonary embolism and infarction (four digits)*
> *Subclassification: 415.11: Iatrogenic pulmonary embolism and infarction (five digits)*

The purpose of the fourth-level and fifth-level diagnosis codes is to reflect the most specific diagnosis documented in the patient medical record. When included in the ICD-9-CM, fourth and fifth digits are not optional; they must be used. For example, current Centers for Medicare and Medicaid Services (CMS) rules state that a Medicare claim will be rejected when the most specific code available is not used.

Annual Updates: The Addenda

The National Center for Health Statistics and the CMS release updates, called the **addenda,** for the ICD-9-CM that are effective as of October 1 and April 1 of every year. New codes must be used, and old codes that have changed or have been removed also become invalid on the effective date of the addenda. The code changes are available early enough that they can be implemented on the effective dates.

The U.S. Government Printing Office (GPO) publishes the official ICD-9-CM on the Internet and in CD-ROM format every year. Various commercial publishers present the updated codes in annual coding books that are also available soon after the addenda are released. Practices must ensure that the current reference is available and that the current codes are in use.

A New Revision: The ICD-10-CM

The tenth edition of the ICD was published by the World Health Organization in the mid-1990s. In the United States, the new *Clinical Modification* (ICD-10-CM) is being reviewed by health care professionals. It is expected to be adopted as the mandatory diagnosis code set before 2010. The major changes include the following:

- The ICD-10 contains over 2,000 categories of diseases, many more than the ICD-9. This creates more codes to permit more specific reporting of diseases and newly recognized conditions.
- Codes are alphanumeric, containing a letter followed by up to five numbers.
- The sixth digit is added to capture clinical details. For example, all codes that relate to pregnancy, labor, and childbirth include a digit that indicates the patient's trimester.
- Codes are added to show which side of the body is affected when a disease or condition can be involved with the right side, the left side, or bilaterally.

For example, separate codes are listed for a malignant neoplasm of right upper-inner quadrant of the female breast and for a malignant neoplasm of left upper-inner quadrant of the female breast.

When ICD-10-CM is mandated for use, a **crosswalk** will also be available. A crosswalk is a printed or computerized resource that connects two sets of data. The crosswalk connecting ICD-10-CM to ICD-9-CM will be used by medical insurance specialists to relate the two coding systems. In fact, although the code numbers look different, the basic systems are very much alike, and people who are familiar with the current codes will find that their training quickly applies to the new system.

Organization of the ICD-9-CM

The ICD-9-CM has three parts:

1. *Diseases and Injuries: Tabular List—Volume 1:* The **Tabular List** is made up of seventeen chapters of disease descriptions and codes, with two supplementary classifications and five appendixes.
2. *Diseases and Injuries: Alphabetic Index—Volume 2:* The **Alphabetic Index** provides (a) an index of the disease descriptions in the Tabular List, (b) an index in table format of drugs and chemicals that cause poisoning, and (c) an index of external causes of injury, such as accidents.
3. *Procedures: Tabular List and Alphabetic Index—Volume 3:* This volume covers procedures performed by physicians and other practitioners, chiefly in hospitals.

Volumes 1 and 2 are used for physician practice (outpatient) diagnostic coding. The use of Volume 3 for hospital coding is covered in Chapter 15.

Although the Tabular List and the Alphabetic Index are labeled Volume 1 and Volume 2, they are related like the parts of a book. First, the Alphabetic Index is used to find a code for a patient's condition or symptom. The index entry provides a pointer to the correct code number in the Tabular List. Then, that code is located in the Tabular List so that its correct use can be checked. This two-step process must be followed in order to code correctly. This chapter follows this order of use, with the Alphabetic Index discussed first, followed by the Tabular List. (Some publishers' versions of the ICD-9-CM place the Alphabetic Index before the Tabular List for the same reason.)

The Alphabetic Index

The Alphabetic Index contains all the medical terms in the Tabular List classifications. For some conditions, it also lists common terms that are not found in the Tabular List. The index is organized by the condition, not by the body part (anatomical site) in which it occurs. For example, the term *wrist fracture* is located by looking under *fracture* (the condition) and then, below it, *wrist* (the location), rather than under *wrist* to find *fracture*.

The medical term describing the condition for which a patient is receiving care is located in the physician's **diagnostic statement**. For each encounter, the diagnostic statement includes the main reason for the patient encounter. It may also provide descriptions of additional conditions or symptoms that have been treated or that are related to the patient's current illness.

Main Terms, Subterms, and Supplementary Terms

The assignment of the correct code begins with looking up the medical term that describes the patient's condition. Figure 4.1 illustrates the format of the Alphabetic Index. Each **main term** is printed in boldface type and is followed by its code number. For example, if the diagnostic statement is "the patient presents with blindness," the main term *blindness* is located in the Alphabetic Index (see Figure 4.1).

Below the main term, any **subterms** with their codes appear. Subterms are essential in the selection of correct codes. They may show the **etiology** of the disease—its cause or origin—or describe a particular type or body site for the main term. For example, the main term *blindness* in Figure 4.1 includes five subterms, each indicating a different etiology or type—such as color blindness—for that condition.

Any **supplementary terms** for main terms or subterms are shown in parentheses on the same line. Supplementary terms are not essential to the selection of the correct code, and are often referred to as nonessential modifiers. They help point to the correct term, but they do not have to appear in the physician's diagnostic statement for the coder to correctly select the code. In Figure 4.1, for

Blepharitis (eyelid) 373.00
  angularis 373.01
  ciliaris 373.00
   with ulcer 373.01
  marginal 373.00
   with ulcer 373.01
  scrofulous (*see also* Tuberculosis) 017.3
    [373.00]
  squamous 373.02
  ulcerative 373.01
Blepharochalasis 374.34
  congenital 743.62
Blepharoclonus 333.81
Blepharoconjunctivitis (*see also* Conjunctivitis)
  372.20
  angular 372.21
  contact 372.22
Blepharophimosis (eyelid) 374.46
  congenital 743.62
Blepharoplegia 374.89
Blepharoptosis 374.30
  congenital 743.61
Blepharopyorrhea 098.49
Blepharospasm 333.81

Blessig's cyst 362.62
Blighted ovum 631
Blind
  bronchus (congenital) 748.3
  eye—*see also* Blindness
   hypertensive 360.42
   hypotensive 360.41
  loop syndrome (postoperative) 579.2
  sac, fallopian tube (congenital) 752.19
  spot, enlarged 368.42
  tract or tube (congenital) NEC—*see* Atresia
Blindness (acquired) (congenital) (Both eyes)
  369.00
  blast 921.3
   with nerve injury—*see* Injury, nerve, optic
  Brightís — *see* Uremia
  color (congenital) 368.59
   acquired 368.55
   blue 368.53
   green 368.52
   red 368.51
   total 368.54
  concussion 950.9
  cortical 377.75

Figure 4.1 Example of Alphabetic Index Entries

example, any of the supplementary terms *acquired, congenital,* and *both eyes* may modify the main term in the diagnostic statement, such as "the patient presents with blindness acquired in childhood," or none of these terms may appear.

Turnover Lines

If the main term or subterm is too long to fit on one line, as is often the case when many supplementary terms appear, turnover (or carryover) lines are used. Turnover lines are always indented farther to the right than are subterms. It is important to read carefully to distinguish a turnover line from a subterm line. For example, under the main term *blindness* (Figure 4.1) in the Alphabetic Index, a long list of supplementary terms appears before the first subterm. Without close attention, it is possible to confuse a turnover entry with a subterm.

Cross-References

Some entries use cross-references. If the cross-reference *see* appears after a main term, the coder *must* look up the term that follows the word *see* in the index. The *see* reference means that the main term where the coder first looked is not correct; another category must be used. In Figure 4.1, for example, to code the last subterm under *blind,* the term *atresia* must be found.

See also, another type of cross-reference, points the coder to additional, related index entries. *See also category* indicates that the coder should review the additional categories that are mentioned. For example, in the following entry, the entries between 633.0 and 633.9 should be checked, as well as 639.0:

Sepsis with
   ectopic pregnancy (see also categories 633.0–633.9) 639.0

Notes

At times, notes are shown below terms. These boxed, italicized instructions are important because they provide information on selecting the correct code. For example, this note appears in the listings for inguinal hernias (category 550):

Note—Use the following fifth-digit subclassification with category 550:
0 unilateral or unspecified (not specified as recurrent)
1 unilateral or unspecified, recurrent
2 bilateral (not specified as recurrent)
3 bilateral, recurrent

This note also illustrates another **convention** that is followed in the index: Numbered items are listed in numerical order from lowest to highest. Conventions are typographic techniques or standard practices that provide visual guidelines for understanding printed material. For example, listing numbered items in numerical order is followed whether the items are pure numbers (1, 2, 3) or words (first, second, third).

The Abbreviation NEC

Not elsewhere classified, or **NEC,** appears with a term when there is no code that is specific for the condition. Use of this abbreviation indicates that regardless of the information available, no code matches the particular situation. For example:

Hemorrhage, brain, traumatic NEC 853.0

Multiple Codes and Connecting Words

Some conditions may require two codes, one for the etiology and a second for the **manifestation**, the disease's typical signs or symptoms. This requirement is indicated when two codes, the second in brackets and italics, appear after a term:

> **Phlebitis**
> *gouty 274.89 [451.9]*

This entry indicates that the diagnostic statement "gouty phlebitis" requires two codes, one for the etiology (gout) and one for the manifestation (phlebitis). The use of italics for codes means that they cannot be used as primary codes; they are listed after the codes for the etiology.

The use of connecting words, such as *due to, during, following,* and *with,* may also indicate the need for two codes, or for a single code that covers both conditions. For example, the main term below is followed by a *due to* subterm:

> **Cowpox (abortive) 051.0**
> **due to vaccination 999.0**

When the Alphabetic Index indicates the possible need for two codes, the Tabular List entry is used to determine whether they are needed. In some cases, a **combination code** describing both the etiology and the manifestation is available instead of two codes. For example:

> **Closed skull fracture with subdural hemorrhage and concussion 803.29**

Common Terms

Many terms appear more than once in the Alphabetic Index. Often, the term in common use is listed, as well as the accepted medical terminology. For example, there is an entry for *flu,* with a cross-reference to *influenza.*

Eponyms

An **eponym** is a condition (or a procedure) named for a person. Some eponyms are named for the physicians who discovered or invented them; others are named for patients. An eponym is usually listed both under that name and under the main term *disease* or *syndrome.* For example, Hodgkin's disease appears as a subterm under *disease* and as a key term.

The Tabular List

The Tabular List received its name from the language of statistics; the word *tabulate* means to count, record, or list systematically. The diseases and injuries in the Tabular List are organized into chapters according to etiology or body system. Supplementary codes and appendixes cover other special situations. The organization of the Tabular List and the ranges of codes each part covers are shown in Table 4.1 on page 116.

Categories, Subcategories, and Subclassifications

Each Tabular List chapter is divided into sections with titles that indicate the types of related disease or conditions they cover. For example, Chapter 9 has seven sections, one of which is

1. The following entry appears in the Alphabetic Index.

   Kimmelstiel(-Wilson) disease or syndrome

   (Intercapillary glomerulosclerosis) 250.4 *[581.81]*

   What type of term is *Kimmelstiel(-Wilson)?*

   _____

   _____

   What type of term is shown indented and in parentheses?

   _____

   _____

   Does this disease require one or two codes?

   _____

   _____

2. Locate the following main terms in the Alphabetic Index. List and interpret any cross references you find next to the entries.

   La grippe

   _____

   Anginoid pain

   _____

   Branchial

   _____

3. Are *see* cross-references in the Alphabetic Index followed by codes? Why?

   _____

4. Locate the main term *Choledocholithiasis* in the Alphabetic Index, and explain the purpose of the note beneath it.

   _____

Hernia of Abdominal Cavity (550–553)

Within each section, there are three levels of codes:

1. A **category** is a three-digit code that covers a single disease or related condition. (See Appendix E of the Tabular List for the complete listing of categories.) For example, the category 551 in Figure 4.2 on page 117 covers "other hernia of abdominal cavity, with gangrene."

TABLE 4.1	Tabular List Organization	
CLASSIFICATION OF DISEASES AND INJURIES		
Chapter		**Categories**
1	Infectious and Parasitic Diseases	001–139
2	Neoplasms	140–239
3	Endocrine, Nutritional, and Metabolic Diseases, and Immunity Disorders	240–279
4	Diseases of the Blood and Blood-Forming Organs	280–289
5	Mental Disorders	290–319
6	Diseases of the Central Nervous System and Sense Organs	320–389
7	Diseases of the Circulatory System	390–459
8	Diseases of the Respiratory System	460–519
9	Diseases of the Digestive System	520–579
10	Diseases of the Genitourinary System	580–629
11	Complications of Pregnancy, Childbirth, and the Puerperium	630–677
12	Diseases of the Skin and Subcutaneous Tissue	680–709
13	Diseases of the Musculoskeletal System and Connective Tissue	710–739
14	Congenital Anomalies	740–759
15	Certain Conditions Originating in the Perinatal Period	760–779
16	Symptoms, Signs, and Ill-Defined Conditions	780–799
17	Injury and Poisoning	800–999
SUPPLEMENTARY CLASSIFICATIONS		
V Codes	Supplementary Classification of Factors Influencing Health Status and Contact with Health Services	V01–V83
E Codes	Supplementary Classification of External Causes of Injury and Poisoning	E800–E999
APPENDIXES		
Appendix A	Morphology of Neoplasms	
Appendix B	Glossary of Mental Disorders	
Appendix C	Classification of Drugs by American Hospital Formulary Services List Number and Their ICD-9-CM Equivalents	
Appendix D	Classification of Industrial Accidents According to Agency	
Appendix E	List of Three-Digit Categories	

2. A **subcategory** is a four-digit subdivision of a category. It provides a further breakdown of the disease to show its etiology, site, or manifestation. For example, the 551 category has six subcategories:

551.0 Femoral hernia with gangrene
551.1 Umbilical hernia with gangrene
551.2 Ventral hernia with gangrene
551.3 Diaphragmatic hernia with gangrene
551.8 Hernia of other specified sites, with gangrene
551.9 Hernia of unspecified site, with gangrene

3. A **subclassification** is a five-digit subdivision of a subcategory. For example, the following fifth digits are to be used with code 551.0:

551.00 Unilateral or unspecified (not specified as recurrent)
551.01 Unilateral or unspecified, recurrent
551.02 Bilateral (not specified as recurrent)
551.03 Bilateral, recurrent

551 **Other hernia of abdominal cavity, with gangrene**
Includes: that with gangrene (and obstruction)
⑤ **551.0** **Femoral hernia with gangrene**
551.00 **Unilateral or unspecified (not specified as recurrent)**
Femoral hernia NOS with gangrene
551.01 **Unilateral or unspecified, recurrent**
551.02 **Bilateral (not specified as recurrent)**
551.03 **Bilateral, recurrent**
551.1 **Umbilical hernia with gangrene**
Parumbilical hernia specified as gangrenous
⑤ **551.2** **Ventral hernia with gangrene**
551.20 **Ventral, unspecified, with gangrene**
551.21 **Incisional, with gangrene**
Hernia:
postoperative   } specified as gangrenous
Recurrent, ventral
551.29 **Other**
Epigastric hernia specified as gangrenous
551.3 **Diaphragmatic hernia with gangrene**
Hernia:
hiatal (esophageal) (sliding)
Paraesophageal   } specified as gangrenous
Thoracic stomach

Excludes: *congenital diaphragmatic hernia (756.6)*

551.8 **Hernia of other specified sites, with gangrene**
Any condition classifiable to 553.8 if specified as gangrenous
551.9 **Hernia of unspecified site, with gangrene**
Any condition classifiable to 553.9 if specified as gangrenous

Figure 4.2 **Example of Tabular List Entries**

Symbols, Notes, Punctuation Marks, and Abbreviations

Coding correctly requires understanding the conventions—the symbols, instructional notes, and punctuation marks—that appear in the Tabular List.

Symbol for Fifth-Digit Requirement

Depending on the publisher of the ICD-9-CM, a section mark (§) or other symbol (such as ⑤ or ✓) appears next to a chapter, a category, or a subcategory that requires a fifth digit to be assigned. (See, for example, the ⑤ that appears next to subcategories 551.0 and 551.2 in Figure 4.2.) These are important reminders to assign the appropriate five-digit subclassification. If the fifth-digit requirement extends beyond the page where this symbol first appears, the symbol is repeated on all other pages where it applies, so that it is easy to notice.

Includes and Excludes Notes

Notes headed by the word *includes* refine the content of the category or section appearing above them. For example, after the three-digit category 461, acute sinusitis, the *includes* note states that the category includes abscess, empyema, infection, inflammation, and suppuration.

Coding Point

Fifth-Digit Requirement
If the ICD-9-CM indicates that a fifth digit is required, it must be included. But if it is not required, a zero or zeroes should not be added to the four-digit or three-digit code. The use of a fifth digit when it is not required makes the code invalid.

Notes headed by the word *excludes* (which is boxed and italicized) indicate conditions that are not classifiable to the code above. In the category 461, for example, the *exclude* note states that the category does not include chronic or unspecified sinusitis. The note may also give the code(s) of the excluded condition(s).

Colons in Includes and Excludes Notes

A colon (:) in an *includes* or *excludes* note indicates an incomplete term. One or more of the entries following the colon is required to make a complete term. Unlike terms in parentheses or brackets, when the colon is used, the diagnostic statement must include one of the terms after the colon to be assigned a code from the particular category. For example, the *excludes* note after the information for *coma* is as follows:

780.0 Alteration of consciousness
> *Excludes: coma:*
> *diabetic (250.2–250.3)*
> > *hepatic (572.2)*
> > *originating in the perinatal period (779.2)*

For the *excludes* note to apply to *coma,* "diabetic," " hepatic," or "originating in the perinatal period" must appear in the diagnostic statement.

Parentheses

Parentheses ( ) are used around descriptions that do not affect the code—that is, supplementary terms. For example, the subcategory 453.9, other venous embolism and thrombosis, of unspecified site, is followed by the entry "thrombosis (vein)."

Brackets

Brackets [ ] are used around synonyms, alternative wordings, or explanations. They have the same meaning as parentheses. For example, category 460, acute nasopharyngitis, is followed by the entry "[common cold]."

Braces

Braces } enclose a series of terms that are attached to the statement that appears to the right of the brace. They are an alternate format for a long list after a colon and also indicate incomplete terms. For example, the information after code 786.59, Chest pain, other, is as follows:

> **Discomfort**
> **Pressure** } **in chest**
> **Tightness**

For this code to be applied to a diagnosis of "chest pain, other," "discomfort," "pressure," or "tightness" must appear in the statement.

Lozenge

The lozenge—▢—next to a code shows that it is not part of the World Health Organization's ICD. It appears only in the ICD-9-CM. This symbol can be ignored in coding diagnostic statements.

Abbreviations

NEC, not elsewhere classified, is found in the Tabular List as well as in the Alphabetic Index. Another abbreviation, **NOS**, or **not otherwise specified**, means **unspecified.** This term or abbreviation indicates that the code above it should be used when a condition is not completely described in the diagnostic statement or elsewhere in the patient medical record. For example, the code 827, other, multiple, and ill-defined fractures of lower limb, includes "leg NOS." If the documentation reads "patient suffered a fractured leg," this code is appropriate, since there is not enough information to determine which bone in the leg is involved. Note, however, that third-party payers may deny claims that use unspecified diagnosis codes. When possible, more specific clinical documentation should be requested of the provider.

Multiple Codes

Some phrases contain instructions about the need for additional codes. The phrases point to situations in which more than one code is required to properly reflect the diagnostic statement. For example, a statement that a condition is "due to" or "associated with" may require an additional code.

Code First Underlying Disease

The instruction *code first underlying disease* appears below a code that must not be used as a primary code. These codes are for symptoms only, never for causes. The codes and their descriptions are in italic type, meaning that the code cannot be listed first even if the diagnostic statement is written that way. The phrase *code first associated disorder* or *code first underlying disorder* may appear below the italicized code and term. At times, a specific instruction is given, such as in this example:

> 366.31 Glaucomatous flecks (subcapsular)
> *Code first underlying glaucoma (365.0–365.9)*

Use Additional Code, Code Also, or Use Additional Code, If Desired

If a code is followed by the instruction *use an additional code* or *code also,* or a note saying the same thing, two codes are required. The order of the codes must be the same as shown in the Alphabetic Index: the etiology comes first, followed by the manifestation code.

The phrase *use additional code, if desired,* also means to use an additional code if it can be determined. This instruction may apply to an entire chapter, or it may appear in a subcategory following a code. When the diagnostic statement has sufficient information, an additional code is determined in the same way as *code first underlying disease.* For example, code 711.00, pyogenic arthritis (site unspecified), is followed by the phrase:

Use additional code, if desired, to identify infectious organisms (041.0–041.8)

In this case, if the documentation indicates it, the infectious organism causing the condition is coded.

Supplementary Classifications

Two supplementary classifications follow the chapters of the Tabular List:

Provide the following information about codes found in the Tabular List.

1. What agent is excluded from subcategory 972.0, cardiac rhythm regulators?

   _____

2. A brace is located under 562.00. What does the brace mean?

   _____

3. What is the meaning of the symbol in front of category 017?

   _____

4. What types of gastric ulcers are included in category 531?

   _____

5. What is the meaning of the phrase that follows subclassification 466.19?

   _____

6. What is the meaning of the phrase that follows subcategory 730.7?

   _____

- **V codes** identify encounters for reasons other than illness or injury.
- **E codes** identify the external causes of injuries and poisoning.

Both V and E codes are alphanumeric; they contain letters followed by numbers. For example, the code for a complete physical examination of an adult is V70.0. The code for a fall from a ladder is E881.0.

V Codes

V codes are used

1. For encounters with healthy patients who receive services other than treatments, such as annual checkups, immunizations, and normal childbirth. This use is coded by a V code that identifies the service, such as

V06.4 Prophylactic vaccination/inoculation against measles-mumps-rubella (MMR)

2. For encounters with patients having known conditions for which they are receiving one of three types of treatment: chemotherapy, radiation therapy, and rehabilitation. In these cases, the encounter is coded first with a V code, and the condition is listed second. For example:

V58.1 Encounter for chemotherapy
233.0 Breast carcinoma

Listing the V code first for these three treatments is an exception to general coding rules. Usually, when patients receive therapeutic treatments for

TABLE 4.2	Terminology Associated with V Codes	
	Example	
Contact	V01.1	Contact with tuberculosis
Contraception	V25.1	Insertion of intrauterine contraceptive device
Counseling	V61.11	Counseling for victim of spousal and partner abuse
Examination	V70	General medical examination
Fitting of	V52	Fitting and adjustment of prosthetic device and implant
Follow-up	V67.0	Follow-up examination following surgery
Health or healthy	V20	Health supervision of infant or child
History (of)	V10.05	Personal history of malignant neoplasm, large intestine
Replacement	V42.0	Kidney replaced by transplant
Screening/test	V73.2	Special screening examination for measles
Status	V44	Artificial opening status
Supervision (of)	V23	Supervision of high-risk pregnancy
Therapy	V57.3	Speech therapy
Vaccination/inoculation	V06	Need for prophylactic vaccination and inoculation against combinations of disease

already diagnosed conditions, the previously diagnosed condition is used for the primary code.

3. For encounters in which a problem not currently affecting the patient's health status needs to be noted. For example, codes V10-V19 cover history. If a person with a family history of colon cancer presents with rectal bleeding, the problem is listed first, and the V code is assigned as an additional code, as is shown here:

569.3 Hemorrhage of rectum and anus
V16.0 Family history of malignant neoplasm

4. For encounters in which patients are being evaluated preoperatively, a code from category V72.8 is listed first, followed by a code for the condition that is the reason for the surgery. For example:

V72.81 Preoperative cardiovascular examination
414.01 Arteriosclerotic heart disease of native coronary artery

A V code can be used as either a primary code for an encounter or as an additional code. It is researched in the same way as other codes, using the Alphabetic Index to point to the term's code and the Supplementary Classification in the Tabular List to verify it. The terms that indicate the need for V codes, however, are not the same as other medical terms. They usually have to do with a reason for an encounter other than a disease or its complications. When found in diagnostic statements, the words listed in Table 4.2 often point to V codes.

E Codes

E (for external) codes are used to classify the injuries resulting from various environmental events, such as transportation accidents, accidental poisoning by drugs or other substances, falls, and fires. E codes are not used alone. They always supplement a code that identifies the injury or condition itself.

E codes are located by first using Section 3 of the Alphabetic Index, Alphabetic Index to External Causes of Injury and Poisoning. This index is organized by main terms describing the accident, circumstance, event, or specific agent

Medical coding specialists work in a number of health care settings, including medical practices, hospitals, government agencies, and insurance companies. Coders who work in practices review patients' medical records and assign diagnosis and procedure codes. They are knowledgeable about the coding rules and procedures for physicians' work, which are different than those for coding hospital services. The position of medical coding specialist is growing in importance in physician practices. Accurate coding is a critical part of ensuring that claims follow the legal and ethical requirements of Medicare and other third-party payers, as well as HIPAA regulations.

Medical office employees may gain required health care work experience and then attain coding positions through coding education from seminars or college classes. Certification as a professional coder offers an excellent route to success as a medical coder in the medical practice setting. Some employers require certification for employment; others state that certification must be earned after a certain amount of time in the position, such as six months. Coding classes followed by examinations are used to obtain certification. Three physician-office coding certifications are available. All require a high school diploma or equivalent.

- The American Health Information Management Association offers the Certified Coding Associate (CCA) credential and the Certified Coding Specialist—Physician-based (CCS-P) credential. The CCA is an entry-level title; completion of either a training program or six months' job experience is recommended. The CCS-P requires at least three years of coding experience.
- The American Academy of Professional Coders also offer an Associate level and the Certified Professional Coder (CPC) credential, which requires both coursework and on-the-job experience.

Those holding these credentials and coding experience may advance to coding management and coding compliance auditor positions. Becoming expert in a specialty such as surgical coding also offers advancement opportunities.

(drug or chemical) that caused the injury. Codes are verified in the Supplementary Classifications section of the Tabular List.

E codes are often used in collecting public health information. These categories are important in medical practices:

- *Accidents:* When patients have accidents, payers check the E codes that are assigned to verify that the services are covered by the medical insurance policy, rather than by an automobile policy or workers' compensation laws.
- *Drug reactions:* The categories E930 to E949 apply to an **adverse effect**, a patient's unintentional, harmful reaction to a proper dosage of a drug. The specific drug is located in the Table of Drugs and Chemicals in the Alphabetic Index. Adverse effects are different from poisoning, which refers to the medical result of the incorrect use of a substance. Poisoning codes are found under categories 960–979.

V Codes
E Codes

Note: If the *Medical Insurance Coding Workbook for Physician Practices* is assigned for coding practice, the student should follow the marginal notes in Chapters 4, 5, and 6 to complete exercises at the appropriate points. For example, the icon at the left means to turn to the *Coding Workbook* for exercises on V codes and E codes.

Coding Steps

The correct procedure for reporting accurate diagnosis codes has three steps.

Coding Point

Correct Coding Procedure Never use only the Alphabetic Index or only the Tabular List to code. Either practice causes coding errors.

Step 1 Determine the Reason for the Encounter

In medical practices, outpatient coding is often based on the patient's chief complaint and the physician's findings; and the **primary diagnosis**, the main reason for the patient encounter, is documented in the patient's medical record. The primary diagnosis is the diagnosis, condition, problem, or other reason that the documentation shows as being chiefly responsible for the services that are provided. This primary diagnosis provides the main term to be coded first. If other conditions or problems are pertinent, they are also coded.

In working with diagnostic statements and physician practice coding, medical insurance specialists follow a different rule than do coding specialists in hospital (inpatient) coding. In the inpatient setting, the reason the patient has been admitted is called the principal (rather than primary) diagnosis, and often it is not known until the end of the hospital stay. (Hospital coding is covered in Chapter 15.)

Step 2 Locate the Term in the Alphabetic Index

The main term for the patient's primary diagnosis is located in the Alphabetic Index. These guidelines should be observed in choosing the correct term:

- Use any supplementary terms in the diagnostic statement to help locate the main term.
- Read and follow any notes below the main term.
- Review the subterms to find the most specific match to the diagnosis.
- Read and follow any cross-references.
- Make note of a two-code (etiology and/or manifestation) indication.

Step 3 Verify the Code in the Tabular List

The code for the main term is then located in the Tabular List. These guidelines are observed to verify the selection of the correct code:

- Read *include* or *excludes* notes, checking back to see if any apply to the code's category, section, or chapter.
- Be alert for and observe fifth-digit requirements.
- Follow any instructions requiring the selection of additional codes (such as "code also" or "code first underlying disease").
- List multiple codes in the correct order.

Key Coding Guidelines

Diagnostic coding in medical practices follows specific guidelines. These are developed by a group made up of CMS advisers and participants from the American Hospital Association, the American Health Information Management Association, and the National Center for Health Statistics. As illustrated in Figure 4.3 (pages 126–127), the guidelines cover all the rules for what is to be coded and in what order the codes should be listed. In this section, three key guidelines are discussed:

1. Code the primary diagnosis first, followed by current coexisting conditions.
2. Code to the highest level of certainty.
3. Code to the highest level of specificity.

Code the Primary Diagnosis First, Followed by Current Coexisting Conditions

The ICD-9-CM code for the primary diagnosis is listed first.

Additional codes are listed to describe all current documented **coexisting conditions**—conditions that affect patient treatment or require treatment during the encounter. Coexisting conditions may be related to the primary diagnosis, or they may involve a separate illness that the physician diagnoses and treats during the encounter.

It is important to note that patients may have diseases or conditions that do not affect the encounter being coded. Some physicians add notes about previous conditions to provide an easy reference to a patient's history. Unless these conditions are directly involved with the patient's treatment, they are not considered in selecting codes. Also, conditions that were previously treated and no longer exist are not coded.

Thinking It Through—4.4

1. Why is it important to use the Alphabetic Index and then the Tabular List to find the correct code? Work through this coding process, and then comment on your result.

   A. Double-underline the main term and underline the subterm.

   patient complains of abdominal cramps

   B. Find the term in the Alphabetic Index, and list its code.

   _____

   C. Verify the code in the Tabular List, reading all instructions. List the code you have determined to be correct.

   _____

   D. Did the result of your research in the Tabular List match the main term's code in the Alphabetic Index? Why?

   _____

2. Place a double underline below the main terms and a single underline below any subterms in each of the following statements, and then determine the correct codes.

   A. cerebral atherosclerosis

   B. spasmodic asthma with status asthmaticus

   C. congenital night blindness

   D. recurrent inguinal hernia with obstruction

   E. incomplete bundle branch heart block

   F. acute bacterial food poisoning

   G. malnutrition following gastrointestinal surgery

   H. skin test for hypersensitivity

   I. frequency of urination at night

If the reason for the visit is a condition other than a disease or illness, the appropriate V code is used to code the encounter:

Coding Acute versus Chronic Conditions

The reasons for patient encounters are often **acute** symptoms—generally, relatively sudden or severe problems. Acute conditions are coded with the specific code that is designated acute, if listed. Many patients, however, receive ongoing treatment for **chronic** conditions—those that continue over a long period of time or recur frequently. For example, a patient may need a regular gold injection for the management of rheumatoid arthritis. In such cases, the disease is coded and reported for as many times as the patient receives care for the condition.

In some cases, an encounter covers both an acute and a chronic condition. Some conditions do not have separate entries for both manifestations, so a single code applies. If both the acute and the chronic illnesses have codes, the acute code is listed first.

Coding Late Effects

A **late effect** is a condition that remains after a patient's acute illness or injury has ended. Often called residual effects, some late effects happen soon after the disease is over, and others occur later. The diagnostic statement may say "late, due to an old . . ." or "due to a previous . . . ." In general, the main term *late* is followed by subterms that list the causes. Two codes are usually required. First reported is the code for the specific late effect (such as muscle soreness), followed by the code for the cause of the late effect (such as the late effect of rickets).

Code to the Highest Level of Certainty

If the physician has not established a diagnosis, the diagnosis codes that cover symptoms, signs, and ill-defined conditions are used. Inconclusive diagnoses, such as those preceded by "rule out," "suspected," or "probable," for example, are not coded. This rule—code only to the highest degree of certainty—exists because an unproven condition reported to a payer could prove damaging to the patient; such a statement could remain in others' records uncorrected. For example, if the diagnostic statement said "rule out aggressive breast carcinoma," a code for that disease was used, and a malignancy was not found, the patient could be denied medical insurance coverage because of the insurer's concern that the patient has cancer.

Coding Signs and Symptoms

Diagnoses are not always established at the first encounter. Two or more visits may be required before the physician determines a primary diagnosis. During this process, although possible diagnoses may appear in a patient's medical record as the physician's work is progressing, these inconclusive diagnoses are not reported for reimbursement of service fees. Instead, the specific signs and symptoms are coded and reported. A *sign* is an objective indication that can be evaluated by the physician, such as weight loss. A *symptom* is a subjective statement by the patient that cannot be confirmed during an examination, such as pain. The following case provides an example of how symptoms and signs are coded:

**Case Example:
Coexisting Condition**

Diagnostic Statement
Patient, a forty-five-year-old male, presents for complete physical examination for an insurance certification. During the examination, patient complains of occasional difficulty hearing; wax is removed from the left ear canal.
Primary Diagnosis
V70.3 Routine physical examination for insurance certification
Coexisting Condition
380.4 Impacted cerumen

**Case Example:
Treated Conditions**

Chart Note
Mrs. Mackenzie, whose previous encounter was for her regularly scheduled blood pressure check, presents today with a new onset of psoriasis.
Primary Diagnosis
696.1 Psoriasis, NOS

**Case Example:
V Codes**

V72.3 Routine gynecological examination with Papanicolaou smear

**Case Example:
Chronic or Acute**

Acute Renal Failure
584.9
Chronic Renal Failure
585

Diagnostic Coding and Reporting Guidelines for Outpatient Services

These coding guidelines for outpatient diagnoses have been approved for use by hospitals/physicians in coding and reporting hospital-based outpatient services and physician office visits.

Information about the use of certain abbreviations, punctuation, symbols, and other conventions used in the ICD-9-CM Tabular List (code numbers and titles), can be found in Section IA of these guidelines, under "Conventions Used in the Tabular List." Information about the correct sequence to use in finding a code is also described in Section I.

The terms encounter and visit are often used interchangeably in describing outpatient service contacts and, therefore, appear together in these guidelines without distinguishing one from the other.

Though the conventions and general guidelines apply to all settings, coding guidelines for outpatient and physician reporting of diagnoses will vary in a number of instances from those for inpatient diagnoses, recognizing that:

The Uniform Hospital Discharge Data Set (UHDDS) definition of principal diagnosis applies only to inpatients in acute, short-term, general hospitals.

Coding guidelines for inconclusive diagnoses (probable, suspected, rule out, etc.) were developed for inpatient reporting and do not apply to outpatients.

A. Selection of first-listed condition

In the outpatient setting, the term first-listed diagnosis is used in lieu of principal diagnosis.

In determining the first-listed diagnosis the coding conventions of ICD-9-CM, as well as the general and disease specific guidelines take precedence over the outpatient guidelines.

Diagnoses often are not established at the time of the initial encounter/visit. It may take two or more visits before the diagnosis is confirmed.

The most critical rule involves beginning the search for the correct code assignment through the Alphabetic Index. Never begin searching initially in the Tabular List as this will lead to coding errors.

B. The appropriate code or codes from 001.0 through V83.89 must be used to identify diagnoses, symptoms, conditions, problems, complaints, or other reason(s) for the encounter/visit.

C. For accurate reporting of ICD-9-CM diagnosis codes, the documentation should describe the patient's condition, using terminology which includes specific diagnoses as well as symptoms, problems, or reasons for the encounter. There are ICD-9-CM codes to describe all of these.

D. The selection of codes 001.0 through 999.9 will frequently be used to describe the reason for the encounter. These codes are from the section of ICD-9-CM for the classification of diseases and injuries (e.g. infectious and parasitic diseases; neoplasms; symptoms, signs, and ill-defined conditions, etc.).

E. Codes that describe symptoms and signs, as opposed to diagnoses, are acceptable for reporting purposes when a diagnosis has not been established (confirmed) by the physician. Chapter 16 of ICD-9-CM, Symptoms, Signs, and Ill-defined conditions (codes 780.0 - 799.9) contain many, but not all codes for symptoms.

F. ICD-9-CM provides codes to deal with encounters for circumstances other than a disease or injury. The Supplementary Classification of factors Influencing Health Status and Contact with Health Services (VO1.0- V83.89) is provided to deal with occasions when circumstances other than a disease or injury are recorded as diagnosis or problems.

G. Level of Detail in Coding

1. ICD-9-CM is composed of codes with either 3, 4, or 5 digits. Codes with three digits are included in ICD-9-CM as the heading of a category of codes that may be further subdivided by the use of fourth and/or fifth digits, which provide greater specificity.

2. A three-digit code is to be used only if it is not further subdivided. Where fourth-digit subcategories and/or fifth-digit subclassifications are provided, they must be assigned. A code is invalid if it has not been coded to the full number of digits required for that code. See also discussion under Section I, General Coding Guidelines, Level of Detail.

(a)

Figure 4.3 ICD-9-CM Guidelines for Coding and Reporting Outpatient Services

H. List first the ICD-9-CM code for the diagnosis, condition, problem, or other reason for encounter/visit shown in the medical record to be chiefly responsible for the services provided. List additional codes that describe any coexisting conditions.

I. Do not code diagnoses documented as "probable," "suspected," "questionable," "rule out," or "working diagnosis." Rather, code the condition(s) to the highest degree of certainty for that encounter/visit, such as symptoms, signs, abnormal test results, or other reason for the visit.

Please note: This differs from the coding practices used by hospital medical record departments for coding the diagnosis of acute care, short-term hospital inpatients.

J. Chronic diseases treated on an ongoing basis may be coded and reported as many times as the patient receives treatment and care for the condition(s).

K. Code all documented conditions that coexist at the time of the encounter/visit, and require or affect patient care treatment or management. Do not code conditions that were previously treated and no longer exist. However, history codes (VIO-V19) may be used as secondary codes if the historical condition or family history has an impact on current care or influences treatment.

L. For patients receiving diagnostic services only during an encounter/visit, sequence first the diagnosis, condition, problem, or other reason for encounter/visit shown in the medical record to be chiefly responsible for the outpatient services provided during the encounter/visit. Codes for other diagnoses (e.g., chronic conditions) may be sequenced as additional diagnoses.

For outpatient encounters for diagnostic tests that have been interpreted by a physician, and the final report is available at the time of coding, code any confirmed or definitive diagnosis(es) documented in the interpretation. Do not code related signs and symptoms as additional diagnoses.

Please note: This differs from the coding practice in the hospital inpatient setting regarding abnormal findings on test results.

M. For patients receiving therapeutic services only during an encounter/visit, sequence first the diagnosis, condition, problem, or other reason for encounter/visit shown in the medical record to be chiefly responsible for the outpatient services provided during the encounter/visit. Codes for other diagnoses (e.g., chronic conditions) may be sequenced as additional diagnoses.

The only exception to this rule is that when the primary reason for the admission/encounter is chemotherapy, radiation therapy, or rehabilitation, the appropriate V code for the service is listed first, and the diagnosis or problem for which the service is being performed listed second.

N. For patients receiving preoperative evaluations only, sequence a code from category V72.8, Other specified examinations, to describe the pre-op consultations. Assign a code for the condition to describe the reason for the surgery as an additional diagnosis. Code also any findings related to the pre-op evaluation.

O. For ambulatory surgery, code the diagnosis for which the surgery was performed. If the postoperative diagnosis is known to be different from the preoperative diagnosis at the time the diagnosis is confirmed, select the postoperative diagnosis for coding, since it is the most definitive.

P. For routine outpatient prenatal visits when no complications are present codes V22.0, Supervision of normal first pregnancy, and V22.l, Supervision of other normal pregnancy, should be used as principal diagnoses. These codes should not be used in conjunction with chapter 11 codes.

(b)

Figure 4.3 (*Continued*)

Diagnostic Statement

Forty-six-year-old male presents with abdominal pain and weight loss. He had to return home from vacation due to acute illness. He has not been eating well because of a vague upper-abdominal pain. He denies nausea, vomiting. He denies changes in bowel habit or blood in stool. Physical examination revealed no abdominal tenderness.

Primary Diagnosis

789.06 Abdominal pain, epigastric region

Coexisting Condition

783.2 Abnormal loss of weight

Coding the Reason for Surgery

Surgery is coded according to the diagnosis that is listed as the reason for the procedure. In some cases, the postoperative diagnosis is available and is different from the physician's primary diagnosis before the surgery. If so, the postoperative diagnosis is coded because it is the highest level of certainty available. For example, if an excisional biopsy is performed to evaluate mammographic breast lesions or a lump of unknown nature, and the pathology results show a malignant neoplasm, the diagnosis code describing the site and nature of the neoplasm is used. (Coding neoplasms is covered later in this chapter.)

Code to the Highest Level of Specificity

A three-digit code is used only if a four-digit code is not provided in the ICD9-CM. Likewise, a four-digit subcategory code is used only when no five-digit subclassification is listed. When a five-digit code is available, it must be used.

The more digits the code has, the more specific it becomes; the additional codes add to the clinical picture of the patient. Using the most specific code possible is referred to as coding to the highest level of specificity.

Thinking It Through—4.5

Provide the diagnostic code(s) for the following cases, and explain the coding guideline that you applied to the case.

1. A thirty-six-year-old female patient presents to the physician's office for her yearly checkup. During the exam, the physician identifies a palpable, solitary lump in the left breast. The physician considers this significant and extends the exam to gather information for diagnosing this problem.

   _____

2. A forty-five-year-old male patient presents to the office complaining of headaches for the past twenty-four hours. Based on the examination, the physician orders an MRI to investigate a possible brain tumor.

   _____

3. An eighty-six-year-old female patient who has a chronic laryngeal ulcer presents for treatment of a painful episode.

   _____

4. A fifty-eight-year-old female patient has muscle weakness due to poliomyelitis in childhood.

   _____

5. A sixty-four-year-old male patient's diagnosis is degenerative osteoarthritis.

   _____

For example, the category code 250 indicates a diagnosis of diabetes mellitus. Under this category, a fourth digit provides information about the cause or site, such as

250.1 Diabetes with ketoacidosis
250.2 Diabetes with hyperosmolarity
250.3 Diabetes with other coma
250.4 Diabetes with renal manifestations

Based on the medical record, a fifth digit must be selected and added to any of the above four-digit codes, according to which of these is documented:

0 Type II or unspecified type, not stated as uncontrolled
1 Type I, not stated as uncontrolled
2 Type II or unspecified type, uncontrolled
3 Type I, uncontrolled

Type I is insulin-dependent; type II is not. *Control* indicates whether the glycemic level (blood sugar) is under control. An uncontrolled diabetic is likely to become blind, lose limbs through amputation because of severely reduced circulation, and experience renal failure. On the other hand, a controlled diabetic usually leads a substantially normal life. The diagnostic code 250.33 indicates diabetes mellitus with other coma, insulin-dependent, and uncontrolled. This diagnosis presents a very different clinical picture than 250.40, diabetes mellitus with renal manifestations, not insulin-dependent, and not stated as being uncontrolled.

Codes 001–139
240–389
460–799

Codes for Circulatory Diseases, Neoplasms, Burns, and Fractures

Some diagnoses require an understanding of additional guidelines for correct coding. This section introduces basic information about three important areas:

1. Circulatory diseases
2. Neoplasms
3. Burns and fractures

Circulatory Diseases

Because the circulatory system involves so many interrelated components, the disease process can create interrelated, complex conditions. Many types of cardio-vascular system disease, such as acute myocardial infarction (heart attack), require hospitalization of patients. A complete description of these diseases is beyond the scope of this chapter. The following introduction covers some frequently coded diagnoses. The notes and *code also* instructions in Chapter 7 of the Tabular List must be carefully observed to code circulatory diseases accurately.

Ischemic Heart Disease and Arteriosclerotic Cardiovascular Disease

Ischemic heart disease conditions—those caused by reduced blood flow to the heart—are coded under categories 410 to 414. Myocardial infarctions that are acute or have a documented duration of eight weeks or less are located in category 410. Chronic myocardial infarctions, or those with duration longer than eight weeks, are coded to subcategory 414.8. An old or healed myocardial infarction without current symptoms is coded 412.

Other chronic ischemic heart diseases are coded under category 414. Coronary atherosclerosis, 414.0, requires a fifth digit for the type of artery involved and includes arteriosclerotic heart disease (ASHD), atherosclerotic heart disease, and other coronary conditions. A diagnosis of angina pectoris—an episode of chest pain from a temporary insufficiency of oxygen to the heart—is coded 413.9, unless it occurs only at night (413.0) or is diagnosed as Prinzmetal (angiospastic) angina (413.1).

Arteriosclerotic cardiovascular disease (ASCVD)—hardening of the arteries affecting the complete cardiovascular system—is coded 429.2. A second code for the arteriosclerosis, 440.9, is also needed for this diagnosis. Likewise, 440.9 is never the primary code when ASCVD is a diagnosis.

Hypertension and Hypertensive Heart Disease

Hypertension is a diagnosis related to high blood pressure. Almost all cases are due to unknown causes. This is called essential hypertension and is the primary diagnosis. In the few cases where the cause is known, the hypertension is called secondary, and its code is listed after the code for the cause.

Within the essential hypertension category, there are three subcategories: malignant (401.0), benign (401.1), and unspecified (401.9). Malignant hypertension is an extremely serious condition, so it is always documented as malignant. Benign hypertension is a relatively mild and often chronic condition. If the diagnostic statement does not contain either word, the hypertension is coded as unspecified. Hypertension can affect the heart and/or the kidneys. Hypertensive heart disease and hypertensive renal disease are coded under the categories 402 to 404.

Note that a diagnosis of hypertension is different from "high (or elevated) blood pressure." If the diagnosis does not include *hypertension,* the statement is coded 796.2, elevated blood pressure reading without diagnosis of hypertension (the Symptoms, Signs, and Ill-Defined Conditions chapter of the ICD-9-CM).

The Alphabetic Index contains a detailed table to point to the various types of hypertensive disease, including its effect on pregnancy. Hypertension is often indicated as a coexisting condition with other conditions, and it may make those more serious. When these diagnoses appear, two codes must be assigned, one for the first condition and one for the hypertension.

Neoplasms

Neoplasms, also called tumors, are growths that arise from normal tissue. (This category does not include a diagnosis statement with the word *mass,* which is a separate main term.)

The Neoplasm Table

The Alphabetic Index contains a Neoplasm Table that points to codes for neoplasms. The table lists the anatomical location in the first column. The next six columns relate to the behavior of the neoplasm, described as

- One of these three types of malignant tumor, each of which is progressive, rapid-growing, life-threatening, and made of cancerous cells:

Case Example

Diagnosis of angina pectoris with essential hypertension: 413.9 and 401.9

Codes 390–459

Primary: The neoplasm that is the encounter's main diagnosis is found at the site of origin.

Secondary: The neoplasm that is the encounter's main diagnosis metastasized (spread) to an additional body site from the original location.

Carcinoma in situ: The neoplasm is restricted to one site (a noninvasive type).

- Benign—slow-growing, not life-threatening, made of normal or near-normal cells
- Uncertain behavior—not classifiable when the cells were examined
- Unspecified nature—no documentation of the nature of the neoplasm.

As an example, the following entries are shown in the Neoplasm Table for a neoplasm of the colon:

In the Tabular List, neoplasms are listed in Chapter 2 under categories 140 to 239.

MALIGNANT						
	Primary	Secondary	Cancer in situ	Benign	Uncertain Behavior	Unspecified
Colon	154.0	197.5	230.4	211.4	235.2	239.0

M Codes

In the regular Alphabetic Index entries, the pointers for neoplasms also show morphology codes, known as M codes. M codes contain the letter M followed by four digits, a slash, and a final digit. M codes (listed in ICD-9-CM, Appendix A) are used by pathologists to report on and study the prevalence of various types of neoplasms. They are not used in physician practice (outpatient) coding. However, pathologists' reports help in selecting the correct code for a neoplasm. In the M code, the digit after the slash indicates the behavior of the neoplasm:

/0 Benign
/1 Uncertain whether benign or malignant/borderline malignant
/2 Carcinoma in situ: intraepithelial, noninfiltrating, or noninvasive
/3 Malignant, primary site
/6 Malignant, metastatic site, secondary site

These codes are related as follows to the Neoplasm Table and the Tabular List:

M Code	Neoplasm Table	Tabular List
/0	Benign neoplasms	210–229
/1	Neoplasm of unspecified nature	239
	Neoplasms of uncertain behavior	235–238
/2	Carcinoma in situ	230–234
/3	Malignant neoplasm, stated or presumed to be primary	140–195
		200–208
/6	Malignant neoplasms, stated or presumed to be secondary	196–198

For example, a pathologist's report might indicate the presence of an endometrioid adenofibroma. If it is benign, the M code is M8381/0, the equivalent of diagnosis code 220. If it is borderline malignant, the M code is M8381/1, and the diagnosis code is 236.2. If it is malignant, the M code is M8381/3, and the diagnosis code is 183.0.

In the case of a metastasized neoplasm, if the secondary site is the main reason for treatment, then the primary site is listed as a coexisting condition if it is still being treated. If the primary site is not documented, the code 199.1, malignant neoplasm without specification of site, other, is used. After the neoplasm is removed or is in remission, a V code for the personal history of malignant neoplasm is used.

Codes 140–239

Burns and Fractures

Diagnostic codes for burns and fractures are located in the Injury and Poisoning chapter of the Tabular List.

Burns

Burns are located in categories 940 to 949, where they are classified according to the cause, such as flames or radiation. They are grouped by severity and by how much of body's surface is involved. Severity is rated as one of three degrees of burns:

1. *First-degree burn:* The epidermis (outer layer of skin) is damaged.
2. *Second-degree burn:* Both the epidermis and the dermis are damaged.
3. *Third-degree burn:* The most severe degree; the three layers of the skin—epidermis, dermis, and subcutaneous—are all damaged.

The total body surface area (TBSA) that is involved determines the extent of the burn for coding purposes (see Figure 4.4). When burns are coded according to extent (category 948), fourth-digit codes are used to show the percentage of TBSA for all of the burns. For third-degree burns, a fifth digit is also required to classify the percentage of third-degree burns:

0 less than 10% or unspecified
1 10%–19%
2 20%–29%

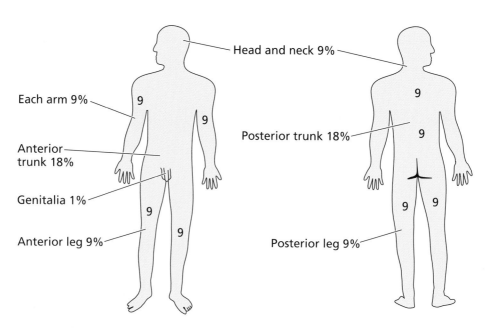

Figure 4.4 Coding Burns

3 30%–39%
4 40%–49%
5 50%–59%
6 60%–69%
7 70%–79%
8 80%–89%
9 90% or more of body surface

Fractures

Fractures are coded using categories 800 to 829. A fourth digit indicates whether the fracture is closed or open. When a fracture is closed, the broken bone does not pierce the skin. An open fracture involves breaking through the skin. If the fracture is not indicated as open or closed, it is coded as closed. A fifth digit is often used for the specific anatomical site. For example:

810 Fracture of clavicle
    The following fifth-digit subclassification is for use with category 810:
    0 unspecified part (Clavicle NOS)
    1 sternal end of clavicle
    2 shaft of clavicle
    3 acromial end of clavicle
    ⑤810.0 Closed
    ⑤810.1 Open

When any of the following descriptions are used, a closed fracture is indicated:

Comminuted
Depressed
Elevated
Fissured
Greenstick
Impacted
Linear
March
Simple
Slipped epiphysis
Spiral
Unspecified

These descriptions indicate open fractures:

Compound
Infected
Missile
Puncture
With foreign body

Codes 800–999

Review

Chapter Summary

1. The ICD-9-CM is the *Clinical Modification* of the World Health Organization's *International Classification of Diseases* used for diagnostic coding in the United States. ICD-9-CM codes are required for reporting patients' conditions on insurance claims and encounter forms. Codes are made up of three, four, or five numbers and a description. The addenda, which are lists of new, changed, or deleted codes, are issued annually. Medical practices must use the current codes because they can affect billing and reimbursement.

2. The ICD-9-CM has two volumes that are used in medical practices, the Tabular List (Volume 1) and the Alphabetic Index (Volume 2). The Alphabetic Index is used first in the process of finding a code. It contains an index of all the diseases that are classified in the Tabular List. These main terms may be followed by related subterms or supported by supplementary terms. The codes themselves are organized into seventeen chapters according to etiology or body system and are listed in numerical order in the Tabular List. Code categories consist of three-digit groupings of a single disease or a related condition. Subcategories have four digits to show the disease's etiology, site, or manifestation. Further clinical detail is supplied by fifth-digit subclassifications.

3. The conventions used in the ICD-9-CM must be observed to correctly select codes. Notes provide details about conditions that are either excluded or included under the code. The cross-reference *see* means that another main term is appropriate. A symbol is used to show a fifth-digit requirement. The abbreviation NOS (not otherwise specified or unspecified) indicates the code to use when a condition is not completely described. The abbreviation NEC (not elsewhere classified) indicates the code to use when the diagnosis does not match any other available code. Parentheses and brackets indicate supplementary terms. Colons and braces indicate that one or more words after the punctuation must appear in the diagnostic statement for the code to be applicable. Codes that are not used as primary appear in italics and are usually followed by an instruction to code first underlying disease or use additional code.

4. V codes identify encounters for reasons other than illness or injury and are used for healthy patients receiving routine services, for therapeutic encounters, for a problem that is not currently affecting the patient's condition, and for preoperative evaluations. E codes, which are never used as primary codes, classify the injuries resulting from various environmental events.

5. The three steps in the coding process are to (a) determine the reason for the encounter that is the patient's primary diagnosis, (b) locate the medical term in the Alphabetic Index, and (c) verify the code in the Tabular List.

6. Three key coding guidelines are (a) code the primary diagnosis first, followed by current coexisting conditions; (b) code to the highest degree of certainty, never coding inconclusive, rule-out diagnoses, and (c) code to the highest level of specificity, using fifth digits or fourth digits when available.

7. Circulatory diseases are often complex and interrelated. Ischemic heart disease includes myocardial infarctions and coronary atherosclerosis. Diagnoses relating to hypertension are located first in the Hypertension Table in the Alphabetic Index. The Alphabetic Index also contains a Neoplasm Table that points to codes for neoplasms listed alphabetically by anatomical location and indicates the code for the type of neoplasm. M codes help point to the correct category. Burns are coded according to the cause, site, and extent; fractures are classified as either open or closed.

Key Terms

acute *page 125*
addenda *page 110*
adverse effect *page 122*
Alphabetic Index *page 111*
category *page 115*
chronic *page 125*
coexisting condition *page 124*
combination code *page 114*
convention *page 113*
crosswalk *page 111*

diagnostic statement *page 112*
E code *page 120*
eponym *page 114*
etiology *page 112*
ICD-9-CM *page 109*
late effect *page 125*
main term *page 112*
manifestation *page 114*
NEC (not elsewhere classified) *page 113*
NOS (not otherwise specified) *page 119*

primary diagnosis *page 123*
subcategory *page 116*
subclassification *page 116*
subterm *page 112*
supplementary term *page 112*
Tabular List *page 111*
unspecified *page 119*
V code *page 120*

Review Questions

Match the key terms in the left column with the definitions in the right column.

A. E code

B. unspecified

C. addenda

D. category

E. V code

F. manifestation

G. eponym

H. convention

I. main term

J. supplementary term

_____ 1. Typographic technique or standard practice that provides visual guidelines for understanding printed material

_____ 2. The medical term in boldfaced type that identifies a disease or condition in the Alphabetic Index

_____ 3. An alphanumeric code used to identify the external cause of an injury or poisoning

_____ 4. A nonessential word or phrase that helps define a diagnosis code

_____ 5. Annual updates to the ICD-9-CM diagnostic coding system

_____ 6. Refers to a code that should be used for an incompletely described condition

_____ 7. An alphanumeric code used for an encounter that is not due to illness or injury

_____ 8. A three-digit code that covers a single disease or related condition

_____ 9. The characteristic signs or symptoms associated with a disease

_____ 10. A condition or procedure that is named for the physician who discovered it

Decide whether each statement is true or false, and write T for true or F for false.

_____ 1. In selecting correct diagnosis codes, the chapters of the Tabular List are first searched, and the code is then verified in the Alphabetic Index.

_____ 2. Subcategories are four-digit diagnosis codes that define the etiology, site, or manifestation of a disease.

_____ 3. In the Alphabetic Index, a *see* cross-reference must be followed.

_____ 4. The etiology of a disease refers to the reason that the patient presents for treatment.

_____ 5. The fifth-digit requirement refers to the need to show a subclassification code for a particular diagnosis.

_____ 6. A code that appears in italics is a secondary code and is not sequenced first.

_____ 7. The coding instruction "use an additional code" means that supplying another code is optional.

_____ 8. A patient has an appointment for a complaint of flulike symptoms. While the patient is in the office, the physician decides to conduct a complete physical examination. A V code is used as the primary diagnosis code for the encounter.

_____ 9. When a diagnosis is being confirmed by tests or other procedures, only the patient's signs, symptoms, or vague condition are coded, not the possible or suspected disease.

_____ 10. A patient's past, cured conditions have no applicability to the coding of current encounters except when late effects are noted.

Write the letter of the choice that best completes the statement or answers the question.

_____ 1. Outpatient coding is based on which volume or volumes of the ICD-9-CM?
A. Volume 1   C. Volumes 1, 2, and 3
B. Volumes 1 and 2   D. Volumes 2 and 3

_____ 2. The medical terms in the Alphabetical Index are arranged by
A. the condition or problem   C. the etiology and the manifestation
B. the anatomical site   D. the signs and symptoms

_____ 3. The unintentional, harmful reaction to a correct dosage of a drug is called
A. a late effect   C. an adverse effect
B. a coexisting condition   D. a manifestation

_____ 4. A condition that remains or recurs after an acute illness has finished is called
A. a late effect   C. an adverse effect
B. a coexisting condition   D. a manifestation

_____ 5. A colon after a term in an *excludes* or *includes* note indicates that
A. the term is not complete without one or more of the additional terms listed
B. the term requires a manifestation code
C. the synonyms, alternative wordings, or explanations that follow may appear in the diagnostic statement
D. the term requires a code for the underlying disease

_____ 6. To code an encounter for chemotherapy, list the codes in the following order:
A. E code, condition code   C. V code, condition code
B. condition code, E code   D. condition code, V code

_____ 7. The diagnostic statement "patient presents for removal of a cast" requires the use of which of the following types of codes?
A. E   C. R
B. V   D. M

_____ 8. If a patient is treated for both an acute and a chronic condition, each of which has a separate code, how should the codes be listed?
A. V code, condition code   C. acute code, V code
B. chronic code, acute code   D. acute code, chronic code

_____ 9. The correct codes for unspecified essential hypertension and elevated blood pressure are
A. 412 and 401.9   C. 401.1 and 796.2
B. 401.9 and 796.2   D. 796.2 and 401.9

_____ 10. The four types of neoplasms are
A. unspecified, malignant, benign, in situ
B. malignant, benign, uncertain, unspecified
C. benign, malignant, primary, secondary
D. none of the above

Provide answers to the following questions in the spaces provided.

1. List the three steps in the diagnostic coding process.

2. List three key coding guidelines for selecting correct diagnosis codes.

Applying Your Knowledge

Case 4.1

Supply the correct ICD-9-CM codes for the following diagnoses.

1. Brewer's infarct

2. conjunctivitis due to Reiter's disease

3. seasonal allergic rhinitis due to pollen

4. cardiac arrhythmia

5. backache

6. sebaceous cyst

7. breast disease, cystic

8. chronic cystitis

9. normal delivery

10. skin tags

11. acute myocarditis due to influenza

12. acute otitis media

13. endocarditis due to Q fever

14. influenza vaccination

15. vertigo

16. essential anemia

17. muscle spasms

18. influenza with acute respiratory infection

19. pneumonia due to Streptococcus, Group B

20. menorrhagia

Case 4.2

Audit the following cases to determine if the correct codes have been reported in the correct order. If a coding mistake has been made, state the correct code and your reason for assigning it.

Case A

Chart note for Henry Blum, date of birth 11/4/53:

Examined patient on 12/6/2006. He was complaining of a facial rash. Examination revealed sebopsoriasis and extensive seborrheic dermatitis over his upper eyebrows, nasolabial fold, and extending to the subnasal region.

The following codes were reported: 696.1, 690.1.

Case B

Physician's notes, 2/24/2005, patient George Kadar, DOB 10/11/1940:

Subjective: This sixty-year-old patient complains of voiding difficulties, primarily urinary incontinence. No complaints of urinary retention.

Objective: Rectal examination: enlarged prostate. Patient catheterized for residual urine of 200 cc. Urinalysis is essentially negative.

Assessment: Prostatic hypertrophy, benign.

Plan: Refer to urologist for cystoscopy.

The following code was reported: 600.0.

Case C

An insulin-dependent diabetic patient is seen for a blood glucose screening.
The following codes were reported: 250.01, V77.1.

Case D

Patient: Gloria S. Diaz:

Subjective: This twenty-five-year-old female patient presents with pain in her left knee both when she moves it and when it is inactive. She denies previous trauma to this area but has had right-knee pain and arthritis in the past.

Objective: Examination revealed the left knee to be warm and slightly swollen compared to the right knee. Extension is 180 degrees; flexion is 90 degrees. Some tenderness in area.

Assessment: Left-knee pain probably due to chronic arthritis.

Plan: Daypro 600 mg 2-QD x 1 week; recheck in one week.

The following codes were reported: 719.48, 716.98.

Computer Exploration

1. Access the Web site of the National Center for Health Statistics:
   http://www.cdc.gov/nchs
   a. Locate information on the current year's ICD-9-CM addenda.
   b. Research and report on the status of ICD-10-CM.
2. Visit the Web site of the Centers for Medicare and Medicaid Services (CMS) that posts information on ICD-9-CM:
   http://cms.hhs.gov/paymentsystems/icd9/default.asp
   Summarize the types of information this site contains. If possible, review the Summary of Updates to ICD-9-CM.

NDCMediSoft Activity

4.1 Diagnosis Code Setup Screens

Diagnosis codes are entered in MediSoft manually or from a database stored on a CD-ROM or other media. MediSoft allows users to enter new codes, edit existing codes, and mark codes that are inactive.

Diagnosis code information is entered manually in MediSoft as follows.

1. Select Diagnosis Codes from the Lists menu. The Diagnosis List dialog box displays the diagnosis codes already entered in the database.

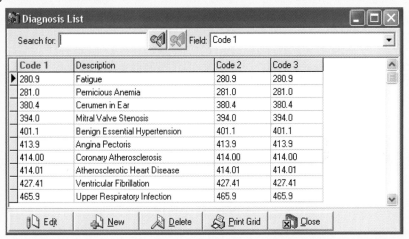

2. Click the New button. The Diagnosis: (new) dialog box appears.

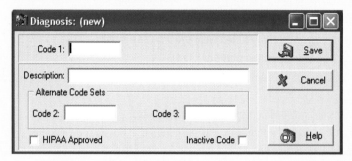

3. The diagnosis code is entered in the box labeled Code 1. A description of the diagnosis code can be entered in the Description box. The two Alternate Code Sets boxes can be used to enter variations of the diagnosis code that are required by different insurance carriers.

4. Click the Cancel button to close the Diagnosis dialog box.

5. Click inside the Search For box at the top left of the Diagnosis List dialog box, and then key "7." Notice that the pointer moves to the first diagnosis code in the list that begins with a 7.

6. Now key "8," and watch the pointer. The first code beginning with 78 is selected. This is an easy way to search for codes in MediSoft.

7. Key "2.1" after the "78" in the Search For box. Rash on Leg should be selected.

8. Click the Edit button. The Diagnosis: Rash on Leg dialog box is displayed. Notice that the code 782.1 is listed in the Code 1 box. The Description field contains the words "Rash on Leg," and since there are no alternate codes required in this case, the same code is entered in the two alternate code boxes.

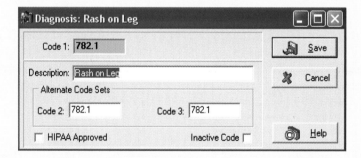

9. Click the Cancel button to exit the Diagnosis dialog box.

10. Click the Close button to close the Diagnosis List dialog box.

4.2 Diagnosis Codes and Transactions

Once diagnosis codes are entered into MediSoft, they can be used to record diagnoses from a patient's encounter form into the patient's records in MediSoft.

1. Click Patients/Guarantors and Cases on the Lists menu. The Patient List dialog box is displayed.

2. Key "NE" in the Search For box to select Isabella Neufeld.

3. Click the Urticaria case on the right side of the dialog box to highlight it. The Case radio button in the upper right corner is automatically selected.

Computer Exploration

4. Click the Edit Case button. The Personal tab of the Case folder for Isabella Neufeld's urticaria condition is displayed.

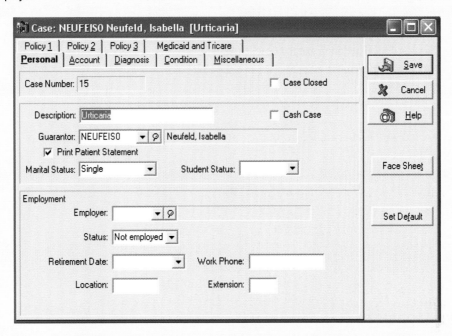

5. Click the Diagnosis tab. Notice that the diagnosis code 708.0, Allergic Urticaria, appears in the Default Diagnosis 1 box. If there were additional diagnoses, they would also be listed (in the Default Diagnosis 2, 3, and 4 boxes).

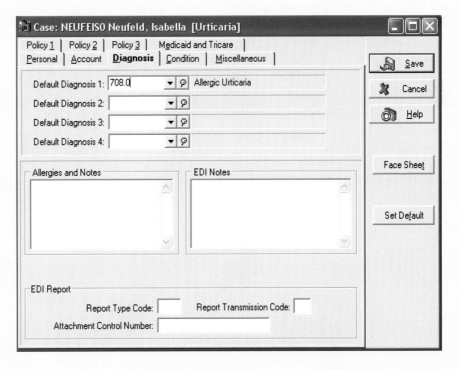

6. Click the triangle button to the right of the Default Diagnosis 1 box to display the full list of diagnosis codes already set up in the current database. Any of these codes could be selected for a patient's record.

7. Scroll up and down through the list to view the range of codes, and then press the Esc key to close the list and return to the 708.0 entry.

8. Click the Cancel button to exit the Case folder.

9. Click the Close button to close the Patient List dialog box.

Procedural Coding: Introduction to CPT and HCPCS

CHAPTER OUTLINE

* All codes are CPT 2004 and are ©2003
American Medical Association.

Objectives

After studying this chapter, you should be able to:

1. Discuss the purpose of CPT and the importance of its annual updates.

2. Describe the structure and content of the index and the main text.

3. Interpret the formats, conventions, and symbols used in CPT.

4. Describe the purpose and correct use of modifiers.

5. List the three general steps for selecting correct procedure codes.

6. Discuss the purpose, structure, and key guidelines associated with each of the six sections of CPT codes.

7. Discuss the key components that are the basis for selection of Evaluation and Management codes and describe the steps for selecting correct codes.

8. Describe the purpose and correct use of HCPCS codes and modifiers.

9. Given procedural statements, apply coding guidelines to determine correct CPT codes.

Introduction to Procedural Coding

Procedure codes, like diagnosis codes, are an important part of the medical billing and reimbursement process. Standard procedure codes are used by physicians in medical practices to report the medical, surgical, and diagnostic services they provide. These codes are used by payers to determine reimbursement levels. Accurate procedural coding ensures that providers receive the maximum appropriate reimbursement for services.

Procedure codes are also used to establish guidelines for the delivery of the best possible care for patients. Researchers at the National Institutes of Health and other medical investigators track various courses of treatment for patients with the same diagnoses and evaluate patients' outcomes. The results are shared with physicians and payers, such as government-sponsored programs and managed care organizations, who help implement improved treatments. For example, this type of analysis has shown that patients who have had heart attacks can reduce the risk of subsequent heart attacks by taking a class of drugs called beta blockers.

Either the physicians, the medical coders, the medical insurance specialists, or an outside company may be responsible for selecting procedure codes in particular practices. Medical insurance specialists verify the procedure codes and use them to report physicians' services. This chapter provides a fundamental understanding of procedural coding principles and guidelines, so that medical insurance specialists can work effectively with insurance claims and encounter forms. Expertise in working with CPT is the baseline for correct physician practice procedural coding. Medical insurance specialists combine this expertise with knowledge about each payer's specific policies and reporting requirements to submit claims efficiently and effectively.

Current Procedural Terminology, Fourth Edition (CPT)

The procedure codes most widely used in the United States are listed in the *Current Procedural Terminology* (referred to as **CPT**). A publication of the American Medical Association (AMA), CPT was first produced in 1966. CPT lists the procedures and services that are commonly used in medical practices and performed by many physicians across the country.

CPT Categtory I codes—which are the majority—have five digits (with no decimals) followed by a **descriptor**, which is a brief explanation of the procedure:

99204   Office visit for evaluation and management of a new patient

Although the codes are grouped into sections, such as Surgery, codes from any section can be used by all types of physicians. For example, a family practitioner might use codes from the Surgery section to describe an office procedure such as the incision and drainage of an abscess.

The wide use of codes began in 1983, when the Health Care Financing Administration (now named the Centers for Medicare and Medicaid, CMS) standardized codes for physician procedures and services reimbursed by government-sponsored programs, especially Medicare. CMS developed the **Healthcare Common Procedure Coding System** (referred to as **HCPCS** and pronounced hick-picks). From the many different coding systems then in use, CMS chose the AMA's codes as its standard for procedure codes. The current HCPCS is discussed in the last section of this chapter.

Within a few years after CMS required HCPCS codes for Medicare claims, most insurance companies that were working with both HCPCS and other systems had also adopted CPT as their standard. Today, codes are required for submitting electronic health care claims to all payers.

Organization and Format

The manual is made up of the main text—sections of codes—followed by appendixes and an index. The main text has the following six sections of procedure codes:

- Evaluation and Management   Codes 99201—99499
- Anesthesia   Codes 00100—01999
- Surgery   Codes 10021—69990
- Radiology   Codes 70010—79999
- Pathology and Laboratory   Codes 80048—89356
- Medicine   Codes 90281—99602

At the back of CPT, an alphabetic index is provided to make the search for the correct code more efficient.

Annual Revisions

Because new procedures and treatments are developed, the AMA publishes a revised CPT each year. In one year, for example, 125 new codes were added and 46 codes were deleted. During the year, practicing physicians, medical specialty societies (such as the American College of Cardiology), and state medical associations send their questions and suggestions for revision to the AMA. This input is reviewed by the AMA's Editorial Panel, which includes physicians as well as representatives from the Health Insurance Association of America, CMS, the American Health Information Management Association (AHIMA), the American Hospital Association (AHA), and Blue Cross and Blue Shield. The panel decides what changes will be made in the annual revision.

HIPAA Tip

Mandated Code Set

CPT is the mandated code set for physician services under HIPAA Electronic Health Care Transactions and Code Sets.

Billing Tip

Keeping Codes Up to Date
When the new and revised procedure codes are received by a medical practice, it is important to implement them on their effective date of January 1. Medical insurance specialists update encounter forms and billing software to reflect the changes. They also inform providers and other professional health care staff of the new codes, because some changes affect billing and reimbursement.

Thinking It Through—5.1

Would you expect to locate codes for the following services or procedures in CPT? What range or series of codes would you investigate?

Service or Procedure Range or Series

1. Routine obstetric care including antepartum care, cesarean delivery, and postpartum care

2. Echocardiography

3. Radiologic examination, nasal bones, complete

4. Home visit for evaluation and management of an established patient

5. Drug test for amphetamines

6. Anesthesia for cardiac catheterization

The new codes and other changes contained in the annual revision are released by the AMA on October 1 and are in effect for procedures and services provided after January 1 of the next year. The CPT annual revision is available in various formats from commercial publishers soon after it is released. Medical specialty societies and the AMA also report the new codes on their Internet Web sites.

The Index

The assignment of a correct procedure code begins by reviewing the physician's statements in the patient's medical record to determine the service, procedure, or treatment that was performed. Then the index entry is located, which provides a pointer to the correct code range in the main text. Using the CPT index makes the process of selecting procedural codes more efficient. The index contains the descriptive terms that are listed in the sections of codes in the CPT.

Main Terms and Modifying Terms

The main terms in the index are printed in boldface type. There are five types of main terms:

1. The name of the procedure or service, such as echocardiography, extraction, and cast
2. The name of the organ or other anatomical site, such as stomach, wrist, and salivary gland
3. The name of the condition, such as abscess, wound, and postpartum care
4. A synonym or an eponym for the term, such as Noble Procedure, Ramstedt operation, and Fowler-Stephens orchiopexy
5. The abbreviation for the term, such as CAT scan and ECMO

Many terms are listed more than one way. For example, the procedure kidney biopsy is listed both as a procedure—Biopsy, kidney—and by the site—Kidney, biopsy.

A main term may be followed by subterms that further describe the entry. These additional indented terms help in the selection process. For example, the procedure repair of tennis elbow is located beneath *repair* under the main term *elbow* (see Figure 5.1).

Code Ranges

A range of codes is shown when more than one code applies to an entry. Two codes, either sequential or not, are separated by a comma:

Cervix
Biopsy 57500, 57520

More than two sequential codes are separated by a hyphen:

Dislocation
Ankle
Closed Treatment 27840-27842

Cross-References and Convention

There are two types of cross-references.

1. *See* is a mandatory instruction. It tells the coder to refer to the term that follows it to find the code. It is used mainly for synonyms, eponyms, and

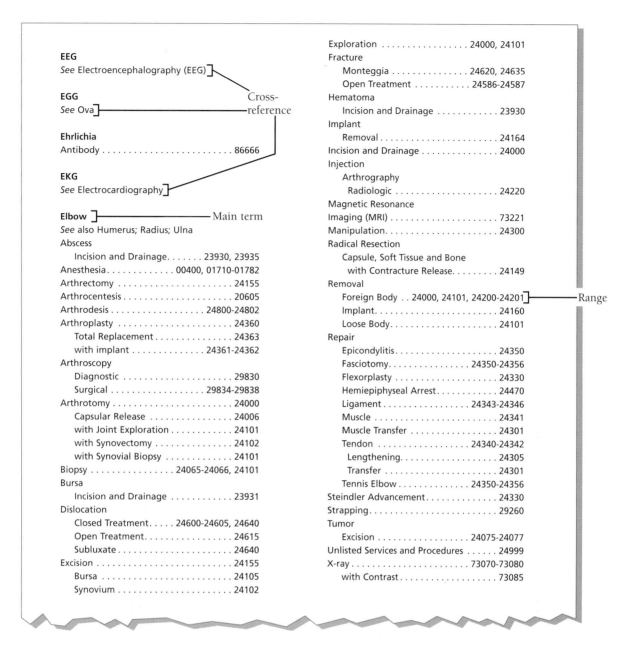

Figure 5.1 Example of Index Entries

abbreviations. For example, the cross-reference "See Electrocardiogram" follows EKG (see Figure 5.1).

2. *See also* tells the coder to look under the term that follows if the procedure is not listed below. For example, under *Elbow*, the cross-reference "See also Humerus; Radius; Ulna" points to those main terms if the entry is not located under *Elbow* (see Figure 5.1).

To save space, some connecting words are left out and must be assumed by the reader. For example:

Ear Cartilage
Graft
to face 21235

should be read "graft of ear cartilage to face." The reader supplies the word *of*.

The Main Text

After the index is used to point to a possible code, the main text is read to verify the selection of the code (see Figure 5.2).

Each of the six sections of the main text lists procedure codes and descriptions under subsection headings. These headings group procedures or services, such as Therapeutic or Diagnostic Injections or Psychoanalysis; body systems, such as Digestive System; anatomical sites, such as Abdomen; and tests and examinations, such as Complete Blood Count (CBC). Following these headings

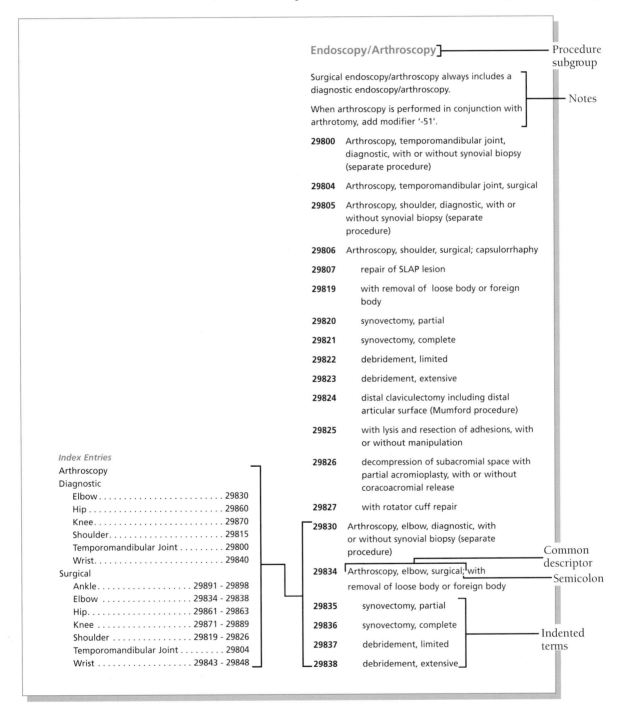

Figure 5.2 Example of Code Listings from the Musculoskeletal System Subsection of the Surgery Section

are additional subgroups of procedures, systems, or sites. For example, Figure 5.2 illustrates the following structure, in which the body system appears as the subsection followed by a procedure subgroup:

> **Surgery Section** <*The Section*>
>> **Musculoskeletal System** <*The Subsection*>
>>> **Endoscopy/Arthroscopy** <*The Procedure Subgroup*>

The section, subsection, and code number range on a page are shown at the top of the page, making it easier to locate a code.

Coding Point

Correct Coding Procedure
A code is never selected on the basis of only the index entry, because often the main text contains additional entries and important guidelines.

Guidelines

Each section begins with **section guidelines** for the use of its codes. The guidelines cover definitions and items unique to the section. They also include special notes about the structure of the section or the rules for its use. The guidelines must be carefully studied and followed in order to correctly use the codes in the section. Some notes apply only to specific subsections. The guidelines list the subsections in which these notes occur, and the notes themselves begin that subsection (see Figure 5.2).

Unlisted Procedures

Most sections' guidelines give codes for **unlisted procedures**—those not completely described by any code in the section. For example, in the Evaluation and Management section, two unlisted codes are provided:

99429 Unlisted preventive medicine service
99499 Unlisted evaluation and management service

Unlisted procedure codes are used for new services or procedures that have not yet been assigned codes in CPT. When these codes are used, which is rare, a written explanation of the procedure or service is needed.

Category II and Category III Codes

The main codes in CPT are called Category I codes, but in common usage are referred to just as CPT codes. There are two other types of CPT codes, Category II and Category III.

Category II codes are used to track performance measures for a medical goal such as reducing tobacco use. These codes are optional and are not part of reimbursement. They help in the development of best practice care and improve documentation. These codes have an alphabetic character for the fifth digit:

0002F Tobacco use, smoking, assessed
0004F Tobacco use cessation intervention, counseling

Category III codes are temporary codes for emerging technology, services, and procedures. If a Category III code exists for a service, it must be used, rather than an unlisted code. These codes also have an alphabetic character for the fifth digit:

0001T Endovascular repair of infrarenal abdominal aortic aneurysm or dissection
0041T Urinalysis infectious agent detection

A temporary code may become permanent and part of the regular codes if the service it identifies proves effective and is widely performed.

New codes are released annually on the American Medical Association Web site and published yearly in the CPT reference.

Special Reports

Some section guidelines suggest the use of **special reports** for rare or new procedures, especially unlisted procedures. These reports, which should be considered mandatory, permit the assessment of the medical appropriateness of the procedure, since it is not considered well-established medical practice. The guidelines cover the information that should be in the report, such as a description of the nature, extent, and need for the procedure, plus additional notes on the symptoms or findings.

Format

Semicolons and Indentions

To conserve space, CPT uses a semicolon and indentions when a common part of a main entry applies to all the indented entries that follow. For example, in the entries listed below, the procedure partial laryngectomy (hemilaryngectomy) is the common descriptor. It applies to the four unique descriptors after the semicolon—horizontal, laterovertical, anterovertical, and antero-latero-vertical. Note that the common descriptor begins with a capital letter, but the unique descriptors after the semicolon do not.

31370	Partial laryngectomy (hemilaryngectomy); horizontal
31375	laterovertical
31380	anterovertical
31382	antero-latero-vertical

This method shows the relationships among the entries without repeating the common word or words. Follow this case example in Figure 5.2:

Index Entry: Arthroscopy, Surgical 29834–29838
Main Text: 29838   Arthroscopy, elbow, surgical; with debridement, extensive

Cross-References

Some codes and descriptors are followed by indented *see* or *use* entries in parentheses, which point to other codes. For example:

82239 Bile acids; total
82240   cholylglycine
(For bile pigments, urine, see 81000–81005)

Examples

Descriptors often contain clarifying examples in parentheses, sometimes with the abbreviation *e.g.* (meaning for example). These provide further descriptions, such as synonyms or examples, but they are not essential to the selection of the code. Here are examples:

87040 Culture, bacterial; blood, with isolation and presumptive identification of isolates (includes anaerobic culture, if appropriate)
50400 Pyeloplasty (Foley Y-pyeloplasty), plastic operation on renal pelvis, with or without plastic operation on ureter, nephropexy, nephrostomy, pyelostomy, or ureteral splinting; simple

50405 complicated (congenital kidney abnormality, secondary pyelosplasty, solitary kidney, calycoplasty)

Symbols for Changed Codes

These symbols have the following meanings when they appear next to CPT codes:

- ● A bullet (a black circle) indicates a new procedure code. The symbol appears next to the code only the year that it is added.
- ▲ A triangle indicates that the code's descriptor has changed. It, too, appears in only the year the descriptor is revised.
- ►◄ Facing triangles (two triangles that face each other) enclose new or revised text other than the code's descriptor.

Symbol for Add-On Codes

A plus sign (+) next to a code in the main text indicates an **add-on code**. Add-on codes describe **secondary procedures** that are commonly carried out in addition to a **primary procedure**. Add-on codes usually use phrases such as *each additional* or *list separately in addition to the primary procedure* to show that they are never used as stand-alone codes. For example, the add-on code +15001 is used after the code for surgical preparation of a free skin graft site (15000) to provide a specific percentage or dimension of body area that was involved beyond the amount covered in the primary procedure.

Thinking It Through—5.2

1. Find the following codes in the index of CPT. Underline the key term you used to find the code.

    A. Intracapsular lens extraction

    B. Coombs test

    C. X-ray of duodenum

    D. Unlisted procedure, maxillofacial prosthetics

    E. DTAP immunization

2. Identify the symbol used to indicate a new procedure code, and list five new codes that appear in CPT.

3. Identify the symbol used to indicate a procedure that is usually done in addition to a primary procedure. Locate code 92981, and describe the unit of measure that is involved with this add-on code.

4. Identify the symbol that indicates that the code's description has been changed, and list five examples of codes with new or revised descriptors that appear in CPT.

5. Identify the symbols that enclose new or revised text other than the code's descriptor, and list five examples of codes with new or revised text that appear in CPT.

CPT Modifiers

A CPT **modifier** is a two-digit number that may be attached to most five-digit procedure codes (see Table 5.1). Modifiers are used to communicate special circumstances involved with a procedure that has been performed. A modifier

TABLE 5.1	CPT Modifiers: Description and Common Use in Main Text Sections						
Code	Description	E/M	Anesthesia	Surgery	Radiology	Pathology	Medicine
−21	Prolonged E/M Service	Yes	Never	Never	Never	Never	Never
−22	Unusual Procedural Service	Never	Yes	Yes	Yes	Yes	Yes
−23	Unusual Anesthesia	Never	Yes				Never
−24	Unrelated E/M Service by the Same Physician During a Postoperative Period	Yes	Never	Never	Never	Never	Never
−25	Significant, Separately Identifiable E/M Service by the Same Physician on the Same Day of the Procedure or Other Service	Yes	Never	Never	Never	Never	Never
−26	Professional Component	—	—	Yes	Yes	Yes	Yes
−32	Mandated Services	Yes	Yes	Yes	Yes	Yes	Yes
−47	Anesthesia by Surgeon	Never	Never	Yes	Never	Never	Never
−50	Bilateral Procedure	—	—	Yes	—	—	—
−51	Multiple Procedures	—	Yes	Yes	Yes	Never	Yes
−52	Reduced Services	Yes	—	Yes	Yes	Yes	Yes
−53	Discontinued Procedure	Never	Yes	Yes	Yes	Yes	Yes
−54	Surgical Care Only	—	—	Yes	—	—	—
−55	Postoperative Management Only	—	—	Yes	—	—	Yes
−56	Preoperative Management Only	—	—	Yes	—	—	Yes
−57	Decision for Surgery	Yes	—	—	—	—	Yes
−58	Staged or Related Procedure/Service by the Same Physician During the Postoperative Period	—	—	Yes	Yes	—	Yes
−59	Distinct Procedural Service	—	Yes	Yes	Yes	Yes	Yes
−62	Two Surgeons	Never	Never	Yes	Yes	Never	—
−63	Procedure Performed on Infants	—	—	Yes	Yes	—	Yes
−66	Surgical Team	Never	Never	Yes	Yes	Never	—
−76	Repeat Procedure by Same Physician	—	—	Yes	Yes	—	Yes
−77	Repeat Procedure by Another Physician	—	—	Yes	Yes	—	Yes
−78	Return to the Operating Room for a Related Procedure During the Postoperative Period	—	—	Yes	Yes	—	Yes
−79	Unrelated Procedure/Service by the Same Physician During the Postoperative Period	—	—	Yes	Yes	—	Yes
−80	Assistant Surgeon	Never	—	Yes	Yes	—	—
−81	Minimum Assistant Surgeon	Never	—	Yes	—	—	—
−82	Assistant Surgeon (when qualified resident surgeon not available)	Never	—	Yes	—	—	—
−90	Reference (Outside) Laboratory	—	—	Yes	Yes	Yes	Yes
−91	Repeat Clinical Diagnostic Laboratory Test	—	—	Yes	Yes	Yes	Yes
−99	Multiple Modifiers	—	—	Yes	Yes	—	Yes

Source: CPT 2004

Key:

Yes = commonly used

— = not usually used with the codes in that section

Never = not used with the codes in that section

indicates to private and government payers that the physician considers the procedure to have been altered in some way. A modifier usually affects the normal level of reimbursement for the code to which it is attached.

For example, the modifier –76, Repeat Procedure by Same Physician, is used when the reporting physician repeats a procedure or service after doing the first one. A situation requiring this modifier to show the extra procedure might be:

Procedural Statement: Physician performed a chest X-ray before placing a chest tube and then, after the chest tube was placed, performed a second chest X-ray to verify its position.

Code: 71020–76   Radiologic examination, chest, two views, frontal and lateral; repeat procedure or service by same physician

The modifiers are listed in Appendix A of CPT. However, not all modifiers are available for use with every section's codes:

- Some modifiers apply only to certain sections. For example, the modifier –21, Prolonged Evaluation and Management Services, is used only with codes that are located in the Evaluation and Management section, as its descriptor implies.
- Add-on codes cannot be modified with –51, Multiple Procedures, because the add-on code is used to add increments to a primary procedure, so the need for multiple procedures is replaced by procedures added on.
- Codes that begin with a circle containing a backslash (⊘) also cannot be modified with –51, "Multiple Procedures."

Modifiers

The use of a modifier indicates that the procedure was different from the listed descriptor, but not in a way that changed the definition or required a different code. Modifiers are used mainly when

- A procedure has two parts—a **technical component** performed by a technician, such as a radiologist, and a **professional component** that the physician performed, usually the interpretation and reporting of the results
- A service or procedure was performed more than once, by more than one physician, and/or in more than one location
- A service or procedure has been increased or reduced
- Only part of a procedure was done
- A bilateral or multiple procedure was performed
- Unusual difficulties occurred during the procedure

Reporting Modifiers

Modifiers are shown by adding a hyphen and the two-digit code to the CPT code. For example, a physician providing therapeutic radiology services in a hospital would report the modifier –26, Professional Component, as follows:

73090-26

This format means professional component only for an X-ray of the forearm. (In effect, it means that the physician who performed the service did not own the equipment used, so the fee is "split" between the physician and the equipment owner.)

Two or more modifiers may be used with one code to give the most accurate description possible. The use of two or more modifiers is shown by reporting –99, Multiple Modifiers, followed by the other modifiers listed with the most essential modifier first.

Procedures: Multitrauma patient's extremely difficult surgery after a car accident; team surgery by orthopedic surgeon and neurosurgeon. The first surgical procedure carries these modifiers:

Modifiers   27236–99, –66, –51, –22

The Appendixes

The five appendixes contain information helpful to the coding process:

1. *Appendix A—Modifiers:* A complete listing of all modifiers with descriptions and, in some cases, examples of usage
2. *Appendix B—Summary of Additions, Deletions, and Revisions:* A summary of the codes added, revised, and deleted in the current version
3. *Appendix C—Clinical Examples:* Case examples of the proper use of the codes in the Evaluation and Management section
4. *Appendix D—Summary of Add-on Codes:* List of supplemental codes used for procedures that are commonly done in addition to the primary procedure
5. *Appendix E—Summary of Codes Exempt from Modifier -51:* Codes to which the modifier showing multiple procedures cannot be attached because they already include a multiple descriptor

Coding Steps

The correct process for reporting accurate procedure codes has three steps. This process applies to the six sections of CPT, as will be discussed in the following sections.

Step 1 Determine the Procedures and Services to Report

The first step is to review the documentation of the patient's visit and decide which procedures and/or services were performed. Then, based on knowledge of the CPT and of the payer's policies, a decision is made about which services can be charged and are to be reported.

Step 2 Identify the Correct Codes

The process for selecting correct codes is as follows:

1. The index is used to locate the main term for each procedure or service. If the term is not found, the organ or body site is looked up, and then the disease or injury. Further checking can be done to locate any synonyms, eponyms, or abbreviations associated with the main term. The entries under the main term are reviewed to see if any apply, and cross-references are checked.
2. If the main term cannot be located in the index, the medical insurance specialist reviews the main term selection with the physician for clarification. In some cases, there is a better or more common term that can be used.
3. The main text listing, including all section guidelines and notes for the particular subsection, is carefully reviewed to make the final code choice.

1. In the CPT, what is the meaning of the symbol in front of code 93501?

2. Based on Appendix A of CPT, what modifiers would you assign in each of the following cases? Why?

CASE 1

Patient has recurrent cancer; surgeon performed a colectomy, which took forty-five minutes longer than the normal procedure due to dense adhesions from the patient's previous surgery.

CASE 2

Surgeon operating on an ingrown toenail administers a regional nerve block.

CASE 3

Patient was scheduled for a total diagnostic colonoscopy, but the patient went into respiratory distress during procedure; surgeon stopped the procedure.

CASE 4

Puncture aspiration of a cyst in the left breast and a cyst in the right breast.

CASE 5

A neurological surgeon and an orthopedic surgeon worked as cosurgeons.

Items that cannot be billed separately because they are covered under another, broader code are eliminated.

4. The codes to be reported for each day's services are ranked in order of highest to lowest rate of reimbursement. The actual order in which they were performed on a particular day is not important. When reporting, the earliest date of service is listed first, followed by subsequent dates of service. For example:

Date	Procedure	Charge
11/17/2006	99204	$202
11/20/2006	43215	$355
11/20/2006	74235	$75

Step 3 Determine the Need for Modifiers

The circumstances involved with the procedure or service may require the use of modifiers. The patient's diagnosis may affect this determination.

Evaluation and Management Codes

The codes in the Evaluation and Management section (**E/M codes**) cover physicians' services that are performed to determine the best course for patient care. The E/M codes are listed first in CPT because they are used so frequently by all types of physicians. Often called the cognitive codes, the E/M codes cover the complex process physicians use to gather and analyze information about a patient's illness and make decisions about the patient's condition and the best treatment or course of management. The actual treatments—such as surgical procedures and injections—are covered in the CPT sections that follow the E/M codes, such as the Anesthesia and Surgery sections.

Although the CPT was first published in 1966, the Evaluation and Management section was introduced much later, in 1992. The E/M coding method came from a joint effort by CMS and the AMA to define ranges of services from simple to very complicated. Patients' conditions require different levels of information gathering, analysis, and decision making by physicians. For example, on the low end of a range might be a patient with a mild case of poison ivy. On the opposite end is a patient with a life-threatening condition. The E/M codes reflect these different levels. There are five codes for an office visit with a new patient, for example, and another five that represent an office visit with established patients. A financial value (fee or prospective payment) is assigned by payers to each code in a range. To justify the use of a higher-level code in the range—one that is tied to a higher value—physicians must perform and document specific clinical facts about patient encounters.

Structure

Most codes in the E/M section are organized by the place of service. A few (for example, consultations) are grouped by type of service. The subsections are as follows:

Office or Other Outpatient Services
Hospital Observation Services
Hospital Inpatient Services
Consultations
Emergency Department Services
Pediatric Critical Care Patient Transport
Critical Care Services
Neonatal and Pediatric Critical Care Services
Pediatric Critical Care
Neonatal Critical Care
Intensive (Non-Critical) Low Birth Weight Service
Nursing Facility Services
Domiciliary, Rest Home, or Custodial Care Services
Home Services
Prolonged Services
Case Management Services
Care Plan Oversight Services
Preventive Medicine Services
Newborn Care
Special/Other E/M Services

New and Established Patients

Many subsections of E/M codes assign different code ranges for new patients and established patients. A new patient has not received any professional services from the physician (or from another physician of the same specialty in the same group practice) within the past three years. An established patient has received professional services under those conditions (see Chapter 3). The distinction is

Billing Tip

New and Established Patients
Some payers have special rules for deciding on the patient's status when the specialty group has subspecialties (for example, a hand surgeon in a surgery practice). Medical insurance specialists need to be familiar with the guidelines for new and established patients of the practice's payers.

important because new patients typically require more effort by the physician and practice staff and should therefore be rated at a higher value.

The term *any professional services* in the definitions of new and established patients means that if a patient had a face-to-face encounter with a physician, the established category is used. The same rule applies to a patient of a physician who moves to another group practice. If the patient then sees the physician (or another of the same specialty) in the new practice, the patient is established. In other words, the patient is new to the practice, but established to the provider. Figure 5.3 presents a decision tree for determining the patient's status.

Consultations

To understand the subsection of E/M codes on consultations requires a review of the difference between a consultation and a referral in coding terminology. A **consultation** occurs when a second physician, at the request of the patient's physician (the attending or treating physician), examines the patient. The second physician usually focuses on a particular issue and reports a written opinion to the first physician. The physician providing a consultation may perform

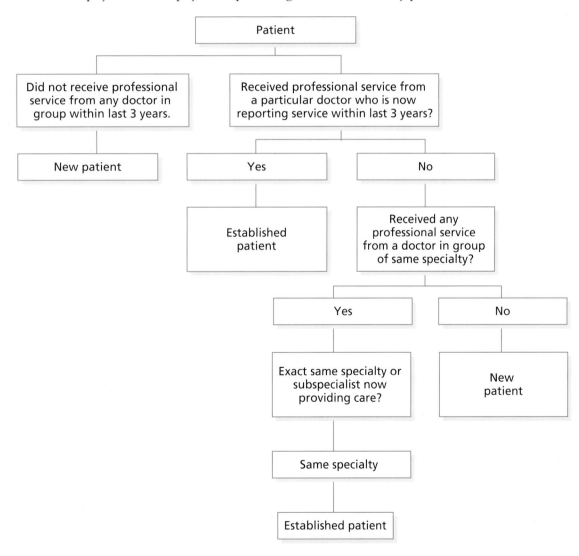

Figure 5.3 Decision Tree for New versus Established Patients

a service for the patient, but does not independently start a full course of treatment (although the consulting physician may recommend one) or take charge of the patient's care. Consultations require use of the E/M consultation codes (the range from 99241 to 99275).

On the other hand, when the patient is given a referral, either the total care or a specific portion of care is transferred to another physician (see Chapter 3). The patient becomes a new patient of that doctor and may not return to the care of the referring physician until the completion of a course of treatment. Referrals require use of the regular office visit E/M service codes.

Modifiers

A number of modifiers are commonly used to indicate special circumstances involved with evaluation and management services.

–21 *Prolonged Evaluation and Management service:* Used when the services are greater than the highest level described for the code range.

–24 *Unrelated Evaluation and Management service by the same physician during a postoperative period:* Used when an E/M service that is not related to the reason for the surgery is provided within the postoperative time period included in the payer's reimbursement.

–25 *Significant, separately identifiable Evaluation and Management service by the same physician on the same day of the procedure or other service:* Used when the physician provides an E/M service in addition to another E/M service or a procedure on the same day. The E/M service to which the modifier is appended must be significant enough to report.

–32 *Mandated services:* Used when the procedure is required by a payer.

–52 *Reduced services:* Used when an E/M service is less extensive than the descriptor indicates.

–57 *Decision for surgery:* Used to indicate the visit where the decision for surgery was made and the patient was counseled about risks and outcomes.

E/M Code Selection

To select the correct E/M code, eight steps are followed (see Figure 5.4).

Step 1 Determine the Category and Subcategory of Service Based on the Location of Service and the Patient's Status

The list of E/M categories, such as office visits, hospital services, and preventive medicine services, is used to locate the appropriate place or type of service in the index. In the main text of the selected category, the subcategory—such as new or established patient—is then chosen.

> **Documentation:** initial hospital visit to established patient
> **Index:** Hospital Services, Inpatient Services, Initial Care, New or
>   Established Patient
> **Code Ranges:** 99221-99223

For most types of service, such as initial hospital care for an established patient, between three and five codes are listed. To select an appropriate code from this range, three key components are considered: (1) the history the physician documented, (2) the examination that was documented, and (3) the medical decisions the physician documented. (The exception to this guideline is selecting a code for counseling or coordination of care, where the

```
STEP 1   Determine the category and subcategory of service based
         on the location of service and the patient's status

STEP 2   Determine the extent of the history that is documented

STEP 3   Determine the extent of the examination that is documented

STEP 4   Determine the complexity of medical decision making that is
         documented

STEP 5   Analyze the requirements to report the service level

STEP 6   Verify the service level based on the nature of the presenting
         problem, time, counseling, and care coordination

STEP 7   Verify that the documentation is complete

STEP 8   Assign the code
```

Figure 5.4 Selecting an Evaluation and Management Code

amount of time the physician spends may be the only key component in some situations.)

Step 2 Determine the Extent of the History That Is Documented

History is the information the physician received by questioning the patient about the chief complaint and other signs or symptoms, about all or selected body systems, and about pertinent past history, family background, and other personal factors. If the patient is incapacitated, the history may be taken from a family member.

The history is documented in the patient medical record as follows:

- *History of present illness (HPI):* The history of the illness is a description of the development of the illness from the first sign or symptom that the patient experienced to the present time. It includes everything related to the illness or condition, such as the severity, location, and timing of pain, and other signs and symptoms.
- *Review of systems (ROS):* The review of systems is an inventory of body systems. These systems are constitutional symptoms (such as fever or weight loss); eyes; ears, nose, mouth, and throat; cardiovascular (CV); respiratory; gastrointestinal (GI); genitourinary (GU); musculoskeletal; integumentary; neurological; psychiatric; endocrine; hematologic/lymphatic; and allergic/immunologic.
- *Past medical history (PMH):* The past history of the patient's experiences with illnesses, injuries, and treatments contains data about other major illnesses and injuries, operations, and hospitalizations. It also covers current medications the patient is taking, allergies, immunization status, and diet.
- *Family history (FH):* The family history reviews the medical events in the patient's family. It includes the health status or cause of death of parents, brothers and sisters, and children; specific diseases that are related to the patient's

chief complaint or the patient's diagnosis; and the presence of any known hereditary diseases.

- *Social history (SH):* The facts gathered in the social history, which depend on the patient's age, include marital status, employment, and other factors.

The histories documented after the HPI are sometimes referred to as PFSH, for past, family, and social history.

The history that the physician decides to obtain is categorized as one of four types on a scale from lesser to greater extent:

1. *Problem-focused:* Determining the patient's chief complaint and obtaining a brief history of the present illness
2. *Expanded problem-focused:* Determining the patient's chief complaint and obtaining a brief history of the present illness, plus a problem-pertinent system review of the particular body system that is involved
3. *Detailed:* Determining the chief complaint; obtaining an extended history of the present illness; reviewing both the problem-pertinent system and additional systems; and taking pertinent past, family, and/or social history
4. *Comprehensive:* Determining the chief complaint and taking an extended history of the present illness, a complete review of systems, and a complete past, family, and social history

Step 3 Determine the Extent of the Examination That Is Documented

The physician may examine a particular body area or organ system or may conduct a multisystem examination. The body areas are divided into the head and face; chest, including breasts and axilla; abdomen; genitalia, groin, and buttocks; back; and each extremity. The organ systems that may be examined are the eyes; the ears, nose, mouth, and throat; cardiovascular; respiratory; gastrointestinal; genitourinary; musculoskeletal; skin; neurologic; psychiatric; and hematologic/lymphatic/immunologic.

The examination that the physician decides to perform is categorized as one of four types on a scale from lesser to greater extent:

1. *Problem-focused:* A limited examination of the affected body area or system
2. *Expanded problem-focused:* A limited examination of the affected body area or system and other related areas
3. *Detailed:* An extended examination of the affected body area or system and other related areas
4. *Comprehensive:* A general multisystem examination or a complete examination of a single organ system

Step 4 Determine the Complexity of Medical Decision Making That Is Documented

The complexity of the medical decisions that the physician makes involves how many possible diagnoses or treatment options were considered; how much information (such as test results or previous records) was considered in analyzing the patient's problem; and how serious the illness is, meaning how much risk there is for significant complications, advanced illness, or death.

The decisions that the physician makes are categorized as one of four types on a scale from lesser to greater complexity:

1. *Straightforward:* Minimal diagnoses options, a minimal amount of data, and minimum risk

2. *Low complexity:* Limited diagnoses options, a low amount of data, and low risk
3. *Moderate complexity:* Multiple diagnoses options, a moderate amount of data, and moderate risk
4. *High complexity:* Extensive diagnoses options, an extensive amount of data, and high risk

Step 5 Analyze the Requirements to Report the Service Level

The descriptor for each E/M code explains the standards for its use. For office visits and most other services to new patients, and for initial care visits, all three of the key component requirements must be met. This is stated as follows:

99203 Office or other outpatient visit for the evaluation and management of a new patient, which require these three key components:

- a detailed history
- a detailed examination
- medical decision making of low complexity

For most services for established patients and for subsequent care visits, two out of three of the key component requirements must be met. For example:

99232 Subsequent hospital care, per day, for the evaluation and management of a patient, which requires at least two of these three key components:

- an expanded problem-focused interval history
- an expanded problem-focused examination
- medical decision making of moderate complexity

Step 6 Verify the Service Level Based on the Nature of the Presenting Problem, Time, Counseling, and Care Coordination

Many descriptors mention two additional components: (1) how severe the patient's condition is, referred to as the nature of the presenting problem, and (2) how much time the physician typically spends directly treating the patient. These factors, while not the key components, help ensure that the correct service level is selected. For example, this statement appears after the 99214 code (office visit for the evaluation and management of an established patient):

> Usually, the presenting problem(s) are of moderate to high severity. Physicians typically spend 25 minutes face-to-face with the patient and/or family.

Counseling is a discussion with a patient regarding areas such as diagnostic results, instructions for follow-up treatment, and patient education. It is mentioned as a typical part of each E/M service in the descriptor, but it is not required to be documented as a key component. Coordination of care with other providers or agencies is also mentioned. When coordination of care is provided but the patient is not present, codes from the case management and care plan oversight services subsections are reported.

Step 7 Verify That the Documentation Is Complete

Meeting the requirements means that the documentation must contain the record of the physician's work. When an E/M code is assigned, the patient's medical record must contain the clinical details to support it. The history, examination, and

The Time Factor

When a patient's visit is predominantly about counseling and/or coordination of care regarding the symptoms or illness, the length of time the physician spends is the controlling factor. If over 50 percent of the visit is spent counseling or coordinating care, time is the main factor. If an established patient's visit is thirty minutes, for example, and twenty minutes are spent counseling, the E/M code is 99214.

medical decision making must be sufficiently documented so that the medical necessity and appropriateness of the service can be understood.

Step 8 Assign the Code

The code that has been selected is assigned. The need for any modifiers, based on the documentation of special circumstances, is also reviewed.

Reporting E/M Codes

Documentation Guidelines for Evaluation and Management

Two sets of guidelines for implementing evaluation and management codes have been published by CMS and the AMA, the 1995 Documentation Guidelines for Evaluation and Management Services and a 1997 version. A new set of guidelines is currently under review. While this process goes on, CMS permits providers to use either the 1995 or the 1997 E/M guidelines.

Office and Hospital Services

Office and other outpatient services are the most often reported E/M services. A patient is an **outpatient** unless admitted to a health care facility, such as a hospital or nursing home, for a twenty-four-hour period or longer.

- When a patient is evaluated and then admitted to a health care facility, the service is reported using the codes for initial hospital care (the range 99221–99223).
- The admitting physician uses the initial hospital care services codes. Only one provider can report these services; other physicians involved in the patient's care, such as a surgeon or radiologist, use other E/M service codes or other codes from appropriate sections.

Confirmatory Consultations

Consultations requested by the patient or family members, not the attending physician, are called confirmatory consultations, and are reported using codes 99271 to 99275.

Emergency Department Services

An emergency department is one that is hospital-based and available to patients 24 hours a day. When emergency services are reported, whether the patient is new or established is not applicable. Time is not a factor in selecting the E/M service code. The code ranges are 99281 to 99288.

Preventive Medicine Services

Preventive medicine services are used to report routine physical examinations in the absence of a patient complaint. These codes, in the range 99381 to 99429, are divided according to the age of the patient. Immunizations and other services, such as lab tests that are normal parts of an annual physical, are reported using the appropriate codes from the Medicine and the Pathology and Laboratory sections (see pages 172–174).

Go to Coding Workbook

Codes 99201–99499
Evaluation and Management

Coding Point

Modifier –25
During a routine physical examination, an illness or clinical sign of a condition may be found that requires the physician to conduct an additional evaluation. In this case, the preventive medicine service code is reported first, followed by the appropriate E/M code for the new problem, adding the -25 modifier, Significant, Separate E/M Service.

1. In which category—problem-focused, expanded problem-focused, detailed, or comprehensive—would you place these statements concerning patient history? Why?

CASE 1

Patient seen for follow-up of persistent sinus problems including pain, stuffiness, and greenish drainage over the past twenty days. She continues to have left-sided pain in the forehead and maxillary areas and feels that her symptoms are worse around dust. She gets drainage into her throat, which causes her to cough. Review of systems reveals no history of diabetes or asthma. She has thyroid problems for which she takes Synthroid®.

CASE 2

Patient presents with a mild case of poison ivy on face and both hands contracted four days ago while gardening; has never been bothered by poison ivy before.

2. Using the office visit E/M codes, which code would you select for each of these cases?

CASE 1

Chart note for established patient:

S: Patient returns for removal of stitches I placed about seven days ago. Reports normal itching around the wound area, but no pain or swelling.

O: Wound at lateral aspect of the left eye looks well healed. Decision made to remove the 5-0 nylon sutures, which was done without difficulty.

A: Laceration, healed.

P: Patient advised to use vitamin E for scar prophylaxis.

CASE 2

Initial office evaluation by oncologist of a sixty-five-year-old female with sudden unexplained twenty-pound weight loss. Comprehensive history and examination performed.

CASE 3

Office visit by established patient for regularly scheduled blood test to monitor long-term effects of Coumadin; nurse spends five minutes, reviews the test, confirms that the patient is feeling well, and states that no change in the dosage is necessary.

Anesthesia Codes

The codes in the Anesthesia section are used to report anesthesia services performed or supervised by a physician. These services include general and regional anesthesia, as well as supplementation of local anesthesia. The main anesthesia codes are **bundled codes**, under which a group of related procedures are covered by a single code. These bundled codes include the usual services of an anesthesiologist:

- Usual preoperative visits for evaluation and planning
- Care during the procedure, such as administering fluid or blood, placing monitoring devices or IV lines, laryngoscopy, interpreting lab data, and nerve stimulation
- Routine postoperative care

Postoperative critical care and pain management requested by the surgeon are not routine and are not included in a bundled code. Such additional procedures done by an anesthesiologist can be reported.

Anesthesia codes are reimbursed according to time. The American Society of Anesthesiologists assigns a base unit value to each code. The anesthesiologist also records the amount of time spent with the patient during the procedure and adds this to the base value. Difficulties, such as a patient with severe systemic disease, also add to the value of the anesthesiologist's services.

Case Example

Anesthesiologist Report:
Initial meeting with seven-year-old patient in good health, determined good candidate for required general anesthesia for tonsillectomy. Surgical procedure conducted April 4, 2006; patient in the supine position; administered general anesthesia via endotracheal tube. Routine monitoring during procedure. Following successful removal of the right and left tonsils, the patient was awakened and taken to the recovery room in satisfactory condition.
00170-P1
Anesthesia for intraoral procedures, including biopsy; not otherwise specified

Structure

The Anesthesia section's subsections are organized by body site. Under each subsection, the codes are arranged by procedures. For example, under the heading *Neck*, codes for procedures performed on various parts of the neck (the integumentary system; the esophagus, thyroid, larynx, trachea; and lymphatic system; and the major vessels) are listed. The body-site subsections are followed by two subsections: (1) radiological procedures—that is, anesthesia services for patients receiving diagnostic or therapeutic radiology—and (2) other or unlisted procedures.

Modifiers

Two types of modifiers are used with anesthesia codes: (1) a modifier that describes the patient's health status and (2) the standard modifiers.

Physical Status Modifiers

Because the patient's health has a large effect on the level of difficulty of anesthesia services, anesthesia codes must be assigned a **physical status modifier**. This modifier is added to the code. The patient's physical status is selected from this list:

P1 Normal, healthy patient
P2 Patient with mild systemic disease
P3 Patient with severe systemic disease
P4 Patient with severe systemic disease that is a constant threat to life
P5 Moribund patient who is not expected to survive without the operation
P6 Declared brain-dead patient whose organs are being removed for donation purposes

For example:

00320-P3 Anesthesia services provided to patient with severe diabetes for procedure on larynx

Modifiers

The following standard modifiers are also commonly used with anesthesia codes:

-22 *Unusual procedural service:* Used with rare, unusual, or variable anesthesia services.

-23 *Unusual anesthesia service:* Used when the procedure normally requires either no anesthesia or local anesthesia but, because of unusual circumstances, general anesthesia is administered.

-32 *Mandated service:* Used when the procedure is required by a payer. For example, a PPO may require an independent evaluation of a patient before procedures are performed.

-51 *Multiple procedures:* Used to identify a second procedure or multiple procedures during the same operation.

-53 *Discontinued:* Used when the procedure is canceled after induction of anesthesia but before the incision is made. If the surgery is canceled after the evaluation of the patient, an E/M code is used rather than this modifier.

-59 *Distinct procedural service:* Used for a different encounter or procedure for the same patient on the same day; also used to describe the requirement for critical care and nonroutine pain management.

Note that modifier -37, Anesthesia by Surgeon, is used only during surgical procedures, not for services performed by anesthesiologists or anesthetists or supervised by surgeons.

For example, an anesthesia code with both types of modifiers appears as:

00320-P3-53 Anesthesia services provided to patient with severe diabetes for procedure on larynx; procedure discontinued because patient experienced a sudden drop in blood pressure

Add-On Codes for Qualifying Circumstances

Four add-on codes are used to indicate that the administration of the anesthesia involved important circumstances that had an effect on how it was performed. As add-on codes, these do not stand alone, but always appear in addition to the primary procedure code. These four codes apply only to anesthesia and are described in the notes for the Anesthesia Section.

+**99100** Anesthesia for patient of extreme age (under one year or over age 70)

+**99116** Anesthesia complicated by utilization of total body hypothermia

+**99135** Anesthesia complicated by utilization of controlled hypotension

+**99140** Anesthesia complicated by specified emergency conditions

Reporting Anesthesia Codes

Anesthesia services for Medicare patients and most other patients are reported using codes from the Anesthesia section. However, medical insurance specialists

---

Billing Tip

Modifier –22
Many payers consider modifier –22 overused (abused). When it is used, the need for the increased service or procedure should be well documented.

Billing Tip

HCPCS Anesthesia Modifiers
Medicare uses additional modifiers for anesthesia services. Part of the HCPCS codes (see Table 5.3 on page 177), these modifiers help clarify special situations when Medicare patient services are reported. For example:
-AA is used when the anesthesiologist directly provides the anesthesia service, instead of directing an assistant anesthetist.

Codes 00100-01999
Anesthesia Section

should be aware that some private payers require anesthesia services to be reported by procedure codes from the Surgery section rather than by codes from the Anesthesia section. The anesthesia modifier is added to the procedure code.

Surgery Codes

The codes in the Surgery section are used for the many hundreds of surgical procedures performed by physicians. This is the largest procedure code section, with codes ranging from 10021 to 69990.

Surgical Package

Most surgical codes are bundled codes. They include:

- After the decision for surgery, one related E/M encounter on the date immediately before or on the date of the procedure
- The operation: preparing the patient for surgery, including injection of local/topical anesthesia (by the surgeon), and performing the operation, including normal additional procedures, such as debridement
- Typical postoperative follow-up care

The case example at the left shows how the procedural elements—the operation, the use of a local anesthetic, and postoperative care—are covered under a single code.

In the Surgery section, the grouping of related activities under a single procedure code is called a **surgical package** or **global surgery concept.** Government and private payers assign a fee to a surgical package code that reimburses all the services provided under it. The period of time that is covered for follow-up care is referred to as the **global period.** For example, the global period for flexor tendon repair may be set at fifteen days. After the global period ends, additional services that are provided can be reported separately for additional payment.

Two types of services are not included in surgical package codes. These services are reported separately and reimbursed in addition to the surgical package fee.

- Complications or recurrences that arise after therapeutic surgical procedures.
- Care for the condition for which a diagnostic surgical procedure is performed. Routine follow-up care included in the code refers only to care related to recovery from the diagnostic procedure itself, not the condition. For example, a diagnostic colonoscopy may be performed to examine a growth in the patient's colon. An office visit after the surgery to evaluate the patient for chemotherapy because the tumor is cancerous is billed separately, not with code 99024 for a postoperative follow-up visit included in global service.

Separate Procedures

Some procedural code descriptors in the Surgery section are followed by the words *separate procedure* in parentheses. **Separate procedure** means that the procedure is usually done as an integral part of a surgical package—usually a larger procedure—but in some situations, it is not. If a separate procedure is performed alone or along with other procedures but for a separate purpose, it may be reported separately. For example:

Case Example

Procedural Statement:
Procedure conducted two weeks ago in office to correct hallux valgus (bunions) on both feet; local nerve block administered, correction by simple exostectomy. Saw patient in office today for routine follow-up; complete healing.
Code: 28290-50
Bunion correction on both feet

42870 Excision or destruction lingual tonsil, any method (separate procedure)

Lingual tonsil excision is a separate procedure. It is usually a part of a routine tonsillectomy, and so cannot be reported separately when a tonsillectomy is performed. When it is done independently, however, this code can be reported.

Structure

Most of the Surgery section's subsections are organized by body system and then divided by body site. Procedures are grouped next under headings followed by specific procedures. For example:

Subsection:	DIGESTIVE SYSTEM
Site:	Lips
Heading—type of procedure:	Excision
Description—specific procedure:	**40490** Biopsy of lip

The exceptions to the usual subsection structure are the Laparoscopy/Hysteroscopy subsection, which groups those operative procedures, and the Maternity Care and Delivery subsection, organized by type of service, such as postpartum care.

Modifiers

A number of modifiers are commonly used to indicate special circumstances involved with surgical procedures.

–22 *Unusual procedural service:* Used with rare, unusual, or variable surgery services; requires documentation.

–26 *Professional component:* Used to report the professional components when a procedure has both professional and technical components.

–32 *Mandated service:* Used when the procedure is required by a payer or governmental, legislative, or regulatory requirement.

–47 *Anesthesia by surgeon:* Used when the surgeon (rather than an anesthesiologist) administers regional or general anesthesia (local/topical anesthesia is bundled in the surgical code).

–50 *Bilateral procedure:* Used to indicate that identical bilateral procedures were performed during the same operation, either through the same incision or on separate body parts, such as left and right bunion correction. Under the guidelines, attaching the bilateral modifier to the code for the first procedure indicates that the procedure was done bilaterally. For example, to report a puncture aspiration of one cyst in each breast:

19100–50 Puncture aspiration of cyst of breast

–51 *Multiple procedures:* Used to identify a second procedure or multiple procedures during the same operation. The additional procedures are the same type and done to the same body system. The modifier is attached to the second procedure code. For example, to report two procedures, a bunionectomy on the great toe and, in the same session, correction of a hammertoe on the fourth toe:

28290 Hallux valgus (bunions) correction
28285–51 Hammertoe operation, one

–52 *Reduced services:* Used to indicate a procedure that is less extensive than described. The modifier is attached to the procedure code. It is not used to identify a reduced or a discounted fee. Instead, usually, the normal fee is listed, and the payer determines the amount of the reduction.

–53 *Discontinued procedure:* Used when the procedure is discontinued due to circumstances that threaten the patient's well-being—for example, surgery discontinued because the patient went into shock during the operation.

–54 *Surgical care only:* Added to the surgery code when the surgeon performs only the surgery itself, without preoperative or postoperative services. The fee is reduced to reflect only that part of the surgical package.

–55 *Postoperative management only:* Added to the surgery code when the physician provides only the follow-up care in the global period after another physician has done the surgery. The fee is reduced to reflect only that part of the surgical package.

–56 *Preoperative management only:* Added to the surgery code when the physician provides only preoperative care. The fee is reduced to reflect only that part of the surgical package.

–58 *Staged or related procedure or service by the same physician during the postoperative period:* Used when the physician performs a postoperative procedure (1) as planned during the surgery to be done later, (2) that is more extensive than the original procedure, or (3) for therapy after diagnostic surgery.

–59 *Distinct procedural service:* Used for a different encounter or procedure for the same patient on the same day. Either a different patient encounter, an unrelated procedure, a different body site or system, or a separate incision or injury must be involved. It may also be used to describe the requirement for critical care and nonroutine pain management. If a separate procedure is performed with other procedures, the modifier -59 is added to the separate code to show that it is a distinct, independent procedure, not part of a surgical package.

–62 *Two surgeons:* Used when a specific surgical procedure requires two surgeons, usually of different specialties; each appends the modifier to the surgical code. Usually each surgeon performs a distinct part of the procedure and dictates a separate operative report. If each surgeon reports different surgical procedure codes, the modifier is not used.

–63 *Procedure performed on infants:* Used when the patient is under twenty-four months of age.

–66 *Surgical team:* Used in very complex procedures that usually require the simultaneous services of physicians of different specialties. Usually used only to report transplant-type procedures.

–76 *Repeat procedure by same physician:* Used when a physician repeats a procedure performed earlier.

–77 *Repeat procedure by another physician:* Used when a physician repeats a procedure done by another physician.

–78 *Return to the operating room for a related procedure during the postoperative period:* Used when the patient develops a complication during the postoperative period that requires an additional procedure by the same physician.

–79 *Unrelated procedure or service by the same physician during the postoperative period:* Used when a second, unrelated surgical procedure is performed by the same physician during the postoperative period.

–80 *Assistant surgeon:* Used when a physician assists another during a surgical procedure. Each physician reports the services using the same code, but the assistant surgeon appends the modifier to the code.

–81 *Minimum assistant surgeon:* Used when an assistant surgeon assists another during only part of a surgical procedure.

–82 *Assistant surgeon (when qualified resident surgeon not available):* Used in teaching hospitals where residents usually assist with surgery but none was available during the reported procedure, so a surgeon performed the assistant's work.

–90 *Reference (outside) laboratory:* Used when laboratory procedures are done by someone other than the reporting physician.

–91 *Repeat clinical diagnostic laboratory test:* Used when laboratory procedures are repeated.

–99 *Multiple modifiers:* Used when more than one modifier is required; the –99 modifier is appended to the basic procedure, followed by the other modifiers in descending order.

Reporting Surgical Codes

Surgical package codes are assigned single fees. Reporting as a separate procedure anything that is included in the surgical package code is considered unbundling, or **fragmented billing**. This practice, as noted earlier, causes denied claims and may result in an audit.

Reporting Sequence

When payers reimburse multiple surgical procedures performed on the same day for the same patient, they pay the full amount of the first listed surgical procedure, but they often pay reduced percentages of the subsequent procedures. For maximum payment when multiple procedures are reported, the most complex or highest-level code—the procedure with the highest reimbursement value—should be listed first. The subsequent procedures are listed with the modifier -51 (indicating multiple procedures).

When warranted, to avoid reduced payment for multiple procedures, the modifier -59 is used to indicate distinct procedures rather than multiple

Thinking It Through—5.5

1. Rank the following codes in order from highest to lowest reimbursement level, and explain your rationale.

   44950–51
   44950–59
   44950-53

2. Compare and contrast the procedural areas that are commonly included in bundled anesthesia codes and global surgical packages. What is the chief difference?

procedures. This is usually done when the surgeon performs procedures on two different body sites or organ systems, such as the excision of a lesion on the chest as well as the incision and drainage (I & D) of an abscess on the leg.

Bilateral Modifier

The bilateral modifier (–50) is attached to unilateral procedures that are done bilaterally. However, there are a few codes that are defined as bilateral procedures. For example:

32853 Lung transplant, double (bilateral sequential or en bloc)

The trend in annual updates is to replace bilateral codes with unilateral codes to which the –50 modifier is attached if needed.

10021–69990
Surgery Section

Billing Tip

Professional Component Requirement
The professional component of a radiologic procedure requires a written interpretation from the physician. This documentation contains the patient's identifying information, the clinical indications for the procedure, the process followed, and the physician's impressions of the findings.

Radiology Codes

The codes in the Radiology section are used to report radiological services performed by or supervised by a physician. Radiology procedures have two parts:

1. *The technical component:* The technologist, the equipment, and processing, including preinjection and postinjection services such as local anesthesia, placement of needle or catheter, and injection of contrast material
2. *The professional component:* The reading of the radiological examination and the written report of interpretation by the physician

Radiology codes follow the same types of guidelines as noted in the Surgery section. For example, some radiology codes are identified as separate procedure codes. These codes are usually part of a larger, more complex procedure and should not be reported as separate codes unless the procedure was done independently. Also, some codes are add-on codes, such as those covering additional vessels that are studied after the basic examination. These codes are used with the primary codes, not alone.

Unlisted Procedures and Special Reports

New procedures are common in the area of radiology services. There are codes for nearly twenty unlisted code areas, such as:

78299 Unlisted gastrointestinal procedure, diagnostic nuclear medicine

When unlisted codes are reported, a special report must be attached that defines the nature, extent, and need for the procedure and describes the time, effort, and equipment necessary to provide it.

Contrast Material

For some radiological procedures, the physician decides whether it is best to perform the procedure with or without contrast material, a substance administered in the patient's blood vessels that helps highlight the area under study. For example, computerized tomography (CT) and magnetic resonance imaging (MRI) each provide different types of information about body parts and may be performed with or without contrast material. The term *with contrast* means

on Careers   Medical Coding Manager

The medical coding manager supervises a staff of medical coders in a medical group practice. In a large organization such as a hospital or managed care organization, the medical coding manager often manages health information technicians who coordinate the retrieval of and preparation of patients' records for the coding team as well as the coders.

Medical coding managers are responsible for the quality and the quantity of the coding work that is done. They must know the regulations imposed by governmental agencies and third-party payers and establish policies and procedures that ensure correct claim reporting. Duties include planning the staff's workload, assigning tasks and following up on completion, and reviewing progress. Excellent communication and human relations skills are also needed; medical coding managers motivate their staff, provide feedback on each person's work, and recommend promotions and salary increases. Managers also educate physicians and other staff members about coding principles, medical record documentation guidelines, and compliance requirements, and keep forms current with annual changes in diagnosis and procedure codes.

Successful experience as a medical coder and continuing education in the medical coding/billing field are required for a medical coding manager position. Additional college education in supervision may also be a plus.

only contrast materials given in the patient's veins or arteries. Contrast materials administered orally or rectally are coded as without contrast.

Structure and Modifiers

The diagnostic radiology, diagnostic ultrasound, and nuclear medicine subsections of the Radiology section are structured by type of procedure, followed by body sites and then specific procedures. For example:

Type: Diagnostic Ultrasound
Body site: Chest
Procedure: Echography, chest, B-scan and/or real time with image documentation

The radiation oncology subsection is organized somewhat differently. The first group of codes covers the planning services oncologists perform to set up a patient's radiation therapy treatment for cancer.

The following modifiers are commonly used in the Radiology section: –22, –26, –32, –51, –52, –53, –58, –59, –62, –66, –76, –77, –78, –79, –80, –90, and –99. Table 5.1 on page 152 has a brief description of each modifier.

> **Coding Point**
>
> **Modifier –26**
> If the physician does not own the equipment used for the radiology procedure, the modifier –26 is appended to the code, such as 76511–26 Ophthalmic biometry by ultrasound echography, A-Scan

Reporting Radiology Codes

Most radiology services are performed and billed by radiologists working in hospital or clinic settings. Medical practices usually do not have radiology equipment and instead refer patients to these specialists. In many cases, the radiologist performs both the technical and the professional components.

Codes 70010–79999
Radiology Section

Pathology and Laboratory Codes

The codes in the Pathology and Laboratory section cover services provided by physicians or by technicians under the supervision of physicians. A complete procedure includes:

- Ordering the test
- Taking and handling the sample
- Performing the actual test
- Analyzing and reporting on the test results.

Panels

Certain tests are customarily ordered together to detect particular diseases or malfunctioning organs. These related tests are grouped under laboratory **panels**. When a panel code is reported, all the listed tests must have been performed. For example, the electrolyte panel requires these tests:

80051 Electrolyte panel
This panel must include the following:
Carbon dioxide (82374)
Chloride (82435)
Potassium (84132)
Sodium (84295)

Panels are considered bundled codes, so that if a panel code is reported, no individual test within it may be additionally reported. Other tests outside that panel may be reported if performed.

Unlisted Procedures and Special Reports

New developments are frequent in pathology and laboratory services. There are codes for twelve unlisted code areas, such as:

86586 Unlisted antigen, each

Any unlisted code must be submitted with a special report that defines the nature, extent, and need for the procedure and describes the time, effort, and equipment necessary to provide it.

Structure and Modifiers

Procedures and services are listed in the Index under the following types of main terms:

- Name of the test, such as urinalysis, HIV, skin test
- Procedure, such as hormone assay
- Abbreviation, such as TLC screen
- Panel of tests, such as Complete Blood Count

The following modifiers are commonly used with pathology and laboratory codes: –22, –26, –32, –52, –53, –59, –90, and –91. Table 5.1 on page 152 has a brief description of each modifier.

Reporting Pathology and Laboratory Codes

Some medical practices have laboratory equipment and perform their own testing. In-office labs are guided by federal safety regulations from OSHA (the Occupational Safety and Health Administration), and the tests that can be performed are regulated by CLIA (the Clinical Laboratory Improvement Amendment of 1988). The CLIA certification program awards one of three levels of certification. The lowest-level in-office certified lab can perform common tests, such as dipstick urinalysis and urine pregnancy.

If the medical practice does not have an in-office lab, the physician may either take the specimen, reporting this service only (for example, using code 36415 for venipuncture to obtain a blood sample), and send it to an outside lab for processing or refer the patient to an outside lab for the complete procedure.

Codes 80048–89399 Pathology and Laboratory Section

Medicine Codes

The Medicine section contains the codes for the many types of evaluation, therapeutic, and diagnostic procedures that physicians perform. (Codes for the Evaluation and Management section described earlier in the chapter, 99201 to 99499, fall numerically at the end of this section, but they appear first in CPT because they are the most frequently used codes.) Medicine codes may be used for procedures and services done or supervised by a physician of any specialty. They include many procedures and services provided by family practice physicians, such as immunizations and injections. The services of many specialists, such as allergists, cardiologists, and psychiatrists are also covered in the Medicine section.

Codes from the Medicine section may be used with codes from any other section. Add-on codes and separate procedure codes are included in the Medicine section. Their use follows the guidelines described for previous sections. Unlisted procedure codes are provided for new procedures; a special report is required with unlisted codes.

Structure and Modifiers

The subsections are organized by type of service. Many subsections have notes containing usage guidelines and definitions. Some services, for example, have subcategories for new and established patients.

The following modifiers are commonly used with codes in the Medicine section: –22, –26, –32, –51, –52, –53, –55, –56, –57, –58, –59, –76, –77, –78, –79, –90, –91, and –99. Table 5.1 on page 152 has a brief description of each modifier.

Reporting Medicine Codes

- Some of the services in the Medicine section are considered Evaluation and Management services, even though they are not listed in the E/M section. For these codes, the -51 modifier, Multiple Procedures, may not be used. For example, if a physician makes a second, brief visit to a patient in the hospital and also provides psychoanalysis, these services are reported separately:

  99231 Subsequent hospital care, problem focused/straightforward or low complexity decision making
  90845 Pschoanalysis

- Immunizations require two codes, one for administering the immunization and the other for the particular vaccine or toxoid that is given. For example, when a patient receives a MMRV vaccine, these two codes are used:

  90471 Immunization administration

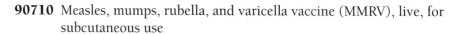

Immunizations and Office Visits
To report a patient's visit for just an immunization, some medical practices use E/M 99211 along with a code for the immunization. This is a misuse of the E/M code, which requires some significant, separate E/M service.

Based on:

1. If a test for ferritin and a comprehensive metabolic panel are both performed, can both be reported?

2. Is it correct to report a comprehensive metabolic panel and an electrolyte panel for the same patient on the same day?

3. Which of these codes, 93000, 93005, or 93010, is used to report the technical component only of a routine ECG? Defend your decision.

90710 Measles, mumps, rubella, and varicella vaccine (MMRV), live, for subcutaneous use

- The descriptors for injection codes also require two codes, one for the injection and one for the substance that is injected (the exception is allergy shots, which have their own codes in the Allergy and Clinical Immunology subsection). For example, to report the intravenous injection of erythromycin:

90784 Therapeutic or diagnostic injection of erythromycin lactobionate; intravenous

99070 Supplies and materials provided by the physician over and above those usually included in the office visit or other services rendered

Codes 90281–99600
Medicine Section

For a Medicare patient, an HCPCS code is used for the material that is injected, instead of the general code 99070.

HCPCS Codes

The Healthcare Common Procedure Coding System (HCPCS) is used to report procedures and services for Medicare patients (see Chapter 11). This system is also used to report most Medicaid services (see Chapter 12). HCPCS has two code levels, referred to as Level I and Level II.

Level I Current Procedural Terminology

Level I repeats the CPT's five-number codes for physician procedures and services. Examples are:

99212 Office or other outpatient visit
00730 Anesthesia for procedures on upper posterior abdominal wall
24006 Arthrotomy of the elbow, with capsular excision for capsular release
70100 Radiologic examination of the mandible
80400 ACTH stimulation panel; for adrenal insufficiency
93000 Electrocardiogram, routine ECG with at least 12 leads; with interpretation and report

Coding Point

Medicare Coding
For a Medicare patient, a HCPCS code from the J series of the Level II codes is used for the material that is injected, instead of the CPT code 99070 (supplies and materials provided by the physician). For example, the J code J1364 is used in place of the CPT code 99070 when the patient receives an injection of erythromycin lactobionate.

Level II National Codes

Level II is made up of more than 2,400 five-digit alphanumeric codes for items that are not listed in CPT. Most of these items are supplies, materials, or injections that are covered by Medicare (see Chapter 11). Some items are new services or procedures that are not covered in CPT.

Level II codes start with a letter followed by four digits, such as J7630. There are twenty-two sections, each covering a related group of items. For example, the E section covers the category of **durable medical equipment (DME)**, reusable medical equipment ordered by the physician for use in the home, such as walkers and wheelchairs. The sections and code ranges are shown in Table 5.2. Examples are:

A0428 Ambulance service; basic life support, nonemergency
E0112 Crutches, underarm, wood, adjustable or fixed; pair, with pads, tips and handgrip

J0120 Injection, tetracycline, up to 250 mg

HCPCS Modifiers

The two-letter modifiers that CMS developed for Medicare claims are useful indicators of other factors than those covered by CPT modifiers. For example, there are HCPCS modifiers for each finger and each toe. Because of their usefulness, many payers accept HCPCS modifiers in addition to CPT modifiers. The examples listed in Table 5.3 are among the most prevalent.

Billing Tip

Using HCPCS Modifiers
When HCPCS modifiers are accepted by a payer, medical insurance specialists apply them if they will better communicate the way the procedure was different from the typical descriptor.

Go to
Coding Workbook

Healthcare Common Procedure Coding System: Level II National Codes and Modifiers

TABLE 5.2   HCPCS Level II Code Sections, Ranges, and Examples

Section	Code Range	Example
Transportation services	A0000-A0999	A0300 Ambulance service; basic life support, nonemergency, all inclusive
Medical and surgical supplies	A4000-A7509	A4211 Supplies for self-administered injections
Miscellaneous and experimental	A9000-A9999	A9150 Nonprescription drugs
Enteral and parenteral therapy	B4000-B9999	B9000 Enteral nutrition infusion pump, without alarm
Temporary hospital Outpatient PPS	C0000-C9999	C1170 Biopsy device, breast, abbi device
Dental procedures	D0000-D9999	D0150 Comprehensive oral exam
Durable medical equipment (DME)	E0000-E9999	E0250 Hospital bed with side rails and mattress
Procedures and services, temporary	G0000-G9999	G0001 Routine venipuncture for collection of specimen(s)
Rehabilitative services	H0000-H9999	H0006 Alcohol and/or drug services; case management
Drugs administered other than oral method	J0000-J8999	J0120 Injection, tetracycline, up to 250 mg
Chemotherapy drugs	J9000-J9999	J9212 Injection, interferon alfacon-1, recombinant, 1 mcg
Temporary codes for DMERCS*	K0000-K9999	K0001 Standard wheelchair
Orthotic procedures	L0000-L4999	L1800 Knee orthosis (KO); elastic with stays
Prosthetic procedures	L5000-L9999	L5050 Ankle, symes; molded socket, SACH foot
Medical services	M0000-M9999	M0064 Brief office visit for the sole purpose of monitoring or changing drug prescriptions used to treat mental psychoneurotic and personality disorders
Pathology and laboratory	P0000-P9999	P3000 Screening papanicolaou smear, cervical or vaginal, up to 3; by technician under physician supervision
Temporary codes	Q0000-Q0099	Q0034 Administration of influenza vaccine to Medicare beneficiaries by participating demonstration sites
Diagnostic radiology services	R0000-R5999	R0070 Transportation of portable X-ray equipment and personnel to home or nursing home, per trip to facility or location; one patient seen
Private payer codes	S0000-S9999	S0187 Tamoxifen citrate, oral, 10 mg
State Medicaid Agency Codes	T0000-T9999	T1001 Nursing assessment/evaluation
Vision services	V0000-V2999	V2020 Frames, purchases
Hearing services	V5000-V5999	V5364 Dysphagia screening

Source: HCPCS 2004

*DMERC=Durable Medical Equipment Regional Carriers

Modifier	Description
–AA	Anesthesia services performed personally by anesthesiologist
–AB	Medical direction of own employee(s) by anesthesiologist (not more than four employees)
–AC	Medical direction of other than own employees by anesthesiologist (not more than four individuals)
–AG	Anesthesia for emergency surgery on a patient who is moribund or who has an incapacitating systemic disease that is a constant threat to life
–AH	Clinical psychologist
–AJ	Clinical social worker
–AM	Physician, team member service
–AS	Physician's assistant, nurse-practitioner, or clinical nurse specialist services for assistant at surgery
–BP	Beneficiary has been informed of the purchase/rental options; purchases the item
–BR	Beneficiary has been informed of the purchase/rental options; rents the item
–BU	Beneficiary has been informed of the purchase/rental options; has not informed supplier of decision after thirty days
–CC	Procedure change code (used to indicate a change in a submitted code)
–E1	Upper left, eyelid
–E2	Lower left, eyelid
–E3	Upper right, eyelid
–E4	Lower right, eyelid
–EJ	Subsequent claim for epoetin alfa-epo-injection claim
–FA	Left hand, thumb
–F1	Left hand, second digit
–F2	Left hand, third digit
–F3	Left hand, fourth digit
–F4	Left hand, fifth digit
–F5	Right hand, thumb
–F6	Right hand, second digit
–F7	Right hand, third digit
–F8	Right hand, fourth digit
–F9	Right hand, fifth digit
–GA	Waiver of liability statement on file
–GC	Service performed in part by resident under the direction of a teaching physician
–GX	Service not covered by Medicare
–LC	Left circumflex, coronary artery
–LD	Left anterior descending coronary artery
–RC	Right coronary artery
–LT	Left side (identifies procedures performed on the left side of the body)
–RT	Right side (identifies procedures performed on the right side of the body)
–QM	Ambulance service provided under arrangement by a provider of services
–QN	Ambulance service furnished directly by a provider of services
–QR	Repeat laboratory test performed on the same day
–TA	Left foot, great toe
–T1	Left foot, second digit
–T2	Left foot, third digit
–T3	Left foot, fourth digit
–T4	Left foot, fifth digit
–T5	Right foot, great toe
–T6	Right foot, second digit
–T7	Right foot, third digit
–T8	Right foot, fourth digit
–T9	Right foot, fifth digit
–TC	Technical component

Source: HCPCS 2004

Review

Chapter Summary

1. CPT, a publication of the American Medical Association, contains the most widely used system of codes for physicians' medical, diagnostic, and procedural services. CPT codes are required for reporting physician practice services on insurance claims and encounter forms. The codes have five digits and a description. Updated versions are released annually. Medical practices must use the current codes because they can affect billing and reimbursement.

2. CPT contains six sections of codes, Evaluation and Management, Anesthesia, Surgery, Radiology, Pathology and Laboratory, and Medicine, followed by the lists of Category II and Category III codes, five appendixes, and an index. The index is used first in the process of selecting a code; it contains alphabetic descriptive main terms and subterms for the procedures and services contained in the main text. The codes themselves are listed in the main text and are generally grouped by body system or site or by type of procedure.

3. Each coding section begins with section guidelines, which discuss definitions and rules for the use of codes, such as for unlisted codes, special reports, and notes for specific subsections. When a main entry has more than one code, a semicolon follows the common part of a descriptor in the main entry, and the unique descriptors that are related to the common description are indented below it. Five symbols are used in the main text: (a) ● (a bullet or black circle) indicates a new procedure code; (b) ▲ (a triangle) indicates that the code's descriptor has changed; (c) ▶◀ (facing triangles) enclose new or revised text other than the code's descriptor; (d) + (a plus sign) before a code indicates an add-on code that is used only along with other codes for primary procedures; and (e) a ⊘ indicates that the code cannot be modified with a -51 modifier.

4. A CPT modifier is a two-digit number that may be attached to most five-digit procedure codes to indicate that the procedure is different from the listed descriptor, but not in a way that changes the definition or requires a different code. Two or more modifiers may be used with one code to give the most accurate description possible.

5. The first step in selecting a procedure code is to determine the procedures and services to report by reviewing the documentation of the patient's visit. Next, after checking the coding system to use, CPT codes are located by finding the procedure in the index and verifying the code in the main text. The reporting order for the procedure codes places the code with the highest rate of reimbursement first. The final step is to determine whether modifiers are needed.

6. A summary of the six sections of codes appears on p. 179.

7. The key components for selecting Evaluation and Management codes are the extent of the history documented, the extent of the examination documented, and the complexity of the medical decision making. The steps for selecting correct E/M codes are to (a) determine the category and subcategory of service, (b) determine the extent of the history, (c) determine the extent of the examination, (d) determine the complexity of medical decision making, (e) analyze the requirements to report the service level, (f) verify the service level based on the nature of the presenting problem, time, counseling, and care coordination, (g) verify that the documentation is complete, and (h) assign the code.

8. HCPCS codes and modifiers are used primarily in the Medicare and Medicaid programs. There are two levels of codes. Level I repeats the codes in CPT. Level II, national codes, cover transportation, supplies, equipment, injections, and procedures not listed in CPT.

Section	Definition of Codes	Structure	Key Guidelines
Evaluation and Management	Physicians' services that are performed to determine the best course for patient care	Organized by place and/or type of service	New/established patients; other definitions Unlisted services, special reports Selecting an E/M service level
Anesthesia	Anesthesia services done by or supervised by a physician; includes general, regional, and local anesthesia	Organized by body site	Time-based Services covered (bundled) in codes Unlisted services/special reports Qualifying circumstances codes
Surgery	Surgical procedures performed by physicians	Organized by body system and then body site, followed by procedural groups	Surgical package definition Follow-up care definition Add-on codes Separate procedures Subsection notes Unlisted services/special reports Starred procedures
Radiology	Radiology services done by or supervised by a physician	Organized by type of procedure followed by body site	Unlisted services/special reports Supervision and interpretation (professional and technical components)
Pathology and Laboratory	Pathology and laboratory services done by physicians or by physician-supervised technicians	Organized by type of procedure	Complete procedure Panels Unlisted services/special reports
Medicine	Evaluation, therapeutic, and diagnostic procedures done or supervised by a physician	Organized by type of service or procedure	Subsection notes Multiple procedures reported separately Add-on codes Separate procedures Unlisted services/special reports

Key Terms

add-on code *page 151*

bundled code *page 164*

Category II codes *page 149*

Category III codes *page 149*

consultation *page 157*

Current Procedural Terminology (CPT) *page 144*

descriptor *page 144*

durable medical equipment (DME) *page 175*

E/M codes *page 155*

fragmented billing *page 169*

global period *page 166*

global surgery concept *page 166*

Healthcare Common Procedure Coding System (HCPCS) *page 144*

modifier *page 152*

outpatient *page 162*

panel *page 172*

physical status modifier *page 164*

primary procedure *page 151*

professional component *page 153*

secondary procedure *page 151*

section guidelines *page 149*

separate procedure *page 166*

special report *page 150*

surgical package *page 166*

technical component *page 153*

unbundling *page 164*

unlisted procedure *page 149*

Review Questions

Match the key terms in the left column with the definitions in the right column.

A. panel

B. professional component

C. separate procedure

D. Category III codes

E. global period

F. bundled code

G. Category II codes

_____ 1. The physician's skill, time, and expertise used in performing a procedure

_____ 2. Temporary codes for emerging technology, services, and procedures

_____ 3. Procedure code that groups related procedures under a single code

_____ 4. A service that is not listed in CPT and requires a special report

_____ 5. The inclusion of postoperative care for a specified period in the charges for a surgical procedure

H. add-on code

I. unlisted procedure

J. modifier

_____ 6. CPT codes that are used to track performance measurement.

_____ 7. In CPT, a single code that groups laboratory tests that are frequently done together

_____ 8. A procedure performed in addition to a primary procedure

_____ 9. A secondary procedure that is performed with a primary procedure and that is indicated in CPT by a plus sign (+) next to the code

_____ 10. A two-digit number indicating that special circumstances were involved with a procedure, such as a reduced service or a discontinued procedure

Decide whether each statement is true or false, and write T for true or F for false.

_____ 1. In selecting correct procedure codes, the main text sections are first searched, and the code is then verified in the index.

_____ 2. HCPCS Level I codes are made up of CPT codes.

_____ 3. In the CPT index, a *see* cross-reference must be followed.

_____ 4. The section guidelines summarize the unlisted codes for the section.

_____ 5. The phrases before the semicolon in a code descriptor define the unique entries; those after the semicolon are common.

_____ 6. Descriptive entries in parentheses are not essential to code selection.

_____ 7. Category III codes end in a letter.

_____ 8. Procedure codes are reported in order of increasing financial value for services performed on the same day.

_____ 9. For new patients, two of the three key factors that are listed must be met.

_____ 10. Because it is an evaluation of a patient, a consultation is coded using Evaluation and Management office services codes.

Write the letter of the choice that best completes the statement or answers the question.

_____ 1. A new patient has not received services from the physician or from another physician of the same specialty in the same group practice for
   A. ninety days   C. two years
   B. one year   D. three years

_____ 2. When a physician asks a patient questions to obtain an inventory of constitutional symptoms and of the various body systems, the results are documented as the
   A. past medical history   C. review of systems
   B. family history   D. comprehensive examination

_____ 3. The abbreviation PFSH stands for
   A. past, family, and/or social history
   B. patient, family, and/or systems history
   C. past, family, and systems history
   D. none of the above

_____ 4. The examination that the physician conducts is categorized as
   A. straightforward, low complexity, moderate complexity, or high complexity
   B. problem-focused, expanded problem-focused, detailed, or comprehensive

C. straightforward, problem-focused, detailed, or highly complex

D. low risk, moderate risk, or high risk

_____ 5. The three key factors in selecting an Evaluation and Management code are

A. time, severity of presenting problem, and history

B. history, examination, and time

C. past history, history of present illness, and chief complaint

D. history, examination, and medical decision making

_____ 6. CPT code 99382 is an example of

A. an emergency department service code

B. a preventive medicine service code

C. a consultation service code

D. a hospital observation code

_____ 7. Anesthesia codes generally include

A. preoperative evaluation and planning, normal care during the procedure, and routine care after the procedure

B. preparing the patient for the anesthetic, care during the procedure, postoperative care, and pain management as required by the surgeon

C. preoperative evaluation and planning, routine postoperative care, but not the administration of the anesthetic itself

D. all procedures that are ordered by the surgeon

_____ 8. Surgery codes generally include

A. all procedures done during the global period that comes before the surgery

B. preoperative evaluation and planning, the operation and normal additional procedures, and routine care after the procedure

C. all aspects of the operation, including preparing the patient for the surgery, performing the operation and normal additional procedures, as well as normal, uncomplicated follow-up

D. preoperative evaluation and planning, routine postoperative care, but not the operation itself

_____ 9. When a Surgery section code has a star next to it, the code descriptor covers

A. all procedures done during the global period that follows the surgery

B. preoperative evaluation and planning, the operation and normal additional procedures, and routine care after the procedure

C. the surgical procedure

D. preoperative evaluation and planning, routine postoperative care, but not the surgical procedure

_____ 10. When a panel code from the Pathology and Laboratory section is reported,

A. all the listed tests must have been performed

B. 90 percent of the listed tests must have been performed

C. 50 percent of the listed tests must have been performed

D. all the listed tests must have been performed on the same day

Provide answers to the following questions in the spaces provided.

1. List the three steps in the procedural coding process.

2. List the three key components used to select E/M codes, and the four levels each component has.

Applying your Knowledge

Case 5.1

Supply the correct E/M service CPT codes for the following procedures and services.

1. Office visit, new patient; detailed history and examination, low complexity medical decision making

2. Hospital visit, new patient; comprehensive history and examination, highly complex case

3. Office consultation for established patient; comprehensive history and examination, moderately complex medical decision making

4. Annual comprehensive physical examination for sixty-four-year-old new patient

5. Medical disability examination by treating physician

6. Hospital visit to previously admitted patient; expanded problem-focused history and examination, twenty-five minutes spent at bedside

7. Hospital emergency department call for established patient with cardiac infarction; detailed history and examination, moderately complex decision making

8. Annual visit to established, stable patient in nursing facility, no change made to medical plan

9. Home visit for new patient, straightforward case, problem-focused history and examination

10. Short telephone call to patient to report laboratory test results

Case 5.2

Supply the correct anesthesia or surgery CPT codes for the following procedures and services.

1. Anesthesia for vaginal delivery only

2. Anesthesia services for patient age seventy-six, healthy, for open procedure on wrist

3. Incision and drainage of infected wound after surgery

4. Destruction of flat wart

5. Closed treatment of acromioclavicular dislocation with manipulation

6. Complicated drainage of finger abscess

7. Paring of three skin lesions

8. Postpartum D & C

9. Excision of chest wall tumor including ribs

10. Transurethral electrosurgical resection of the prostate (TURP); patient has mild systemic disease; payer requires surgery codes

11. Amniocentesis, diagnostic

12. Ureterolithotomy on lower third of ureter

13. Tonsillectomy and adenoidectomy, patient age fifteen

14. Flexible sigmoidoscopy with specimen collection, separate procedure

15. Kidner type procedure

16. Application of short leg splint

17. Unilateral transorbital frontal sinusotomy

18. Puncture aspiration of three cysts in breast

19. Posterior arthrodesis for scoliosis patient, eleven vertebral segments

20. Routine obstetrical care, vaginal delivery

Case 5.3

Supply the correct radiology, pathology and laboratory, or medicine CPT codes for the following procedures and services.

1. Subcutaneous chemotherapy administration

2. Material (sterile tray) supplied by physician

3. Routine ECG with fifteen leads, with the physician providing only the interpretation and report of the test

4. CRH stimulation panel

5. Automated urinalysis for glucose, without microscopy

6. Aortography, thoracic, without serialography, radiological supervision and interpretation

7. Bone marrow smear interpretation

8. Physical therapy evaluation

9. Ingestion challenge test

10. Electrocorticogram at surgery, separate procedure

Case 5.4

1. What is the meaning of each of the modifiers used in the following case example? A multitrauma patient had a bilateral knee procedure as part of team surgery following a motorcycle crash. The orthopedic surgeon also reconstructed the patient's pelvis and left wrist.

   A. –99

   B. –66

C. –51

D. –50

Supply the correct codes and modifiers for these cases.

2. A surgeon administers a regional Bier block and then monitors the patient and the block while repairing the flexor tendon of the forearm.

3. Primary care provider performs a frontal and lateral chest X-ray and observes a mass. The patient is sent to a pulmonologist, who, on the same day, repeats the frontal and lateral chest X-ray. How should the pulmonologist report the X-ray service?

4. A day after surgery for a knee replacement, the patient develops an infection in the surgical area and is returned to the operating room for debridement. Which modifier is attached to the second procedure?

Computer Exploration

Internet Activity

1. The American Academy of Professional Coders (AAPC) is a coding association that certifies medical coders and provides information on coding issues. Point your Web browser at

   http://www.aapc.com

   and investigate the ways this association keeps its members up to date about changes in procedural coding. Also review the activities of this group in your local area.

2. The American College of Cardiology (ACC) is the association for physicians in the specialty of cardiology. As a service to its members, the ACC reports the addenda items that apply to their specialty each year. For example, point your Web browser at

   http://www.acc.org

   and explore the procedure coding updates related to cardiology. Report on how many new cardiology codes have been added for this year.

3. Current HCPCS codes are available on the CMS Web site. Visit this location:

   http://cms.hhs.gov/medicare/hcpcs/default.asp

   and locate examples of temporary codes and effective dates for their use.

NDCMediSoft Activity

5.1 Review Procedure Code Setup Screens in MediSoft

Procedure codes are entered in MediSoft manually or from a database of codes stored on a CD-ROM or other media. MediSoft allows users to enter new codes, edit existing codes, and mark codes that are no longer used as inactive.

To examine the type of information that is stored in MediSoft for procedure codes:

1. Select Procedure/Payment/Adjustment Codes on the Lists menu. The Procedure/Payment/Adjustment List dialog box displays all existing codes in the program. Scroll through the list to view the range of codes.

Computer Exploration

2. Depending on what option is selected in the Field box, the codes may be listed numerically by code number, alphabetically by description, or grouped according to type of code. For now, make sure that Code 1 is selected in the Field box.

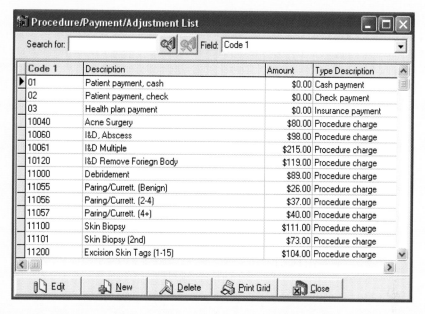

3. Click inside the Search For box to activate it, and then key 10120. Procedure code 10120, I&D Remove Foreign Body, is selected.

4. With code 10120 selected, click the Edit button. The Procedure/ Payment/ Adjustment dialog box is displayed with information on code 10120. The dialog box contains three tabs: General, Amounts, and Allowed Amounts.

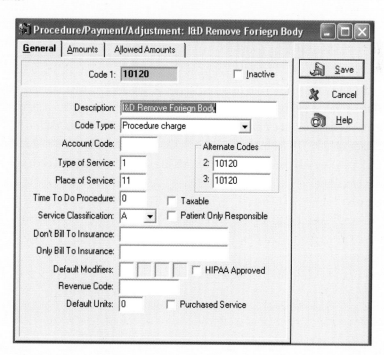

5. Review the information listed in the General tab that is currently displayed. Notice that there are options for entering a description for the procedure code, the type of service and place of service connected with the procedure, and the time normally required to complete the procedure (this can be used when scheduling appointments in an electronic scheduling program).

   There are also fields to indicate whether the code should be excluded from certain claims or used only for certain claims, depending on the carrier. If the code requires a modifier or modifiers, these can be entered also. A modifier entered in the General tab is automatically entered in the Transaction Entry dialog box every time this procedure code is entered in a transaction.

   Click the Amounts tab.

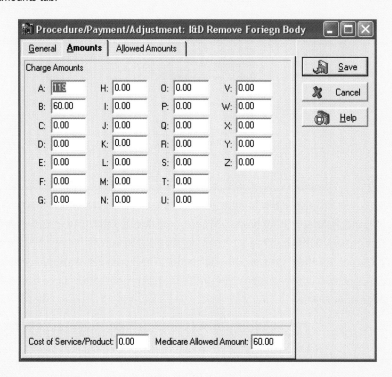

6. In the Amounts tab there are 26 boxes, labeled A through Z, in which different charge amounts can be entered. This is very useful when different insurance plans allow different amounts for the same procedure. In this example, Charge Amount A is for a commercial plan, such as Anthem BCBS Traditional, while Charge Amount B is for Medicare. The dollar amount entered in box B is from the Medicare Fee Schedule.
7. Click the Allowed Amounts tab. This tab lists the allowed amount that each insurance carrier will pay for this procedure.

Computer Exploration

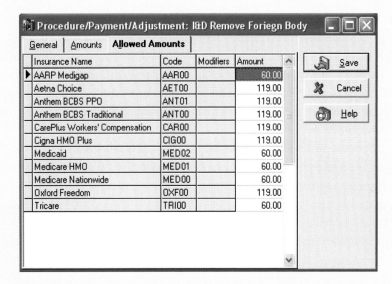

8. Click the Cancel button to exit the Procedure/Payment/Adjustment dialog box.
9. Click the Close button to close the Procedure/Payment/Adjustment List dialog box.

5.2 Review Procedure Code Entries for a Patient

Once procedure codes are entered in MediSoft, they can be used to record procedures from a patient's encounter form into the appropriate MediSoft database. Procedures in MediSoft are recorded in the Transaction Entry dialog box.

1. Select Enter Transactions on the Activities menu. The Transaction Entry dialog box is displayed. The box is blank until a patient is selected in the Chart box at the top of the dialog box.
2. Key "H" and notice that the dropdown list highlights the first patient whose chart number begins with "H," in this case Alan Harcar. Press Enter to select Alan Harcar.

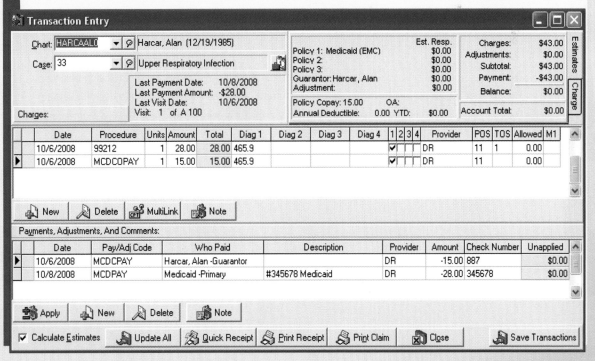

3. Study the fields in the middle portion of the Transaction Entry dialog box, which is labeled Charges. This section of the dialog box is used for recording procedures and their corresponding charges. Notice that two procedures have already been recorded.

4. Click inside the Procedure box for the first transaction (containing code 99212), and then click the triangle button to the right of the code to display the dropdown list of codes and code descriptions.

5. A complete list of all procedure codes and descriptions is displayed, the same list that was examined in the previous activity.

6. In this example, the procedure code led us to the code's description (EP Problem Focused). If you knew the description of a procedure, but not the exact code number, you could use the Search feature inside the Procedure box to locate the code number. Click the small magnifying glass icon that is located just to the right of the triangle button inside the Procedure box. The Procedure Search Window is displayed.

7. In the Field box in the top right corner of the window, click the triangle button to display the dropdown list of fields. MediSoft can search for a procedure by its code number, description, or type. In this case, select Description.

8. Click inside the Search For box to activate it, and then key the description "ecg."

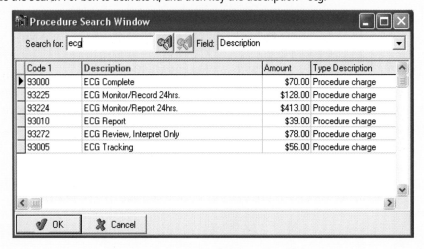

9. MediSoft locates the procedure code (93000 ECG Complete) in the list of codes and descriptions in the database. To display this code in the Procedure box of Alan Harcar's Transaction Entry dialog box, you would click the OK button. However, as Harcar's current transaction does not need to be edited at the point, click the Cancel button.

10. The Procedure Search Window dialog box closes.

11. Click the Close button to close the Transaction Entry dialog box without saving your work.

Coding Linkage and Compliance

Objectives

After studying this chapter, you should be able to:

1. Explain the importance of properly linking diagnoses and procedures when reporting services for reimbursement.
2. Discuss the major laws and guidelines that regulate coding compliance.
3. Describe actions that are considered fraudulent, and discuss the major types of errors medical practices make in reporting codes.
4. Identify the parts of a compliance plan, and discuss how they help avoid errors.
5. Compare and contrast external audits and internal audits.
6. Discuss the use of audit tools to verify code selection.

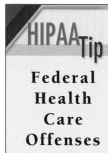

Introduction

Physicians have the ultimate responsibility for proper documentation and correct coding, as well as for compliance with regulations. Medical insurance specialists help ensure that medical practices promptly receive maximum appropriate reimbursement for reported services by submitting correct health care claims. These claims, as well as the process used to create them, must comply with the rules imposed by federal and state law and with payer requirements. Correct claims help reduce the chance of an investigation of the practice and the risk of liability if an investigation does occur.

The possible consequences of inaccurate coding and incorrect billing include

- Denied claims
- Delays in processing claims and receiving payments
- Reduced payments
- Fines and other sanctions
- Loss of hospital privileges
- Exclusion from payers' programs
- Prison sentences
- Loss of the physician's license to practice medicine

Code Linkage

On correct claims, each reported service is connected to a diagnosis that supports the procedure as necessary to investigate or treat the patient's condition. Payers analyze this connection between the diagnostic and the procedural information, called **code linkage**, to evaluate the medical necessity of the reported charges. Correct claims also comply with the many other requirements issued by government or private payers. Some regulations involve the place, frequency, or level of services. For example, Medicare reimburses one treatment for routine foot care and for mycotic nail treatment every sixty days. Other regulations address specific documentation that must be prepared. Authorization to use a new drug therapy for osteoarthritis, for instance, often requires a special report covering the patient's continued high level of pain despite a regimen of other, established drugs.

Linkage and Compliance Review

In the linkage and compliance review step in the claims processing sequence, medical insurance specialists work with patients' encounter forms and medical records to verify the services that should be billed. (Refer to the ten-step billing and reimbursement sequence in Chapter 3.) The codes and the documentation are also reviewed to make sure errors have not been made. The review checks these key points:

- Are the codes appropriate to the patient's profile (age, gender, condition; new or established), and is each coded service billable?
- Is there a clear and correct link between each diagnosis and procedure?
- Have the payer's rules about the diagnosis and the procedure been followed?
- Is the documentation in the patient's medical record adequate to support the reported services?
- Do the reported services comply with all regulations?

This chapter discusses the general topic of coding compliance. Chapters 10 through 14 explain the particular regulations and requirements of the major payers.

- Chapter 10 covers typical rules issued by private payers, including the payers in the Blue Cross and Blue Shield Association.
- Chapters 11 and 12 discuss Medicare and Medicaid regulations.
- Chapter 13 covers the other major government-sponsored program, TRICARE.
- Chapter 14 explains the special requirements for handling disability and workers' compensation claims.

Insurance Fraud and Abuse

Almost everyone involved in the delivery of health care is a trustworthy person devoted to patients' welfare. However, some people are not. For example, according to the Department of Health and Human Services (HHS), in 2002 the federal government recovered more than $1.8 billion in judgments, settlements, and other fees in health care fraud cases.

Definition of Fraud and Abuse

Fraud is an act of deception used to take advantage of another person or entity. For example, it is fraudulent for people to misrepresent their credentials or to forge another person's signature on a check. If a person pretends to be a physician and treats patients without a valid medical license, this is fraudulent. Fraudulent acts are intentional; they are made because the individual knows that some illegal or unauthorized benefit will probably result.

Claims fraud occurs when health care providers or others falsely represent their services or charges to payers. For example, a provider may bill for services that were not performed, overcharge for services, or fail to provide complete services under a contract. A patient may exaggerate an injury to get a settlement from an insurance company or ask a medical insurance specialist to change a date on a chart so that a service is covered by a health plan.

In federal law, **abuse** means an action that misuses the money that the government has allocated, such as Medicare funds. Abuse is illegal because taxpayers' dollars are misspent. An example of abuse is an ambulance service that billed Medicare for transporting a patient to the hospital when the patient did not need ambulance service. This abusive action resulted in improper payment for the ambulance company. In this example, the key difference between fraud and abuse is: to bill when the task was not done is fraud; to bill when it was not necessary is abuse.

Fraud and abuse charges are one of two types, according to the laws that apply. Most medical cases involve civil law, which regulates crimes against individuals' rights and the remedies for them. Examples of civil law cases are trespassing, divorce proceedings, and breach of contract. The punishment for those found guilty in a civil suit is typically a monetary fine. However, some cases of medical fraud and abuse involve criminal law. Criminal law typically regulates what are considered crimes against the state, such as kidnapping, robbery, and arson. The punishment for criminal acts is most often imprisonment as well as fines.

Examples of Fraudulent or Abusive Acts

A number of billing practices are fraudulent or abusive. Investigators reviewing physicians' billing work look for patterns like these:

- Reporting services that were not performed
  Example: A lab bills Medicare for a general health panel (CPT 80050), but the thyroid stimulating hormone (TSH) test was not done.

- Reporting services at a higher level than was carried out
  Example: After a visit for a flu shot, the provider bills the encounter as an Evaluation and Management service (CPT 99213) plus a vaccination (90471/90657).

- Performing and billing for procedures that are not related to the patient's condition and therefore not medically necessary
  Example: After reading an article about Lyme disease, a patient is worried about having worked in her garden over the summer, and she requests a Lyme disease diagnostic test. Although no symptoms or signs have been reported, the physician orders and bills for the *Borrelia burgdorferi* (Lyme disease) confirmatory immunoblot test (CPT 86617).

- Billing separately for services that are bundled in a single procedure code
  Example: When a primary care physician (PCP) orders a comprehensive metabolic panel (CPT 80053), the pathologist bills for the panel as well as for a quantitative glucose test (CPT 82947).

- Reporting the same service twice
  Example: On claims for a new patient who has been hospitalized for cardiac infarction, the cardiologist's office billed for initial observation care (CPT 99220) twice on the same date of service.

Thinking It Through—6.1

Mary Kelley, a patient of the Good Health Clinic, asked Kathleen Culpepper, the medical insurance specialist, to help her out of a tough financial spot. Her medical insurance authorized her to receive four radiation treatments for her condition, one every thirty-five days. Because she was out of town, she did not schedule her appointment for the last treatment until today, which is one week beyond the approved period. The insurance company will not reimburse Mary for this procedure. She asks Kathleen to change the date on the record to last Wednesday so that it will be covered, explaining that no one will be hurt by this change and, anyway, she pays the insurance company plenty.

What type of action is Mary asking Kathleen to do?

_____

How should Kathleen handle Mary's request ?

_____

Compliance Regulations

Coding compliance is a part of the overall effort of medical practices to comply with regulations in many areas, such as protecting PHI. In this sense, coding compliance creates correct claims that are an indication of a compliant medical practice. On the other hand, claims that contain errors raise the question of whether the practice is generally acting in a fraudulent or abusive manner. Medical practice staff as well as physicians must be aware of, understand, and comply with applicable regulations and laws.

Federal Law

A number of federal laws have made compliance with government regulations vital for medical practices.

HIPAA

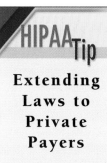

The Health Insurance Portability and Accountability Act of 1996 (HIPAA) created the **Health Care Fraud and Abuse Control Program** to uncover fraud and abuse in the Medicare and Medicaid programs, as well as among private payers. Under this law, the **Office of the Inspector General (OIG)** has the task of detecting health care fraud and abuse and enforcing all laws relating to them. This focus has become a high national priority for federal law enforcement. The OIG works with the U.S. Department of Justice (DOJ), which includes the Federal Bureau of Investigation (FBI), under the direction of the U.S. Attorney General to investigate and prosecute those suspected of medical fraud and abuse.

OIG has the authority to investigate suspected fraud cases and to **audit** the records of physicians and third-party payers. In an audit, investigators review selected records for compliance with accepted documentation standards, such as the signing and dating of entries by the responsible health care professional and the linkage between the diagnosis and the procedures. The accounting records are often reviewed as well. When problems are found, the investigation proceeds and may result in charges of fraud or abuse against the practice.

Federal False Claims Act (31 USC § 3729)

The federal False Claims Act (FCA) prohibits submitting a fraudulent claim or making a false statement or representation in connection with a claim. It also encourages reporting of suspected fraud and abuse against the government by protecting and rewarding people involved in *qui tam*, or whistle-blower, cases. The person who makes the accusation of suspected fraud is called the **relator**. Under the law, the relator is protected against employer retaliation. If the lawsuit results in a fine paid to the federal government, the whistle-blower may be entitled to 15 to 25 percent of the amount paid. People who blow the whistle are current or former employees of insurance companies or medical practices, program beneficiaries, and independent contractors.

Additional Laws

- An antikickback statute makes it illegal to knowingly offer incentives to induce referrals of items or services that are reimbursable by government health care programs. Many financial actions are considered to be incentives, including illegal direct payments to other physicians and routine waivers of coinsurance and deductibles.

Case Example

Whistle-Blower Action
Winning a competition for referrals cost one health system $3,750,000. A hospital allegedly violated the law by granting below-market leases and other incentives to physician groups in return for patient referrals. The defendants will pay the fine in exchange for a release of liability under the False Claims Act.

**Compliance
Guideline**

**Ongoing Compliance
Education**

As explained in detail later
in the chapter, medical
office staff receive ongoing
training and education in
current rules, so they can
avoid even the appearance
of fraud.

- Self-referral prohibitions (Stark Law I and II, 1992 and 1995) make it illegal for physicians to own (wholly or in part) clinics to which they refer their patients, such as radiology service clinics and clinical laboratory services. (Note, however, that there are many legal exceptions to this prohibition under various business structures.)
- Laws mandating coverage for various screening tests are often passed. For example, the 1998 Women's Health and Cancer Rights Act requires all health insurance plans that provide coverage for mastectomies to also provide coverage for associated treatments, such as breast reconstruction after surgery.
- The Sarbanes-Oxley Act of 2002 requires publicly traded corporations to attest that their financial management is sound. These provisions apply to for-profit health care companies. The act includes whistle-blower protection so that employees can report wrongdoing without fear of retaliation.

Government Investigations and Advice

Most billing-related accusations are based on the False Claims Act and on HIPAA, which states that providers who *knew or should have known* that a claim for service was false can be held liable. This means that the intent to commit fraud does not have to be proved by the accuser in order for the provider to be found guilty. Actions that might be viewed as errors or occasional slips might also be seen as establishing a pattern of violations, which constitute the knowledge meant by "providers knew or should have known."

These penalties can be imposed for those guilty of fraud and abuse:

- *Under civil law:* The maximum penalty for medical fraud is $10,000 for each item or service for which fraudulent payment has been received. An amount up to three times the amount of the claim can also be fined.
- *Under criminal law:* Since medical fraud can have criminal aspects, those found guilty can receive jail sentences of up to ten years as well as fines. If a patient is seriously injured or dies, longer jail sentences—up to life imprisonment—are probable.
- *Under administrative law:* Physicians can also be subject to administrative remedies, such as exclusion from participation as providers in all government health care programs.

Example

Overbilling

A physician paid
$185,000 to resolve
government claims that
he overbilled Medicare.
Based on its investiga-
tion, the government
alleged that the doctor
overbilled Medicare ap-
proximately fourteen
hundred times by charg-
ing for higher-paid con-
sultation services, when
he was actually perform-
ing lower-reimbursed
regular patient visits. As
part of the settlement,
the government recov-
ered all amounts that
were overbilled, plus
additional sums to offset
the cost of investigating
the case. The doctor also
entered into a **corporate
integrity agreement**
with the Office of the
Inspector General; this
helps the government
monitor his compliance
with Medicare billing
guidelines.

Although the OIG says that "under the law, physicians are not subject to civil, administrative, or criminal penalties for innocent errors, or even negligence," decisions about whether there are clear patterns and inadequate internal procedures can be subjective at times, making the line between honest mistakes and fraud very thin. Medical practice staff must avoid any action that could be perceived as noncompliant.

The OIG Work Plan

Each year, as part of a Medicare Fraud and Abuse Initiative, the OIG announces the **OIG Work Plan**. The Work Plan lists the year's planned projects for sampling particular types of billing to see if there are problems. These are some of the physician services areas targeted in 2004:

- *Consultations:* Determine the appropriateness of billings for physician consultation services and the financial impact of inaccurate billings on the Medicare program.
- *Coding of Evaluation and Management Services:* Examine whether physicians accurately coded Evaluation and Management services, for which Medicare paid over $23 billion in 2001.

- *Use of Modifier –25:* Determine whether providers used modifier –25 appropriately. In general, a provider should not bill evaluation and management codes on the same day as a procedure or other service unless the evaluation and management service is unrelated to such procedure or service. A provider reports such a circumstance by using modifier –25.
- *Services and supplies incident to physicians' services:* Evaluate the conditions under which physicians bill **incident-to** services and supplies. Physicians may bill for the services provided by allied health professionals, such as nurses, technicians, and therapists, as incident to their professional services. Most incident-to services must be provided by an employee of the physician under the physician's direct supervision.

OIG Work Plans point to the areas on which government investigations will focus. Medical practices, and particularly the compliance officers many practices appoint to keep current with changing regulations, study these initiatives and make sure their procedures comply with the existing rules.

Advisory Opinions

At times, the effort to be in compliance can be problematic for practices. Some regulations are contradictory or unclear, and some are too new to be well understood. For help, both the OIG and CMS issue **advisory opinions** on various questions. These opinions are legal advice only for the requesting parties, who, if they act according to the advice, cannot be investigated on the matter.

To receive an advisory opinion, an individual, such as a physician, or a legal entity, such as a hospital, formally presents a situation and asks whether the way they intend to handle it is fraudulent. CMS or the OIG responds with an opinion. Although taking this advice legally protects only the party that asks the question, the answers are valuable to everyone who has an interest in the subject.

The following example is taken from an OIG advisory opinion. (When advisory opinions are published, the names of the parties are redacted—removed from the public document—to keep that information private.) In this situation, the parties asked for the OIG's opinion on a business arrangement that they were concerned might be investigated as fraud.

> We are writing in response to your request for an advisory opinion, in which you asked whether an arrangement whereby an independent physician association would acquire an equity interest in a managed care organization would constitute grounds for the imposition of sanctions under the anti-kickback statute. . . . [Conclusion] we conclude that the Proposed Arrangement . . . poses no more than a minimal risk of fraud and abuse. Accordingly . . . the OIG will not subject the Proposed Agreement to sanctions arising under the anti-kickback statute.

Advisory opinions are considered the best way to be sure that an intended action will not be subject to investigation. They are published on the OIG's Web site (oig.hhs.gov).

Audit Reports

The OIG also issues **audit reports**, which summarize the department's findings after it has investigated a potentially problematic situation. These reports are also posted to the Web site. Here is an example:

> The HHS Office of Inspector General has posted an Audit Report to its website. A summary of the report follows . . . Review of the Medicaid Drug Rebate

Program, State of Minnesota, Minnesota Department of Human Services, St. Paul, Minnesota . . . The objective of this audit was to evaluate whether the Minnesota Department of Human Services had established adequate accountability and internal controls over the Medicaid drug rebate program. In our opinion, the State had established adequate accountability and internal controls. The financial management system used to provide the necessary information complies with Federal regulations.

Special Fraud Alerts and Advisory Bulletins

OIG Fraud Alerts are issued periodically to inform providers of problematic actions that have come to the OIG's attention. With CMS, the OIG also issues CMS advisory bulletins that alert providers and government-sponsored program beneficiaries of potential problems. Examples include:

- An advisory bulletin explained how Medicare-participating hospitals are to handle Medicare and Medicaid patients enrolled in managed care plans when they seek treatment of possible emergency medical conditions.
- A fraud alert warned physicians to be sure that home health care and durable medical equipment (DME) they order is medically necessary. It also urged physicians and medical practice staff to report suspicious activity about false certification of patients' needs for these services. A certificate of medical necessity (see Chapter 11) is needed for Medicare reimbursement of home health services or some types of medical equipment, such as wheelchairs. The alert came after audits showed that some physicians signed certificates of medical necessity without even knowing the patients.

Excluded Parties

If employees, physicians, and contractors have been found guilty of fraud, they may be excluded from work for government programs. An OIG exclusion has national scope and is important to many institutional health care providers because Congress established a Civil Monetary Penalty for institutions that knowingly hire **excluded parties**. The OIG maintains the List of Excluded Individuals/Entities (LEIE), a database that provides the public, health care providers, patients, and others with information about parties excluded from participation in Medicare, Medicaid, and federal health care programs. As shown in Figure 6.1, this list is available on the OIG's Web site.

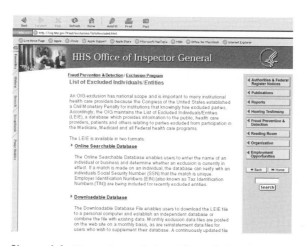

Figure 6.1 Home Page of the Office of the Inspector General List of Excluded Individuals/Entities

Medicare Regulations

The Medicare program has two parts, one for hospitals (Part A) and one for most physician services (Part B). (These programs are covered in Chapter 11.) **Medicare carriers** are insurance companies hired as independent contractors to administer claims for CMS in particular geographical areas. They are paid per claim to receive the claims from medical practices, check and review them, and process them for payment.

Medicare Manuals

The proposed and approved rules from CMS about the Medicare program are published in the *Federal Register*, the main documentation of all proceedings of the federal government. In addition, CMS issues a number of manuals with rules and interpretations of Medicare program guidelines. Medicare carriers implement these rules for the geographical areas they administer and also issue local policies. Figure 6.2 shows an example of a Medicare Coverage decision.

National Correct Coding Initiative

Medicare's national policy on correct coding is called the Medicare **National Correct Coding Initiative (NCCI)**. The NCCI is an ongoing process to standardize bundled codes and control improper coding that would lead to inappropriate payment for Medicare claims for physician services. The NCCI list, which is updated every quarter, contains more than two hundred thousand CPT-4 code combinations used by Medicare carriers' computers to check claims. These code combinations, called **NCCI edits**, make up the computerized screening process used by Medicare to examine claims.

The NCCI edits explain what procedures and services cannot be billed together for the same patient on the same day of service. There are three types of edits for coding errors:

- *Comprehensive versus component edits:* In this group, the first column of codes contains the comprehensive code, and the second column shows the component code. According to the NCCI, the comprehensive code includes all the services that are described by the component code, so the component code cannot be billed together with the comprehensive code for the same patient on the same day of service.

Compliance Guideline

Medicare Fraud Watch
Under a special program, Medicare beneficiaries can earn a reward of up to $1,000 if they turn in providers who are proven to have committed fraud against the program. A Medicare beneficiary has the right to ask a provider for an itemized statement for any item or service for which Medicare has paid. The program instructs Medicare recipients to check their Medicare Summary Notice, which the Medicare program sends them to explain the benefits they have received, and verify that they received listed services.

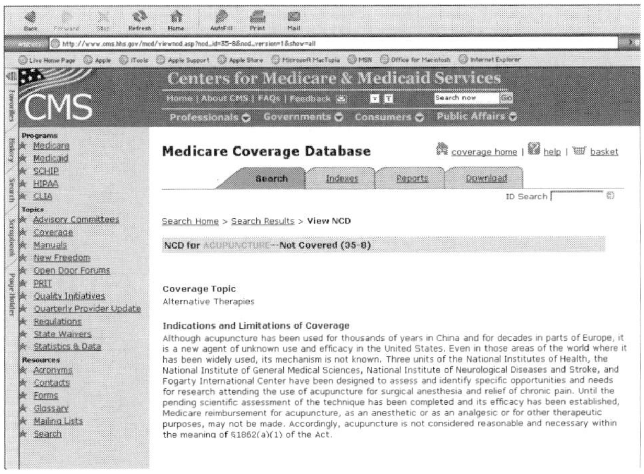

Figure 6.2 Example of CMS Coverage Issues Manual

Example

Comprehensive	Component
27370	20610, 76000, 76003

- *Mutually exclusive edits:* This group also lists codes in two columns. According to CMS regulations, the services represented by these codes could not have both reasonably been done during a single patient encounter, so they cannot be billed together. If the provider reports both codes from both Column 1 and Column 2 for a patient on the same day, Medicare pays only the lower-paid code.

Example

Column 1	Column 2
50021	49061, 50020

- *Modifier indicators:* This type of NCCI modifier is a number appearing alongside the comprehensive and component code list and the mutually exclusive code list. A provider may include an NCCI modifier to allow payment for both services within the code pair under certain circumstances.

Private Payer Regulations

Private payers develop code edits similar to the NCCI. Although private payers give medical practices information about their payment policies in their policy handbooks and bulletins, the exact code edits may not be shared with physicians. At times, their claims-editing software does not follow CPT guidelines

Thinking It Through—6.2

1. A hospital and a large multispecialty practice are considering a business merger. They are concerned that they may be targeted for a fraud investigation because they both have Medicare patients. What action would you recommend that they take?

2. What type of code edit could be used for the following rule? Medicare Part B covers a screening Pap smear for women for the early detection of cervical cancer but will not pay for an E/M service for the patient on the same day.

3. An OIG project found that during one month in a single state, there were 23,000 billings for an E/M service with the modifier –25 reported with one of these CPT codes: 11055, 11056, 11057, 11719, and HCPCS code G0127 (trimming of dystrophic nails).

   Look up the descriptors for the CPT codes. Do you think the procedures appear to be simple or complicated?

   _____

   Why do you think that this billing combination continues to be under scrutiny by CMS?

   _____

and bundles distinct procedures or does not accept properly used modifiers. In these cases, medical insurance specialists must follow up with the payer for clarification (see Chapters 9 and 10).

Policy handbooks usually contain additional regulations, such as the documentation required for certain procedures. Generally, the use of unlisted procedure codes requires a description of the services. Other services may also have special requirements. For example, a state Blue Cross and Blue Shield manual contains the requirement that the reporting of CPT code 90730, hepatitis A immunization, must be documented with the name of the serum, the dosage, and the route of administration.

Compliance Errors

Health care payers often base their decisions to pay or deny claims only on the diagnosis and procedure codes. The integrity of the request for payment rests on the accuracy and honesty of the coding. Incorrect coding may simply be an error, or it may represent deliberate efforts to obtain fraudulent payment. Some compliance errors are related to medical necessity; others are a result of incorrect code selection or billing practices. Other fraudulent activities are business arrangements that violate referral law, fee waivers for professional courtesy and other discounts not uniformly applied, and employment of people who have been excluded from federal programs.

Errors Relating to Code Linkage and Medical Necessity

To establish medical necessity, the payer must understand the severity of the patient's condition and the signs, symptoms, or history that relate to the reason for care. To be appropriately linked, diagnosis and procedure codes must pass the test of clinical consistency. For example, if a condition has been diagnosed, other reported symptoms must be related to it—shortness of breath should have a logical primary diagnosis, such as lung disease, heart failure, or anxiety. Treatments should be related to functional impairments and disabilities. And clinically, the overall coding of the case should be reasonable. These facts must be documented in the patient's medical record as well as in the codes (see Chapters 2 and 3).

Claims are denied due to lack of medical necessity when the reported services are not consistent with the symptoms or the diagnosis or not in keeping with generally accepted professional medical standards. Correctly linked codes that support medical necessity meet these conditions:

- The CPT procedure codes match the ICD-9-CM diagnosis codes.
  Example: A procedure to drain an abscess of the external ear or auditory canal should be supported by a diagnosis of disorders of the external ear or an ear carbuncle or cyst.

- The procedures are not elective, experimental, or nonessential.
  Example: Cosmetic nasal surgery performed to improve a patient's appearance is typically excluded. However, a cosmetic procedure may be considered medically necessary when it is performed to repair an accidental injury or to improve the functioning of a malformed body member. A diagnosis of deviated septum, nasal obstruction, acquired facial deformity, or the late effects of facial bone fracture supports the medical necessity for cosmetic nasal surgery.

HIPAATip

PHI and the Minimum Necessary Standard

PHI from the patient's medical record must be available for the payer to review if it is requested. Be sure to release only the minimum necessary information to answer the payer's questions.

- The procedures are furnished at an appropriate level.
  Example: A high-level Evaluation and Management code for an office visit (such as 99204/99205 and 99214/99215) must be matched by a serious, complex condition such as a sudden, unexplained large loss of weight.

Medical necessity edits are established by each payer. For example, each Medicare carrier has its own rules for particular procedures and the diagnoses that must be linked for payment. Private payers at times have different edits, and inconsistency among payers is not uncommon.

Errors Relating to the Coding Process

To avoid coding errors, it is essential that all codes are currently correct and complete. **Truncated coding**, in which diagnosis codes are not reported at the highest level of specificity available, causes rejected claims, as does using codes that are out of date. The gender or age of the patient must match the selected code when the code involves selection for either criterion. Documentation must clearly support the codes. Following are other incorrect practices:

- **Assumption coding**—reporting items or services that are not actually documented, but that the coder assumes were performed
- Altering documentation after services are reported
- Coding without proper documentation
- Reporting services provided by unlicensed or unqualified clinical personnel
- Not having all necessary documentation available at the time of coding
- Not satisfying the conditions of coverage for a particular service, such as the physician's direct supervision of a radiologist's work
- Not complying with the billing requirements for a service, such as the rules for global surgical period coverage.

Errors Relating to the Billing Process

A number of errors are related to the billing process. These errors include reporting services that are not covered or have limited coverage, and using modifiers incorrectly. Another error involves either **upcoding** or **downcoding**—using a procedure code that provides a higher or lower reimbursement rate than the code that actually reflects the service provided. (Some physicians downcode to be "safe," especially E/M codes.) When upcoding is found by the payer, the code is changed to a lower-value code that the payer thinks is correct.

Unbundling—billing the parts of a bundled procedure as separate procedures—must also be avoided. For clarity on the procedures that bundled surgical codes contain, medical practices should be specific about their descriptions of these codes. Many practices adopt Medicare's NCCI list of bundling rules for such codes, and others adopt the slightly different list from the American Medical Association. Practices communicate their standard to the private payers with whom they work.

Strategies for Medical Insurance Specialists and Coders

For medical insurance specialists and medical coders, strategies for avoiding fraud and abuse are especially important. This can be a difficult and complex assignment. Coding claims in order to generate payment at the highest possible level is a critical goal of the billing staff's responsibilities. Sometimes, however, regulations can be unclear or even disagree with each other.

1. Medical necessity must be shown for emergency department visits for physicians' patients. If a four-year-old wakes at 3 A.M. with an earache and a temperature of 103°, in what order should the following diagnosis codes be listed to show the urgent reason for an emergency department visit by the child's pediatrician: 381.00, 780.6, 388.71?

2. The following diagnosis and procedure codes were rejected for payment. What is the probable reason for the payer's decision in each case?

   A. 881.1

   B. V50.3, 69090

   C. 054.79, 69145

   D. V70.0, 80050, 80053

The best defense against fraud investigations is to prevent them from happening in the first place. These measures help prevent problems:

- Keep coding knowledge up to date through ongoing continuing education in changing codes
- Read third-party payer bulletins and regulatory publications and update the written policies and procedures.
- Review coding accuracy by asking:
  Do the diagnosis codes relate correctly to the procedure codes?
  Are reported codes supported by documentation in the patient medical record?
  Are there any unusual coding patterns, such as using only the highest reimbursement level of codes rather than the expected range of levels?
- File all written correspondence with government-sponsored and other payers, and be sure that any recommendations from them on billing matters are in writing
- Clarify coding and billing questions with physicians, and be sure that the physician adds any needed clarification to the documentation
- Use the information from claims that are denied or paid at a lesser rate to modify procedures as needed

Part 3 Coding Linkage and Compliance

Strategies for Compliance: The Compliance Plan

Because of the risk of fraud and abuse liability, medical practices must be sure that reimbursement regulations are followed by all staff members. In addition to responsibility for their own actions, physicians are liable for the professional actions of employees they supervise. This responsibility is a result of the law of *respondeat superior,* which states that an employer is responsible for an employee's actions. Physicians are held to this doctrine, so they can be charged for the fraudulent behavior of any staff member.

Coding compliance auditors, often also called compliance specialists or compliance officers, are responsible for accurate, compliant coding and reporting. Because of continuing fraud and abuse initiatives by agencies of the federal government and oversight by other payers, correct coding is increasingly important for medical practices. Coding compliance auditors function as internal auditors to confirm the accuracy of coding and the completeness of documentation. They establish the auditing tools that will be used, and analyze and audit patients' medical records for correct clinical documentation. They also review reimbursements and recommend changes in billing policies. In a large practice, a separate compliance and auditing department may perform this role, staffed by a manager of coding and compliance to whom the coding compliance auditors report.

Coding compliance auditors also help monitor the practice's compliance plan. They recommend compliance policies and procedures such as the correct way to handle overpayments, and train physicians and medical office staff in correct procedures. They are also usually responsible for directing inquiries and helping handle external audits.

Advancement to the position of coding compliance auditor requires experience, computer literacy, education (preferably with certification) in both ICD and CPT coding, a good understanding of health care institutions, and thorough knowledge of regulations.

A wise slogan is, "the best defense is a good offense." For this reason, a medical practice writes and implements a **compliance plan** to find compliance problems and correct them to avoid risking liability. A compliance plan is a process for finding, correcting, and preventing illegal medical office practices. Its goals are to:

- Prevent fraud and abuse through a formal process to identify, investigate, fix, and prevent repeat violations relating to reimbursement for health care services provided
- Ensure compliance with applicable federal, state, and local laws, including employment laws and environmental laws as well as antifraud law
- Help defend the practice if it is investigated or prosecuted for fraud by substantiating the desire to behave compliantly and thus reduce any fines or criminal prosecution

When a compliance plan is in place, it demonstrates to outside investigators that honest, ongoing attempts have been made to find and fix weak areas of compliance with regulations. Development of this written plan is led by a compliance officer and committee to (1) audit and monitor compliance with government regulations, especially in the area of coding and billing, (2) develop written policies and procedures that are consistent, (3) provide for ongoing staff training and communication, and (4) respond to and correct errors.

Although coding and billing compliance are the plan's major focus, it covers all areas of government regulation of medical practices, such as Equal Employment Opportunity (EEO) regulations (for example, hiring and promotion policies) and Occupational Safety and Health Administration (OSHA) regulations (for example, fire safety and handling of hazardous materials such as bloodborne pathogens).

OIG Compliance Program Guidance for Individual and Small Group Physician Practices

Compliance plans vary according to the type of practice and its range of services, its location, and its business structure. Generally, according to the **OIG Compliance Program Guidance for Individual and Small Group Physician Practices**, voluntary plans should contain seven elements:

1. Consistent written policies and procedures
2. Appointment of a compliance officer and committee
3. Training
4. Communication
5. Disciplinary systems
6. Auditing and monitoring
7. Responding to and correcting errors

Following the OIG's guidance can help in the defense against a false claims accusation. Having a plan in place shows that efforts are made to understand the rules and correct errors. This indicates to the OIG that the problems may not add up to pattern or practice of abuse, but may simply be errors.

Compliance Officer and Committee

To establish the plan and follow up on its provisions, most medical practices appoint a compliance officer who is in charge of the ongoing work. The compliance officer may be one of the practice's physicians, the practice manager, or the billing manager. A compliance committee is also usually established to oversee the program. It may be made up of the governing board of the practice, members of the professional and administrative staff, or others. The compliance officer and the committee analyze all areas that present a risk for out-of-compliance behavior in the practice by reviewing:

- Federal and state statutes
- Government-sponsored program regulations (Medicare and Medicaid)
- Medicare Carriers Manual and Coverage Issues Manual
- Current and past years' OIG Work Plans
- OIG Fraud Alerts and audit reports

Code of Conduct

The practice's compliance plan emphasizes the procedures that are to be followed to meet existing documentation, coding, and medical necessity requirements. It also has a code of conduct for the members of the practice, which covers:

- Procedures for ensuring compliance with laws relating to referral arrangements.
- Provisions for discussing compliance during employees' performance reviews and for disciplinary action against employees, if needed.
- Mechanisms to encourage employees to report compliance concerns directly to the compliance officer. These provisions reduce the risk of whistle-blower actions.

Promoting ethical behavior in the practice's daily operations can also reduce employee dissatisfaction and turnover by showing employees that the practice has a strong commitment to honest, ethical conduct.

Compliance Guideline

Medical Liability Insurance
Medical liability cases for fraud often result in lawsuits. Professional liability insurance is purchased by physicians to cover such legal expenses. Although covered under the physician's policy, other medical professionals often purchase their own liability insurance. Medical coders and medical insurance specialists who perform coding tasks are also advised to have professional liability insurance called error and omission (E&O) insurance, which protects against financial loss due to intentional or unintentional failure to perform work correctly.

Ongoing Training

Physician Training

Part of the compliance plan is a commitment to keep physicians trained in pertinent coding and regulatory matters. Often the medical insurance specialist or medical coder is assigned the task of briefing physicians on changed codes or medical necessity regulations. The following guidelines are helpful in conducting physician training classes:

- Keep the presentation as brief and straightforward as possible.
- In a multispecialty practice, issues should be discussed by specialty; all physicians do not need to know changed rules on dermatology, for example.
- Use actual examples, and stick to the facts when presenting material.
- Explain the benefits of coding compliance to the physicians, and listen to their feedback to improve job performance.
- Set up a way to address additional changes during the year, such as an office newsletter or compliance meetings.

Staff Training

An important part of the compliance plan is a commitment to train medical office staff members who are involved with coding and billing. Ongoing training also requires having the current annual updates, reading health plans' bulletins and periodicals, and researching changed regulations. Compliance officers often conduct refresher classes in proper coding and billing techniques.

Correct Preparation of Job Reference Aids and Documentation Templates

Many medical practices develop **job reference aids**, also known as cheat sheets, to help the coding process. These aids usually list the procedures and CPT codes that are most frequently reported by the practice. Some also list frequently used diagnoses with ICD codes. Although job reference aids can be helpful during the coding process, they may also lead to questions about compliance. Are codes assigned by selecting one that is close to the patient's condition on the aid, rather than by researching the precise code based on the documentation?

If job reference aids are used in a practice, these guidelines should be followed:

- Job reference aids should be dated, to be sure that current codes are in use, and reissued every year with updated codes.
- The job reference aid for CPT codes must contain all the codes in a range that the practice may assign. For example, if the medical practice includes office visit codes on a CPT aid, all ten codes should be listed (five levels for both new and established patients).
- An aid for ICD-9-CM codes should be presented in one of two ways: (1) The aid should have only the ICD categories (three-digit numbers) to speed the code selection process, and the manual should be reviewed for the proper usage and highest degree of specificity; or (2) If three-, four-, and five-digit codes are listed, the complete range should be shown, not one or two codes from the group. For example, if heartburn is to be listed, the complete range of symptoms involving the digestive system (787.0–787.99) should be shown, with the correct level of specificity shown as well.

Many practices also list CPT and ICD codes on the office's encounter form. In some cases, these are the only codes listed; in others, these standard codes are shown next to the accounting codes the practice uses. Encounter forms, like job reference aids, must not select from various codes in a range; all the possibilities should be listed, so that it is clear that all have been considered before the code is checked on the encounter form.

Some physician practices develop forms called **documentation templates** to assist physicians as they document each examination of a patient. Templates prompt the physician to document a complete review of systems (ROS) when done and note the medical necessity for the planned treatment. Like other forms used in medical coding, these templates must be compliant and clearly illustrate the services that were rendered. If filed in the medical record, the template should be signed and dated by the physician.

Compliance
Guideline

**Compliant Job
Reference Aids**
Job reference aids or encounter forms should never link diagnoses and procedures. This would give the appearance that coding is based on reimbursement rather than on the patient's condition.

Handling Overpayments

Overpayments (also called credit balances), from the payer's point of view, are improper or excessive payments resulting from billing errors for which a refund is owed by the provider. Examples include duplicate billing of Medicare and another insurer, and being paid for services that are not covered by Medicare. Because overpayments are a major Medicare fraud and abuse initiative, it is important to actively find and refund overpayments. The compliance plan should state the procedure to follow when an overpayment is discovered. Usually, there is a standard refund procedure for the voluntary refund of overpayments to payers or to remedy overbilling. This procedure should also apply to cases in which the payer has caused the error, such as paying the same claim twice.

Ongoing Monitoring

Another major aspect of the compliance plan is monitoring the coding and billing process. Monitoring is done either by the practice's compliance officer or by a staff member who is knowledgeable about coding and compliance regulations. The responsible person establishes a routine system for internal monitoring and regular compliance checks to ensure adherence to established policies and procedures. The plan covers all the steps in the claims processing sequence from the point of collecting patient data to the transmission of a claim for payment.

One monitoring method is to compare the codes that the practice reports with national averages for those codes. Medical coding consulting firms as well as CMS have developed computer programs to profile average billing patterns

Thinking It Through—6.4

1. Should a job reference aid include blank spaces for writing diagnoses and procedures? Why?

2. In what ways do you think that improving physicians' diagnostic and procedural statements might help ensure compliance?

for various types of codes. For example, a practice that reported only the top two of a five-level E/M code range for new or established patient office visits would not fit a normal pattern of office visit codes. The normal pattern has codes at all levels, with more codes in the middle and fewer at the first and the fifth levels. While reporting outside of the normal range is sometimes justified by a practice's circumstances, most often it is evidence of a compliance problem and, when known to a payer, a cause for investigation. Part of the monitoring effort is to be aware of code-reporting patterns and to watch for patterns that do not seem normal. Another part of the monitoring system is conducting regular internal audits, as discussed in the next section.

Audits

An audit is a formal examination or review. Income tax audits are performed to find out if a person's or a firm's income or expenses were misreported. Similarly, compliance audits judge whether the practice's physicians and coding and billing staff comply with regulations for correct coding and billing.

An audit does not involve reviewing every claim and document. Instead, a representative sample of the whole is studied to reveal whether erroneous or fraudulent behavior exists. For instance, an auditor might make a random selection, such as a percentage of the claims for a particular date of service, or a targeted selection, such as all claims in a period that have a certain procedure code. If the auditor finds indications of a problem on the sample, more documents and more detail are usually reviewed.

External Audits

In an **external audit**, private payers' or government investigators review selected records of a practice for compliance. Coding linkage, completeness of documentation, and adherence to documentation standards, such as the signing and dating of entries by the responsible health care professional, may all be studied. The accounting records are often reviewed as well.

Payers use computer programs of code edits to review claims before they are processed. This process is referred to as a prepayment audit. For example, the Medicare NCCI edits perform computer checks before processing claims. Some prepayment audits check only to verify that documentation of the visit is on file, rather than investigating the details of the coding.

Audits conducted after payment has been made are called postpayment audits. Most payers conduct routine postpayment audits of physicians' practices to ensure that claims correctly reflect performed services, that services are billed accurately, and that the physicians and other health care providers who participate in the plan comply with the provisions of their contracts.

In routine private-payer audits, the payer's auditor usually makes an appointment in advance and may conduct the review either in the practice's office or by taking copies of documents back to the payer's office. (Note that patient authorization must be current for any records that are reviewed or photocopied.) Often, the auditor requests the complete medical records of selected plan members for a specified period. The claims information and documentation might include all office and progress notes, laboratory test results, referrals, X-rays, patient sign-in sheets, the office appointment books, and billing records. When problems are found, the investigation proceeds farther and may result in charges of fraud or abuse against the practice.

Case Example

Medically Unnecessary Procedures

Tenet Healthcare Corporation paid the federal government a record-setting $54 million as part of an ongoing criminal and civil investigation of alleged unnecessary cardiac procedures and surgeries at Redding Medical Center in California. The case involved allegations of unnecessary procedures, tests, lab studies, and surgeries. Tenet also agreed to random audits of cardiology procedures to be held twice yearly and other measures to ensure compliance.

Internal Audits

To reduce the chance of an investigation or external audit and to reduce potential liability when one occurs, most practices' compliance plans require **internal audits** to be conducted regularly, either by the medical practice staff or by a hired consultant. These audits are routine and are performed periodically without a reason to think that a compliance problem exists. They help the practice determine whether coding is being done appropriately and whether all performed services are being reported for maximum revenue. The goal is to uncover problems so that they can be corrected. They also help:

- Determine whether new procedures or treatments are correctly coded and documented
- Analyze the skills and knowledge of the personnel assigned to handle medical coding in the practice
- Locate areas where training or additional review of practice guidelines is needed
- Improve communications among the staff members involved with claims processing—medical coders, medical insurance specialists, and physicians

Internal audits are done either prospectively or retrospectively. A **prospective audit** (also called a concurrent audit), like a prepayment audit, is done before the claims that are being examined are reported to a payer for reimbursement. Some practices audit a percentage of claims each day. Others select claims for routine auditing according to other criteria, such as new or especially complex types of procedures. These audits reduce the number of rejected or downcoded claims by verifying compliance before billing.

Retrospective audits are conducted after the claims have been submitted for payment and the remittance advice (RA) has been received. Auditing at this point in the process has two advantages: (1) The complete record, including the RA, is available, so the auditor knows which codes have been rejected or downcoded, and (2) claim problems can be analyzed by specific payer. Retrospective audits are helpful in analyzing the explanations of rejected or reduced charges and making changes to the coding approach if needed.

Auditing Tools to Verify E/M Code Selection

Compliance plans focus on training physicians to use the joint CMS/AMA Documentation Guidelines for Evaluation and Management Services, as well as to know current codes, in order to code correctly. As explained in Chapter 5, the key components for selecting Evaluation and Management codes are the extent of the history documented, the extent of the examination documented, and the complexity of the medical decision making. The CMS/AMA guidelines reduce the amount of subjectivity in making judgments about E/M codes, such as one person's opinion of what makes an examination extended. They do this by describing the specific items that may be documented for each of the three key E/M components. They also explain how many items are needed to place the E/M service at the appropriate level.

The documentation guidelines have precise number counts of these items, and these counts can be used to audit as well as to initially code services. The audit double-checks the selected code based on the documentation in the patient medical record. The auditor looks at the record and, usually using an auditing tool such as that shown in Figure 6.3 (pages 208–209), independently analyzes the services that are documented. The auditor then compares the code

Coding Point

Importance of Documentation
Because of their importance, E/M codes are an ongoing focus of audits. According to CMS, most E/M codes that failed audits did so because they were found to have been up-coded in relation to documentation. The problem is not that E/M services are coded at a higher level than was actually performed by physicians. In fact, many physicians who do their own E/M coding report that they code lower than the service they performed because they are fearful of an audit and hope this avoids one. However, many times the documentation does not justify even the lower code levels they select, so their actions both curtail revenue they should have received and do not protect them from investigation.

HISTORY

HPI (history of present illness)				Brief	Brief	Extended	Extended
❑ Location ❑ Severity ❑ Timing ❑ Modifying factors ❑ Quality ❑ Duration ❑ Context ❑ Associated signs and symptoms					*1-3 elements*	≥ 4 elements or status of ≥ 3 chronic or inactive conditions	

ROS (review of systems)					None	Pertinent to problem	Extended	Complete
❑ Constitutional (wt loss, etc) ❑ Eyes	❑ Ears, nose, mouth, throat ❑ Card/vasc ❑ Resp	❑ GI ❑ GU ❑ Musculo	❑ Integumentary (skin, breast) ❑ Neuro ❑ Psych	❑ Endo ❑ Hem/lymph ❑ All/imm ❑ "All others negative"		*1 system*	*2-9 systems*	≥ 10 systems, or some systems with statement "all others negative"

PFSH (past family and social history) ❑ Past medical history ❑ Family history ❑ Social history		None	None	One history area	Two or three history areas
	Established/ Subsequent				
No PFSH required: 99231-33, 99261-63, 99311-33	New/Initial	None	None	One or two history area(s)	Three history areas

Circle the entry farthest to the right for each history area. To determine history level, draw a line down the column with the circle farthest to the left.	**PROBLEM FOCUSED**	**EXP. PROB. FOCUSED**	**DETAILED**	**COMPRE-HENSIVE**

EXAM

General Multi-system Exam		Single Organ System Exam
1-5 elements	PROBLEM FOCUSED	1-5 elements
≥6 elements	EXPANDED PROBLEM FOCUSED	≥6 elements
≥ 2 elements from 6 areas/systems OR	DETAILED	≥ 12 elements EXCEPT
≥12 elements from at least 2 areas/systems		≥9 elements for eye and psychiatric exams
≥2 elements from 9 areas/systems	COMPREHENSIVE	Perform and document all elements

COMPLEXITY

A Number of Diagnoses or Treatment Options

Problems to Exam Physician	Number X Points = Result
Self-limited or minor (stable, improved or worsening)	Max = 2 · 1
Est. problem (to examiner); stable, improved	1
Est. problem (to examiner); worsening	2
New problem (to examiner); no additional workup planned	Max = 1 · 3
New prob. (to examiner); add. workup planned	4
	TOTAL

Bring total to line A in final Result for Complexity

B Amount and/or Complexity of Data to Be Reviewed

Data to Be Reviewed	Points
Review and/or order of clinical lab tests	1
Review and/or order of tests in the radiology section of CPT	1
Review and/or order tests in the medicine section of CPT	1
Discussion of test results with performing physician	1
Decision to obtain old records and/or obtain history from someone other than patient	1
Review and summarization of old records and/or obtaining history from someone other than patient and/or discussion of case with another health care provider	2
Independent visualization of image, tracing or specimen itself (not simply review of report)	2
	TOTAL

Bring total to line B in final Result for Complexity

Draw a line down the column with 2 or 3 circles and circle decision making level OR Draw a line down the column with the center circle and circle the decision making level.

A	Number diagnoses or treatment options	≤1 Minimal	2 Limited	3 Multiple	≥4 Extensive
B	Amount and complexity of data	≤1 Minimal or low	2 Limited	3 Moderate	≥4 Extensive
C	Highest risk	Minimal	Low	Moderate	High
	Type of decision making	STRAIGHT-FORWARD	LOW COMPLEX.	MODERATE COMPLEX.	HIGH COMPLEX.

C Risk of Complications and/or Morbidity or Mortality

Level of risk	Presenting Problem(s)	Diagnostic Procedure(s) Ordered	Management-Options Selected
MINIMAL	• One self-limited or minor problem, *e.g. cold, insect bite, tinea corporis*	• Laboratory tests requiring venipuncture • Chest xrays • EKG/EEG • Urinalysis • Ultrasound • KOH prep	• Rest • Gargles • Elastic bandages • Superficial dressings
LOW	• Two or more self-limited or minor problems • One stable chronic illness (*well-controlled hypertension or non-insulin dependent diabetes, cataract, BPH*) • Acute uncomplicated illness or injury (*cystitis, allergic rhinitis, simple sprain*)	• Physiological tests not under stress, *e.g. PFT* • Noncardiovascular imaging studies with contrast (*barium enema*) • Superficial needle biopsies • Clinical lab tests requiring arterial puncture • Skin biopsies	• Over-the-counter drugs • Minor surgery w/no identified risk factors • Physical therapy • Occupational therapy • IV fluids without additives
MODERATE	• One or more chronic illnesses with mild exacerbation, progression or side effects of tx • Two or more stable chronic illnesses • Undiagnosed new problem with uncertain prognosis (*breast lump*) • Acute illness with systemic symptoms (*pyelonephritis, pneumonia, colitis*) • Acute complicated injury (*head injury with brief loss of consciousness*)	• Physiologic tests under stress (*cardiac stress test, fetal contraction test*) • Diagnostic endoscopies with no identified risk factors • Deep needle or incisional bx • Cardiovascular imaging studies w/contrast and no identified risk factors (*arteriogram, cardiac cath*) • Obtain fluid from body cavity (*lumbar puncture, thoracentesis, culdocentesis*)	• Minor surgery with identified risk factors • Elective major surgery (open, percutaneous or endoscopic) with no identified risk factors • Prescription drug management • Therapeutic nuclear medicine • IV fluids w/additives • Closed tx of fracture or dislocation without manipulation
HIGH	• One or more chronic illnesses with severe exacerbation, progression or side effects of tx • Acute or chronic illnesses or injuries that may pose a threat to life or bodily function (*multiple trauma, acute MI, pulmonary embolus, severe respiratory distress, progressive severe rheumatoid arthritis, psychiatric illness with potential threat to self or others, peritonitis, acute renal failure*) • A sudden change in neurological status (*seizure, TIA, sensory loss*)	• Cardiovascular imaging studies with contrast with identified risk factors • Cardiac electrophysiological tests • Diagnostic endoscopies w/identified risk factory • Discography	• Elective major surgery (open, percutaneous or endoscopic) with identified risk factor • Emergency major surgery (open, percutaneous or endoscopic) • Parenteral controlled substances • Drug therapy requiring intensive monitoring for toxicity • Decision not to resuscitate or to de-escalate care because of poor prognosis

Figure 6.3 Example of Evaluation and Management Code Assignment Audit Form

Transfer the history, exam and medical decision making results to the appropriate chart below and follow the specific instructions for that chart.

OUTPATIENT, CONSULTS (OUTPATIENT, INPATIENT & CONFIRMATORY) AND ER

	New/Consults/ER					Established				
	If a column has 3 circles, draw a line down the column and circle the code OR find the column with the circle farthest to the left, draw a line down the column and circle the code.					If a column has 2 or 3 circles, draw a line down the column and circle the code OR draw a line down the column with the center circle and circle the code.				
History	PF	EPF	D ER: EPF	C ER: D	C	Minimal problem that may	PF	EPF	D	C
Examination	PF	EPF	D ER: EPF	C ER: D	C	not require presence	PF	EPF	D	C
Complexity of medical decision	SF	SF ER: L	L ER: M	M	H	of physician	SF	L	M	H
	99201 99241 99251 99271 99281	99202 99242 99252 99272 99282	99203 99243 99253 99273 99283	99204 99244 99254 99274 99284	99205 99245 99255 99275 99285	99211	99212	99213	99214	99215

INPATIENT

	Initial Hospital/Observation			Subsequent Inpatient/Follow-up Consult		
	If a column has 3 circles, draw a line down the column and circle the code OR find the column with the circle farthest to the left, draw a line down the column and circle the code.			If a column has 2 or 3 circles, draw a line down the column and circle the code OR draw a line down the column with the center circle and circle the code.		
History	D or C	C	C	PF interval	EPF interval	D interval
Examination	D or C	C	C	PF	EPF	D
Complexity of medical decision	SF/L	M	H	SF/L	M	H
	99221 99218 99234	99222 99219 99235	99223 99220 99236	99231 99261	99232 99262	99233 99263

NURSING FACILITY

	Annual Assessment/Admission			Subsequent Nursing Facility		
	Old Plan Review	New Plan	Admission			
	If a column has 3 circles, draw a line down the column and circle the code OR find the column with the circle farthest to the left, draw a line down the column and circle the code.			If a column has 2 or 3 circles, draw a line down the column and circle the code OR draw a line down the column with the center circle and circle the code.		
History	D interval	D interval	C	PF interval	EPF interval	D interval
Examination	C	C	C	PF	EPF	D
Complexity of medical decision	SF/L	M to H	M to H	SF/L	M	M to H
	99301	99302	99303	99311	99312	99313

DOMICILIARY (REST HOME, CUSTODIAL CARE)

	New			Established		
	If a column has 3 circles, draw a line down the column and circle the code OR find the column with the circle farthest to the left, draw a line down the column and circle the code.			If a column has 2 or 3 circles, draw a line down the column and circle the code OR draw a line down the column with the center circle and circle the code.		
History	PF	EPF	D	PF interval	EPF interval	D interval
Examination	PF	EPF	D	PF	EPF	D
Complexity of medical decision	SF/L	M	H	SF/L	M	H
	99321	99322	99323	99331	99332	99333

LEVEL OF SERVICE

PF = Problem focused   EPF = Expanded problem focused   D = Detailed   C = Comprehensive
SF = Straightforward   L = Low   M = Moderate   H = High

TIME

If the physician documents total time and suggests that counseling or coordinating care dominates (more than 50%) the encounter, time may determine level of service. Documentation may refer to: prognosis, differential diagnosis, risks, benefits of treatment, instructions, compliance, risk reduction or discussion with another health care provider.

If all answers are "yes," may select level based on time.

Does documentation reveal total time	Time: Face-to-face in outpatient setting / Unit/floor in inpatient setting	❏ Yes	❏ No
Does documentation describe the content of counseling or coordinating care		❏ Yes	❏ No
Does documentation reveal that more than half of time was counseling or coordinating care		❏ Yes	❏ No

Figure 6.3 (*Continued*)

that should be selected with the code that has been reported. When the resulting codes are not the same, the auditor has uncovered a possible problem in interpreting the documentation guidelines.

Many practices use this type of audit tool to help them conduct audits in a standard way. These tools are distributed to physicians and staff members to develop internal audits, not to make initial code selections. An experienced medical insurance specialist may be responsible for using the audit tool to monitor completed claims and audit selected claims before they are released.

Auditing Example: Is It a Brief or Extended History of the Present Illness?

Selecting the Code

As part of selecting the correct E/M code, the coder (the physician or medical coder) determines the extent of history. The overall history is problem-focused, expanded problem-focused, detailed, or comprehensive. Part of determining this extent is based on the history of present illness (HPI). The HPI may include from none to eight factors in the patient's medical record:

- Location (where on the body the symptom is occurring)
- Quality (the character of the pain)
- Severity (the rank of the symptom or pain on a scale, such as 1 to 10)
- Duration (how long the symptom or pain has been present or how long it lasts when it occurs)
- Timing (when the symptom or pain occurs)
- Context (the situation that is associated with the pain or symptom, such as eating dairy products)
- Modifying factors (things done to make the pain or symptom change, such as using an ice pack for a headache)
- Associated signs and symptoms (other things that happen when this symptom or pain happens, such as "my chest pain makes me feel short of breath").

Depending on the count, the HPI is either brief or extended. A brief HPI has one to three of the elements. An extended HPI has at least four of the eight elements. The coder should make this judgment on the evidence in the patient's medical record, not on recollecting or making assumptions about what was actually done. (Remember, if it is not documented, it did not happen.)

Auditing the Code Selection

After the coding is done, the auditor examines the patient's medical record and analyzes the documentation. The HPI section at the top of Figure 6.3, which matches the Documentation Guidelines counts for HPI, is as follows:

HPI (history of present illness)				Brief	Extended
❏ Location	❏ Severity	❏ Timing	❏ Modifying factors	*1–3 elements*	*4–8 elements*
❏ Quality	❏ Duration	❏ Context	❏ Associated signs and symptoms		

Using this tool, the auditor checks off the appropriate items for HPI:

Patient's chief complaint: Right shoulder pain

History: The patient noted a sharp pain in the right shoulder about three days ago. The pain is worse when he lies on the arm.

Auditor's analysis: The HPI is extended; four elements are documented, as follows:

Location: Right shoulder

Quality: Sharp pain

Duration: Three days ago

Context: Worse when lies on arm

The auditor follows the form through all its elements to verify the overall selection of the Evaluation and Management code.

Thinking It Through—6.5

Refer to Figure 6.3(b) and read the instructions for Outpatient, Consults, and ER at the top and for the established patient section at the right. The instructions state: "If a column has 2 or 3 circles, draw a line down the column . . . and circle the code." In other words, for the established patient, it is not necessary to document the same level for all three components—history, examination, and decision making—to verify the code.

1. Why is this the case?

2. What code is correct for an established patient with a PF (problem-focused) result in the History column, an EPF (expanded problem-focused) result in the Examination column, and a L (low) result in the Complexity of Medical Decision Making column?

Review

Chapter Summary

1. Diagnoses and procedures must be correctly linked when services are reported for reimbursement, because payers analyze this connection to determine the medical necessity of the charges. Correct claims also comply with all applicable regulations and requirements. Codes should be appropriate and documented as well as compliant with each payer's rules.

2. The major laws and guidelines that regulate coding compliance include (a) federal laws, such as the False Claims Act (FCA) and HIPAA (Health Insurance Portability and Accountability Act); (b) the annual OIG Work Plan that pursues the goals of the Medicare Fraud and Abuse Initiative; (c) the advisory opinions, fraud alerts, and bulletins from OIG and CMS; (d) national Medicare regulations and code edits contained in the NCCI and local carriers' rules; and (e) private payers' code edits and regulations.

3. A number of billing practices are considered fraudulent when they are part of a repeated pattern, such as reporting services that were not performed, reporting at a higher level than performed, billing for procedures that were not medically necessary to treat the patient's condition, unbundling services, and repeat billing for the same service. Claims are rejected or downcoded because of (a) medical necessity errors, including poor linkage between procedures and conditions, services at an inappropriate level, and billing for experimental procedures; (b) coding errors such as truncated diagnosis codes and codes that lack proper documentation; and (c) errors related to billing, such as reporting uncovered services, using incorrect modifiers, and upcoding.

4. A medical practice compliance plan includes (a) the appointment of a compliance officer and committee, (b) a code of conduct for physicians' business arrangements and employees' compliance, (c) training plans, (d) properly prepared and updated coding tools such as job reference aids, encounter forms, and documentation templates, (e) rules for prompt identification and refunding of overpayments, and (f) ongoing monitoring and auditing of claim preparation. Each part of the plan addresses compliance concerns of government and private payers, and having a formal process in place is a sign that the practice has made a good-faith effort to achieve compliance in coding.

5. Payer audits are routine external audits that are conducted to ensure practice compliance with coding and billing regulations. Prospective internal audits help the practice reduce the possibility that claims will be rejected or downcoded due to coding compliance errors. Retrospective internal audits are used to analyze feedback from payers, identify problems, and address problems with additional training and better communication. E/M codes, because they are so frequently used, are an ongoing audit focus.

6. Practices should conduct internal audits of their E/M claims using audit tools based on the joint CMS/AMA Documentation Guidelines for Evaluation and Management Services. This audit process highlights possible problems the practice has with interpretation of the guidelines or with its documentation approach.

Key Terms

abuse *page 191*

advisory opinion *page 195*

assumption coding *page 200*

audit *page 193*

audit report *page 195*

code linkage *page 190*

compliance plan *page 202*

corporate integrity agreement *page 194*

documentation template *page 205*

downcode *page 200*

excluded parties *page 196*

external audit *page 206*

fraud *page 191*

Health Care Fraud and Abuse Control Program *page 193*

incident-to *page 195*

internal audit *page 207*

job reference aid *page 204*

Review Questions

Match the key terms in the left column with the definitions in the right column.

A. upcode

B. NCCI edits

C. truncated coding

D. advisory opinion

E. prospective audit

F. overpayment

G. code linkage

H. retrospective audit

I. downcode

J. OIG Work Plan

_____ 1. A payer's review and reduction of a procedure code to a lower value than reported by the provider

_____ 2. The OIG's annual list of planned projects under the Medicare Fraud and Abuse Initiative

_____ 3. The connection between the service or procedure that was performed and the patient's condition or illness

_____ 4. An internal audit conducted before claims are reported to payers

_____ 5. An improper or excessive payment to a provider as a result of billing or claims processing errors for which a refund is owed by the provider

_____ 6. An internal audit conducted after claims are processed by payers

_____ 7. Use of a procedure code that provides a higher reimbursement rate than the code for the service actually provided

_____ 8. A computerized screening system used to identify Medicare billing errors

_____ 9. Diagnosis codes that are not reported at the highest level of specificity available

_____ 10. An opinion issued by CMS or the OIG that becomes legal advice for the requesting party

Decide whether each statement is true or false, and write T for true or F for false.

_____ 1. Code linkage is analyzed to assess the patient's response to treatments.

_____ 2. The False Claims Act prohibits making a false statement to get a false claim paid by a government program.

_____ 3. Intent to commit fraud does not have to be proven in a False Claims Act case.

_____ 4. Under Medicare rules, no modifiers can be used with code combinations listed in the NCCI.

_____ 5. It is fraudulent to bill Medicare for a service that was not done.

_____ 6. Because the work was actually done, it is acceptable to change a date of service on a claim for a patient so that the charge is covered.

_____ 7. Federal agencies consider a compliance plan a sign of good-faith efforts by a practice to properly create claims.

_____ 8. Overpayments do not have to be repaid if they were received in the previous ninety-day period.

_____ 9. During an audit, all the claims from a particular period are usually examined.

_____ 10. Internal audits are a routine aspect of compliance plans.

Write the letter of the choice that best completes the statement or answers the question.

_____ 1. An OIG Fraud Alert
   A. informs practices about upcoming audits
   B. explains the Department of Justice's regulations
   C. advises practices about compliance problems the OIG has uncovered
   D. provides advice to individuals or business entities

_____ 2. The OIG Work Plan describes
   A. planned projects for investigating possible fraud in various billing areas
   B. legislative initiatives under HIPAA
   C. the FBI's investigations
   D. the current cases that are being prosecuted by the OIG's attorneys

_____ 3. Under Medicare's code edits, mutually exclusive codes
   A. can be billed together if they are component codes
   B. can be billed together if they have a -1 modifier code attached
   C. cannot be billed together for the same patient on the same day
   D. cannot be billed more than once by a single provider on the same date of service

_____ 4. Intentionally reporting a service at a higher level than was performed is a clear example of
   A. auditing   C. assumption coding
   B. poor coding linkage   D. fraud

_____ 5. Possible consequences of incorrect billing are
   A. downcoded claims   C. unlinked claims
   B. upcoded claims   D. code edits

_____ 6. A compliance plan often includes
   A. code edits, code of conduct, and advisory opinions
   B. code of conduct, ongoing training programs, and documentation procedures
   C. previous years' code reference manuals, encounter forms, and black box edits
   D. fraud alerts, regulations, and bulletins

_____ 7. Retrospective internal audits help determine
   A. patterns of rejected or downcoded claims
   B. problems with documentation
   C. training needs
   D. all the above

_____ 8. An encounter form containing E/M codes should list
   A. the most frequently billed codes
   B. just blanks, so the correct E/M code can be entered
   C. complete ranges of codes for each type or place of service listed
   D. none of the above

_____ 9. The E/M code audit tools are based on
   A. the documentation guidelines published by CMS and the AMA
   B. the advisory opinions published by the OIG
   C. the federal laws
   D. the OIG Work Plan

_____ 10. If a coder selects codes on the basis of the documentation, the auditor's findings generally should _____ the coder's.

A. disagree with
B. agree with
C. downcode
D. have no relationship to

Provide answers to the following questions in the spaces provided.

1. The abbreviation OIG stands for

2. The abbreviation NCCI stands for

Applying Your Knowledge

Case 6.1

Are the following procedure and diagnostic codes appropriately linked? If not, what is (are) the error(s)?

CPT	ICD-9-CM	LINKED?
1.	76091	V76.12
2.	99214	V54.8
3.	57284	601.1, 041.1
4.	96408	V58.1, 233.0
5.	99203, 72040, 73600	824.2, 847.0, E888, E849.4

Case 6.2

A forty-year-old established female patient is having an annual checkup. During the examination, her physician identifies a lump in her left breast. The physician considers this a significant finding and performs the key components of a problem-focused E/M service. These four codes and modifier should be reported. In what order should they be listed?

CPT codes: 99212, 99396
ICD codes: V70.0, 611.72
Modifier: –25

Computer Exploration

Internet Activity

1. The American Compliance Institute provides a forum for compliance officers to exchange information on compliance-related issues. Point your Web browser at
    http://www.compliance.com
   and research this site. What types of publications and newsletters are available?

2. Point your Web browser at the OIG Web site at

http://oig.hhs.gov/

a. Click "What's New." Select a recent audit and prepare a report summarizing its major points.

b. Using the search feature, locate the OIG Work Plan for either the current or the coming year. Report on five points listed under "Medicare Physicians and Other Health Professionals."

3. Visit the Web site that offers information and training on the National Correct Coding Initiative at

http://cms.hhs.gov/medlearn/ncci.asp

Research the frequently asked questions about Correct Coding Principles and Edits. How often are the NCCI edits updated?

4. Check the format of the NCCI edits as listed on the CMS Web site:

http://cms.hhs.gov/physicians/cciedits/default.asp

NDCMediSoft Activity

6.1. MultiLink Codes

The MultiLink feature allows several related procedure codes to be grouped into a single entry to speed data entry. For example, physical examinations typically include procedures such as blood work, urine analysis, and an ECG. Without MultiLink, the procedure codes for each of these services would have to be entered individually. MultiLink sets up one code that represents all these activities. Rather than entering each CPT code individually, the MultiLink code is selected, and the program automatically enters all the individual codes.

1. To view an example of a MultiLink code that is already set up in the Valley Associates, P.C., database, click MultiLink Codes on the Lists menu. The MultiLink List dialog box is displayed.

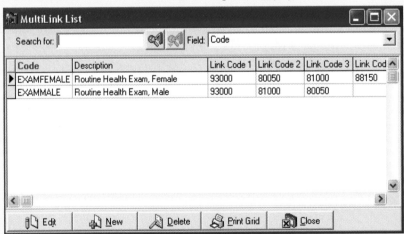

2. With the code EXAMFEMALE selected, click the Edit button. The MultiLink Code dialog box for EXAMFEMALE appears. This MultiLink code can be used to enter procedures commonly performed together when a woman visits the office for a routine physical examination. The procedure codes that are included in this MultiLink code are listed under the Link Codes section of the dialog box. In this example, the CPT codes are 93000, 80050, 81000, and 88150.

Computer Exploration

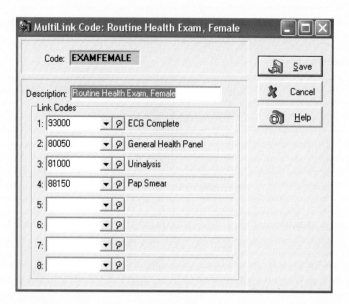

3. Click the Cancel button to exit the MultiLink Code dialog box.
4. Click the Close button to close the MultiLink List dialog box.
5. To see how a MultiLink code is entered in the Transaction Entry dialog box, click Enter Transactions on the Activities menu.
6. Key "JANSSR" in the Chart box, so that Robyn Janssen's chart number is highlighted, and then press Enter.
7. Notice Robyn Janssen's insurance (Tricare) and case (Absence of Menstruation) information are displayed in the top section of the Transaction Entry dialog box. No transactions have been entered yet in the Charges section.

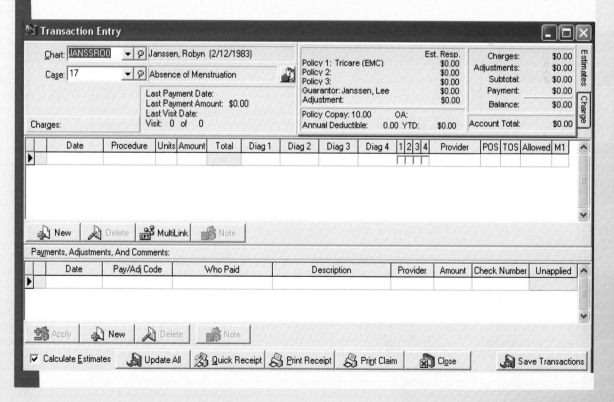

8. In the Charges section of the dialog box, click the MultiLink button. The MultiLink dialog box appears.

9. Click the triangle button to the right of the MultiLink Code box. The list of available MultiLink codes is displayed.

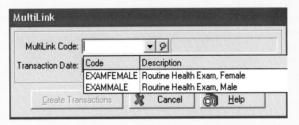

10. Click the EXAMFEMALE code. The EXAMFEMALE code appears in the MultiLink Code box. To enter the procedure codes associated with this code, click the Create Transactions button.

11. An Information dialog box appears, reminding you that a $10 copay is required for the visit. Click OK.

12. The program automatically enters CPT codes 93000, 80050, 81000, and 88150, saving you the time it would take to enter all four codes individually. This is the main advantage of using MultiLink codes when entering patient transactions.

13. Click the Close button to close the Transaction Entry dialog box without saving the transactions. When an Information dialog box displays the message, "There are transactions that are not saved. Save now?" click No.

6.2 Linking Procedure Codes and Diagnosis Codes

1. Select Enter Transactions on the Activities menu. The Transaction Entry dialog box is displayed.

2. Key "E" in the Chart box to highlight Wilma Estephan's chart number, and then press Enter.

3. Transaction information for Wilma Estephan is displayed. Notice that her case description, Hypertension, is displayed in the Case box.

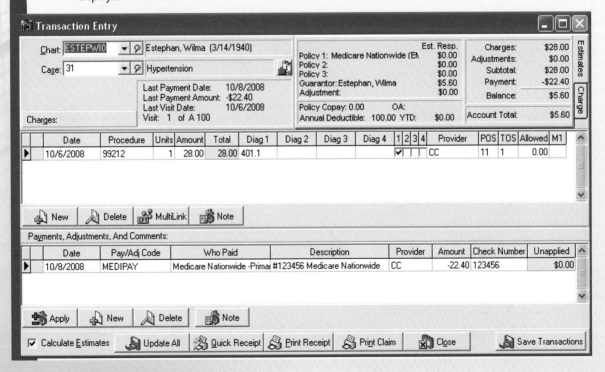

Computer Exploration

4. Look in the Charges section of the dialog box to locate the boxes labeled Diag 1, Diag 2, Diag 3, and Diag 4. This is where diagnosis codes are listed. MediSoft copies the information entered in the Diagnosis tab of the Case folder and displays it here in the Transaction Entry dialog box.
5. Notice that code 401.1 (Benign Essential Hypertension) is listed in the first diagnosis box, Diag 1. In the same transaction line, locate the CPT code for this charge, 99212 (EP Problem Focused).
6. To the right of the Diag 1, Diag 2, Diag 3, and Diag 4 boxes are four corresponding boxes labeled 1, 2, 3, and 4. A check mark in box 1 indicates that diagnosis code 1 is the diagnosis associated with procedure code 99212 in this transaction. If a patient had more than one diagnosis, whichever diagnosis was associated with a given procedure would be checked in the corresponding 1, 2, 3, or 4 box. If multiple diagnoses were connected to that procedure, more than one box would be checked. This is how MediSoft links procedure code entries with diagnosis codes in the Transaction Entry dialog box.
7. Click the Close button to close the Transaction Entry dialog box.

Part 3 Claims Processing

Provider Charges and Payment Methods

Objectives

After studying this chapter, you should be able to:

1. Compare the usual, customary, and reasonable (UCR) and the resource-based relative value scale (RBRVS) methods of determining fees for providers' services.

2. Describe the steps used to calculate RBRVS payments under the Medicare Fee Schedule.

3. Identify the three provider payment methods most payers use.

4. Discuss the calculation of payments for participating and nonparticipating providers, and describe how balance-billing regulations affect the charges that can be collected from patients.

5. List the types of charges for which patients may be responsible.

6. Describe the calculations and billing procedures for patient payments that are due at the time of service.

Introduction

"How much will my insurance pay?" "How much will I owe?" "Why are these doctor's fees different from my previous doctor's fees?" Questions such as these are handled by medical insurance specialists every day. Not only must they correctly prepare health care claims and encounter forms, but they often must also review patients' insurance coverage, estimate what charges payers will cover, review patients' insurance forms, and file claims on behalf of patients. To do these tasks, they need to be familiar with the way providers establish their fees and how payers set the maximum charges they pay for providers' services. Medical insurance specialists also collect some types of patient payments at the time of service—that is, when the patient and the provider have completed an encounter. This task involves knowledge of patients' financial responsibilities for services, how to calculate the charges that are due from patients, and how to communicate effectively with patients.

This chapter describes the types of providers' fee structures and the payment methods used by government and private payers. (Specific payers' policies are discussed in Chapters 10–14.) The chapter also covers how to calculate the charges that are collected from patients at the time of service and how to estimate those for which the patient will be billed.

Fee Structures

There are two main methods for determining fees: charge-based and resource-based. **Charge-based fee structures** are based on the fees that providers of similar training and experience have charged for similar services. **Resource-based fee structures** are built by comparing three factors: (1) how difficult it is for the provider to do the procedure, (2) how much office overhead the procedure involves, and (3) the relative risk that the procedure presents to the patient and to the provider.

Providers' Usual Fees

Physicians establish a list of their **usual fees** for the procedures and services they frequently perform. The usual fees are those that they charge to most of their patients most of the time under typical conditions. Exceptions to usual fees may be made. For example, workers' compensation patients often must be charged according to a state-mandated fee schedule (see Chapter 14).

The typical ranges of physicians' fees nationwide are published in commercial databases. For example, Figure 7.1 on page 224 shows the fees for a group of CPT codes from the surgical section. The first and second columns list the CPT code and a brief description of the service. The third, fourth, and fifth columns show the following amounts:

- *Column 3:* Half (50 percent) of the reported fees were higher than this fee, and the other half were lower. This is called the *midpoint* of the range.
- *Column 4:* One-quarter (25 percent) of the fees were higher than this fee, and three-quarters (75 percent) were lower.
- *Column 5:* Ten percent of the fees were higher than this fee, and 90 percent were lower.

For example, in Figure 7.1, CPT 29085, Application of hand/wrist cast, columns 3, 4, and 5 show the values $86, $111, and $136. This means that half

(1) CODE	(2) SHORT DESCRIPTION	(3) 50TH	(4) 75TH	(5) 90TH	(6) MFS	(7) RVU
APPLICATION OF CASTS AND STRAPPING						
29000	APPLICATION OF BODY CAST. HALO TYPE	478	617	753	151	4.12
29010	APPLY BODY CAST. RISSER JACKET	376	485	591	167	4.56
29015	APPLY BODY/HEAD CAST. RISSER JACKET	439	567	692	179	4.87
29020	APPLY BODY CAST, TURNBUCKLE JACKET	359	463	565	146	3.98
29025	APPLY BODY/HEAD CAST. TURNBUCKLE	384	496	605	113	3.09
29035	APPLY BODY CAST. SHOULDER TO HIPS	255	329	401	143	3.98
29040	APPLY BODY CAST. SHOULDER TO HIPS	339	438	534	160	4.36
29044	APPLY BODY CAST. SHOULDER TO HIPS	299	386	471	160	4.37
29046	APPLY BODY CAST. SHOULDER TO HIPS	324	419	511	176	4.80
29049	APPLY SHOULDER CAST. FIGURE-EIGHT	126	163	199	48	1.30
29055	APPLY SHOULDER CAST. SHOULDER SPICA	239	308	376	110	3.00
29058	APPLY SHOULDER CAST. VELPEAU	150	193	236	71	1.94
29065	APPLICATION OF LONG ARM CAST	122	157	191	63	1.73
29075	APPLICATION OF FOREARM CAST	95	121	147	52	1.42
29085	APPLICATION OF HAND/WRIST CAST	86	111	136	51	1.38
29105	APPLICATION OF LONG ARM SPLINT	82	106	129	51	1.38
29125	APPLY FOREARM SPLINT. STATIC	63	81	99	35	.96
29126	APPLY FOREARM SPLINT. DYNAMIC	109	140	171	43	1.17

Figure 7.1 Sample Physician Fee Database

Thinking It Through—7.1

Based on Figure 7.1:

1. Fifty percent of surveyed providers charged less than what amount for CPT 29044?

2. If four thousand providers were surveyed about their charges for CPT 29000, how many reported that they charged more than $617?

of the reporting providers charged less than $86 for this service, and half charged more. Three-quarters of the reporting providers charged less than $86 for this service, and half charged more. Three-quarters of the reporting providers charged less than $111 for this service, and 25 percent charged more. Ninety percent of the reporting providers charged less than $136, while only 10 percent charged more. (The sixth and seventh columns contain Medicare data, which is discussed in the RBRVS section below. That section also describes reasonable fees.)

In every geographic area, there is a normal range of fees for each procedure that is commonly performed. Different practices set their fees at some point along this range. For example, if the practice's physicians think that patients are willing to pay higher fees for their services—perhaps because of their unique qualifications or the equipment they have—they may set all fees at the high end of the ranges. Another practice may decide to set fees at the midpoint of each range. A practice that set its fees in the past and has not updated them may fall at the low end of the payment scale.

Usual, Customary, and Reasonable (UCR) Payment Structures

Third-party payers, too, must establish the rates they pay providers. Payers using a charge-based fee structure also analyze charges using one of the national databases. Each payer creates a schedule of UCR (for **usual, customary, and reasonable**) fees by determining the percentage of the published fee ranges that they will pay. For example, a payer may decide to pay all surgical procedures reported in a specific geographical area at the midpoint of each range.

These UCR fees, for the most part, accurately reflect prevailing charges. However, fees may not be available for new or rare procedures. Lacking better information, a payer may set too low a fee for such procedures.

Relative Value Scale (RVS)

Another payment structure is called a **relative value scale (RVS)**. Historically, the idea behind an RVS was that fees should reflect the relative difficulty of procedures. If most providers agreed that procedure A took more skill, effort, or time than procedure B, procedure A could be expected to have a higher fee than procedure B.

Although it is no longer used, the California Medical Association's *California Relative Value Studies*, published from 1956 to 1974, was the foundation for the RVS approach. Providers were interviewed to determine the amounts they had charged for each procedure. They were also asked how difficult each procedure was and how much risk the procedure presented to the patient and the provider. The results of the interviews were organized into a relative value scale.

In an RVS, each procedure in a group of related procedures is assigned a *relative value* in relation to a *base unit*. For example, if the base unit is 1 and these numbers are assigned—limited visual field examination 0.66; intermediate visual field examination 0.91; and extended visual field examination 1.33—the first two procedures are less difficult than the unit to which they are compared. The third procedure is more difficult. The relative value that is assigned is called the **relative value unit**, or **RVU**.

To calculate the price of each service, the relative value is multiplied by a **conversion factor**, which is a dollar amount that is assigned to the base unit. The conversion factor is increased or decreased each year so that it reflects changes in the cost of living index.

The *California Relative Value Studies* eventually came under federal scrutiny and ceased to be published. It was accused of being a price-fixing book created by providers for providers. Despite the problems with this study, the relative value scale is a useful concept. Unlike providers, software companies and publishers are not restricted from gathering and publishing fee information, so the national fee databases they produce now list both UCR fees and a relative value for each procedure. Payers and providers may use the RVS factor in setting their fees.

Case Example

The year's conversion factor is $35.27.
The relative value of an extended visual field examination is 1.33.
This year's price for the extended visual field examination = $35.27 × 1.33 = $46.90.

Resource-Based Relative Value Scale (RBRVS)

The payment system used by Medicare is called the **resource-based relative value scale (RBRVS)**. The RBRVS establishes relative value units for services. Medicare payments had been based on a Medicare-developed **reasonable fee** schedule that used historical charges. The RBRVS replaces providers' consensus on fees—the historical charges—with a relative value that is based on resources—what each service really costs to provide.

Below are sample relative value units and geographic practice cost indices from a Medicare Fee Schedule. The conversion factor for this particular year is $34.7315.

Sample RVUs

CPT/HCPCS	Description	Work RVU	Practice Expense RVU	Malpractice Expense RVU
33500	Repair heart vessel fistula	25.55	30.51	4.07
33502	Coronary artery correction	21.04	15.35	1.96
33503	Coronary artery graft	21.78	26	4.07
99203	OV new	1.34	0.64	0.05
99204	OV new	2.00	0.96	0.06

Sample GPCIs

Locality	Work GPCI	Practice Expense GPCI	Malpractice Expense GPCI
San Francisco, CA	1.067	1.299	0.667
Manhattan, NY	1.093	1.353	1.654
Columbus, Ohio	0.990	0.939	1.074
Galveston, TX	0.988	0.970	1.386

Calculate the expected payments for:

1. Office visit, new patient, detailed history/examination, low-complexity decision making, in Manhattan, NY _____

2. Coronary artery graft in San Francisco, CA _____

3. Repair heart vessel fistula in Columbus, OH _____

4. Coronary artery correction in Galveston, TX _____

There are three parts to an RBRVS fee:

1. *The nationally uniform relative value:* The relative value is based on three cost elements—the physician's work, the practice cost (overhead), and the cost of malpractice insurance. Another way of stating this is that every $1.00 of charge is made up of x cents for the physician's work, x cents for office expenses, and x cents for malpractice insurance. For example, the relative value for a simple office visit, such as to receive a flu shot, is much lower than the relative value for a complicated encounter such as the evaluation and management of uncontrolled diabetes in a patient. (Column 7 in Figure 7.1 lists the RVUs for procedures in Column 1.)

2. *A geographic adjustment factor:* A geographic adjustment factor called the **geographic practice cost index (GPCI)** is a number that is used to multiply each relative value element so that it better reflects a geographical area's relative costs. For example, the cost of the provider's work is

affected by average physician salaries in an area. The cost of the practice depends on things such as office rental prices and local taxes. Malpractice expense is also affected by where the work is done. The factor may either reduce or increase the relative values. For example, the GPCI lowers relative values in a rural area, where all costs of living are lower. A GPCI from a major city, where everything costs more, raises the relative values. In some states, a single GPCI applies; in others, different GPCIs are listed for large cities and other areas.

3. *A nationally uniform conversion factor:* A uniform conversion factor is a dollar amount used to multiply the relative values to produce a payment amount. It is used by Medicare to make adjustments according to changes in the cost of living index.

Note that when RBRVS fees are used, providers receive considerably lower payments than when UCR fees are used. On average, according to a study done by the Medicare Payment Advisory Commission, a nonpartisan federal advisory panel, private health plans' fees are about 15 percent higher than Medicare fees. (For example, compare Columns 3, 4, and 5 with Column 6 in Figure 7.1.)

Each part of the RBRVS—the relative values, the GPCI, and the conversion factor—is updated each year by CMS (Centers for Medicare and Medicaid Services). The year's **Medicare Fee Schedule (MFS)** is published by CMS in the *Federal Register.* The goal is for the net effect of all changes to be budget-neutral, meaning that the total that Medicare pays will not go over its budget for that year. If fees for family practitioners go up, for example, because the practice-expense component is valued at a higher level, this increase needs to be offset, such as by reducing practice-expense fees for surgeons.

Figure 7.2 illustrates the formula for calculating a Medicare payment. The following steps are involved:

Billing Tip

A Move to Resource-Based Fee Structures
Other payers consider resource-based fees that Medicare has implemented to be a fairer representation of the real costs involved in providing a medical service or procedure than charge-based fees. Charge-based fees represent what has historically been done, not a rationale for the way charges are set. For this reason, resource-based fee structures are increasingly used by many payers in addition to Medicare to establish what they pay for each CPT code. Because of this widespread use, providers are also changing from using a charge-based to a resource-based method to set or modify their practices' fee schedules.

Work RVU x Work GPCI = *W*
Practice-Expense RVU x Practice-Expense GPCI = *PE*
Malpractice RVU x Malpractice GPCI = *M*
Conversion Factor = *CF*

(*W* + *PE* + *M*) x *CF* = Payment

Example:

Work RVU = 6.39
Work GPCI = 0.998
6.39 x 0.998 = *W* = 6.37

Practice-Expense RVU = 5.87
Practice-Expense GPCI = 0.45
5.87 x 0.45 = *PE* = 2.64

Malpractice RVU = 1.20
Malpractice GPCI = 0.721
1.20 x 0.721 = *M* = 0.86

Conversion Factor = 34.54

(6.37 + 2.64 + 0.86) x 34.54 = $340.90 Payment

Figure 7.2 Medicare Physician Fee Schedule Formula

1. Determine the procedure code for the service.
2. Use the Medicare Fee Schedule to find the three RVUs—work, practice expense, and malpractice—for the procedure.
3. Use the Medicare GPCI list to find the three geographic practice cost indices (also for work, practice expense, and malpractice).
4. Multiply each RVU by its GPCI to calculate the adjusted value.
5. Add the three adjusted totals, and multiply the sum by the conversion factor to determine the payment.

Payment Methods

Most payers use one of three methods of paying providers:

1. Allowed charges
2. Contracted fee schedule
3. Capitation

Allowed Charges

Many payers set an **allowed charge** for each procedure or service. This amount is the most the payer will pay any provider for that work. The allowed charge is also called a maximum allowable fee, maximum charge, allowed amount, allowed fee, or allowable charge.

Whether a provider actually receives the allowed charge depends on three things:

1. *The provider's usual charge for the procedure or service:* The usual charge may be higher, equal to, or lower than the allowed charge.
2. *The provider's status in the particular plan or program:* The provider is either participating or nonparticipating (see Chapter 3). A participating provider (PAR) agrees to accept allowed charges—which are usually 25 to 50 percent lower than the provider's usual fees—in return for incentives to be part of the plan. For example, providers who are Medicare participants are paid faster than nonparticipating (nonPAR) providers.
3. *The payer's rules:* These rules govern whether the provider is permitted to bill a patient for the part of the charge that the payer does not cover.

When a payer has an allowed charge, it never pays more than this amount to a provider. If a provider's usual fee is higher, only the allowed charge is paid. If a provider's usual fee is lower, the payer reimburses that lower amount. The payer's payment is always the lower of the two amounts: the provider's charge or the allowable charge.

Example The payer's allowed charge for a new patient's evaluation and management (E/M) service (CPT 99204) is $160.

Provider A Usual Charge = $180   Payment = $160
Provider B Usual Charge = $140   Payment = $140

Whether a participating provider can bill the patient for the difference between a higher usual fee and a lower allowed charge—called **balance billing**—depends on the payer's rules. In most cases, participating providers may not balance bill the patient for the difference. Instead, the provider must **write off** the difference, meaning that the amount of the difference is subtracted from the patient's bill and never collected.

For example, Medicare-participating providers (see Chapter 11) may not receive an amount greater than the Medicare allowed charge that is based on the

Medicare Fee Schedule. Medicare is responsible for paying 80 percent of this allowed charge (after patients have met their annual deductible; see Chapter 11). Patients are responsible for the other 20 percent.

Example   A Medicare PAR provider reports a usual charge of $200 for a diagnostic flexible sigmoidoscopy (CPT 45330), and the Medicare allowed charge is $84. The provider must write off the difference between the two charges. The patient is responsible for 20 percent of the allowed charge, not of the provider's usual charge:

Provider's usual fee:	$200.00
Medicare allowed charge:	$ 84.00
Medicare pays 80 percent	$ 67.20
Patient pays 20 percent	$ 16.80

The total the provider can collect is $84. The provider must write off the difference between the usual fee and the allowed charge, $116.

A provider who does not participate in a private plan can usually balance bill patients. In this situation, if the provider's usual charge is higher than the allowed charge, the patient must pay the difference. However, Medicare and other government-sponsored programs have different rules for nonparticipating providers, as explained in Chapters 11–13.

Example

Payer policy: There is an allowed charge for each procedure. The plan provides a benefit of 100 percent of the provider's usual charges, up to this maximum fee. Provider A is a participating provider; Provider B does not participate and can balance bill. Provider A and Provider B both perform abdominal hysterectomies (CPT 58150). The policy's allowed charge for this procedure is $2,880.

Provider A (PAR)

Provider's usual charge	$3,100.00
Policy pays its allowed charge	$2,880.00
Provider writes off the difference between the usual charge and the allowed charge:	$ 220.00

Provider B (nonPAR)

Provider's usual charge	$3,000.00
Policy pays its allowed charge	$2,880.00
Provider bills patient for the difference between the usual charge and the allowed charge	$ 120.00 ($3,000.00 – $2,880.00)
There is no write-off	

Coinsurance provisions in many private plans provide for patient cost-sharing. Rather than paying the provider the full allowed fee, for example, a plan may require the patient to pay 25 percent, while the plan pays 75 percent. In this case, if a provider's usual charges are higher than the plan's allowed charge, the patient owes more for a service from a nonparticipating provider than from a participating provider. The calculations are explained below.

Example

Payer policy: A policy provides a benefit of 75 percent of the provider's usual charges, and there is a maximum allowed charge for each procedure. The patient is responsible for 25 percent of the maximum allowed charge. Balance billing is not permitted for plan participants.

Provider A is a participating provider, and Provider B is a nonparticipant in the plan. Provider A and Provider B both perform total abdominal hysterectomies (CPT 58150). The policy's allowed charge for this procedure is $2,880.00.

Provider A (PAR)	
Usual charge	$3,100.00
Policy pays 75 percent of its allowed charge	$2,160.00 (75% of $2,880.00)
Patient pays 25 percent of the allowed charge	$ 720.00 (25% of $2,880.00)
Provider writes off the difference between the usual charge and the allowed charge:	$ 220.00
Provider B (nonPAR)	
Usual charge	$3,000.00
Policy pays 75 percent of its allowed charge	$2,160.00 (75% of $2,880.00)
Patient pays for:	
(1) 25 percent of the allowed charge +	$ 720.00 (25% of $2,880.00)
(2) the difference between the usual charge and the allowed charge	$ 120.00 ($3,000.00 – $2,880.00)

Patient pays $840.00 ($720.00 + $120.00)
The provider has no write-off

Contracted Fee Schedule

Some payers, particularly PPOs and other types of managed care plans that contract directly with providers, establish fixed fee schedules with their participating providers. Based on their review of national databases of providers' fees and the Medicare Fee Schedule, they decide what they will pay for services in particular geographical areas. Their contracts stipulate these fixed fees for the procedures and services that the plan covers. In a particular geographical area, for example, the PPO sends practices a list of fixed fees for them to consider. If the providers join the PPO network, they enter into a contract to charge patients who are enrolled in that PPO according to that fee schedule. Large group practices may negotiate some changes to the fixed fees. Smaller practices usually must either accept the fees or not join the PPO.

When a provider is working under a contracted fee schedule, the payer's allowed charge and the provider's charge are the same. The terms of the plan determine what percentage of the charges, if any, the patients owe, and what percentage the payer covers. Participating providers can typically bill patients their usual charges for procedures and services that are not covered by the plan.

Capitation

The fixed prepayment for each plan member in capitation contracts (see Chapter 1), called the **capitation rate** or **cap rate**, is determined by the managed care plan that initiates contracts with providers. The plan first decides on the allowed charges for the contracted services and then analyzes the health-related characteristics of the plan's members. The plan calculates the number of times each age group and gender group of members is likely to use each of the covered services. For example, if the primary care provider (PCP) contract covers obstetrics and a large percentage of the group's members are young women who are likely to require services related to childbirth, the cap rate is higher than for a group of members containing a greater percentage of men, or of women in their forties or fifties who are not as likely to require obstetrics services.

The plan's contract with the provider lists the services and procedures that are covered by the cap rate. For example, a typical contract with a primary care provider might include the following services:

Preventive care: well-child care, adult physical exams, gynecological exams, eye exams, and hearing exams

Counseling and telephone calls

Office visits

Medical care: medical care services such as therapeutic injections and immunizations, allergy immunotherapy, electrocardiograms, and pulmonary function tests

Local treatment of first-degree burns, application of dressings, suture removal, excision of small skin lesions, removal of foreign bodies or cerumen from external ear

These services are covered in the per-member charge for each plan member who selects the PCP. This cap rate, usually a prepaid monthly payment (per member per month, or PMPM), may be a different rate for each category of plan member, as shown in Table 7.1, or an average rate. To set an average rate, the monthly capitation rate for each member profile is added, and the total is divided by the number of member profiles.

TABLE 7.1	Example of a Capitation Schedule
Member Profile	**Monthly Capitation Rate**
0–2 Years, M/F	$30.10
2–4 Years, M/F	$ 8.15
5–19 Years, M/F	$ 7.56
20–44 Years, M	$ 8.60
20–44 Years, F	$16.66
45–64 Years, M	$17.34
45–64 Years, F	$24.76
Over 65 Years, M, Non-Medicare	$24.22
Over 65 Years, F, Non-Medicare	$27.32
Over 65, M, Medicare Primary	$10.20
Over 65, F, Medicare Primary	$12.05

1. In Table 7.1, which category of plan member does the plan consider likely to use the most medical services in a given period? The fewest services?

2. If the capitation schedule in Table 7.1 is used to calculate an average payment per patient, what is the average cap rate?

Noncovered services can be billed to patients using the provider's usual rate. Plans often require the provider to notify the patient in advance that a service is not covered and to state the fee for which the patient will be responsible. Some managed care plans may also require a **provider withhold** from their participating providers. Under this provision of their contract with the provider, the plan withholds a percentage, such as 20 percent, from every payment to the provider. The amount withheld is supposed to be set aside in a fund to cover unanticipated medical expenses of the plan. At the close of a specified period, such as a year, the amount withheld is returned to the provider if the plan's financial goals have been achieved. Some plans pay back withholds depending on the overall goals of the plan, and some pay according to the individual provider's performance against goals.

Calculations of Patient Charges

The patients of medical practices have a variety of health plans, including managed care organizations (MCOs). Practices receive payments in various ways from patients and from this mixture of payers.

The Insured's Financial Responsibilities

Insured individuals have a variety of financial responsibilities (see Chapter 1) under their insurance plans. Usually, a periodic premium payment is required. There are five other types of payments that patients may be obligated to pay: deductibles, copayments, coinsurance, excluded and over-limit services, and balance billing.

Deductibles

Most payers require policyholders to pay a certain amount of covered expenses to providers before the insurance benefits begin. This amount is called the deductible, since it in effect is deducted from the benefits the insured receives (see Chapter 1). The deductible is due per time period, usually annually, starting at the beginning of the year. For example, a plan may require a patient to pay the first $200 of physician charges each year. Payments for **excluded services**—those that the policy does not cover—do not count toward a deductible. Some plans require an **individual deductible**, which must be met for each individual—whether the policyholder or a covered dependent—who has an encounter. In other cases, there is a **family deductible** that can be met by the combined payments to providers for any covered member(s) of the insured's family.

Copayments

Many health care plans require a patient copayment (copay). Copayments are always due and collected at the time of service. Copayments may be different for various types of services. Usually, they are stated as a dollar amount, such as $15 for an office visit or $10 for a prescription drug.

Coinsurance

Many payers require coinsurance, a specific ratio (percentage) of benefits that the insured pays to the provider after the deductible is met. For example, the coinsurance may be stated as a ratio of 80–20. In that case, after the deductible is met, the insured must pay 20 percent of the covered medical benefits to the provider, and the payer pays the other 80 percent. Noncapitated health care plans such as PPOs usually require patients to pay a greater percentage of the charges of out-of-network providers than of plan providers.

Excluded and Over-Limit Services

All payers require patients to pay for excluded (noncovered) services. Providers generally can charge their usual fees for these services. Likewise, in managed care plans that set limits on the annual (or other period) usage of covered services, patients are responsible for usage beyond the allowed number. For example, if one preventive physical examination is permitted annually, additional preventive examinations are paid for by the patient.

Balance Billing

Patients may be responsible for the amount of the usual charge that exceeds the payer's allowed charge.

Limits on Patients' Charges and Possible Reimbursements

The deductibles, coinsurance, and copayments that patients pay to providers in relation to covered expenses are referred to as the insured's out-of-pocket expenses. Some insurance plans state a maximum amount that an insured has to pay before the plan begins to cover 100 percent of the charges. This protects the insured against catastrophic loss—a financially ruinous charge. For example, a plan may state that it pays all out-of-pocket expenses of the insured that are more than $2,500.

On the other hand, most payers' plans set a **maximum benefit limit**, which is a total amount that will be paid for each covered person's covered expenses over the course of the person's lifetime. For example, the plan may state that the maximum benefit limit is $2,000,000, meaning that the plan will not make payments totaling more than this amount on behalf of the insured. Beyond this total, the insured is responsible for payment.

Charges Due at Time of Service Versus Charges Billed

Medical practices must succeed in two ways: They must satisfy their patients, and they must make a profit. From a business point of view, the sooner fees are collected—from both patients and payers—the better the practice's cash flow. That is, in order to pay ongoing expenses, such as rent for the office and the salaries of everyone who works in the practice, cash must be available. For this

Billing Tip

Collecting Copays
Many offices tell patients who are scheduling a visit what copays they will owe at the time of service.

Billing Tip

Multiple Copayments
When patients receive more than one covered service in a single day, their health plan may permit multiple copayments. For example, copays for an annual physical exam and for lab tests may both be due from the patient. The health plan contract or policy should be reviewed to determine whether multiple copays can be collected on the same day of service.

reason, practices collect patient charges at the time of service when it is possible to do so. (As covered in Chapter 8, they also process claims as quickly and efficiently as possible.)

These types of patient charges are customarily collected at the time of service:

- Copayments
- Usual fees for services that are excluded under the patient's plan
- Usual fees for services to patients performed by nonparticipating providers (except for government-sponsored programs) and HMO out-of-network providers

To collect other patient charges, each practice has to determine the best way to handle the process. There are two options:

1. *Collect at the time of service:* Calculate charges based on the usual fees, and collect payment from patients before insurance claims are adjudicated and the payers' reimbursements are received.
2. *Bill after claims processing:* Submit insurance claims for charges based on the usual fees, and bill patients after insurance claims are adjudicated and reimbursements are received.

The first option has the advantage of producing payments from patients faster. It has two drawbacks, however. First, to calculate an accurate amount due from the patient, the medical insurance specialist must spend considerable time researching whether the patient's deductible has been met, the coinsurance rate, and the policy's exclusions. There may not be enough time to do this research while the patient is in the office. Second, even when this information is obtained, the eventual reimbursement may differ from the amount expected; the payer may, in fact, reduce or deny the claim. If patients' payments are collected before claims adjudication, the patient must often be billed again (or sent a refund) after the payer's explanations of what it paid or rejected are received, requiring more staff time and risking irritating or frustrating the patient.

The second option ensures that patients are billed correctly. Although it delays the patient's payment, it also reduces the amount of staff time required to create the claim and does not create the need to send a refund to the patient.

For these reasons, most practices do not collect patient coinsurance charges at the time of service. Usually, patients are billed after payers' reimbursements are received (see Chapter 9). However, some practices do collect patient deductibles. This policy creates some overbilling situations during the first months of the year. Because a patient often sees more than one provider in the time period, the deductible may be collected by each provider and need to be refunded after the claims for the period are adjudicated.

Communications with Patients About Charges

When patients have encounters with a provider who participates in the plan under which they have coverage—such as a Medicare-participating (PAR) provider—they generally sign an assignment of benefits statement (see Chapter 3). When this occurs, the provider agrees to **acceptance of assignment** for the patients, which is usually expressed as "we accept assignment." The provider files insurance claims for patients, receives payments directly from the payers, and agrees to accept a payer's allowed charge. Patients are billed for charges that payers deny or do not pay. When patients have encounters with nonparticipating (nonPAR) providers, the procedure is usually different. To avoid the difficulty of collecting payments at a later date from a patient, practices may either

(1) require the patient to assign benefits or (2) require payment in full at the time of services.

Many times, patients want to know what their bills will be. To estimate these charges, the medical insurance specialist verifies:

- The patient's deductible amount and whether it has been paid in full, the covered benefits, and coinsurance or other patient financial obligations
- The payer's allowed charges for the services that the provider anticipates providing

If the patient's request comes after the encounter, the medical insurance specialist can use the encounter form to tell the payer what CPT codes are going to be reported on the patient's claim to learn the likely payer reimbursement.

Patients should always be reminded of their financial obligations under their plans, including claim denials, according to practice procedures. The practice's financial policy regarding payment for services is usually either displayed on the wall of the reception area or included in a new patient information packet. The policy should explain what is required of the patient and when payment is due. For example, the policy may state:

> *For unassigned claims:* Payment for the physician's services is expected at the end of your appointment, unless you have made other arrangements with our practice manager.
>
> *For assigned claims:* After your insurance claim is processed by your insurance company, you will be billed for any amount you owe. You are responsible for any part of the charges that are denied or not paid by the carrier. All patient accounts are due within thirty days of the date of the invoice you receive.
>
> *For HMO members:* Copayments must be paid before patients leave the office.

If patients have large bills that they must pay over time, a financial arrangement for a series of payments may be made (see Figure 7.3 on page 236). Such arrangements usually require the approval of the practice manager. They may also be governed by state laws.

It is also good practice to notify patients in advance of the probable cost of procedures that are not going to be covered by their plan. For example, many private plans, as well as Medicare, do not pay for most preventive services, such as annual physical examinations (see Chapters 10–14). Many patients, however, consider preventive services a good idea and are willing to pay for them. Patients should be asked to agree in writing to pay for such noncovered services. A letter of agreement (see Figure 7.4 on page 237) should also specify why the service will not be covered and the cost of the procedure.

Payment Methods: Cash, Check, Credit or Debit Card

The medical insurance specialist handles patients' payments as follows:

- *Cash:* If payment is made by cash, a receipt is issued.
- *Check:* If payment is made with a check, the amount of the payment and the check number are entered on the encounter form, and a receipt is offered.
- *Credit or debit card:* If payment is made with a credit or debit card, the card slip is filled out, and the card is passed through the card reader. A transaction authorization number is received from the card issuer, and the approved card slip is signed by the person paying the bill. Patients are usually offered a receipt in addition to the copy of the credit card sales slip. Telephone approval may be needed if the amount of payment is over a specified limit.

Compliance Guideline

Collecting Charges
Some managed care plans and some private payers do not permit providers to collect any charges except copayments from patients until insurance claims are adjudicated.

Billing Tip

Charging When Patients Have Not Received the Service
A participating provider may not charge a patient for a product used to set up a procedure when the patient cancels and does not have the procedure. A physician may bill only for a rendered service, not for an anticipated service that is not delivered, including cancellations and no-shows. In nonparticipating situations, having patients agree in writing to pay before scheduling procedures gives them appropriate advance warning of their responsibility for payment. Usually, however, the likelihood of actually collecting the fee is small, and most practices therefore do not bill for no-shows or cancellations.

Patient Name and Account Number

Total of All Payments Due

FEE $_____
PARTIAL PAYMENT $_____
UNPAID BALANCE $_____
AMOUNT FINANCED $_____   (amount of credit we have provided to you)
FINANCE CHARGE $_____   (dollar amount the interest on credit will cost)
ANNUAL PERCENTAGE RATE $_____   (cost of your credit as a yearly rate)
TOTAL OF PAYMENTS DUE $_____   (amount paid after all payments are made)

Rights and Duties

I (we) have reviewed the above fees. I agree to make _____ payments in monthly
installments of $ _____, due on the _____ day of each month payable to _____,
until the total amount is paid in full. The first payment is due on _____. I may
request an itemization of the amount financed.

Delinquent Accounts

I (we) understand that I am financially responsible for all fees as stated. My account
will be overdue if my scheduled payment is more than 7 days late. There will be a
late payment charge of $_____ or _____% of the payment, whichever is less. I
understand that I will be legally responsible for all costs involved with the collection
of this account including all court costs, reasonable attorney fees, and all other expenses
incurred with collection if I default on this agreement.

Prepayment Penalty

There is no penalty if the total amount due is paid before the last scheduled payment.

I (we) agree to the terms of the above financial contract.

_____   _____
Signature of Patient, Parent or Legal Representative   Date

_____   _____
Witness   Date

_____   _____
Authorizing Signature   Date

Figure 7.3 Financial Arrangement for Professional Services Rendered Form

Some practices ask patients who want to use a credit or debit card to complete a preauthorization form (see Figure 7.5). The authorization should be renewed according to practice policy.

Walkout Receipts

If the provider has not accepted assignment and is not going to file a claim for a patient, the billing program is used to create a walkout receipt for the patient. The walkout receipt summarizes the services and charges for that day, as well as any payment the patient made (see Figure 7.6 on page 238). Practices generally handle unassigned claims in one of two ways:

Service to be performed: _____

Estimated charge: _____

Date of planned service: _____

Reason for exclusion: _____

_____

I, _____, a patient of _____, understand the service described above is excluded from my health insurance. I am responsible for payment in full of the charges for this service.

Figure 7.4 Sample Agreement for Patient Payment of Excluded Services

Provider's name:_____

Provider's tax ID no.: _____

I assign my insurance benefits to the provider listed above. This credit card authorization form is valid for one year unless I cancel the authorization through written notice to the provider.

_____   _____
Patient name   Cardholder name

_____
Billing address

_____   _____ _____
City   State   Zip

_____   _____
Credit card account number   Expiration date

_____   _____
Cardholder signature   Date

I authorize _____ (provider) to keep my signature/account number on file and to charge my American Express/ Discover/Visa/Mastercard/Other credit card account number listed above for the balance of charges not paid by insurance within 90 days and not to exceed $_____.

Figure 7.5 Preauthorized Credit Card Payment Form

1. The payment is collected from the patient at the time of service (at the end of the encounter), and the walkout receipt is used by the patient to report the charges and payments to the insurance company. The insurance company repays the patient (or insured) after the deductible is met, according to the terms of the plan.

Valley Associates, P.C.
1400 West Center Street
Toledo, OH 43601-0123
(555)321-0987

Page: 1

10/1/2008

Patient:	Walter Williams
	17 Mill Rd
	Brooklyn, OH 44144-4567
Chart #:	WILLIWA0
Case #:	8

Instructions:
Complete the patient information portion of your insurance claim form. Attach this bill, signed and dated, and all other bills pertaining to the claim. If you have a deductible policy, hold your claim forms until you have met your deductible. Mail directly to your insurance carrier.

Date	Description	Procedure	Modify	Dx 1	Dx 2	Dx 3	Dx 4	Units	Charge
10/1/2008	EP Problem Focused	99212		401.1	780.7			1	46.00
10/1/2008	ECG Complete	93000		401.1	780.7			1	70.00
10/1/2008	Aetna Copayment Charge	AETCOPAY		401.1	780.7			1	15.00
10/1/2008	Aetna Copayment	AETCPAY						1	-15.00

Provider Information	
Provider Name:	Christopher Connolly M.D.
License:	37C4629
Commercial PIN:	
SSN or EIN:	16-1234567

Total Charges:	$ 131.00
Total Payments:	-$ 15.00
Total Adjustments:	$ 0.00
Total Due This Visit:	**$ 116.00**
Total Account Balance:	$ 116.00

Assign and Release: I hereby authorize payment of medical benefits to this physician for the services described above. I also authorize the release of any information necessary to process this claim.

Patient Signature: _____   Date: _____

Figure 7.6 Example of Walkout Receipt

2. The payment is collected from the patient at the time of service, and the practice sends a claim to the insurance company on behalf of the patient. The insurance company sends a check to the patient with an explanation of benefits, and sends a copy of the EOB to the provider.

In some cases, patients arrange to be billed for payments due. In this case, the billing program issues an invoice when the practice's bills are generated (see Chapter 9).

When patients' charges and payments have been entered, the billing program updates the patient ledger (see Chapter 3). When insurance payments are received by the medical practice for patients with reimbursement plans, those payments are posted to the patient's account, and necessary write-offs are handled. This process is covered in Chapter 9.

Management of the Fee Schedule

Medical practices are challenged to set fees that are both competitive for their area—that is, in line with patients' expectations—and at the maximum permitted by government and private payers. Setting and maintaining a practice's

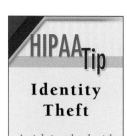

HIPAA Tip

Identity Theft

A risk involved with credit card use is identity theft. The HIPAA Security Rule requires medical practices to protect patients' credit card information when this payment method is used.

Medical billing managers, also called billing supervisors, supervise a staff of medical billers and collections specialists. Billing managers may be employed by medical group practices, hospitals, managed care organizations, and other facilities.

Medical billing managers are responsible for the quality and quantity of the billing work that is done. They must have excellent supervisory skills, including interviewing, hiring, and evaluating staff as well as planning the staff's workload, assigning tasks, and following up on completion and reviewing progress. Billing managers need strong computer applications skills and analytical ability in order to monitor accounts receivable. They are also required to know collection procedures, diagnostic and procedural coding, and reimbursement under both fee-for-service and capitation contracts. Excellent communication and human relations skills are needed to resolve payer-related issues. Managers also educate physicians and other staff members about reimbursement issues and compliance requirements. They may be assigned to monitor fee schedules and to check the reimbursement sections of managed care contracts.

Successful experience as a medical biller and additional college education in accounting, management, and supervision are often required for the position of billing manager. Employers in specialized areas such as ophthalmology or radiology billing prefer candidates with a billing background in the medical specialty.

list of fees is a complex and ongoing process. The physicians or practice managers analyze the rates charged by other providers in the area, what government programs pay, and the payment policies of insurance carriers and managed care plans in order to develop the list of fees.

To keep track of whether the practice's fees are correctly set, the practice manager may analyze reports from the billing program. These reports indicate the most frequently performed services (say, the top twenty procedures) and the providers' fees for them. This list is compared to the charges that payers pay. If the providers' fees are always paid in full, that is an indication that the fees are set too low—below payers' maximum allowable charges. If all fees are reduced by payers, this may indicate that the fees are set too high. When the practice feels that fees are regularly too high or too low, the usual fee structure can be adjusted accordingly.

Medical insurance specialists update the practice's fee schedules when new codes are released. When new or altered CPT codes are among those the practice reports, the fees related to them must be updated, too. For example, if the definition of a surgical package changes, a surgeon's fees need to be altered to tie exactly to the revised elements of the package. Or a new procedure may need to be included. Providers may refer to the UCR national databases or, more likely, review those databases and the Medicare Fee Schedule in order to establish the needed new fees.

1. A patient's insurance policy states:

   Annual deductible: $300.00

   _____

   Coinsurance: 70–30

   _____

   This year, the patient has made payments totaling $533.00 to all providers. Today, the patient has an office visit (fee: $80.00). The patient presents a credit card for payment of today's bill. What is the amount that the patient should pay?

2. A patient is a member of a health plan with a 15 percent discount from the provider's usual fees and a $10.00 copay. The days' charges are $480.00. What are the amounts that the HMO and the patient each pay?

3. A patient is a member of a health plan that has a 20 percent discount from the provider and a 15 percent copay. If the day's charges are $210.00, what are the amounts that the HMO and the patient each pay?

4. In your opinion, how should providers go about setting their usual fees? What factors might justify setting charges at the upper end of the fee range?

Review

Chapter Summary

1. Fee structures for providers' services are either charge-based or resource-based. Charge-based structures, such as UCR (usual, customary, and reasonable), are based on the fees that many providers have charged for similar services. Relative value scales (RVS) account for the relative difficulty of procedures by comparing the skill involved in each of a group of procedures. An RVS is charge-based if the charges that are attached to the relative values are based on historical fees. Resource-based relative value scales (RBRVS), such as the Medicare Fee Schedule, are built by comparing three cost factors: (a) how difficult it is for the provider to do the procedure, (b) how much office overhead the procedure involves, and (c) the relative risk that the procedure presents to the patient and the provider. Both charge-based and resource-based fee structures are affected by the geographical area in which the service is provided.

2. The following steps are used to calculate RBRVS payments under the Medicare Fee Schedule: (a) determine the procedure code for the service; (b) use the Medicare Fee Schedule to find the three RVUs—work, practice expense, and malpractice—for the procedure; (c) use the Medicare GPCI list to find the three geographic practice cost indices (also for work, practice expense, and malpractice); (d) multiply each RVU by its GPCI to calculate the adjusted value; (e) add the three adjusted totals, and multiply the sum by the annual conversion factor to determine the payment.

3. Most third-party payers use one of three provider payment methods: allowed charges, contracted fee schedules, or capitation. When a maximum allowed charge is set by a payer for each service, if a provider's usual fee is greater, the provider does not receive the difference from the payer. If the provider participates in the patient's plan, the difference is written off; if the provider does not participate, the plan's rules on balance billing determine whether the patient is responsible for the amount. Under a contracted fee schedule, the allowed charge for each service is all that the payer or the patient pays; no additional charges can be collected. Under capitation, the health care plan sets a capitation rate that pays for all contracted services to enrolled members for a given period.

4. Payments to participating providers are limited to the allowed charge. Some part of that amount is paid by the payer and some part by the patient according to the coinsurance provisions of the plan. Nonparticipating providers in most private plans (but not government-sponsored plans) can collect their usual fees, even when they are higher than the allowed charge, by receiving the specified part of the allowed charge from the payer and the rest of the allowed charge, plus the balance due resulting from a lower allowed charge and a higher usual charge, from the patient.

5. Patients may be responsible for copayments, excluded services, over-limit usage, and coinsurance. Patients often must meet deductibles before receiving benefits. Under some conditions, patients may also be obligated to pay the difference between a higher provider usual fee and a lower payer allowed charge.

6. Although collecting charges from patients at the time of service improves cash flow, many practices do not do so because calculation is complicated and prone to error. Some types of payments, however, such as copayments and charges when a patient has not assigned benefits or for excluded services, are often collected at the time of service. Practices inform patients about their financial responsibilities in general, and usually notify patients in writing about the costs of procedures that are not covered by a payer. Patients' payments are entered into the patient billing system to update the patient ledger.

Key Terms

acceptance of assignment *page 234*
allowed charge *page 228*
balance billing *page 228*
capitation rate (cap rate) *page 231*
charge-based fee structure *page 223*
conversion factor *page 225*
excluded service *page 232*
family deductible *page 232*

geographic practice cost index (GPCI) *page 226*
individual deductible *page 232*
maximum benefit limit *page 233*
Medicare Fee Schedule (MFS) *page 227*
provider withhold *page 232*
reasonable fee *page 225*
relative value scale (RVS) *page 225*

relative value unit (RVU) *page 225*
resource-based fee structure *page 223*
resource-based relative value scale (RBRVS) *page 225*
usual, customary, and reasonable (UCR) *page 225*
usual fee *page 223*
write off *page 228*

Review Questions

Match the key terms in the left column with the definitions in the right column.

A. provider withhold

B. excluded service

C. capitation rate

D. usual fee

E. allowed charge

F. acceptance of assignment

G. balance billing

H. write-off

I. conversion factor

J. individual deductible

_____ 1. Fee for a service or procedure that is charged by a provider for most patients under typical circumstances

_____ 2. The maximum charge allowed by a payer for a specific service or procedure

_____ 3. If the provider's usual fee is higher than the payer's allowed charge, the provider collects the difference from the insured, rather than writing it off

_____ 4. The amount that a participating provider must deduct from a patient's account because of a contractual agreement to accept a payer's allowed charge

_____ 5. The contractually set periodic prepayment amount to a provider for specified services to each enrolled plan member

_____ 6. A participating physician's agreement to accept the allowed charge as payment in full

_____ 7. A service specified in a medical insurance contract as not covered

_____ 8. Amount that each insured person must pay annually before receiving benefits from a payer

_____ 9. An amount withheld from a provider's payment by a managed care plan under contractual terms; may be repaid to the provider after a specified period if stated requirements are met

_____ 10. Dollar amount used to multiply a relative value unit to arrive at a charge

Decide whether each statement is true or false, and then write T for true or F for false.

_____ 1. Resource-based fee structures are based on the procedure's difficulty, the practice expense it involves, and the risk it entails.

_____ 2. The Medicare Fee Schedule is based on the UCR method of setting charges.

_____ 3. The geographic practice cost index (GPCI) is used to adjust each of the cost elements when a Medicare charge is calculated.

_____ 4. The Medicare Fee Schedule's conversion factor is set for a one-year period.

_____ 5. If a provider's usual fee is higher than a payer's allowed charge, the higher of the two fees is paid.

_____ 6. If a payer's allowed charge is higher than a provider's usual fee, the higher of the two fees is paid.

_____ 7. If a payer does not permit a provider to balance bill a patient, the provider must write off the difference between the usual fee and the amount paid.

_____ 8. Managed care capitation rates are based on the services that the group of members is likely to use.

_____ 9. Providers send bills to patients for copayments.

_____ 10. Insurance plans may protect insured individuals against catastrophic loss by setting a limit on out-of-pocket expenses.

Write the letter of the choice that best completes the statement or answers the question.

_____ 1. Usual, customary, and reasonable (UCR) fees are based on
   A. relative values
   B. historical charges
   C. practice expense
   D. malpractice

_____ 2. A provider's usual fees are those that are charged to
   A. patients who pay cash
   B. managed care patients
   C. most patients
   D. workers' compensation patients

_____ 3. Based on the RVU table on page 226, the smallest cost element in most Medicare RBRVS fees is
   A. malpractice expense
   B. practice expense
   C. work expense
   D. customary expense

_____ 4. In calculations of RBRVS fees, the three relative value units are multiplied by
   A. their respective geographic practice cost indices
   B. the neutral budget factor
   C. the national conversion factor
   D. the UCR factor

_____ 5. Medicare typically pays for what percentage of the allowed charge?
   A. 50 percent
   B. 60 percent
   C. 70 percent
   D. 80 percent

_____ 6. If a participating provider's usual fee is $400 and the allowed amount is $350, what amount is written off?
   A. zero
   B. $25
   C. $50
   D. $75

_____ 7. If a nonparticipating provider's usual fee is $400, the allowed amount is $350, and balance billing is permitted, what amount is written off?
   A. zero
   B. $25
   C. $50
   D. $75

_____ 8. If a nonparticipating provider's usual fee is $400, the allowed amount is $350, and balance billing is not permitted, what amount is written off?
   A. zero
   B. $25
   C. $50
   D. $75

_____ 9. The usual fees for excluded services are
   A. written off
   B. collected at the time of service
   C. subtracted from the annual deductible
   D. subject to balance billing rules

10. Types of charges that patients are responsible for include
    A. copayments, malpractice expense, balance bills, deductibles, and coinsurance
    B. copayments, deductibles, coinsurance, balance bills, and excluded services
    C. copayments, capitation rates, practice expense, malpractice expense, and excluded services
    D. copayments, withholds, deductibles, coinsurance, and excluded services

Provide answers to the following questions in the spaces provided.

1. What is the formula for calculating a RBRVS charge using the Medicare Fee Schedule?

_____

_____

_____

2. Define the following abbreviations:

A. GPCI _____

B. MFS _____

C. UCR _____

D. RVS _____

E. RBRVS _____

Applying your Knowledge

Case 7.1

Using the sample relative value units and GPCIs shown on page 226, and the conversion factor of $34.7315, calculate the expected charge for each of the following services:

A.   CPT 99204 in Galveston, TX

B.   CPT 33502 in Manhattan, NY

C.   CPT 99203 in Columbus, OH

Case 7.2

Dr. Mary Mandlebaum is a PAR provider in Medicare and in Mountville Health Plan, which has allowed charges for services and does not permit balance billing of plan members. She is not a PAR provider in the Ringdale Medical Plan. Based on the following table of charges, calculate the charges that the payer and the patient will pay in each of the situations. Show your calculations.

Service	CPT	Usual Charge	Mountville Health Plan Allowed Charge	Medicare Allowed Charge
Office/Outpatient Visit, New, Min.	99201	$54	$48	$43
Office/Outpatient Visit, New, Low	99202	$73	$65	$58
Office/Outpatient Visit, New, Mod.	99203	$100	$89	$80
Office/Outpatient Visit, New, Mod.	99204	$147	$129	$116
Office/Outpatient Visit, New, High	99205	$190	$168	$151
Office/Outpatient Visit, Est., Min.	99211	$29	$26	$22
Office/Outpatient Visit, Est., Low	99212	$44	$39	$35
Office/Outpatient Visit, Est., Mod.	99213	$60	$54	$48
Office/Outpatient Visit, Est., Mod.	99214	$87	$78	$70
Office/Outpatient Visit, Est., High	99215	$134	$119	$107
Rhythm ECG with Report	93040	$30	$36	$30
Breathing Capacity Test	94010	$83	$69	$58
DTAP Immunization	90700	$102	$87	$74

A. Insurance Plan: Mountville Health Plan; patient has met annual deductible of $250; 80–20 coinsurance

Services: CPT 99203, 90700

Payer Reimbursement:_____ Patient Charge:_____

B. Insurance Plan: Mountville Health Plan; patient has paid $125 toward an annual deductible of $500; 80–20 coinsurance

Services: CPT 99215, 93040, 94010

Payer Reimbursement:_____ Patient Charge:_____

C. Insurance Plan: Ringdale Medical Plan A; no deductible or coinsurance; copayment of $5/PAR; $25/NonPAR

Services: CPT 99212

Payer Reimbursement:_____ Patient Charge:_____

D. Insurance Plan: Ringdale Medical Plan B; patient has met annual deductible of $300; 80–20 coinsurance

Services: CPT 99215

Payer Reimbursement:_____ Patient Charge:_____

E. Insurance Plan: Medicare; annual deductible has been met by patient

Services: CPT 99213, 93040

Payer Reimbursement:_____ Patient Charge:_____

Computer Exploration

1. Point your Web browser at the CMS Web site at
     http://www.cms.hhs.gov/physicians/mpfsapp
   Read and accept the CPT copyright notice and then click start on the Medicare Physician Payment Systems page.
     After selecting Single HCPC Code and RVU, accept Default on the next screen. When prompted, enter 10021 for the code and select All Modifiers. You should view three records. Report on your findings. Confirm that the RVUs for the modifiers "TC" and –26" add to the total RVUs for the code.

2. Visit the CMS Web site that describes the process involved with setting the annual conversion factor at
     http://www.cms.hhs.gov/providers/sgr
   Research the current year's Conversion Factor for the Medicare Fee Schedule. (*Hint:* The conversion factor is shown near the end of the document.) Using this current factor, recalculate the math in Figure 7.2 to find the payment for this year.

3. The American Medical Association is a part of the process involved with setting the relative value units (RVUs) for CPT codes. Visit the organization's Web site at
     http://ama-assn.org/
   Using the Search feature, find "Fees" and locate "Opinions on Fees and Charges." Research and report on a topic of your selection.

NDCMediSoft Activity

7.1 Review Setup of Payment Codes in MediSoft

A number of different codes are used to enter payments in MediSoft. Different codes are used for entering payments made by insurance carriers and payments made by patients. These codes are set up in the Procedure/Payment/Adjustment dialog box—the same dialog box that lists all the procedures currently in the database.

1. Select Procedure/Payment/Adjustment Codes on the Lists menu. The Procedure/Payment/Adjustment List dialog box appears.
2. The Search For box at the top can be used to search for a specific code or a specific set of codes that begin with the same prefix. From an earlier activity, the Field box to the right of the Search For box may be set to Description. If so, click the triangle button in the Field box, and then select Code 1 from the dropdown list so that MediSoft will search by code.
3. Key "ANT" in the Search For box. A list of four accounting codes for Anthem BCBS Traditional is selected: ANTADJ (Adjustment), ANTDED (Deductible), ANTPAY (Payment), and ANTWIT (Withhold).

Computer Exploration

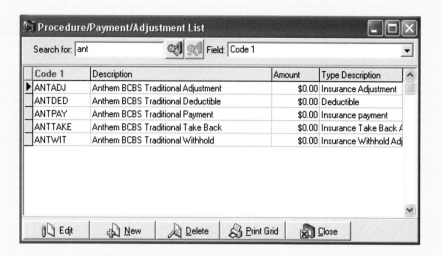

4. Key "P" after "ANT" in the Search For box to select ANTPAY. This is the code that is used when a payment from Anthem BCBS Traditional is entered.

5. Click the Edit button. The Procedure/Payment/Adjustment dialog box for the Anthem BCBS Traditional Payment code appears.

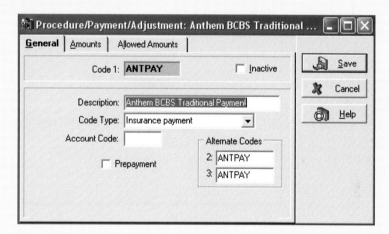

6. Notice that the Code Type is Insurance payment. The Code Type tells the program that this is a payment entry from an insurance carrier. Click the Cancel button to exit the dialog box.

7. Delete the previous entry in the Search For box (highlight the text and press the Delete key) and key "T." Six accounting codes are selected for Tricare—the usual adjustment, deductible, payment, and withhold codes plus two other codes. Because the Tricare insurance plan requires the patient to make a copayment at each visit, two additional codes are listed—a code for the copayment charge and a code for the copayment itself.

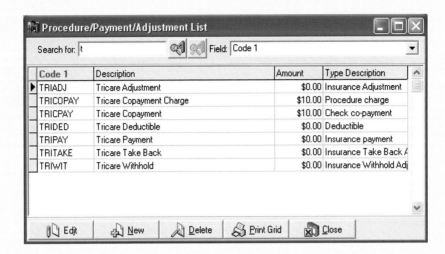

8. Click the code for TRICPAY (Tricare Copayment) to highlight it, and then click the Edit button.

9. The Procedure/Payment/Adjustment dialog box for the TRICPAY code is displayed. Notice that the Code Type is Check copayment. This is the code used to enter patient copayments that are in the form of checks.

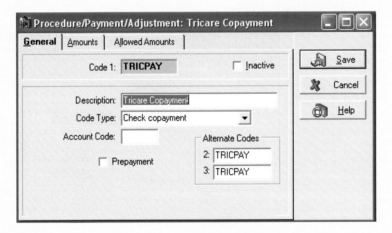

10. Click the Cancel button to close the Procedure/Payment/Adjustment dialog box.

11. Click the Close button to close the Procedure/Payment/Adjustment List dialog box.

7.2 Review Copayment Entries in the Transaction Entry Dialog Box

Copayments made by patients are entered in MediSoft in the Transaction Entry dialog box.

1. Select Enter Transactions on the Activities menu.

2. Enter "KOPELM" in the Chart box to highlight Mary Anne Kopelman. Press the Enter key. Transactions for Mary Anne Kopelman's fatigue case are displayed.

Computer Exploration

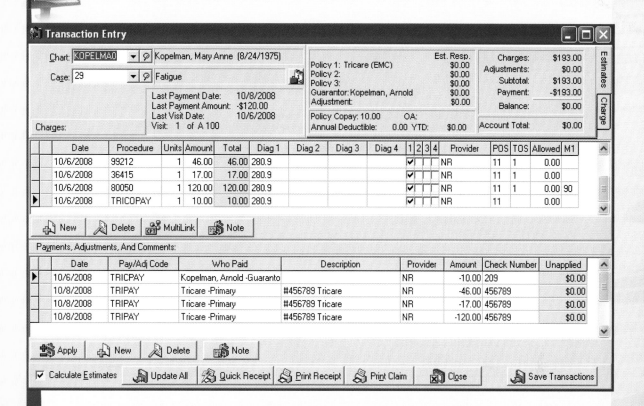

Transaction Entry

Chart: KOPELMA0 ▼ 🔍 Kopelman, Mary Anne (8/24/1975)

Case: 29 ▼ 🔍 Fatigue

Policy 1: Tricare (EMC)		Est. Resp.		Charges:	$193.00
Policy 2:		$0.00		Adjustments:	$0.00
Policy 3:		$0.00		Subtotal:	$193.00
Guarantor: Kopelman, Arnold		$0.00		Payment:	-$193.00
Adjustment:		$0.00		Balance:	$0.00

Last Payment Date: 10/8/2008
Last Payment Amount: -$120.00
Last Visit Date: 10/6/2008
Charges: Visit: 1 of A 100

Policy Copay: 10.00   OA:
Annual Deductible: 0.00 YTD: $0.00

Account Total: $0.00

Date	Procedure	Units	Amount	Total	Diag 1	Diag 2	Diag 3	Diag 4	1	2	3	4	Provider	POS	TOS	Allowed	M1
10/6/2008	99212	1	46.00	46.00	280.9				✓				NR	11	1	0.00	
10/6/2008	36415	1	17.00	17.00	280.9				✓				NR	11	1	0.00	
10/6/2008	80050	1	120.00	120.00	280.9				✓				NR	11	1	0.00	90
▶ 10/6/2008	TRICOPAY	1	10.00	10.00	280.9				✓				NR	11		0.00	

[New] [Delete] [MultiLink] [Note]

Payments, Adjustments, And Comments:

Date	Pay/Adj Code	Who Paid	Description	Provider	Amount	Check Number	Unapplied
▶ 10/6/2008	TRICPAY	Kopelman, Arnold -Guaranto		NR	-10.00	209	$0.00
10/8/2008	TRIPAY	Tricare -Primary	#456789 Tricare	NR	-46.00	456789	$0.00
10/8/2008	TRIPAY	Tricare -Primary	#456789 Tricare	NR	-17.00	456789	$0.00
10/8/2008	TRIPAY	Tricare -Primary	#456789 Tricare	NR	-120.00	456789	$0.00

[Apply] [New] [Delete] [Note]

☑ Calculate Estimates   [Update All] [Quick Receipt] [Print Receipt] [Print Claim] [Close] [Save Transactions]

3. In the Payments, Adjustments, and Comments section of the dialog box, locate the payment transaction that displays TRICPAY in the Pay/Adj Code box. This entry refers to the patient copayment (–10.00) made by Mary Anne Kopelman during her 10/6/2008 visit. The minus sign indicates that the amount is a payment and not a charge. Notice the check number is also displayed in the Check Number box.

4. Now look at the list of charge transactions in the Charges section of the dialog box. You will see a number of procedure code charges, including 99212, 36415, 80050–90, and then TRICOPAY. The TRICOPAY entry (10.00) refers to the corresponding $10 copayment charge for the visit.

5. Click the Close button to close the Transaction Entry dialog box without saving any changes.

7.3 The Calculate Estimates Feature

1. Select Enter Transactions on the Activities menu.

2. Key "E" in the Chart box to highlight Wilma Estephan. Press the Enter key. Transactions for Wilma Estephan's Hypertension case are displayed.

Computer Exploration

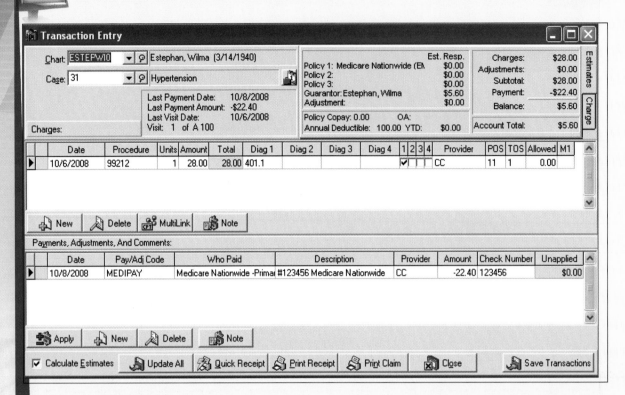

3. Locate the Calculate Estimates check box in the bottom left corner of the dialog box. By default, this box contains a check mark, indicating the feature is activated. If the Calculate Estimates check box on your screen does not contain a check mark, please click in it now to display the check mark. When activated, this feature regularly updates and displays all affected sums in the account detail section of the Transaction dialog box, including the estimated responsibility column.

4. Locate the account detail section in the top right panel of the Transaction Entry dialog box. It contains two tabs, Estimates and Charge. When the Estimates tab is open, two rows of figures are displayed, one labeled "Est. Resp." and the other unlabeled but summed up in an "Account Total" box. Locate this information in Wilma Estephan's Transaction Entry dialog box.

5. The estimated responsibility column estimates how much each responsible party currently owes on the account. This feature provides a quick way to estimate how much a patient owes on his or her account.

   Notice Wilma Estephan currently owes $5.60. Out of the total charges of $28, Medicare has paid 80% (see the payment for $22.40 from Medicare on 10/8/2008). Wilma Estephan owes the remaining 20% ($5.60). These estimates are based on the fact that her Medicare Nationwide plan pays 80 percent of charges, and the beneficiary pays 20 percent—information that can be verified in the Policy 1 tab of the Case dialog box.

6. The Calculate Estimates feature is activated by default. However, it can be disabled by unchecking the Calculate Estimates check box. When this feature is disabled, MediSoft will not display any figures in the account detail portion of the dialog box. This may be required in certain situations to protect the privacy of the information.

7. Click the Close button to close the Transaction Entry dialog box.

Health Care Claim Preparation and Transmission

Objectives

After studying this chapter, you should be able to:

1. Describe the health care claim preparation process using a medical billing program.

2. Discuss the data elements that are required in the five major sections of the HIPAA electronic health care claim.

3. Describe the purpose of and source for the taxonomy codes that are reported on health care claims.

4. Compare billing provider, pay-to provider, rendering provider, and referring provider.

5. Distinguish between a claim control number and a line item control number.

6. Explain how claim attachments and credit–debit information are handled.

7. Identify the three major methods of electronic claim transmission.

8. Describe three of the measures that are used to provide security when protected health information is transmitted.

Introduction to Health Care Claims

Health care claims are a critical communication between providers and payers on behalf of patients. Claims may be created by many different types of providers, such as physician practices, hospitals, outpatient clinics, hospices, home health organizations, and laboratories. In this chapter, the focus is on physician practice claims. The way claims are prepared and transmitted greatly affects the medical insurance specialist's job. Claim processing is a major task, and the numbers can be huge. For example, a forty-physician group practice with fifty-five thousand patients typically processes a thousand claims daily.

The information for claims is gathered from the various databases of the medical billing program, such as provider information and patient information. After a visit, a claim can be completed when the medical insurance specialist enters the visit transactions—the services, charges, and payments—that are indicated on the encounter form. Any missing elements or information are added after the claim editing process. The typical flow of the claim is shown in Figure 8.1.

HIPAA Claims and Paper Claims

Two types of claims, HIPAA and paper, are in use. The HIPAA claim is an electronic transaction named the HIPAA X12 837 Health Care Claim or Equivalent Encounter Information. This electronic claim is usually called the "837 claim" or the "HIPAA claim." The paper format is known as the CMS-1500 claim form (previously the HCFA-1500). Most of the claims handled by medical insurance specialists are HIPAA claim transactions, so this chapter covers these in depth. Basic instructions for completing the CMS-1500 are also included.

Background

The CMS-1500 was originally a typed or computer-generated printed form that was mailed or faxed to payers. For a few years before HIPAA, the Centers for Medicare and Medicaid Services (CMS) asked providers, on a voluntary basis, to use an electronic version of the 1500 form for Medicare claims. Today, CMS mandates electronic transmission of Medicare claims using the 837 format, except for very small practices and for those that never send any kind of electronic health care transactions. These excepted offices are the only providers that can still use paper claims. The HIPAA 837 claim is mandated for all other providers.

Before the HIPAA mandate for standard transactions (covered in Chapters 2 and 3), some payers required additional records, such as their own information sheets, when providers billed them. Some payers also used their own coding systems in place of the ICD-9-CM and CPT/HCPCS. The HIPAA 837 mandate means that health plans are required to accept the standard claim submitted electronically. Payers may not require providers to make changes or additions to it. Further, they cannot refuse to accept the standard transaction or delay payment of a proper standard transaction.

Claim Content

The **National Uniform Claim Committee (NUCC)**, led by the American Medical Association, determines the content of both 837 and CMS-1500 claims. The 837 requires more information than does the CMS-1500. The CMS-1500 requires about 150 discrete items, while the 837 requires over 1,000. For example, when a patient is referred by another physician, the medical specialty

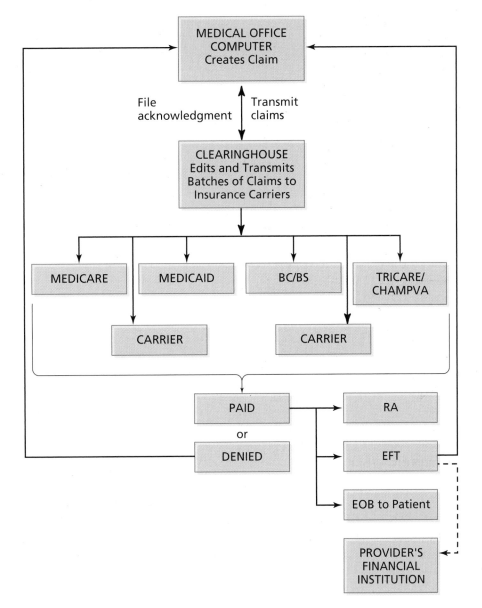

Figure 8.1 Claim Flow Using a Clearinghouse

code and date of referral must be reported on the 837; these elements are not required on the CMS-1500 claim. The addition of information that is captured makes claim processing faster and more accurate.

HIPAA Claim Data Elements

The HIPAA 837 claim contains many **data elements**. Examples of data elements are a patient's first name, middle name/initial, and last name. These elements are reported in the five major sections, or levels, of the claim. Table 8.1 on pages 254–255 shows the data elements that can be reported. An explanation of the major elements begins on page 256.

Billing Tip

Electronic Claims Cut Costs
It costs a practice from $7 to $12 to file a paper-based claim, but it only costs $1.50 to $3 to file the same claim electronically

TABLE 8.1   HIPAA Claim Data Elements

PROVIDER, SUBSCRIBER, PATIENT, PAYER

Billing Provider

Last or Organization Name
  First Name
  Middle Name
  Name Suffix
Primary Identifier: NPI
Address 1
Address 2
City Name
State/Province Code
ZIP Code
Country Code
Secondary Identifiers, such as State License Number
Contact Name
Communication Numbers
  Telephone Number
  Fax
  E-mail
  Telephone Extension
Taxonomy Code
Currency Code

Pay-to Provider

Last or Organization Name
  First Name
  Middle Name
  Name Suffix
Primary Identifier: NPI
Address 1
Address 2
City Name
State/Province Code
ZIP Code
Country Code
Secondary Identifiers, such as State License Number
Taxonomy Code

Subscriber

Insured Group or Policy Number
Group or Plan Name
Insurance Type Code
Claim Filing Indicator Code
Last Name
First Name
Middle Name
Name Suffix
Primary Identifier
  Member Identification Number
  National Individual Identifier
  IHS/CHS Tribe Residency Code
Secondary Identifiers
  HIS Health Record Number
  Insurance Policy Number
  SSN
Patient's Relationship to Subscriber
Other Subscriber Information
Birth Date
Gender Code
Address Line 1
Address Line 2

City Name
State/Province Code
Zip Code
Country Code

Patient

Last Name
First Name
Middle Name
Name Suffix
Primary Identifier
  Member ID Number
  National Individual Identifier
Address 1
Address 2
City Name
State/Province Code
Zip Code
Country Code
Birth Date
Gender Code
Secondary Identifiers
  IHS Health Record Number
  Insurance Policy Number
  SSN
Death Date
Weight
Pregnancy Indicator

Responsible Party

Last or Organization Name
First Name
Middle Name
Suffix Name
Address 1
Address 2
City Name
State/Province Code
Zip Code
Country Code

Payer

Payer Responsibility Sequence Number Code
Organization Name
Primary Identifier
  Payer ID
  National Plan ID
Address 1
Address 2
City Name
State/Province Code
Zip Code
Secondary Identifiers
  Claim Office Number
  NAIC Code
  TIN
Assignment of Benefits
Release of Information Code
Patient Signature Source Code
Referral Number
Prior Authorization Number

TABLE 8.1	HIPAA Claim Data Elements (*Continued*)

CLAIM

Claim Level

Claim Control Number (Patient Account Number)
Total Submitted Charges
Place of Service Code
Claim Frequency Code
Provider Signature on File
Medicare Assignment Code
Participation Agreement
Delay Reason Code
Onset of Current Symptoms or Illness Date
Similar Illness/Symptom Onset Date
Last Menstrual Period Date
Admission Date
Discharge Date
Patient Amount Paid
Claim Original Reference Number
Investigational Device Exemption Number
Medical Record Number
Note Reference Code
Claim Note
Diagnosis Code 1–8
Accident Claims
   Accident Cause
      Auto Accident
      Another Party Responsible
      Employment Related
      Other Accident
   Auto Accident State/Province Code
   Auto Accident Country Code
   Accident Date
   Accident Hour

Rendering Provider

Last or Organization Name
First Name

Middle Name
Name Suffix
Primary Identifier
   EIN
   NPI
   SSN
Taxonomy Code
Secondary Identifiers

Referring/PCP Providers

Last or Organization Name
First Name
Middle Name
Name Suffix
Primary Identifier
   EIN
   NPI
   SSN
Taxonomy Code
Secondary Identifiers
Proc

Service Facility Location

Type Code
Last or Organization Name
Primary Identifier
   EIN
   NPI
   SSN
Address 1
Address 2
City Name
State/Province Code
Zip Code
Country Code
Secondary Identifiers

SERVICE LINE INFORMATION

Procedure Type Code
Procedure Code
Modifiers 1–4
Line Item Charge Amount
Units of Service/Anesthesia Minutes
Place of Service Code
Diagnosis Code Pointers 1–4
Emergency Indicator
Copay Status Code
Service Date Begun
Service Date End

Shipped Date
Onset Date
Similar Illness or Symptom Date
Referral/Prior Authorization Number
Line Item Control Number
Ambulatory Patient Group
Sales Tax Amount
Postage Claimed Amount
Line Note Text
Rendering/Referring/PCP Provider at the Service Line Level
Service Facility Location at the Service Line Level

Claim Sections

The HIPAA 837 claim has these major sections:

1. Provider
2. Subscriber (guarantor/insured/policyholder) and patient (the subscriber or another person)
3. Payer
4. Claim details
5. Services

These levels are set up as a hierarchy, starting at the provider level, so that data elements have to be included only when they are not a repeat of previous data. For example, if the subscriber and the patient are the same, then the patient data is not needed. If the subscriber and the patient are different people, information about both is reported on the claim.

Many data elements are required. Others are situational and are used only when certain conditions apply. For example, if a claim involves pregnancy, the date of the last menstrual period is required. If the claim does not involve pregnancy, that date should not be reported.

Billing Tip

Knowledge of Claim Data Elements
Medical insurance specialists become familiar with the claim data elements most often used on the claims their practice prepares, so that they can efficiently research missing information and respond to payers' questions. Memorization is not required, but good thinking and organizational skills are.

Provider Information

Information in the first section of the claim covers the provider. The **billing provider** is the organization or person transmitting the claim to the payer. This term is used to distinguish between a billing provider and the **pay-to provider**, the organization or person that should receive payment.

This distinction is necessary because physician practices often hire other firms, such as a billing service or a clearinghouse, to send their claims. When this is done, the outside organization is the billing provider, and the practice is the pay-to provider receiving the payment from the insurance carrier. If a practice sends claims directly to the payer, it is both the billing provider and the pay-to provider, so there is no additional pay-to provider to report.

Another term associated with claim preparation is **rendering provider.** It is common to have a billing provider (a clearinghouse), a pay-to provider (a practice), and a rendering provider, such as a laboratory.

Billing Provider Data Elements

The name, address, city, state, and Zip code are reported for the billing entity. If the entity is a person, the first name, middle name or initial, and name suffix (such as Jr. or II) are also required. A contact name and telephone number must be supplied.

An identifying number called the **National Provider Identifier** (NPI) is required as a **primary provider identifier.** NPIs are obtained both for organizatons (such as practices) and individuals (such as physicians).

A **secondary provider identifier** number is required by various payers for physicians that participate in their plans (see Chapter 10). Examples of possible secondary identifiers are listed in Table 8.2.

HIPAA Tip

HIPAA National Provider Identifier

The Department of Health and Human Services (HHS) has adopted a standard provider identifier called the National Provider Identifier (NPI), effective in 2005.

Pay-to Provider Data Elements

Pay-to provider data elements are reported when the pay-to provider is a different person or organization than the billing provider. The elements include the name and address information. If the entity is a person, the complete name is also reported.

TABLE 8.2	Secondary Identification Numbers
State license number	
Blue Plan number—required by most Blue Cross/Blue Shield Plans	
Medicaid number	
CHAMPUS ID number—required for TRICARE claims	
Facility ID number	
PPO number	
HMO number	
Clinic number	
Commercial number	
Site number	
Location number	
USIN (Unique Supplier Identification Number)	
State Industrial Accident provider number	

HIPAA Tip

*The taxonomy codes are an example of a nonmedical **administrative code set**. These code sets, which are maintained by the NUCC, are business-related, in contrast to medical code sets such as the ICD and CPT. Under HIPAA, they may be referred to as nonclinical or nonmedical code sets.*

The National Provider Identifier is entered for the pay-to provider. Secondary provider identification numbers are required by various payers for their participants (see Table 8.2).

Other Provider Elements

There are other data elements about the billing or the pay-to provider that are reported in certain situations.

Taxonomy Code

A **taxonomy code** is a ten-digit number that stands for a physician's medical specialty. This code is reported on the claim when the type of specialty affects the physician's pay, usually because of the payer's contract with the physician (see Chapter 10 for information on payers' participation contracts). For example, nuclear medicine is usually a higher-paid specialty than internal medicine. An internist who is also certified in nuclear medicine would report the nuclear medicine taxonomy code when billing for that service and use the internal medicine taxonomy code when reporting internal medicine claims.

Many medical billing programs store a taxonomy-code database (see Figure 8.2 on page 258). The user selects the correct specialty, and the code is correctly selected for reporting on the claim. Appendix A contains a list of taxonomy codes for physicians.

Currency Code; Country Code

A currency code is required only if financial amounts submitted in the claim file are in a currency not normally used by the receiver for processing claims, such as euros instead of dollars. The country code is used when an address is outside the United States.

Billing Tip

Taxonomy Codes
Physicians select the taxonomy code that most closely matches their education, license, or certification.

Compliance Guideline

Correct Code Sets
The correct medical code sets are those valid at the time the health care is provided. The correct nonmedical code sets are those valid at the time the transaction—such as the claim—is started.

Thinking It Through—8.1

1. If a physician practice uses a billing service to prepare and transmit its health care claims, which entity is the pay-to provider and which the billing provider?

2. What type of data element is a physician's PPO number?

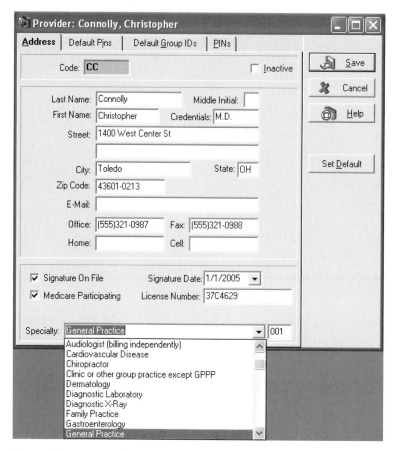

Figure 8.2 Example of MediSoft Screen for Taxonomy Code Selection

Subscriber, Patient, or Responsible Party Information

The next section of data elements describes the **subscriber**, who is the insurance policyholder or guarantor. The subscriber may be the patient or someone other than the patient. If the subscriber and patient are not not the same person, data elements about the patient are also required. Data about any **responsible party**—an entity or person other than the subscriber or patient who has financial responsibility for the bill—may be reported if applicable.

Subscriber Data Elements

The subscriber's complete name is reported, as well as a number of data elements about the subscriber's insurance plan.

Insurance Coverage

The subscriber's health plan member number is required when the subscriber's primary identifier with the payer is a member identification number. When the National Patient ID is mandated for use, that number will be required instead.

The subscriber's insurance policy number is required when a second insurance policy number is needed to identify the subscriber. The subscriber's Social

Security number may be supplied if a secondary identification number is necessary to identify the subscriber. For Indian Health Services, the subscriber IHS/CHS Tribe Residency Code/Health Record Number is reported.

The insured's group or policy number, group or plan name, and a claim filing indictor code are also reported. One of the following claim filing indicator codes identifies the type of health plan for the claim, such as a PPO. These codes are valid until a National Payer ID system is HIPAA-mandated.

Code	Definition
09	Self-pay
10	Central certification
11	Other nonfederal programs
12	Preferred provider organization (PPO)
13	Point of service (POS)
14	Exclusive provider organization (EPO)
15	Indemnity insurance
16	Health maintenance organization (HMO) Medicare risk plan
AM	Automobile medical
BL	Blue Cross and Blue Shield
CH	CHAMPUS (TRICARE)
CI	Commercial insurance company
DS	Disability
HM	Health maintenance organization
LI	Liability
LM	Liability medical
MB	Medicare Part B
MC	Medicaid
OF	Other federal program
TV	Title V
VA	Department of Veteran's Affairs plan
WC	Workers' compensation health claim
ZZ	Unknown

Relationship of Patient to Subscriber

If the subscriber is the patient, the billing program enters the correct code when the relationship of patient to subscriber of "self" is selected by the medical insurance specialist. When the patient and the subscriber are not the same person, a code is required to specify the patient's relationship to the subscriber. The complete list of choices follows. (Note that many billing programs used to limit the options to "self," "spouse," "child," and "other;" the programs must be updated for HIPAA requirements so that the particular relationship can be correctly reported.)

Code	Definition
01	Spouse
04	Grandfather or grandmother
05	Grandson or granddaughter
07	Nephew or niece
09	Adopted child
10	Foster child
15	Ward

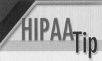

HIPAA Tip

Verifying Information About Subscribers and Patients

Early in the claim-processing sequence, the HIPAA Eligibility for a Health Plan transaction (the provider's inquiry and the payer's response) is used to verify insurance coverage and eligibility for benefits. If that transaction turns up new or different information, the changes are correctly posted in the billing program, so that the 837 contains accurate, updated data elements.

HIPAA Tip

HIPAA Individual Identifier

Under HIPAA, HHS must adopt a standard system for a National Patient ID, an individual identifier. This identifier is also referred to as National Individual Identifier (NII) or as the HealthCare ID.

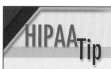

Under HIPAA, HHS must adopt a standard health plan identifier system. Each plan's number will be its **National Payer ID.** *It is also called the* **National Health Plan ID.**

Code	Definition
17	Stepson or stepdaughter
19	Child
20	Employee
21	Unknown
22	Handicapped dependent
23	Sponsored dependent
24	Dependent of a minor dependent
29	Significant other
32	Mother
33	Father
34	Other adult
36	Emancipated minor
39	Organ donor
40	Cadaver donor
41	Injured plaintiff
43	Child where insured has no financial responsibility
53	Life partner
G8	Other relationship

Other Subscriber Data Elements

These data elements are required when another payer may be involved in paying the claim.

- Other Subscriber Birth Date
- Other Subscriber Gender Code (The codes are F (female), M(male), and U (unknown).
- Other Subscriber Address

Billing Tip

Patient Address
If the patient's address is not known, "Unknown" should be entered, because it is a required data element.

Patient Data Elements

The patient's complete name, address, gender, date of birth (using eight digits), and primary identifier are reported (see Figure 8.3). The patient's member ID number is required if it is different from the subscriber's. (The patient National Individual Identifier will be required when the national individual identifier is mandated for use.) Secondary identifiers, such as IHS Health Record Number, insurance policy number, or Social Security number, may be required for claim adjudication.

Other data elements are used to report specific information about the patient. Some of these are:

- Patient Death Date: The date of death is required when the patient is known to be deceased and the provider knows the date on which the patient died.
- Weight
- Pregnancy Indicator Code: If the patient is pregnant, a Y used for "yes" is required when mandated by law.

Responsible Party Data Elements

If there is a "responsible party" for the charges, the entity's name and address are reported. If the responsible party is a person, the complete name is supplied.

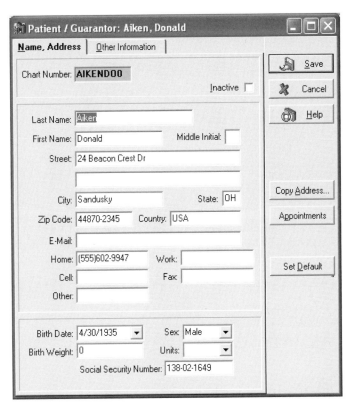

Figure 8.3 Example of MediSoft Screen for Patient Information

---

Thinking It Through—8.2

Joan McNavish, a sixty-one-year-old retiree, is covered by her husband's insurance policy. Her husband is still working and receives health benefits through his employer, Rockford Valley Concrete, which has a PPO plan.

1. What code describes Joan's relationship to the subscriber?

2. What claim filing indicator code is reported?

3. What claim filing indicator code is likely to be used if the insurance is TRICARE?

Payer Information

This section contains information about the payer to which the claim is going to be sent, called the **destination payer** (see Figure 8.4 on page 262).

Level of Payment Responsibility

A payer responsibility sequence number code identifies whether the insurance carrier is the primary (P), secondary (S), or tertiary (T) payer. This code is used when more than one insurance plan is responsible for payment. The T code is used for the payer of last resort, such as Medicaid (see Chapter 12 for an explanation of "payer of last resort").

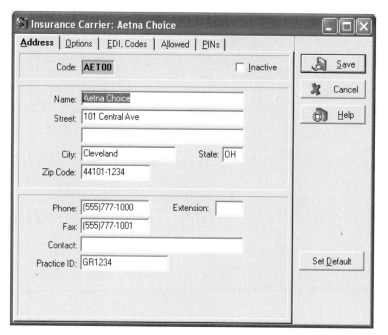

Figure 8.4 Example of MediSoft Screen for Payer Information

Identification

The payer's name and ID are required data elements (the National Payer ID will be used when mandated). Another number may be required to identify the destination payer. Options include the payer claim office number for correct electronic routing of the claim, the payer's NAIC (National Association of Insurance Commissioners) code, and the payer's tax ID number.

Other Data Elements

An assignment of benefits code indicates whether the insured or authorized person authorizes benefits to be paid to the provider. A release of information code/signature source code indicates whether the provider has on file a signed statement by the patient authorizing the release of medical data to other organizations.

A referral number or prior authorization number is required when services on the claim involve a referral or preauthorization. The number used should be the one that was assigned by the payer to which the claim is being sent. If the claim requires referral numbers from more than one payer, a number should be recorded for each payer.

Claim Information

The claim information section reports information related to the particular claim. For example, if the patient's visit is the result of an accident, a description of the accident is included. Data elements about the rendering provider—if not the same as the billing provider or the pay-to provider—are supplied. If another provider referred the patient for care, the claim reports data elements about the referring physician or primary care physician (PCP).

Claim-Level Data Elements

There are various data elements that are reported at the claim level. A **claim control number**, unique for each claim, is assigned by the sender. The maximum number of characters is twenty. The claim control number will appear on payments that come from payers (see Chapter 9), so it is very important for tracking purposes.

In the claim information, the total submitted charges must be reported. If the patient made any payment for the claim, this dollar amount is also supplied.

The **place of service (POS) code**, also called the facility type code, identifies where the services reported on the claim were performed. Table 8.3 on page 264 shows typical codes for physician practice claims. The complete list is provided in Appendix B. This code is important, because payers may authorize different payments for different locations. For example, Medicare regulations provide for different levels of payments to physicians depending on where the service is performed. Higher payments are made for physician office services, and lower for ambulatory surgical centers and hospital outpatient departments.

The **claim frequency code**, which is also called the **claim submission reason code**, for physician practice claims indicates whether this claim is one of the following.

HIPAA Tip

Coordination of Benefits

The 837 claim transaction is also used to send data elements regarding coordination of benefits to other payers on the claim.

TABLE 8.3	Selected Place of Service Codes	
Code	**Definition**	
11	Office	
12	Home	
22	Outpatient hospital	
23	Emergency room—hospital	
24	Ambulatory surgical center	
31	Skilled nursing facility	
81	Independent laboratory	

Code	Definition
1	Original claim: The initial claim sent for the patient/date of service/procedure.
7	Replacement of prior claim: Used if an original claim is being replaced with a new claim.
8	Void/cancel of prior claim: Used to completely eliminate a submitted claim.

Billing Tip

Billing for Capitated Visits
If the claim is to report an encounter under a MCO capitation contract, a value of zero (0) may be used.

First claims are always a "1." Payers do not usually allow for corrections to be sent after a claim has been submitted; instead, an entire new claim is transmitted. However, some payers cannot process a claim with the frequency code 7 (replace a submitted claim). In this situation, submit a void/cancel of prior claim (frequency code 8) to cancel the original incorrect claim, and then submit a new, correct claim.

When a claim is replaced, the original claim number (Claim Original Reference Number) is reported.

Diagnosis codes from the ICD-9-CM are reported. The 837 permits up to eight ICD-9-CM codes to be reported. The order of entry is not regulated. Each diagnosis code must be directly related to the patient's treatment. Up to four of these codes can be linked to each procedure code that is reported.

Other data elements include:

Coding Point

Diagnosis Codes
At least one diagnosis code must appear on a claim.

Primary Diagnosis Codes
An E code cannot be used as a primary diagnosis. Some V codes are also allowed only for secondary classifications.

- Provider Signature on File: To indicate whether the provider's signature is on file.
- Medicare Assignment Code: For Medicare claims, a code is used to indicate if the patient has authorized payments directly to the physician (see Chapter 11).
- Onset of Current Symptoms or Illness Date: Required when information is available and when the date is different than the date of service. If not used, the payer assumes that the claim service date is the date of onset of illness or symptoms.
- Similar Illness or Symptom Onset Date: Required when the claim involves services to a patient experiencing symptoms similar or identical to previously reported symptoms. Up to ten dates can be reported.
- Last Menstrual Period Date: Required when the claim involves pregnancy.
- Claim Note: Used when a statement needs to be included, such as to satisfy a state requirement or to substantiate the patient's medical treatment that is not reported elsewhere in the claim.

Rendering Provider Data Elements

When the rendering provider is a different person or organization than the billing provider or the pay-to provider, the provider's name and NPI are required. The taxonomy code is required when the claim payment will be based on the specialty of the provider. Secondary provider identification numbers are also required by various payers, or may be required to identify the provider to the receiver (see Table 8.2).

Referring/PCP Provider Data Elements

When the visit involves a referral from another physician, data elements about the **referring provider** or primary care physician are required to report this fact. The referring provider's name and NPI are required. The taxonomy code is required when the claim payment will be based on the specialty of the provider. Secondary provider identification numbers are also required by various payers, or may be required to identify the provider to the receiver (see Table 8.2).

Service Facility Location

Sometimes physicians treat patients in locations that are not usual for their practice, such as a hospice for a dermatologist. If the location of the health care services is other than that associated with the normal operation of the billing or pay-to provider, the facility's place of service code, name, tax identification number, and address are reported, along with secondary identifiers if required by the payer.

Thinking It Through—8.3

1. What type of code shows the location where the patient was treated?

2. What type of code shows whether a claim is the original claim, a replacement, or being cancelled?

3. What type of code is used to report the medical specialty of a referring or rendering physician?

Service Line Information

The term **service line information** describes the part of the claim that reports the procedures—that is, the services—performed for the patient (see Figure 8.5 on page 266). Each service line has a procedure code and a charge, with additional information as detailed below. The date of service is required. If the end date is different from the date service began, this date is also reported.

Note that different information for a particular service line, such as a prior authorization number that applies only to that service, can be supplied at the service line level.

Procedure Code

For physician practices, the procedure code is usually identified as HC for HCPCS, which contains the CPT codes and modifiers as Level I codes (see Chapter 5). State-defined procedure and supply codes are needed for workers' compensation claims.

Modifier(s)

From one to four modifiers can be appended to the procedure code to clarify the reported procedure.

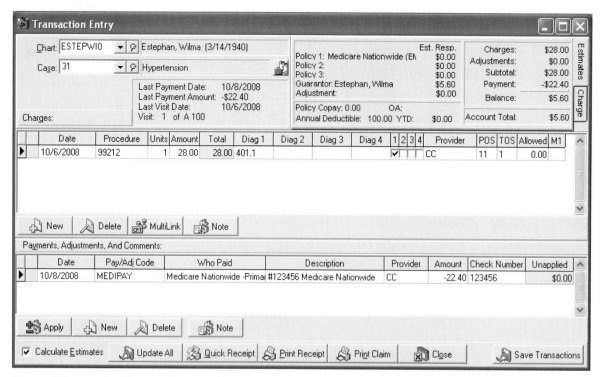

Figure 8.5 Example of MediSoft Screen for Service Line Information

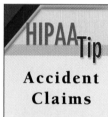
Line Item Charge Amount

A charge for each service line must be reported. If the claim reports an encounter with no charge, such as a capitated visit, a value of zero (0) may be used. If units of service such as minutes are involved, this is also reported here; the billing program calculates the charge.

Diagnosis Code Pointers

A total of four diagnosis codes can be linked to each service line procedure. At least one diagnosis code must be linked to the procedure code. Codes two, three, and four may also be linked, in declining level of importance regarding the patient's treatment, to the service line.

Line Item Control Number

A **line item control number** is a unique number assigned by the sender to each service line. Like the claim control number, it is used to track payments from the insurance carrier, but for a particular service rather than the entire claim.

Claim Attachments

A **claim attachment** is an additional printed form or electronic record needed to process a claim. A HIPAA transaction standard for electronic health care claim attachments is under development. When it is adopted, payers will be required to accept all attachments that are submitted by providers according to the standard.

Until a HIPAA electronic claim attachment standard is mandated, health plans have the right to require providers to submit claim attachments in the format they specify. Attachments that are sent separately from the main claim file may be paper or electronically based.

While driving to his son's soccer game, Leonard Rush had a minor automobile accident. He was treated in the emergency room of the Mount Horeb Regional Medical Center by Dr. Arun Govindarajan and released. Several days later, his ankle began to swell, and he was treated by his internist, Dr. Rhoda Lowenstein.

1. In what section is the automobile accident reported on the HIPAA claim?

2. What place of service code is reported?

3. Using Table 8.4 (pages 268–269) and Figure 8.6 (page 270), identify the form locator(s) where this situation is reported on the CMS-1500 claim.

HIPAA Tip

PHI on Attachments

Claim payers should receive only what they need to process a claim. If an attachment has PHI related to another patient, those data must be marked over or deleted. Information about other dates of service or conditions not pertinent to the claim should also be crossed through or deleted.

Credit–Debit Information

When federal or state privacy regulations do not prohibit it, the use of credit or debit cards is a popular payment option. (Note that the use of this payment option is currently prohibited in conjunction with federal health plans such as Medicaid and TRICARE, covered in Chapters 12 and 13.)

Providers typically offer patients a variety of service payment options when the patient's portion of the cost is known either before or at the time of service. Examples of payment options include cash, check, being billed, and using a credit or debit card. A credit or debit card may also be used to pay the patient or subscriber portion of a claim when that amount is not known at the time of service. In this case, the patient or subscriber authorizes payment via a consent form up to a maximum amount, allowing the provider to bill the credit card after the claim has been adjudicated. The patient's consent form also authorizes the transmission of credit or debit card information over a health care EDI network. The consent form must identify how the transaction will be used and who will receive the information. When this option is used, the amount charged to the patient's credit or debit card is reported after the claim is adjudicated.

Compliance Guideline

Emergency Indicator
A Y is reported when the service line reports an emergency situation in which the patient required immediate medical intervention as a result of severe, life-threatening, or potentially disabling conditions. An N is used to report a nonemergency service.

Paper Claims: The CMS-1500

If a CMS-1500 (HCFA-1500) paper claim is required, it is prepared as summarized in Table 8.4 on pages 268–269. Figure 8.6 on page 270 shows an example of this claim form. The CMS-1500 contains thirty-three form locators, which are numbered items. Form locators 1 through 13 refer to the patient and the patient's insurance coverage. Form locators 14 through 33 contain information about the provider and the transaction information, including the diagnoses, procedures, and charges.

The Future of Paper Claims

With the exception of Medicare, which accepts paper claims from small providers only, payers usually accept paper transactions. But practices that elect to use paper claims must have two versions of their medical billing software, one to capture the necessary data elements for HIPAA-compliant electronic Medicare claims and an older version to generate CMS-1500s. It is anticipated that, for cost reasons, all payers will eventually require electronic submission and add this provision to their contracts with providers.

TABLE 8.4	CMS-1500 Completion
Locator Form	**Content**
1	Type of Insurance: Medicare, Medicaid, CHAMPUS/TRICARE, CHAMPVA, FECA Black Lung, Group Health Plan, or Other.
1a	Insured's ID Number: The insurance identification number that appears on the insurance card of the policyholder.
2	Patient's Name: As it appears on the insurance card.
3	Patient's Birth Date/Sex: Date of birth in eight-digit format; appropriate selection for male or female.
4	Insured's Name: The full name of the person who holds the insurance policy (the insured). If the patient is a dependent, the insured may be a spouse, parent, or other person. If the insured is the patient, enter "Same."
5	Patient's Address: Address includes the number and street, city, state, and ZIP code.
6	Patient's Relationship to Insured: Self, spouse, child, or other. Self means that the patient is the policyholder.
7	Insured's Address: Address of the person who is listed in form locator 4. If the insured's address is the same as the patient's, enter "Same" in form locator 7. This form locator does not need to be completed if the patient is the insured person.
8	Patient Status: Marital status—single, married, or other—as well as the patient's employment status—employed, full-time student, or part-time student.
9	Other Insured's Name: If there is additional insurance coverage, the insured's name.
9a	Other Insured's Policy or Group Number: The policy or group number of the other insurance plan.
9b	Other Insured's Date of Birth: Date of birth and sex of the other insured.
9c	Employer's Name or School Name: Other insured's employer or school.
9d	Insurance Plan Name or Program Name: Other insured's insurance plan or program name.
10a–10c	Is Patient Condition Related to: To indicate whether the patient's condition is the result of a work injury, an automobile accident, or another type of accident. If the services provided are related to one of these occurrences, indicate this by marking yes. If the services are related to an automobile accident, enter the two-character abbreviation of the name of the state where the accident occurred. Other refers to injuries or conditions that can be reported to a liability insurance carrier or no-fault insurance program.
10d	Reserved for Local Use: Varies with the insurance plan.
11	Insured's Policy Group or FECA Number: As it appears on the insurance identification card.
11a	Insured's Date of Birth/Sex: The insured's date of birth and sex if the patient is not the insured.
11b	Employer's Name or School Name: Insured's employer or school.
11c	Insurance Plan Name or Program Name: Of the insured.
11d	Is There Another Health Benefit Plan? Yes if the patient is covered by additional insurance. If yes, form locators 9a-9d and/or 11-11c must also be completed. If the patient does not have additional insurance, select No. If not known, leave blank.
12	Patient's or Authorized Person's Signature: If the patient's or authorized representative's signature authorizing release of information is on file, the words "Signature on file" or "SOF" are entered in form locator 12. If an authorized representative is used because the patient is unable to sign, the representative's relationship to the patient and the reason the patient cannot sign are also entered in form locator 12.
13	Insured or Authorized Person's Signature: Indicating that the patient or patient's representative authorizes payments from the insurance carrier to be made directly to the provider of the services listed on the claim form.
14	Date of Current Illness or Injury or Pregnancy: The date that symptoms first began for the current illness, injury, or pregnancy. For pregnancy, enter the date of the patient's last menstrual period (LMP). If the actual date is not known, leave blank.
15	If Patient Has Had Same or Similar Illness: Date when the patient first consulted the provider for treatment of the same or a similar condition. If the patient has not had a same or similar illness, or if it is not known, leave blank.
16	Dates Patient Unable to Work in Current Occupation: Dates the patient has been unable to work in form locator 16. If not known, leave blank.

| TABLE 8.4 | CMS-1500 Completion (*Continued*) |

Locator Form	Content
17	Name of Referring Physician or Other Source: Name of the physician or other source who referred the patient to the billing provider.
17a	ID Number of Referring Physician: Identifying number for the referring physician.
18	Hospitalization Dates Related to Current Services: If the services provided are needed because of a related hospitalization, the admission and discharge dates are entered. For patients still hospitalized, the admission date is listed in the From box, and the To box is left blank.
19	Reserved for Local Use
20	Outside Lab? Varies with carrier.
21	Diagnosis or Nature of Illness or Injury: ICD-9-CM codes in priority order.
22	Medicaid Resubmission: Medicaid-specific.
23	Prior Authorization Number: If required by the carrier.
24A	Dates of Service: If the same service is provided multiple times, list the To and From dates once and indicate the number of days or units in form locator 24G. If services were provided on a single day, the entry in form locator 24A varies with each carrier; some require the date in both the To and From columns; some require just the To column to be completed, and others require just the From column to be completed.
24B	Place of Service: A place of service (POS) code describes the location at which the service was provided.
24C	Type of Service: Carrier-specific code.
24D	Procedures, Services, or Supplies: CPT/HCPCS codes for services provided. Up to three modifiers can be listed next to each code. If there are more than three modifiers, enter -99 and list the additional modifiers in form locator 19.
24E	Diagnosis Code: Using the numbers (1, 2, 3, 4) listed to the left of the diagnosis codes in form locator 21, enter the diagnosis for the each service listed in form locator 24D.
24F	$ Charges: For each service listed in form locator 24D, enter charges without dollar signs and decimals.
24G	Days or Units: The number or days or units.
24H	EPSDT Family Plan: Medicaid-specific.
24I	EMG (Emergency): If services were provided in an emergency room.
24J	COB (Coordination of Benefits): Some insurance plans require a check in this box if the patient has other insurance coverage in addition to the primary plan.
24K	Reserved for Local Use
25	Federal Tax ID Number: Physician's or supplier's Federal Tax ID number (for incorporated practices), Social Security number (for unincorporated practices), or Employer Identification Number (EIN).
26	Patient's Account No.: Patient account number used by the practice's accounting system.
27	Accept Assignment? If the physician accepts assignment, select Yes.
28	Total Charge: Total of all charges in form locator 24F.
29	Amount Paid: Amount of the patient payment that is applied to the services listed on this claim in form locator 29. If there is also payment from another insurance carrier, a copy of the remittance advice or claim denial should be forwarded. If no payment was made, enter none or 0.00.
30	Balance Due: Balance resulting from subtracting the amount in form locator 29 from the amount in form locator 28.
31	Signature of Physician or Supplier Including Degrees or Credentials: For claims that are sent using a computer, the provider's electronic signature appears. On claims that are printed and mailed, the provider's or supplier's signature, the date of the signature, and the provider's credentials (such as MD) are entered.
32	Name and Address of Facility Where Services Were Rendered (If Other Than Home or Office): If the facility and address where services were performed is the same as the one listed in form locator 33, enter Same. If services were provided at a location other than the office or home, enter the name and address of the facility in form locator 32.
33	Physician's, Supplier's Billing Name, Address, ZIP code, and Telephone Number.

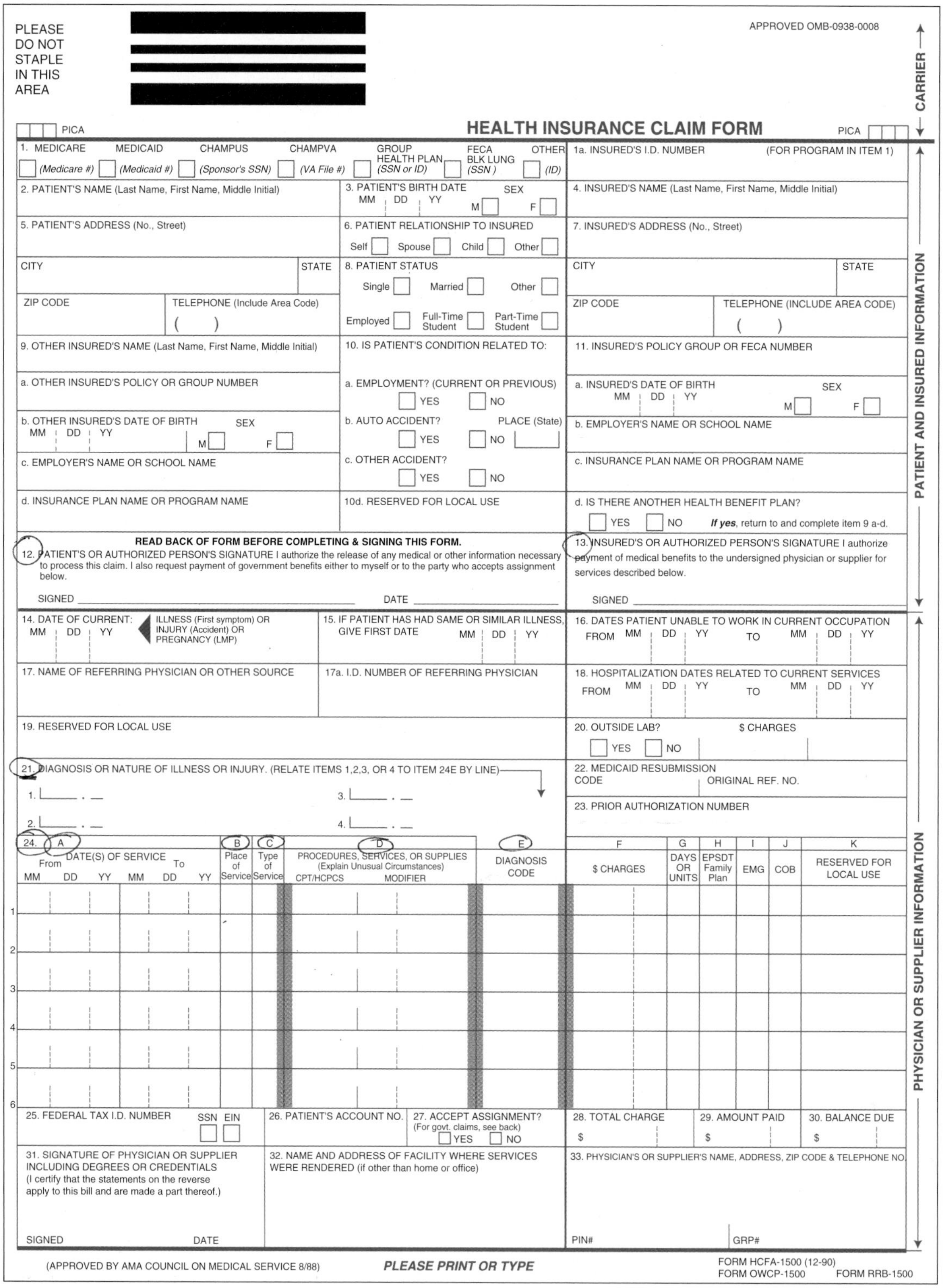
PLEASE DO NOT STAPLE IN THIS AREA

APPROVED OMB-0938-0008

CARRIER

PICA HEALTH INSURANCE CLAIM FORM PICA

1. MEDICARE (Medicare #) MEDICAID (Medicaid #) CHAMPUS (Sponsor's SSN) CHAMPVA (VA File #) GROUP HEALTH PLAN (SSN or ID) FECA BLK LUNG (SSN) OTHER (ID)

1a. INSURED'S I.D. NUMBER (FOR PROGRAM IN ITEM 1)

2. PATIENT'S NAME (Last Name, First Name, Middle Initial)

3. PATIENT'S BIRTH DATE MM DD YY SEX M F

4. INSURED'S NAME (Last Name, First Name, Middle Initial)

5. PATIENT'S ADDRESS (No., Street)

6. PATIENT RELATIONSHIP TO INSURED Self Spouse Child Other

7. INSURED'S ADDRESS (No., Street)

CITY STATE

8. PATIENT STATUS Single Married Other

CITY STATE

ZIP CODE TELEPHONE (Include Area Code) ( )

Employed Full-Time Student Part-Time Student

ZIP CODE TELEPHONE (INCLUDE AREA CODE) ( )

9. OTHER INSURED'S NAME (Last Name, First Name, Middle Initial)

10. IS PATIENT'S CONDITION RELATED TO:

11. INSURED'S POLICY GROUP OR FECA NUMBER

a. OTHER INSURED'S POLICY OR GROUP NUMBER

a. EMPLOYMENT? (CURRENT OR PREVIOUS) YES NO

a. INSURED'S DATE OF BIRTH MM DD YY SEX M F

b. OTHER INSURED'S DATE OF BIRTH MM DD YY SEX M F

b. AUTO ACCIDENT? PLACE (State) YES NO

b. EMPLOYER'S NAME OR SCHOOL NAME

c. EMPLOYER'S NAME OR SCHOOL NAME

c. OTHER ACCIDENT? YES NO

c. INSURANCE PLAN NAME OR PROGRAM NAME

d. INSURANCE PLAN NAME OR PROGRAM NAME

10d. RESERVED FOR LOCAL USE

d. IS THERE ANOTHER HEALTH BENEFIT PLAN? YES NO *If yes*, return to and complete item 9 a-d.

READ BACK OF FORM BEFORE COMPLETING & SIGNING THIS FORM.

12. PATIENT'S OR AUTHORIZED PERSON'S SIGNATURE I authorize the release of any medical or other information necessary to process this claim. I also request payment of government benefits either to myself or to the party who accepts assignment below.

SIGNED DATE

13. INSURED'S OR AUTHORIZED PERSON'S SIGNATURE I authorize payment of medical benefits to the undersigned physician or supplier for services described below.

SIGNED

PATIENT AND INSURED INFORMATION

14. DATE OF CURRENT: MM DD YY ILLNESS (First symptom) OR INJURY (Accident) OR PREGNANCY (LMP)

15. IF PATIENT HAS HAD SAME OR SIMILAR ILLNESS, GIVE FIRST DATE MM DD YY

16. DATES PATIENT UNABLE TO WORK IN CURRENT OCCUPATION FROM MM DD YY TO MM DD YY

17. NAME OF REFERRING PHYSICIAN OR OTHER SOURCE

17a. I.D. NUMBER OF REFERRING PHYSICIAN

18. HOSPITALIZATION DATES RELATED TO CURRENT SERVICES FROM MM DD YY TO MM DD YY

19. RESERVED FOR LOCAL USE

20. OUTSIDE LAB? YES NO $ CHARGES

21. DIAGNOSIS OR NATURE OF ILLNESS OR INJURY. (RELATE ITEMS 1,2,3, OR 4 TO ITEM 24E BY LINE)

1. ___ . __ 3. ___ . __

2. ___ . __ 4. ___ . __

22. MEDICAID RESUBMISSION CODE ORIGINAL REF. NO.

23. PRIOR AUTHORIZATION NUMBER

24. A DATE(S) OF SERVICE From MM DD YY To MM DD YY	B Place of Service	C Type of Service	D PROCEDURES, SERVICES, OR SUPPLIES (Explain Unusual Circumstances) CPT/HCPCS MODIFIER	E DIAGNOSIS CODE	F $ CHARGES	G DAYS OR UNITS	H EPSDT Family Plan	I EMG	J COB	K RESERVED FOR LOCAL USE
1										
2										
3										
4										
5										
6										

25. FEDERAL TAX I.D. NUMBER SSN EIN

26. PATIENT'S ACCOUNT NO.

27. ACCEPT ASSIGNMENT? (For govt. claims, see back) YES NO

28. TOTAL CHARGE $

29. AMOUNT PAID $

30. BALANCE DUE $

31. SIGNATURE OF PHYSICIAN OR SUPPLIER INCLUDING DEGREES OR CREDENTIALS (I certify that the statements on the reverse apply to this bill and are made a part thereof.)

SIGNED DATE

32. NAME AND ADDRESS OF FACILITY WHERE SERVICES WERE RENDERED (if other than home or office)

33. PHYSICIAN'S OR SUPPLIER'S NAME, ADDRESS, ZIP CODE & TELEPHONE NO.

PIN# GRP#

PHYSICIAN OR SUPPLIER INFORMATION

(APPROVED BY AMA COUNCIL ON MEDICAL SERVICE 8/88) *PLEASE PRINT OR TYPE* FORM HCFA-1500 (12-90) FORM OWCP-1500 FORM RRB-1500

Figure 8.6 CMS-1500 Claim Form

Claim Transmission

Practices handle transmission of electronic claims—which may be called electronic media claims, or EMC—in a variety of ways. Some practices transmit claims themselves; others hire outside vendors to handle this task for them. No matter who handles the electronic data interchange (EDI) transactions, patients' protected health information (PHI) must remain secure and private.

Claims are prepared for transmission after all required data elements have been posted to the medical billing software program. The data elements that are transmitted are not seen physically, as they would be on a paper form. Instead, these elements are in a computer file.

Checking the Claim

An important step comes before claim transmittal—checking the claim. Most billing programs provide a way for the medical insurance specialist to review claims for accuracy and to create a record of the claims that are about to be sent. For example, NDCMedisoft has a **verification report**. Review the sample of this report in Figure 8.7 below. It permits validation that the correct data elements appear. After the verification report has been checked, it should be printed and kept on file.

Transmission Methods

There are three major methods of transmitting claims electronically: direct transmission to the payer, clearinghouse use, and direct data entry.

Compliance Guideline

Disclosing Information for Payment Purposes Under HIPAA, covered entities such as physician practices may disclose PHI for payment purposes. For example, a provider may disclose a patient's name to a financial institution in order to cash a check or to a clearinghouse to initiate electronic transactions.

Valley Associates, P.C.
EMC Verification
EMC Batch Verification Report

Filename: C:\MediData\VAPC\EMC\ndcreq.dat   Billing Code Range: ALL
Chart Number Range: ALL   Provider: ALL
Date Created Range: ALL   Insurance Carrier Range: ALL

| Claim# | Chart# | Patient Name | | Policy# | | | Group# | Referring Provider | Facility |
| | | Date From | Proc. Code | Modifiers | Pos | Tos | Units | Diagnoses | Amount |

Provider: Christopher Connolly (CC)

| 53 | WILLIWA0 | Walter Williams | | ABC103562239 | BDC1001 | | Not Found | | Not Found |

Primary Carrier: Aetna Choice (AET00)
Diagnoses: 1: 401.1   Benign Essential Hypertension
           2: 780.7   Fatigue

| | 10/01/2008 | 99212 | | | 11 | 1 | 1 | Diagnosis: 1, 2 | $46.00 |
| | 10/01/2008 | 93000 | | | 11 | 1 | 1 | Diagnosis: 1, 2 | $70.00 |

Claim 53 Total: $116.00

| 52 | PEREZCA0 | Carmen Perez | | 140603312X | | | Not Found | | Not Found |

Primary Carrier: Cigna HMO Plus (CIG00)
Diagnoses: 1: 493.00   Extrinsic Asthma

| | 10/01/2008 | 99213 | | | 11 | 1 | 1 | Diagnosis: 1 | $62.00 |

Claim 52 Total: $62.00

| 48 | PORCEJE0 | Jennifer Porcelli | | 7123408080X | G0119 | | Not Found | | Not Found |

Primary Carrier: Oxford Freedom (OXF00)
Diagnoses: 1: 465.9   Upper Respiratory Infection

| | 10/13/2008 | 99212 | | | 11 | 1 | 1 | Diagnosis: 1 | $46.00 |
| | 10/13/2008 | 87081 | | | 11 | 1 | 1 | Diagnosis: 1 | $30.00 |

Claim 48 Total: $76.00

Provider Christopher Connolly (CC) Total: $254.00

Total Transaction(s):   5
Total Claim(s):   3   Batch Total: $254.00

Figure 8.7 Example of MediSoft Verification Report

Transmit Claims Directly

In the direct transmission approach, providers and payers exchange transactions directly. To conduct electronic data interchange (EDI), they need information systems, including a translator and communications technology. The provider must meet HIPAA data elements content and X12 formatting rules.

Use a Clearinghouse

Billing Tip

Clearinghouses
There are many electronic claims and transaction processing firms in the health care industry. Two of the largest are NDC Health and WebMD Envoy. Other firms include ProxyMed, Medifax-EDI, MedUnite, and Electronic Network Systems.

Providers whose medical billing software vendors do not have translation software must use a clearinghouse to send and receive data in the correct EDI format (see Figure 8.8 on page 273). Under HIPAA, clearinghouses can take in nonstandard formats and translate them into the standard format. Clearinghouses must receive all required data elements from the provider, because they are prohibited from creating or modifying data content.

Practices may choose to use a clearinghouse to transmit all claims, or to use a combination of direct transmission and a clearinghouse. For example, they may send claims directly to Medicare, Medicaid, and a few other major commercial payers, and use a clearinghouse to send claims to other payers.

Use Direct Data Entry (DDE)

Some payers offer online direct data entry (DDE) to providers. DDE involves using an Internet-based service into which employees key the standard data elements. Although the data elements must meet the HIPAA standards regarding content, they do not have to be formatted into the standard X12N transaction. Instead, they are loaded directly into the health plans' computer.

Clean Claims

Although health care claims require many data elements and are complex, simple errors often prevent physician practices from generating **clean claims**—that is, those with the proper HIPAA content. Following are common errors.

- Missing or incomplete service facility name, address, and identification for services rendered outside the office or home. This includes invalid Zip codes or state abbreviations.
- Missing Medicare assignment indicator or benefits assignment indicator.
- Invalid provider identifier (when present) for rendering provider, referring provider, or others.
- Missing part of the name or the identifier of the referring provider.
- Missing or invalid subscriber's birth date.
- Missing insurance type code for secondary coverage. This information, such as a spouse's payer, is important for filing primary claims in addition to secondary claims.
- Missing payer name and/or payer identifier, required for both primary and secondary payers.
- Missing attachment transmission code on claims with attachments.
- Incomplete other payer information. This is required in all secondary claims and all primary claims that will involve a secondary payer.
- Invalid procedure codes.

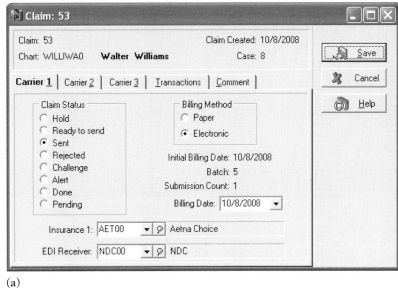

(a)

Claim	Chart	Date Created	Primary	Batch 1	#1 Bill Date	Secondary	Batch 2	#2 Bill Date	Tertiary	Batch 3	#3 Bill Date
					Valley Associates, P.C.						
					Claim List						
					10/08/08						
52	PEREZCA0	10/8/2008	CIG00	5	10/08/08	MED00	0			0	
53	WILLIWA0	10/8/2008	AET00	5	10/08/08	MED00	0			0	

(b)

Figure 8.8 Example of MediSoft Screen for Claim Transmission

Claim Security

The HIPAA Security rule sets standards for protecting individually identifiable health information (PHI) when it is maintained or transmitted electronically. Providers, as well as health plans and clearinghouses, must establish ways to protect the confidentiality, integrity, and availability of PHI.

Local Area Networks and Firewalls

Electronic data about patients are stored on the practice's computer systems. Most physician practices use computer networks in which personal computers are connected to a local area network (LAN), so users can exchange and share information and hardware. The central component of the LAN is a server, a powerful computer that acts as an intermediary between PCs on the network and provides a large volume of disk storage for shared information, such as patients' files. The server controls access to the data through the use of access controls that limit user access to various files and programs stored on the server.

Billing Tip

Editing
Editing software programs called claim scrubbers make sure that all required fields are filled and that only valid codes are used, and perform other checks. Some providers use a clearinghouse for editing, and others use claim scrubbers in their billing department before they send claims.

The LAN is linked to remote networks such as the Internet by a router, which determines the best route for data to travel across the network. Packets of data traveling between the LAN and the Internet—such as electronic claims—usually must pass through a **firewall**, a security device that examines information, such as e-mail, entering and leaving a network, and determines whether to forward it to its destination. A firewall acts as a gatekeeper, deciding who has legitimate access to a network and what sorts of materials should be allowed in and out.

Security Measures

A number of security measures are used by providers to enforce the HIPAA Security Rule. These include

- Access control, passwords, and log files to keep intruders out
- Backups to replace items after damage
- Security policies to handle violations that do occur

Access Control, Passwords, and Log Files

Most practices use role-based access, meaning that those who need information are the only people who can access it. Once access rights have been assigned, each user is given a key to the designated databases. To initiate a session on the network, users at a PC must provide a user ID and **password** (the key). They are then able to use the files to which they have been granted access rights. Physician practices use software to create activity logs of who has accessed—or tried to access—information, and passwords prevent unauthorized users from gaining access to information on a computer or network.

Backups

Backing up is the activity of copying files to another medium so that they will be preserved in case the originals are no longer available. A successful backup plan is critical in recovering from either a minor or major security incident that jeopardizes critical data.

Security Policy

A practice develops a security policy, including being sure that employees are informed about their own responsibilities for protecting the practice's electronically stored information. Many practices include this information in handbooks distributed to all employees when they are hired and when the handbooks are revised. These handbooks set forth general information about the organizations, their structures, and their policies as well as specific information about employee responsibilities.

Thinking It Through—8.5

1. Imagine that you are employed as a medical insurance specialist for Valley Associates, P.C. Make up a password that you will use to keep your files secure.

2. As an employee, how would you respond to another staff member who asked to see your latest claim files in order to check out how you handled a particular situation?

Good Passwords

There are a number of tips to observe in creating a good password:

1. Always use a combination of letters and numbers that are not real words and also not obvious, such as a number string like 123456 or a birth date.
2. Do not use a user ID (log-on, sign-on) as a password. Even if an ID has both numbers and letters, it is not secret.
3. Select a mixture of uppercase and lowercase letters if the system can distinguish between them, and include special characters, such as @, $, or &, if possible.
4. Use a minimum of six alphanumeric characters. The optimal minimum lengths vary by system, but most security experts recommend at least six or seven characters.
5. Change passwords periodically, but not too often. Forcing frequent changes can make security worse because users are more likely to write down passwords.

Review

Chapter Summary

1. The data elements on claims are gathered from the information in the medical billing program's databases. First, data about the patient, guarantor (subscriber), insurance coverage, and demographics are entered based on the patient information form. After the patient's visit, the transactions—the charges and payments—are entered, as detailed on the encounter form. The software program combines the elements from its relevant databases and prepares the claim that has been specified, either the HIPAA claim (837) or a paper claim (CMS-1500). Any missing elements or information are added after the claim editing process.

2. The HIPAA 837 claim has five major sections. The main data elements reported in each section are as follows.

   - The provider section: The billing provider and pay-to provider name, primary identifier (National Provider Identifier), address; and possibly secondary identifier(s) and taxoomy code.

   - The subscriber/patient section: The subscriber (insured/policyholder) name, relationship to patient, member identifier (future National Patient ID), policy number and plan name; claim filing indicator code (future National Payer ID); if different, the patient name, member identifier (future National Patient ID), address, date of birth, gender, possibly secondary identifier(s), and in some cases date of death, weight, or pregnancy indicator.

   - The payer section: Level of payment responsibility for the payer; payer name, identifier (future National Payer ID), secondary identifier(s), assignment of benefits/release of information code/signature source code, and referral/authorization number.

   - The claim information section: Data elements about the claim itself: Claim control number, total submitted charges, patient payment, place of service code, claim frequency code, provider signature on file, diagnosis code(s) and possibly onset data, similar illness date, or last menstrual date; note. Additional data elements include: If appropriate, name, primary and secondary identifier(s), and taxonomy code(s) of rendering provider/referring provider; accident data; and additional service facility location.

   - The service line information section: For each service line, a line item control number, procedure code, modifier, associated charge amounts, units of service, diagnosis code pointers, and date begun/ended; data elements covering attachments and credit—debit information.

3. Taxonomy codes, ten-digit numbers representing physicians' medical specialties, are an administrative code set maintained by the National Uniform Claim Committee (NUCC).

4. The billing provider is the entity that is transmitting the claim to the payer, usually a billing service or a clearinghouse. The pay-to provider receives the payment from the insurance carrier. A rendering provider is a physician who provides the patient's treatment but is not the pay-to provider entity. A referring provider has sent the patient for treatment.

5. A claim control number is a unique number given to each claim that is used to track the claim's payments. A line item control number is another unique number assigned to each service line. Like the claim control number, it is used to track payments from the insurance carrier, but for a particular service rather than the entire claim.

6. Claim attachments may be electronic or paper. A claim attachment number is assigned, and the type of attachment is reported with a code. Patient credit—debit information for future payment of the amount due after the carrier pays can also be reported using the health care claim transaction.

7. Three methods for claim transmittal are (a) direct transmission, in which the claim is sent by EDI directly to the payer's computer system, (b) via a clearinghouse, in which the clearinghouse takes nonstandard formats, translates

them to HIPAA-standard transactions, and transmits this data file to the payer, and (c) direct data entry, in which the provider keys data elements directly into the payer's computer system, rather than transmitting them via EDI.

8. A number of measures are used to provide security for PHI. Computer networks have firewalls that govern access to the LAN and prevent unauthorized data from leaving it. Physician practices control access to PHI by restricting information to those who need it to perform their work. Passwords and activity logs also control use. When problems do occur, practices have made regular backups, so that the PHI is available for use. Finally, these security measures are mandated and monitored through the practice's overall security policy, which sets forth employees' responsibilities for protecting the practice's information.

Key Terms

administrative code set *page 257*
billing provider *page 256*
claim attachment *page 267*
claim control number *page 262*
claim frequency code (claim submission reason code) *page 263*
claim scrubber *page 273*
clean claim *page 272*
data elements *page 253*
destination payer *page 261*
firewall *page 274*

line item control number *page 266*
National Patient ID (National Individual Identifier; NII) *page 259*
National Payer ID (National Health Plan ID) *page 260*
National Provider Identifier (NPI) *page 257*
National Uniform Claim Committee (NUCC) *page 252*
password *page 274*
pay-to provider *page 256*

place of service (POS) code *page 263*
primary provider identifier *page 257*
referring provider *page 265*
rendering provider *page 257*
responsible party *page 258*
secondary provider identifier *page 257*
service line information *page 265*
subscriber *page 258*
taxonomy code *page 257*
verification report *page 271*

Review Questions

Match the key terms in the left column with the definitions in the right column.

A. billing provider
B. claim control number
C. destination payer
D. line item control number
E. pay-to provider
F. POS code
G. referring provider
H. rendering provider
I. subscriber
J. taxonomy code

_B_ 1. Unique number assigned by the sender to a claim.

_D_ 2. Unique number assigned by the sender to each service line on a claim.

_G_ 3. Physician who has sent the patient to the billing/pay-to provider.

_J_ 4. Stands for the type of provider specialty.

_H_ 5. Entity providing patient care for this claim if other than the billing/pay-to provider.

_E_ 6. Entity that is to receive payment for the claim.

_F_ 7. Stands for the type of facility in which services reported on the claim were provided.

_C_ 8. Insurance carrier that is to receive the claim.

_A_ 9. Entity that is sending the claim to the payer.

_I_ 10. The insurance policyholder or guarantor for the claim.

Decide whether each statement is true or false, and write T for true or F for false.

_____ 1. When a claim is created, the medical insurance specialist enters information about the charges and payments for a patient's visit.

_____ 2. The five major sections of the HIPAA claim are provider, patient, payer, history, and services.

_____ 3. Some data elements are always required on a claim, such as the patient's full name, address, date of birth, and gender.

_____ 4. The billing provider and the rendering provider are usually the same person or organization.

_____ 5. If the services reported on a claim involve a referral, a referral number should be reported.

_____ 6. Claim control number, place of service code, and total submitted charges are data elements reported in the claim-level section of the HIPAA claim.

_____ 7. Neither diagnosis codes nor procedure codes are required data elements.

_____ 8. Claim attachments can be submitted in paper or electronic form.

_____ 9. HIPAA standard claims may be transmitted by mail, fax, or the Internet.

_____ 10. A password is an example of a security measure used to protect patients' health information.

Write the letter of the choice that best completes the statement or answers the question.

_A_ 1. The NPI is used to report the _____ on a claim.
   A. provider identifier   C. payer identifier
   B. patient identifier   D. employer identifier

_AB_ 2. The National Individual Identifier will be used to report the _____ on a claim.
   A. provider identifier   C. payer identifier
   B. patient identifier   D. employer identifier

_A_ 3. The Health Plan ID will be used to report the _____ on a claim.
   A. provider identifier   C. payer identifier
   B. patient identifier   D. employer identifier

_D_ 4. How many diagnosis code pointers can be assigned to a procedure code?
   A. one   C. three
   B. two   D. four

_B_ 5. The content of claims and the taxonomy codes are set by
   A. HIPAA   C. ICD-9-CM
   B. NUCC   D. CPT/HCPCS

_C_ 6. The number of the HIPAA claim transaction is
   A. CMS-1500   C. X12 837
   B. HCFA-1500   D. X12 834

_D_ 7. If a physician practice sends claims directly to a payer, which of these entities is *not* additionally reported?
   A. referring provider   C. billing provider
   B. rendering provider   D. pay-to provider

_____ 8. The POS code for a military treatment facility is
   A. 12   C. 42
   B. 26   D. 72

_B_ 9. Which of the following may be the same person as the patient?
   A. referring provider   C. pay-to provider
   B. subscriber   D. destination payer

10. Which of the following is *not* a commonly used transmission method for HIPAA claims?
   - A. fax
   - B. direct data entry
   - C. direct transmission
   - D. clearinghouse

Provide answers to the following questions in the spaces provided.

1. List the five major sections of the HIPAA claim.
   - A. *PROVIDER*
   - B. *SUBSCRIBER*
   - C. *PAYER*
   - D. *Claim details*
   - E. *Services*

2. Describe how the following security measures help protect patients' private information:
   - A. Firewall _____
   - B. Password _____
   - C. Activity log _____
   - D. Backups _____
   - E. Security policy _____

Applying Your Knowledge

In this exercise, you play the role of a medical insurance specialist who is preparing HIPAA claims for transmission. Assume you are working with the practice's medical billing software to enter the transaction to be reported, based on the patient information form and the encounter form.

- Claim control numbers are created by adding the eight-digit date to the patient account number, as in PORCEJE0-01012008.

- A copayment of $15 is collected from each Oxford PPO patient at the time of the visit. A copayment of $10 is collected for Oxford HMO. These copayments are *not* subtracted from the charges; the payer's allowed amounts have already taken the copayment into account.

- The practice uses the services of NDC for its clearinghouse to transmit claims.

- The necessary data for the payer and the clearinghouse are stored in the program's databases.

Provider Information

Practice Name:	Valley Associates, PC
Address:	1400 West Center Street
	Toledo, OH 43601-0213
National Provider Identifier:	16-1234567
Oxford PPO Provider Number:	1011
Oxford HMO Provider Number:	2567

Physician Name: Christopher M. Connolly, MD
Medicare: Accepts Assignment
Physician Signature on File

Answer the questions that follow each case.

Case 8.1

From the Patient Information Form:

Name   Jennifer Porcelli
Sex   Female
Birth Date   07/05/1965
Address   310 Sussex Turnpike
              Shaker Heights, OH
              44118-2345
Employer   24/7 Inc.
SSN   712-34-0808
Insurance Policy Group Number   G0119
Insurance Plan/Program Name   Oxford Freedom PPO
Member ID   712340808X
Assignment of Benefits   Y
Signature on File   Y

Encounter Form: See page 281.

Questions

1. What is the name of the pay-to provider?

2. List the pay-to provider's primary and secondary identification numbers for this claim.

3. Are the subscriber and the patient the same person?

4. What copayment is collected?

5. What amount is being billed on the claim?

VALLEY ASSOCIATES, P.C.
Christopher M. Connolly, M.D. - Internal Medicine
555-967-0303
NPI16-1234567

PATIENT NAME	APPT. DATE/TIME	
Jennifer Porcelli	10/06/2008	12:30pm

PATIENT NO.	DX
PORCEJE0	**1.** 465.9 upper respiratory infection **2.** **3.** **4.**

DESCRIPTION	✓	CPT	FEE	DESCRIPTION	✓	CPT	FEE
EXAMINATION				**PROCEDURES**			
New Patient				Diagnostic Anoscopy		46600	
Problem Focused		99201		ECG Complete		93000	
Expanded Problem Focused		99202		I&D, Abscess		10060	
Detailed		99203		Pap Smear		88150	
Comprehensive		99204		Removal of Cerumen		69210	
Comprehensive/Complex		99205		Removal 1 Lesion		17000	
Established Patient				Removal 2-14 Lesions		17003	
Minimum		99211		Removal 15+ Lesions		17004	
Problem Focused	✓	99212	46	Rhythm ECG w/Report		93040	
Expanded Problem Focused		99213		Rhythm ECG w/Tracing		93041	
Detailed		99214		Sigmoidoscopy, diag.		45330	
Comprehensive/Complex		99215					
				LABORATORY			
PREVENTIVE VISIT				Bacteria Culture		87081	
New Patient				Fungal Culture		87101	
Age 12-17		99384		Glucose Finger Stick		82948	
Age 18-39		99385		Lipid Panel		80061	
Age 40-64		99386		Specimen Handling		99000	
Age 65+		99387		Stool/Occult Blood		82270	
Established Patient				Tine Test		85008	
Age 12-17		99394		Tuberculin PPD		85590	
Age 18-39		99395		Urinalysis		81000	
Age 40-64		99396		Venipuncture		36415	
Age 65+		99397					
				INJECTION/IMMUN.			
CONSULTATION: OFFICE/ER				DT Immun		90702	
Requested By:				Hepatitis A Immun		90632	
Problem Focused		99241		Hepatitis B Immun		90746	
Expanded Problem Focused		99242		Influenza Immun		90659	
Detailed		99243		Pneumovax		90732	
Comprehensive		99244					
Comprehensive/Complex		99245		**TOTAL FEES**			

Encounter Form for Case 8.1

Case 8.2

From the Patient Information Form:

Name	Kalpesh Shah
Sex	M
Birth Date	01/21/1998
SSN	330-42-7928
Assignment of Benefits	Y
Signature on File	Y

Primary Insurance

Insured	Raj Shah
Patient Relationship to Insured	Son
Insured's Birth Date	02/16/1970
Insured's Sex	M
Insured's Address	1433 Third Avenue
	Cleveland, OH
	44101-1234
Insured's Employer	Cleveland Savings Bank
Insured's SSN	330-21-1209
Insurance Policy Group Number	G0904
Insurance Plan/Program Name	Oxford Freedom PPO
Member ID	3302112090X

Encounter Form: See page 283.

Questions

1. Are the subscriber and the patient the same person?

2. What is the code for the patient's relationship to the insured?

3. What is the claim filing indicator code?

4. What amount is being billed on the claim?

5. What claim control number would you assign to the claim?

VALLEY ASSOCIATES, P.C.
Christopher M. Connolly, M.D. - Internal Medicine
555-967-0303
NPI16-1234567

PATIENT NAME			APPT. DATE/TIME		
Kalpesh Shah			10/06/2008 3:30pm		
PATIENT NO.			**DX**		
SHAHKAL0			1. 380.4 cerumen in ear 2. 3. 4.		

DESCRIPTION	✓	CPT	FEE	DESCRIPTION	✓	CPT	FEE
EXAMINATION				**PROCEDURES**			
New Patient				Diagnostic Anoscopy		46600	
Problem Focused		99201		ECG Complete		93000	
Expanded Problem Focused		99202		I&D, Abscess		10060	
Detailed		99203		Pap Smear		88150	
Comprehensive		99204		Removal of Cerumen	✓	69210	15
Comprehensive/Complex		99205		Removal 1 Lesion		17000	
Established Patient				Removal 2-14 Lesions		17003	
Minimum	✓	99211	30	Removal 15+ Lesions		17004	
Problem Focused		99212		Rhythm ECG w/Report		93040	
Expanded Problem Focused		99213		Rhythm ECG w/Tracing		93041	
Detailed		99214		Sigmoidoscopy, diag.		45330	
Comprehensive/Complex		99215					
				LABORATORY			
PREVENTIVE VISIT				Bacteria Culture		87081	
New Patient				Fungal Culture		87101	
Age 12-17		99384		Glucose Finger Stick		82948	
Age 18-39		99385		Lipid Panel		80061	
Age 40-64		99386		Specimen Handling		99000	
Age 65+		99387		Stool/Occult Blood		82270	
Established Patient				Tine Test		85008	
Age 12-17		99394		Tuberculin PPD		85590	
Age 18-39		99395		Urinalysis		81000	
Age 40-64		99396		Venipuncture		36415	
Age 65+		99397					
				INJECTION/IMMUN.			
CONSULTATION: OFFICE/ER				DT Immun		90702	
Requested By:				Hepatitis A Immun		90632	
Problem Focused		99241		Hepatitis B Immun		90746	
Expanded Problem Focused		99242		Influenza Immun		90659	
Detailed		99243		Pneumovax		90732	
Comprehensive		99244					
Comprehensive/Complex		99245		**TOTAL FEES**			

Encounter Form for Case 8.2

Case 8.3

From the Patient Information Form:

Name	Josephine Smith
Sex	F
Birth Date	05/04/1977
SSN	610-32-7842
Address	9 Brook Rd.
	Alliance, OH
	44601-1812
Employer	Central Ohio Oil
Referring Provider	Dr. Mark Abelman, MD, Family Medicine
Insurance Policy Group Number	G0404
Insurance Plan/Program Name	Oxford Choice HMO
Member ID	610327842X
Assignment of Benefits	Y
Signature on File	Y

Encounter Form: See page 285.

Questions

1. List the pay-to provider's primary and secondary identification numbers for this claim.

2. What amount is being billed on the claim?

3. What two data elements should be reported since a referral is involved?

4. What claim control number would you assign to the claim?

5. What claim filing indicator code would you assign?

VALLEY ASSOCIATES, P.C.
Christopher M. Connolly, M.D. - Internal Medicine
555-967-0303
NPI16-1234567

PATIENT NAME	APPT. DATE/TIME	
Jospehine Smith	10/10/2008	1:00pm
PATIENT NO.	**DX**	
SMITHJO0	**1.** 401.1 benign essential hypertension **2.** **3.** **4.**	

DESCRIPTION	✓	CPT	FEE	DESCRIPTION	✓	CPT	FEE
EXAMINATION				**PROCEDURES**			
New Patient				Diagnostic Anoscopy		46600	
Problem Focused		99201		ECG Complete	✓	93000	125
Expanded Problem Focused		99202		I&D, Abscess		10060	
Detailed		99203		Pap Smear		88150	
Comprehensive		99204		Removal of Cerumen		69210	
Comprehensive/Complex		99205		Removal 1 Lesion		17000	
Established Patient				Removal 2-14 Lesions		17003	
Minimum		99211		Removal 15+ Lesions		17004	
Problem Focused		99212		Rhythm ECG w/Report		93040	
Expanded Problem Focused	✓	99213	56	Rhythm ECG w/Tracing		93041	
Detailed		99214		Sigmoidoscopy, diag.		45330	
Comprehensive/Complex		99215					
				LABORATORY			
PREVENTIVE VISIT				Bacteria Culture		87081	
New Patient				Fungal Culture		87101	
Age 12-17		99384		Glucose Finger Stick		82948	
Age 18-39		99385		Lipid Panel		80061	
Age 40-64		99386		Specimen Handling		99000	
Age 65+		99387		Stool/Occult Blood		82270	
Established Patient				Tine Test		85008	
Age 12-17		99394		Tuberculin PPD		85590	
Age 18-39		99395		Urinalysis		81000	
Age 40-64		99396		Venipuncture		36415	
Age 65+		99397					
				INJECTION/IMMUN.			
CONSULTATION: OFFICE/ER				DT Immun		90702	
Requested By:				Hepatitis A Immun		90632	
Problem Focused		99241		Hepatitis B Immun		90746	
Expanded Problem Focused		99242		Influenza Immun		90659	
Detailed		99243		Pneumovax		90732	
Comprehensive		99244					
Comprehensive/Complex		99245		**TOTAL FEES**			

Encounter Form for Case 8.3

Computer Exploration

1. Visit the Web site of the National Uniform Claim Committee (NUCC) to locate information on taxonomy codes:

   http://www.nucc.org

2. The Washington Publishing Company is a designated publishing company specializing in distributing EDI information from organizations that develop, maintain, and implement EDI standards. Visit this site to briefly review the X12 837 professional Implementation Guidelines and Addenda:

   http://www.wpc-edi.com/Default_40.asp

NDCMediSoft Activity

8.1 HIPAA Identifiers

The HIPAA claim form contains data elements for three new identifiers—a national provider identifier (NPI), payer identifier, and patient identifier. The NPI system is to be used as of 2005. The payer and patient identifier systems are expected in the near future. MediSoft contains three fields to be used for these identifiers once they are adopted. This activity examines these fields.

HIPAA National Provider Identifier (NPI)

1. The field for the national identifier for providers is located in the PINs tab of the Provider dialog box. The Provider dialog box is used to set up the records for all providers in the practice. Click the Providers option on the List menu.

2. The Provider List dialog box appears with the names of the providers in the Valley Associates, P.C., database. Click Dr. Connolly's name to highlight it, and then click the Edit button.

3. The Provider dialog box appears with Dr. Connolly's information displayed. The Provider dialog box is used to enter data on a new provider or to edit the information already stored in the database on an existing provider. Open the Default Pins tab of the Provider dialog box.

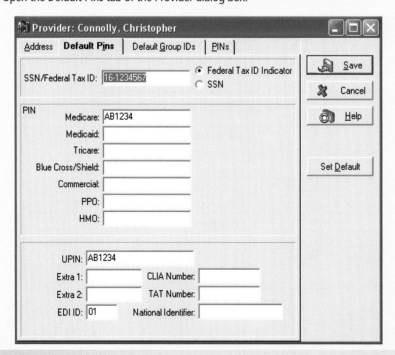

Computer Exploration

4. Notice the name of the last field—National Identifier. This field is used to enter a provider's national identifier, a ten-digit alphanumeric code provided and administered through CMS. NPIs will be assigned for life.

5. Currently, the HIPAA claim requires a Social Security number or Federal Tax ID instead of the NPI. Notice that the first data entry box in the Provider dialog box contains this information.

   Before closing the Default PINS tab, view the other types of PINs available. Any PINs assigned to the provider by the various types of insurance carriers are entered in the PIN section of the tab. Notice there are boxes for recording PINs from the following types of carriers: Medicare, Medicaid, Tricare, Blue Cross/Shield, Commercial, PPO, and HMO. If the physician is part of a group practice that has been assigned a group number by Medicare, that number is recorded here.

6. Before closing the Provider dialog box, open the Address tab.

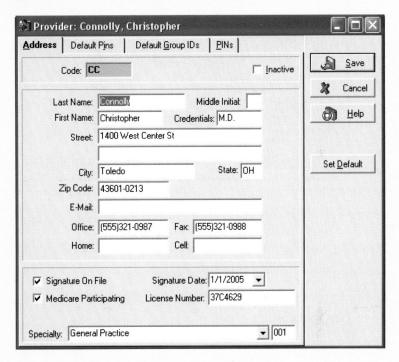

7. Notice that the Address tab contains other information about each provider that is required on most HIPAA claims. The top section is used to record the provider's name, address, and various phone numbers. The bottom section contains the following boxes: Signature On File, Signature Date, Medicare Participating, License Number, and Specialty.

8. Click the drop-down list in the Specialty box to view the list of specialties and corresponding codes. The selection in the Specialty box defines the taxonomy code required for certain HIPAA claims.

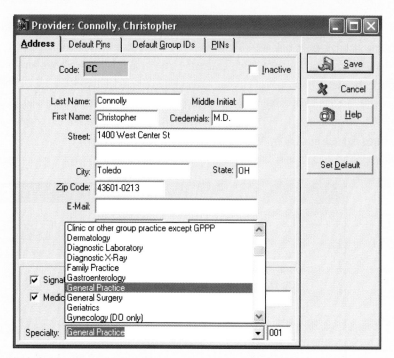

9. Click the Cancel button to close the Provider dialog box.
10. Click the Close button to close the Provider List dialog box.

Tip:

The Referring Provider dialog box is used in the same way as the Provider dialog box to set up the records for all referring providers in the practice. Therefore, it contains the same NPI field.

HIPAA National Plan Identifier

11. A second HIPAA identifier field is found in the Insurance Carrier dialog box. Under HIPAA, each insurance carrier will be required to adopt a standard health plan identifier, which will be implemented by insurance carriers. Click Insurance Carriers on the Lists menu.
12. The Insurance Carrier List dialog box is displayed. Click AARP Medigap to highlight it, and then click the Edit button.

13. The Insurance Carrier dialog box appears with AARP Medigap's information displayed. Open the Options tab.

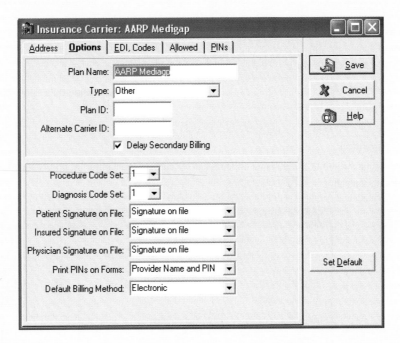

14. Notice the third box is labeled Plan ID. This field will be used to record a ten-digit HIPAA national plan identifier, also known as the National Payer ID. Once mandated, the information in the Type box above this field will no longer be used. Click the triangle button in the Type box to display the drop-down list of insurance carrier types.

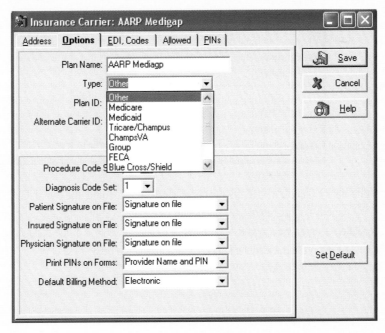

15. Scroll though the list to view all the options. At present, a clearinghouse translates the option selected in the Type box into the corresponding type-of-claim code required for the HIPAA claim. Click the Cancel button to close the Insurance Carrier dialog box.

16. Click the Close button to close the Insurance Carrier List dialog box.

HIPAA Individual Identifier

17. The third HIPAA identifier field is located in the Patient/Guarantor dialog box. Click Patients/Guarantors and Cases on the Lists menu.

18. The Patient List dialog box appears. Click Donald Aiken's name to highlight it, and then click the Edit Patient button.

19. The Patient/Guarantor dialog box appears with Donald Aiken's information displayed. Open the Other Information tab.

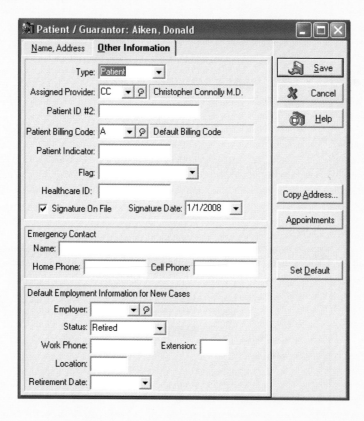

20. Locate the Health Care ID field in the top panel. Once implemented, the Health Care ID field will be used to record the patient's or guarantor's unique health care identification code, also known as a National Patient ID. Legislation is under way to specify protections regarding the use of the code.

21. Click the Cancel button to close the Patient/Guarantor dialog box.

22. Click the Close button to close the Patient List dialog box.

Computer Exploration

8.2 Electronic Claims Transmission

This activity takes you through the steps of transmitting a claim electronically in MediSoft. Under HIPAA, Medicare claims must be submitted electronically using the HIPAA electronic claim format, rather than on paper. The only exceptions are paper claims submitted from the smallest of providers. MediSoft is set up to transmit claims to a clearinghouse using the electronic version of the CMS-1500 (still referred to in MediSoft as the HCFA-1500). The clearinghouse then translates the data in the CMS-1500 to the required electronic HIPAA format and submits the claim to the payer.

Because most instructional environments are not actually set up to transmit electronic claims in MediSoft, in this activity you will go through the process of transmitting a claim electronically, but will not send it.

1. Click Claim Management on the Activities menu. The Claim Management dialog box is displayed.
2. Highlight the claim for Chart Number PORCEJE0. This is Jennifer Porcelli's claim, which was created for the purpose of this activity. Notice the Status 1 column for the claim reads "Ready to Send," and the Media 1 column displays the initials "EMC" for electronic media claim. (Remember from the chapter that EMC is an alternative term for electronic claim.)

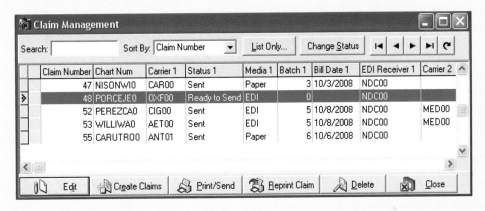

3. Click the Print/Send button.

4. The Print/Send Claims dialog box appears. As Jennifer Porcelli's claim was created as an electronic media claim, click the Electronic radio button to change the billing method to electronic. Leave the Electronic Claim Receiver box set to NDC, which stands for National Data Corporation.

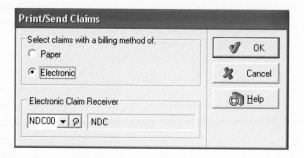

5. Click the OK button.

6. The Send Electronic Claims dialog box is displayed, with National Data Corporation displayed as the receiver. Click the Send Claims Now button.

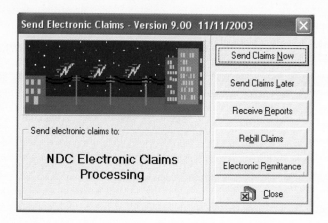

Computer Exploration

7. The Data Selection Questions dialog box appears. The various range boxes provide options for filtering the claims. In the first Chart Number Range box, key PO to select Jennifer Porcelli, and then press Enter. Follow the same steps to fill in the second Chart Number Range box.

8. For the purposes of this activity, delete the date displayed in the second Date Created Range box.

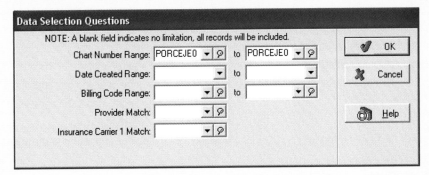

9. Click the OK button.

10. An Information dialog box appears, asking if you want to view a Verification report. Click the Yes button.

11. The Preview Report window appears with a copy of an EMC Verification report displayed. The report contains all the details of Jennifer Porcelli's claim, which is the only claim in the batch. Normally, in a

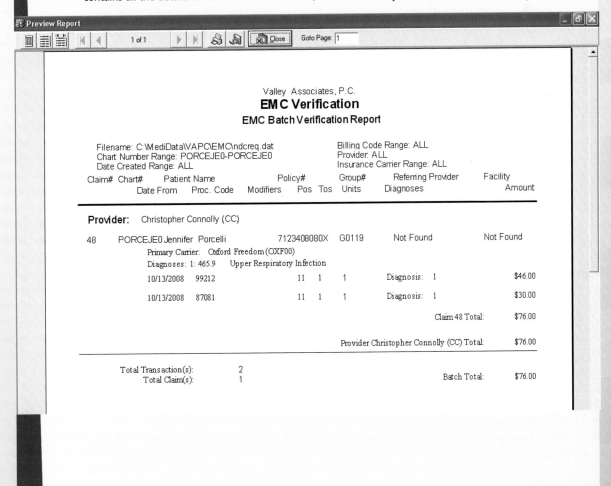

medical office, more than one claim would be transmitted at a time. For example, all claims created during the day might be transmitted regularly at the end of the day. The Verification report is designed to display the details of each claim in a given batch.

12. Click the Close button when finished viewing the report. The Preview Report window closes, and an Information dialog box appears, asking you if you want to continue with the transmission.

13. If you were in a medical office, you would click the Yes button and the claim would be sent via cable lines, telephone lines, or satellite from your computer to a computer at the clearinghouse. However, because you are in a school setting and are not actually set up to submit electronic claims at this time, click the No button.

14. The Information dialog box disappears and the Claim Management dialog box appears as before. Because Jennifer Porcelli's claim was not actually sent, the "Ready to Send" status still appears. If the claim had actually been sent electronically, the status column would now read "Sent."

15. Click the Close button to close the Claim Management dialog box and return to the main MediSoft window.

MediSoft TIP:

When a claim is sent electronically, an attachment that needs to accompany the claim, such as radiology films, must be referred to in the claim. In MediSoft, the EDI Report panel is used to indicate to the payer when an attachment will accompany the claim, and how the attachment will be transmitted. The EDI Report panel is located in the Diagnosis tab of the Case dialog box.

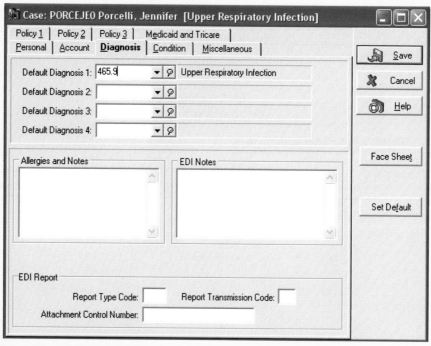

The EDI Report panel contains three boxes:

- The Report Type Code box indicates the type of report that is to be attached (for example, a diagnostic report).
- The Report Transmission Code indicates how the report will be transmitted to the payer (for example, via mail or e-mail).
- The Attachment Control Number box records the attachment's reference number (up to seven digits, assigned by the practice).

Refer to the MediSoft Help feature for a list of Report Type and Report Transmission codes.

Claim Adjudication, Follow-Up, and Collections

Objectives

After studying this chapter, you should be able to:

1. Describe the steps payers follow to adjudicate claims.

2. List ten checks that automated medical edits perform.

3. Describe the methods used to monitor and follow up claims with payers, including the use of the HIPAA 276/277 status inquiry/response.

4. Explain how the HIPAA 835 payment and remittance advice is processed by medical insurance specialists.

5. Discuss how appeals, postpayment audits, and overpayments may affect claim payments.

6. Describe the importance of accounts receivable billing and collections to medical practices.

7. Describe the purpose of a retention schedule.

Introduction

A major responsibility of the medical insurance specialist is the preparation of clean claims that will be paid in full and on time. Rejected claims can cost the practice twice as much to handle and result in reduced cash flow. Claims that payers decide not to pay, or to reduce, also have a negative effect on the practice's financial success.

To follow up on claims, medical insurance specialists need to understand what happens during third-party payer adjudication—the process that payers follow to examine claims and determine payments. Besides explaining the process, this chapter covers the process of entering payers' payments in the medical billing system, billing patients, and collecting overdue accounts. To complete the billing and reimbursement cycle, the retention of patient records is also briefly described.

Claim Adjudication

Initial processing of a claim occurs when it first enters the payer's computer system. Following that, adjudication begins. Although adjudication varies somewhat depending on the payer's policies, the essential steps—edits, reviews, and a payment decision—are the same.

Initial Processing or Claim Rejection

During the initial processing, each claim's data elements are checked by computer edits. This initial processing rejects claims with missing or incorrect information. The review might find such problems as the following.

- The numbers of a group policy number may have been transposed when they were entered, creating an invalid number.
- A valid diagnosis code has not been reported.
- A reporting provider in a PPO is not currently under contract or certified.
- A charge has not been given for a procedure (most payers require a fee to be listed for each service).
- The patient is not the correct sex for a reported gender-specific procedure code.

When information needs to be supplied or corrected as a result of initial processing, the payer's claims examiner asks the sender to fix and resubmit the claim. The medical insurance specialist should respond to these requests as quickly as possible by supplying the correct information and, if necessary, submitting another claim. The actual adjudication process begins when the complete and factually correct claim is accepted by the payer for processing.

Automated Medical Edits

A payer's medical edit review is done by complex screening edits that reflect the payer's payment policies for the plan. For example, Medicare's National Correct Coding Initiative (NCCI) edits cover all of its payment rules (Chapters 6 and 11). Failure to pass an edit may cause the claim's reported services, or some part of them, to be automatically denied. Failing other edits causes the claim to be removed from automated processing. These edits flag situations that must be looked at closely by a claims examiner before a payment decision is made.

The automated medical edits check for the following.

1. *Patient eligibility for benefits:* Edits check that the patient is eligible for the services provided. The patient must be enrolled in the plan for the date of service, and the premium payment must be current. Some group plans, for example, require a **waiting period**: they do not provide coverage until an employee has been on the job for a specified time period, such as thirty or sixty days. A **preexisting condition**—an illness or disorder that existed before the medical insurance contract went into effect—may not be covered under some plans. Under individual plans, coverage usually ends thirty days after a premium remains unpaid.

2. *Time limits for filing claims:* Claims must be submitted within the payer's time limits for filing claims. One payer may require claims to be filed no later than the end of the calendar year following the year in which services were provided. Other payers may have a shorter timetable, such as six months. Claims filed after the payer's deadline are either paid at a reduced rate or not reimbursed. Providers are not permitted to bill patients for these claims if they have missed the payer's submission deadline.

3. *Preauthorization and referral:* If a reported service requires preauthorization or a referral under the payer's policies, the edits verify that the claim contains a valid preauthorization or referral number.

4. *Duplicate dates of service:* Edits check for repeat billing of the same service. Dates of service for a patient should not be the same as those submitted on previous claims.

5. *Noncovered services:* Edits screen for services that are not covered under the patient's policy.

6. *Valid codes:* Diagnosis and procedure codes must be valid for the year of service. Outdated codes are rejected.

7. *Bundled codes:* The edits check for unbundling of surgical codes and other bundled codes (see Chapter 5).

8. *Medical review:* A **medical review program** is established by the payer's medical director and other professional medical staff. The program's stated goal is to ensure that providers give patients the most appropriate care in the most cost-effective manner. Under the automated review, the basic medical review screens are conducted. These edits check whether, according to the payer's rules, the services that were provided were appropriate and necessary. Medical necessity edits check that

- Procedure codes match the diagnosis codes.

- Procedures are not elective.

- Procedures are not experimental.

- Procedures are essential for treatment.

- Procedures are furnished at an appropriate level.

For example, a payer's guidelines may reimburse an acid perfusion test for esophagitis only when the diagnosis is esophagitis, esophageal reflux, or chest pain. This review also checks the approved usage—known as the frequency limits—of certain services, such as the number of times a service can be provided in a time period or for a specified condition. For example, in the Medicare program, one nursing home visit each month is a covered benefit, and chiropractic care is covered up to twelve visits in a year.

9. *Utilization review:* A **utilization review** determines the appropriateness of hospital-based health care services delivered to a member of a plan.
10. *Concurrent care:* **Concurrent care** refers to medical situations in which a patient receives extensive care from two or more providers on the same date of service. For example, both a nephrologist and a cardiologist would attend a hospitalized patient with kidney failure who has had a myocardial infarction. Instead of one provider's working under the direction of another, such as the relationship between a supervising surgeon and an anesthesiologist, in concurrent care each provider has an independent role in treating the patient. When two providers report services as attending physicians, rather than one as one attending and one consulting provider, a review is done to determine whether the concurrent care makes sense given the diagnoses and the providers' specialties.

Manual Review

When a claim is removed from the system, it is sent for manual review by the medical review department. A claims examiner in that department reviews the claim and any attachments. The examiner may decide that payment is justified or should be denied and will process the claim accordingly. The examiner may instead decide to hold the claim and ask the provider for additional clinical information before making a payment determination. In this case, the examiner may request documentation to check

- Where the service took place
- Whether the treatments were appropriate and a logical outcome of the facts and conditions shown in the medical record
- That services provided were accurately reported

Claims examiners are trained in the payer's payment policies, but they usually have little or no clinical medical background. In some cases, examiners choose to have claims reviewed by staff medical professionals—nurses or physicians—in the medical review department. For example, an examiner may not feel qualified to determine the medical necessity of an unlisted procedure and will turn the claim over to the professional for a decision.

Example

As an example, the following table shows the benefit matrix—a grid of benefits and policies—for a preferred provider organization's coverage of mammography.

BENEFIT MATRIX

Female Patient Age Group	In-Network	Out-of-Network
35–39		
One baseline screening	No charge	20 percent per visit after deductible
40–49		
One screening every two years, or more if recommended	No charge	20 percent per visit after deductible
50 and older		
One screening every year	No charge	10 percent per visit after deductible

- *Initial processing:* The payer's initial claims processing would check, among other points, that the patient for whom a screening mammogram is reported is a female over age thirty-five.

- *Automated medical edits:* The payer's edits reflect its payment policy for female patients in each of the three age groups. If a claim reports a single screening mammogram for a forty-five-year-old in-network patient within a twenty-four-month period, it passes the edit. If the claim contains two mammograms in fewer than twenty-four months, the edit would flag it for review by the claims examiner.
- *Manual review:* If two mammograms are reported within a two-year period for a patient in the forty to forty-nine year age range, the claims examiner would require documentation that the extra procedure was recommended and then review the reason for the recommendation. If an X-ray is included as a claim attachment, the claim examiner would probably ask a staff medical professional to evaluate the patient's condition and judge the medical necessity for the extra procedure.

Claim Payment, Denial, or Reduction

For each service line on a claim, the payer makes a payment **determination**—a decision whether to (1) pay it, (2) deny it, or (3) pay it at a reduced level. If the claims examiner decides that the claim falls within normal guidelines and is complete, the claim is paid. If it is not reimbursable, the claim is denied. If the examiner determines that the services the patient received were at too high a level for the diagnosis, the examiner may assign a lower-level code to the service line. When the level of service is reduced, the examiner has downcoded the service (see also Chapter 6). Claims may also be denied for lack of medical necessity, called a **medical necessity denial.**

Claims may be denied or downcoded because the procedure code does not match the diagnosis. Perhaps the procedure's place of service is an emergency department, but the patient's problem is not considered an emergency. Claims may also be denied or downcoded because the documentation fails to support the level of service claimed. For example, if the provider has coded a high-level evaluation and management service for a patient who presents with an apparently straightforward problem, the claims examiner is likely to request the encounter documentation. The medical record should contain information about the type of medical history and examination done as well as the complexity of the medical decision making that was performed. If the documentation does not support the service, the examiner downcodes the E/M code to a level considered appropriate.

Claim Monitoring and Follow-Up

After claims have been accepted for processing by payers, medical insurance specialists should communicate with payers to check on claim status and reply to any requests for information quickly.

Claim Status

Knowing when to follow up on transmitted claims requires two types of information. First, just as providers are required to file claims within a certain number of days after the date of service, payers also agree to process claims within a certain time period, referred to as the **claim turnaround time.** In support of this, most states have prompt-payment laws that obligate carriers to pay clean claims within a certain time period, typically forty-five days. Second, the medical billing program can generate a report that lists the claims transmitted each day

Billing Tip

Medical Necessity Denials
Medical insurance specialists should understand payers' regulations covering medical necessity denials. Often, claims denied for lack of medical necessity cannot be recovered from patients. For example, the payer's policy may state that participating providers cannot balance bill plan members when a claim is denied for lack of medical necessity, unless the patient agreed in advance to pay.

Billing Tip

Monitoring Changes in Coding Rules
Successful billers routinely check payers' Web sites to research changes in their rules regarding codes and reimbursement. The objective is to prevent third-party denials and speed claim payment.

A payer's utilization guidelines for preventive care and medical services benefits are shown below.

SERVICE	UTILIZATION
Pediatric:	
Birth–1 year	Six exams
1–5 years	Six exams
6–10 years	One exam every two years
11–21 years	One exam
Adult:	
22–29 years	One exam every 5 years
30–39 years	One exam every 3 years
40–49 years	One exam every 2 years
+50 years	One exam every year
Vision Exam	Covered once every 24 months
Gynecological	Covered once every year
Medical Office Visit	No preset limit
Outpatient Therapy	60 consecutive days per condition/year
Allergy Services	Maximum benefit: 60 visits in 2 years

If a provider files claims for each of the following cases, what is the payer's likely response? (Research the CPT codes in the current CPT before answering.) Explain your answers. An example is provided.

PATIENT	AGE	CPT CODE	DOS	PAYER RESPONSE?
Case Example:				
Patient X	45	99212	11/09/2008	*Pay the claim, because unlimited medical office visits are covered.*
1. Guy Montrachez	25	92004	11/08/2008	
2. Carole Regalle	58	99385	12/04/2008	
3. Mary Hiraldo	25	99385 and 88150; 88150	11/08/2008 12/10/2008	
4. George Gilbert	48	99386 99386	10/20/2007 11/02/2008	

and whether they have been paid. The report, called an **insurance aging report**, shows how long a payer has taken to respond to each claim. A typical report, shown in Figure 9.1, shows claims that have been sent fewer than thirty days ago, between thirty and sixty days ago, and so on.

```
                              Valley Associates, P.C.
                            Primary Insurance Aging
                                 As of 11/30/2008


Date of                         -- Past --   -- Past --   -- Past --   -- Past --   -- Past --    Total
Service    Procedure            0  -  30     31  -  60    61  -  90    91  - 120    121 ----->   Balance

Aetna Choice  (AET00)                                                                          (555)777-1000

WILLIWA0      Walter  Williams              SS: 401-26-9939      Policy: ABC103562239   Group: BDC1001
Birthdate: 9/4/1936
Claim: 53          Initial Billing Date: 10/8/2008     Last Billing Date: 10/8/2008
   10/1/2008    99212                         46.00                                              46.00
   10/1/2008    93000                         70.00                                              70.00
                                    0.00      116.00        0.00        0.00        0.00        116.00

             Insurance Totals    $0.00      $116.00       $0.00       $0.00       $0.00       $116.00


Anthem BCBS PPO  (ANT01)                                                                      (555)888-1000

CARUTRO0      Robin  Caruthers               SS: 331-24-0789       Policy: GH331240789    Group: OH4071
Birthdate: 3/29/1979
Claim: 49          Initial Billing Date: 10/6/2008     Last Billing Date: 10/6/2008
   10/6/2008    99212                         46.00                                              46.00
                                    0.00       46.00        0.00        0.00        0.00         46.00

             Insurance Totals    $0.00       $46.00       $0.00       $0.00       $0.00        $46.00


Cigna HMO Plus  (CIG00)                                                                       (555)666-3001

PEREZCA0      Carmen  Perez                  SS: 140-24-6113       Policy: 140603312X
Birthdate: 5/15/1934
Claim: 52          Initial Billing Date: 10/8/2008     Last Billing Date: 10/8/2008
   10/1/2008    99213                         62.00                                              62.00
                                    0.00       62.00        0.00        0.00        0.00         62.00

             Insurance Totals    $0.00       $62.00       $0.00       $0.00       $0.00        $62.00
```

Figure 9.1 Sample MediSoft Insurance Aging Report

HIPAA Health Care Claim Status Inquiry/Response

Aware of the claim turnaround time for the practice's major payers, the medical insurance specialist examines the report and selects claims for follow-up. Most practices follow up on claims that are under thirty days old in seven to fourteen days from the date of the claim. The medical insurance specialist contacts the payer to ensure that the claims have been received and are in process.

The HIPAA Health Care Claim Status Inquiry/Response is the standard electronic transaction used for this purpose. The inquiry that is sent is called the 276, and the response that is returned by the payer is called the 277. Figure 9.2 on page 302 shows how this exchange is sent between provider and payer. The 276/277 contain codes for the main types of responses:

- A codes indicate an acknowledgment.
- P codes indicate that a claim is pending; that is, the payer is waiting for information before making a payment decision.
- F codes indicate that a claim has been finalized.
- R codes indicate a request for more information.
- E codes indicate that an error has occurred in transmission, such as the payer does not understand the data, or the payer's computer system is not operating properly.

Billing Tip

Automated Claim Status Requests
Some medical billing programs can be set up to automatically track how many days claims have been unpaid and to send a claim status inquiry after a certain number of days. For example, if a particular payer pays claims on the twentieth day, the program transmits a 276 for any unpaid claims aged day twenty-one.

Valley Associates, P.C.

Patient Account Ledger

As of October 31, 2008

Entry	Date	POS	Description	Procedure	Document	Provider	Amount
GIROUKA0	Karen Giroux			(555)683-5364			
	Last Payment: -96.00		On: 10/8/2008				
6	10/7/2008			99396	0310060000	NR	149.00
7	10/7/2008			93000	0310060000	NR	70.00
8	10/7/2008			88150	0310060000	NR	29.00
9	10/7/2008			81000	0310060000	NR	17.00
10	10/7/2008			80050	0310060000	NR	120.00
40	10/8/2008		#234567 Anthem BCBS Traditiona	ANTPAY	0310060000	NR	-119.20
41	10/8/2008		#234567 Anthem BCBS Traditiona	ANTPAY	0310060000	NR	-56.00
42	10/8/2008		#234567 Anthem BCBS Traditiona	ANTPAY	0310060000	NR	-23.20
43	10/8/2008		#234567 Anthem BCBS Traditiona	ANTPAY	0310060000	NR	-13.60
44	10/8/2008		#234567 Anthem BCBS Traditiona	ANTPAY	0310060000	NR	-96.00
	Patient Totals						77.00
	Ledger Totals						77.00

Figure 9.2 General Claim Status Request/Response Information Flow

Working with Payers

In order to have claims processed as quickly as possible, medical insurance specialists must be familiar with the policies and procedures of the practice's payers. They should establish good working relationships with payer representatives. The following information should be available for each payer.

- The policies and procedures manuals for the standard plans the payer offers (including both the national and the local carrier for Medicare)
- The timetable for filing primary claims after the date of service and for submitting corrected claims, as well as for filing secondary claims (usually a period of time from the date of payment by the primary payer)
- How to resubmit corrected claims that are denied for missing or incorrect data (some payers, such as Medicare, may have an automated telephone procedure that can be used to resubmit a claim after missing information has been supplied)
- How to handle claim attachments

Some payers' manuals indicate that certain services will be reimbursed only if specific information accompanies the claim when it is filed. The 837 data element called "Claim Note" or a claim attachment is used to provide the required description. (Notes and attachments are described in Chapter 8.)

> *Example:* Allergy practices must supply proof of tests, submitting: skin testing sheets, test dates, test type (prick or intradermal), the name of the nurse who performed the test, and the doctor's signature.

Requests for information from payers should be answered as quickly as possible. Communications with payers' representatives should also be courteous and complete. Medical insurance specialists should use proper medical terminology to show that they understand what the payer is asking. In many cases,

Compliance Guideline

Claim Data: Correct and Documented
The best way to avoid queries from payers is to properly prepare and check claims. When payers' queries on claims are received, however, medical insurance specialists must ensure that the information they provide is correct and documented in the patient medical record and that any needed authorization to release information is current.

the medical insurance specialist must justify the reported procedures. For example, a payer often questions a problem-oriented evaluation and management (E/M) service that is reported on the same date of service as a procedure or a preventive physical examination, on the grounds that the E/M should not be reimbursed separately. Saying "well, the doctor did do both" is less persuasive than saying "the patient's presenting problems required both the level of E/M as indicated as well as the reported procedure; note that we attached the modifier –25 to indicate the necessity for this separate service."

Remittance Advice (RA) Processing

The remittance advice (RA) summarizes the results of the payer's adjudication process. If the provider has accepted assignment, the provider receives the RA and payment, and the patient receives an explanation of benefits (EOB). If the patient has not assigned benefits to the provider, the provider collects payment from the patient, preferably at the time of service, and the EOB and payment are sent directly to the patient.

The HIPAA Health Care Payment and Remittance Advice

RAs cover groups of claims and various service lines on those claims, not just a single claim. The claims that are paid are not consecutive or logically grouped; they are usually for different patients' claims and different dates of service (see Figure 9.3 on page 304). The EOBs that patients receive, on the other hand, list just the information for the recipient.

The HIPAA standard electronic transaction for RAs is the 835. An RA has the following types of information.

- A remittance document number (voucher number) assigned by the payer
- Name, address, and identification number of the pay-to provider
- Patient identification numbers, patient names, and names of the insured, if not the patient
- Dates of service
- Procedure codes
- Benefit plans
- Provider charges
- Allowed amounts
- Patient liability
- Benefit amounts
- Paid amount
- Claim adjustments
- Total amount of the payment accompanying the RA

Billing Tip

Reduced Payments for CPT Codes
Medical insurance specialists should be alert and compare the payer's payment for each CPT with the payer's fee schedule. Some payers downcode by paying the fee for a lesser CPT code but do not show that they have reduced the code itself to a lower-paid service.

Review and Processing

An RA contains an important piece of information—the claim control numbers that the provider assigned to claims when sending them. The RA contains this number for each claim so that the payment can be matched to a claim. Using the medical billing program, each claim listed on the RA is located, either manually or automatically by the computer system. The following procedure is followed.

PROVIDER REMITTANCE
THIS IS NOT A BILL
A PAYMENT SUMMARY AND AN EXPLANATION OF
CODES ARE AT THE END OF THIS STATEMENT

(1) MICHAEL A. JONES, MD
414 ISLAND RD.
PAVE, OH 43068-1101

(2) PAGE: 1 OF 1
(3) DATE: 01/13/2003
(4) ID NUMBER: 0100004820H01

PAR PROVIDER

(5) PATIENT: SMITH   MARY   (6) CLAIM: 99999999999   (7) ID. NO: 0001234567   (8) PLAN CODE: P-PAR   (9) MFD. REC. NO: 0555-99

(10) PROC CODE	(11) FROM DATE	(12) THRU DATE	(13) TREAT-MENT	(14) STATUS CODE	(15) AMOUNT CHRGD	(16) AMOUNT ALLWD	(17) COPAY/ DEDUCT	(18) COINS	(19) OTHER REDUCT	(20) AMOUNT APPRVD	(21) PATIENT BALANCE
99213-00	01/13/03	01/13/03	1	A	55.00	54.00	.00	5.00	.00	49.00	5.00
93000-00	01/13/03	01/13/03	1	A	40.50	39.50	.00	.00	.00	39.50	.00
81000-00	01/13/03	01/13/03	1	A	8.00	5.85	.00	.00	.00	5.85	.00
CLAIM TOTALS					103.50	94.35	.00	5.00	.00	89.35	5.00

PATIENT: ALLEN   ALLAN   CLAIM: 89999999999   ID. NO: 0000234567   PLAN CODE: C2000   MFD. REC. NO: 0444-88

PROC CODE	FROM DATE	THRU DATE	TREAT-MENT	STATUS CODE	AMOUNT CHRGD	AMOUNT ALLWD	COPAY/ DEDUCT	COINS	OTHER REDUCT	AMOUNT APPRVD	PATIENT BALANCE
99201-00	02/17/03	02/17/03	1	A	90.00	82.00	.00	10.00	.00	63.80	10.00
CLAIM TOTALS					90.00	82.00	.00	10.00	.00	63.80	10.00

PATIENT: JAMES   JAMES   CLAIM: 79999999999   ID. NO: 0001034567   PLAN CODE: STATE   MFD. REC. NO:

PROC CODE	FROM DATE	THRU DATE	TREAT-MENT	STATUS CODE	AMOUNT CHRGD	AMOUNT ALLWD	COPAY/ DEDUCT	COINS	OTHER REDUCT	AMOUNT APPRVD	PATIENT BALANCE
99214-00	01/07/03	01/07/03	1	A	101.00	58.00	.00	5.00	.00	68.00	5.00
CLAIM TOTALS					101.00	68.00	.00	5.00	.00	68.00	5.00

PAYMENT SUMMARY		TOTAL ALL CLAIMS		CHECK INFORMATION	
TOTAL AMOUNT PAID	224.35	AMOUNT CHARGES	294.50	NUMBER	00000XXXXXX
PRIOR CREDIT BALANCE	.00	AMOUNT ALLOWED	244.35	DATE	02/27/03
CURRENT CREDIT DEFERRED	.00	DEDUCTIBLE	.00	AMOUNT	224.35
PRIOR CREDIT APPLIED	.00	COPAY/COINS	20.00		
NEW CREDIT BALANCE	.00	OTHER REDUCTION	.00		
NET DISBURSED	224.35	AMOUNT APPROVED	224.35		
		PATIENT BALANCE	20.00		
		TOTAL CREDITS	.00		

(22) STATUS CODES:
A - APPROVED   AJ - ADJUSTMENT   IP - IN PROCESS   R - REJECTED   V - VOID

Codes

1. Name and address of provider who rendered medical services.
2. Number of pages for the provider remittance.
3. Date the provider remittance was issued.
4. 13-digit identification number of provider who rendered medical services.
5. Name of the patient.
6. Claim number.
7. Identification number we assign to the claim.
8. Name of the member's benefit plan.
9. Number the provider's office has assigned to the patient; will be reflected only if submitted in box 26 of the red HCFA-1500 claim form.
10. Procedure code(s) describing medical services rendered.
11. Date on which medical services began.
12. Date on which medical services ended.
13. Number reflected in box 24g of the red HCFA-1500 claim form; describes the number of days or units related to the medical service.
14. The status of the claim; see box 22 for more information.
15. The amount charged by provider for performing the medical service(s).
16. The amount that we will pay.
17. The amount that has been applied to the member's deductible.
18. The amount of the copayment or the coinsurance for which the member is responsible.
19. Any plan-specific reduction for which the member may be financially responsible.
20. The amount that we will pay.
21. Any amount for which the member is financially responsible.
22. Describes the abbreviations of the status codes reflected in item 14.

Figure 9.3 Example of a Payer's Remittance Advice

1. The patient data, plan, date of service, and listed procedures are checked against the claim.

2. Mismatched or missing information is noted, so that the claim can be corrected.

3. The payment for each procedure is reviewed against the expected amount.

4. The total paid by the patient and all third-party payers (the primary insurance and any other insurance) should equal the expected total payment.

5. The payer's explanations for unpaid, downcoded, or denied claims are reviewed. If the payer's action is not warranted, the claim is resubmitted or appealed.

Claims may be resubmitted or appealed under a number of circumstances.

- *Rejected or partially paid claims:* If the payer has not paid a claim because of missing information, the claim is corrected and resubmitted. If a procedure has been overlooked, a new claim is created to report that procedure. If resubmitted claims are again rejected, the medical insurance specialist (or perhaps the practice manager or provider) determines if an **appeal**, a request for reconsideration of the determination, should be filed. (The appeal process is discussed below.)

- *Denied claims:* If the payer has denied payment because a procedure is not a covered benefit or if the patient is not eligible for other reasons, the patient is billed for the uncovered amount. If the claim is denied for lack of medical necessity, the medical insurance specialist checks with the provider or practice manager for a decision on whether to appeal. If the practice decides not to appeal, the patient is billed for the amount.

- *Downcoded claims:* A payer's claims examiner may have downcoded a claim based on the screening edits or a medical review. As in the case of a denied claim, the provider may decide to appeal the decision. If no appeal is made, the patient may be responsible for the balance due.

Posting Payments

The medical insurance specialist enters the payments that are documented on the RA in the patient billing program. The claim adjustments are shown as **claim adjustment reason codes**. Examples are provided in Table 9.1 on pages 306–307. As is shown in Figure 9.3, the amount the patient owes for charges under a required deductible, copayment, or coinsurance is subtracted from the reimbursement to the provider. The provider then bills the patient for the amount owed. The due date for the patient's payment is set by the practice; usually it is thirty days from the invoice date.

In some offices, the medical billing program has an **auto-posting** feature. Instead of posting payments manually, this feature takes the payment data in the RA and uses the information to automatically post to the correct account. The software allows the user to establish posting rules, such as "only post a payment automatically if the claim is paid at 100 percent," so that the medical insurance specialist can examine those that are not paid as expected.

Medical insurance specialists may need to resolve payment issues with a payer. For example, a check may have been received for someone who is not a patient of the provider, or the payment and the RA may not match. In these cases, communications with the claims department by phone, mail, fax, or e-mail are required to resolve the discrepancy or error.

Denial Logs
Logs help determine problem areas for denied claims. Keeping a log of claims denials can help the practice track the most common denial reasons and find solutions to prevent similar denials in the future. Pay attention to the following problem areas:
- Coding errors, such as incorrect bundling or diagnosis codes inconsistent with procedure codes
- Front desk mistakes, such as errors during the preauthorization process
- Billing errors, such as duplicate claims
- Payer requests for more information or general delays in claims processing

TABLE 9.1 | Claim Adjustment Reason Codes

1 Deductible Amount

2 Coinsurance Amount

3 Copayment Amount

4 The procedure code is inconsistent with the modifier used or a required modifier is missing.

5 The procedure code/bill type is inconsistent with the place of service.

6 The procedure/revenue code is inconsistent with the patient's age.

7 The procedure/revenue code is inconsistent with the patient's gender.

8 The procedure code is inconsistent with the provider type/specialty (taxonomy).

9 The diagnosis is inconsistent with the patient's age.

10 The diagnosis is inconsistent with the patient's gender.

11 The diagnosis is inconsistent with the procedure.

12 The diagnosis is inconsistent with the provider type.

13 The date of death precedes the date of service.

14 The date of birth follows the date of service.

15 Payment adjusted because the submitted authorization number is missing, invalid, or does not apply to the billed services or provider.

16 Claim/service lacks information which is needed for adjudication. Additional information is supplied using remittance advice remarks codes whenever appropriate.

17 Payment adjusted because requested information was not provided or was insufficient/incomplete. Additional information is supplied using the remittance advice remarks codes whenever appropriate.

18 Duplicate claim/service.

19 Claim denied because this is a work-related injury/illness and thus the liability of the workers' compensation carrier.

20 Claim denied because this injury/illness is covered by the liability carrier.

21 Claim denied because this injury/illness is the liability of the no-fault carrier.

22 Payment adjusted because this care may be covered by another payer per coordination of benefits.

23 Payment adjusted because charges have been paid by another payer.

24 Payment for charges adjusted. Charges are covered under a capitation agreement/managed care plan.

25 Payment denied. Your stop loss deductible has not been met.

26 Expenses incurred prior to coverage.

27 Expenses incurred after coverage terminated.

29 The time limit for filing has expired.

30 Payment adjusted because the patient has not met the required eligibility, spend down, waiting, or residency requirements.

31 Claim denied as patient cannot be identified as our insured.

32 Our records indicate that this dependent is not an eligible dependent as defined.

33 Claim denied. Insured has no dependent coverage.

36 Balance does not exceed copayment amount.

37 Balance does not exceed deductible.

38 Services not provided or authorized by designated (network/primary care) providers.

39 Services denied at the time authorization/precertification was requested.

40 Charges do not meet qualifications for emergency/urgent care.

41 Discount agreed to in preferred provider contract.

42 Charges exceed our fee schedule or maximum allowable amount.

45 Charges exceed your contracted/legislated fee arrangement.

47 This (these) diagnosis(es) is (are) not covered, is (are) missing, or is (are) invalid.

49 These are noncovered services because this is a routine exam or screening procedure done in conjunction with a routine exam.

50 These are noncovered services because this is not deemed a "medical necessity" by the payer.

| TABLE 9.1 | Claim Adjustment Reason Codes (*continued*) |

51 These are noncovered services because this is a preexisting condition

52 The referring/prescribing/rendering provider is not eligible to refer/prescribe/order/perform the service billed.

55 Claim/service denied because procedure/treatment is deemed experimental/investigational by the payer.

56 Claim/service denied because procedure/treatment has not been deemed "proven to be effective" by the payer.

57 Payment denied/reduced because the payer deems the information submitted does not support this level of service, this many services, this length of service, this dosage, or this day's supply.

58 Payment adjusted because treatment was deemed by the payer to have been rendered in an inappropriate or invalid place of service.

62 Payment denied/reduced for absence of, or exceeded, precertification/authorization.

63 Correction to a prior claim.

65 Procedure code was incorrect. This payment reflects the correct code.

96 Noncovered charge(s).

97 Payment is included in the allowance for another service/procedure.

109 Claim not covered by this payer/contractor. You must send the claim to the correct payer/contractor.

110 Billing date predates service date.

111 Not covered unless the provider accepts assignment.

112 Payment adjusted as not furnished directly to the patient and/or not documented.

114 Procedure/product not approved by the Food and Drug Administration.

115 Payment adjusted as procedure postponed or canceled.

123 Payer refund due to overpayment.

124 Payer refund amount—not our patient.

125 Payment adjusted due to a submission/billing error(s). Additional information is supplied using the remittance advice remarks codes whenever appropriate.

138 Claim/service denied. Appeal procedures not followed or time limits not met.

140 Patient/insured health identification number and name do not match.

145 Premium payment withholding

146 Payment denied because the diagnosis was invalid for the date(s) of service reported.

150 Payment adjusted because the payer deems the information submitted does not support this level of service.

151 Payment adjusted because the payer deems the information submitted does not support this many services.

152 Payment adjusted because the payer deems the information submitted does not support this length of service.

155 This claim is denied because the patient refused the service/procedure.

160 Payment denied/reduced because injury/illness was the result of an activity that is a benefit exclusion.

A0 Patient refund amount.

A1 Claim denied charges.

B12 Services not documented in patients' medical records.

B13 Previously paid. Payment for this claim/service may have been provided in a previous payment.

B14 Payment denied because only one visit or consultation per physician per day is covered.

B15 Payment adjusted because this procedure/service is not paid separately.

B16 Payment adjusted because "New Patient" qualifications were not met.

B17 Payment adjusted because this service was not prescribed by a physician, not prescribed prior to delivery, the prescription is incomplete, or the prescription is not current.

B18 Payment denied because this procedure code/modifier was invalid on the date of service or claim submission.

B22 This payment is adjusted based on the diagnosis.

D7 Claim/service denied. Claim lacks date of patient's most recent physician visit.

D8 Claim/service denied. Claim lacks indicator that "x-ray is available for review."

W1 Workers' Compensation State Fee Schedule Adjustment.

Patient ID	Patient Name	Plan	Date of Service	Procedure	Provider Charge	Allowed Amount	Patient Payment (Coinsurance and Deductible)	Claim Adjusment Reason Code	Benefit Amount
537-88-5267	Ramirez, Gloria B.	R-1	02/13/2008–02/13/2008	99214	$105.60	$ 59.00	$ 8.85	2	$ 50.15
348-99-2537	Finucula, Betty R.	R-1	01/15/2008–01/15/2008	99292	$ 88.00	$ 50.00	$ 7.50	2	$ 42.50
537-88-5267	Ramirez, Gloria B.	R-1	02/14/2008–02/14/2008	90732	$ 38.00	0	$ 38.00	49	0
760-57-5372	Jugal, Kurt T.	R-1	02/16/2008–02/16/2008	93975	$580.00	$261.00	$139.15	1	$121.85
				99204	$178.00	$103.00	$ 15.45	2	$ 87.55
875-17-0098	Quan, Mary K.	PPO-3	02/16/2008–02/16/2008	20004	$192.00	$156.00	$ 31.20	2	$124.80
								TOTAL	$426.85

The RA shown above has been received by a provider.

1. What is the patient coinsurance percentage required under plan R-1?

2. What is the patient coinsurance percentage required under plan PPO-3?

3. What is Gloria Ramirez's balance due for the two dates of service listed?

4. Kurt Jugal's first visit of the year is the encounter shown for DOS 2/16/2008. What is the patient deductible under plan R-1? (*Hint:* Since the deductible was satisfied by the patient's payment for the first charge, that payment was made up of the deductible and the coinsurance under the plan.)

Electronic Funds Transfer

Many practices that receive RAs establish bank accounts that can receive electronically transmitted funds. In this case, the practice authorizes the payer to provide an **electronic funds transfer (EFT)** of the payment. The funds are deposited by the payer's bank directly into the practice's bank account. These funds are immediately available for use, and the transfer costs less than checks to process. If an EFT is not set up, the payer sends a check to the practice, and the check is taken to the practice's bank for deposit. In this case, the funds are available several days after the deposit date.

Appeals, Postpayment Audits, and Refunds

After RAs are processed, a number of events may affect the payments received. When a claim has been denied or payment reduced, an appeal may be filed with the payer for reconsideration. Postpayment audits, such as those conducted by Medicare (see Chapters 6 and 11), may result in a change in the payment determination. Under certain conditions, refunds may be due to either the payer or the patient.

The Appeal Process

A provider who accepts assignment may decide to request a review of the payer's denial or reduced payment of a claim. (NonPARs do not appeal; rather, they collect the payment from the patient.) Patients, too, have the right to request an appeal. Whether the provider or the patient, the person filing the appeal is the **claimant**. Payers have a consistent process for providers' appeals and for their internal procedures to review them. Before starting an appeal, the practice's staff reviews the payer's appeal process and plans its actions according to the rules.

When providers file an appeal, they are acting to secure compensation both for themselves and for the patient. For this reason, some providers add a limited power of attorney clause to the patient release of information form that authorizes them to handle claim-related financial matters for the patient.

Basic Steps

Appeals must be filed within a specified time after the claim has been returned. Most payers have an escalating structure of appeals, such as (1) a complaint, (2) an appeal, and (3) a grievance. The claimant must move through the three levels in pursuing an appeal, starting at the lowest and continuing to the highest, final level. Some payers also have rules about the minimum amount of the charge that must be involved for an appeal to be processed.

Options after Appeal Rejection

Claimants can take another step if the payer has rejected all the appeals on a claim. State insurance commissions regulate the payers that are licensed to offer insurance coverage to the state's citizens, and one of their functions is to review appeals that have been rejected by payers. If a claimant decides to pursue an appeal with the state insurance commission, copies of the complete case file—all documents that relate to the initial claim determination and the appeals process—are sent, along with a letter of explanation.

Postpayment Audits

Most postpayment reviews are used to build clinical information. Payers use their audits of practices, for example, to study the treatments and their outcomes for

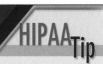
Compliance Guideline

Medicare NonPAR

Under Medicare, if a nonparticipating provider collected a fee at the time of service and the claim is denied or reduced, the provider must refund to the patient the difference between what was collected and what the patient was reimbursed. In this situation, the provider must write off the uncollected charge.

Thinking It Through—9.3

In a large practice of forty providers, the staff responsible for creating claims and billing is located in one building, and the staff members who handle RAs work at another location. In your opinion, what difficulties might this separation present? What strategies can be used to ensure that complete and compliant claims are submitted?

---

patients with similar diagnoses. The patterns that are determined are used to confirm or alter best practice guidelines.

At times, however, the postpayment audit is done to verify the medical necessity of reported services or to uncover fraud and abuse. The audit may be based on the detailed records about each provider's services that are kept by payers' medical review departments. Some payers keep records that go back for many months or years. The payer analyzes these records to assess patterns of care from individual providers and to flag outliers—those that differ from other providers. A postpayment audit might be conducted to check the documentation of these providers' cases or, in some cases, to check for fraudulent practices (see Chapter 6).

Refunds of Overpayments

Medicare and other payers' postpayment audits may determine that the documentation does not support a paid claim. In this case, the auditor may downcode or deny the claim. Some or all of the reimbursement that the provider has received for the claim is then considered an overpayment, and the payer will ask for a refund. If the audit shows that the claim was for a service that was not medically necessary, the provider also must refund any payment collected from the patient. Occasionally, the payer may overpay a claim by mistake. When an overpayment is received, the medical insurance specialist arranges for a refund check to be sent to the payer.

Patient Billing

A medical practice's financial viability depends on a sufficient cash flow to cover the cost of doing business. For this reason, practices closely track their **accounts receivable (A/R)**—the money that is owed for services rendered. Because medical insurance specialists are responsible for generating and following up on insurance claims and payments, they play an important role in accounts receivable collection.

Accounts Receivable and Billing

The accounts receivable is made up of payments due from third-party payers and from patients. It is maintained in the medical billing program.

Patient Encounter Transaction Data and Claim Data

When the patient completes an office visit, the medical insurance specialist uses the encounter form and the practice's fee schedule to enter the charges for the services. The billing program updates the patient's ledger (the record of a patient's financial transactions; also called the patient account record) to show the patient's balance due. If the patient makes any payment, such as a copayment, that amount is entered and subtracted from the balance due. Then the insurance claim for the service is created and transmitted to the payer.

Third-Party Payment Data

After the payer adjudicates the claims and sends an RA listing the patient's claim to the practice, the medical insurance specialist posts the payer's payment amount, either manually or using an auto-posting feature. These steps are followed:

1. The payer's payment for each reported procedure is posted.
2. The amount the patient owes for each reported procedure is posted.
3. If any part of a charge must be written off, this amount is also entered.

The billing program uses this information to update the **day sheet**, which is a summary of the financial transactions that occur each day. The patient ledger is also updated.

Coordination of Benefits

When additional insurance coverage applies to a claim, the information on an RA is used to create a claim (837) for a secondary (or tertiary) payer. The medical insurance specialist sends the secondary payer the adjudication data from the RA for the first claim. The payer determines what additional benefits are due, then sends payment with an RA to the provider.

Patient Statements

Periodically, according to practice procedures, the billing program is used to generate bills called **patient statements.** Most practices mail patient statements at least twice a month, such as billing half of the patients in the middle of the month and the other half at the end of the month. Larger practices usually bill more often. Patient statements show the balance patients owe; payers' payments have been subtracted from the accounts.

Example

On pages 312–313, this process is illustrated for a patient. Study the billing program computer screen, the patient account ledger, and the patient statement for this case:

> Patient: Karen Giroux
> Date of Service: 10/7/08
> Date of RA: 10/8/08

Compliance Guideline

Avoid Deleting Posted Data
Transactions should not be deleted in the patient billing program, because this could be interpreted by an auditor as a fraudulent act. Instead, corrections, changes, and write-offs are made with adjustments to the existing transactions. The adjusting entries provide the practice and the patient with a history of events in case there is a billing inquiry or an audit.

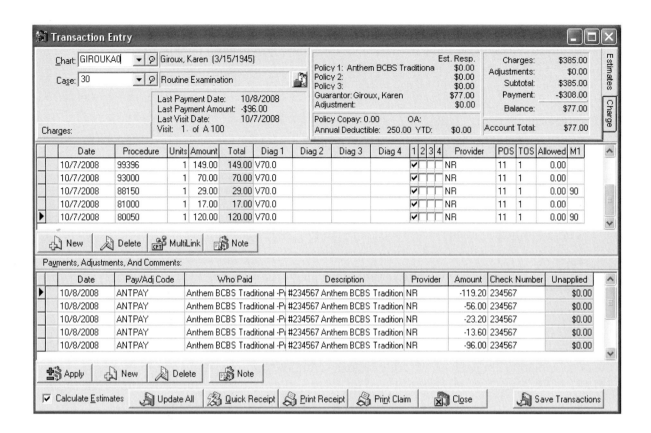

Encounter information and insurance payment The computer screen above illustrates the entry of the transaction for Karen Giroux's office visit on 10/7/2008 and a payment received from the health plan on 10/8/2008. The report below shows these charges and the receipt of the payment on the patient's ledger. The patient statement on page 313 is sent to the patient or guarantor and shows the balance that is owed.

Valley Associates, P.C.
Patient Account Ledger
As of October 31, 2008

Entry	Date	POS	Description	Procedure	Document	Provider	Amount
GIROUKA0		Karen Giroux		(555)683-5364			
			Last Payment: -96.00 On: 10/8/2008				
6	10/7/2008			99396	0310060000	NR	149.00
7	10/7/2008			93000	0310060000	NR	70.00
8	10/7/2008			88150	0310060000	NR	29.00
9	10/7/2008			81000	0310060000	NR	17.00
10	10/7/2008			80050	0310060000	NR	120.00
40	10/8/2008		#234567 Anthem BCBS Traditiona	ANTPAY	0310060000	NR	-119.20
41	10/8/2008		#234567 Anthem BCBS Traditiona	ANTPAY	0310060000	NR	-56.00
42	10/8/2008		#234567 Anthem BCBS Traditiona	ANTPAY	0310060000	NR	-23.20
43	10/8/2008		#234567 Anthem BCBS Traditiona	ANTPAY	0310060000	NR	-13.60
44	10/8/2008		#234567 Anthem BCBS Traditiona	ANTPAY	0310060000	NR	-96.00
		Patient Totals					77.00
		Ledger Totals					77.00

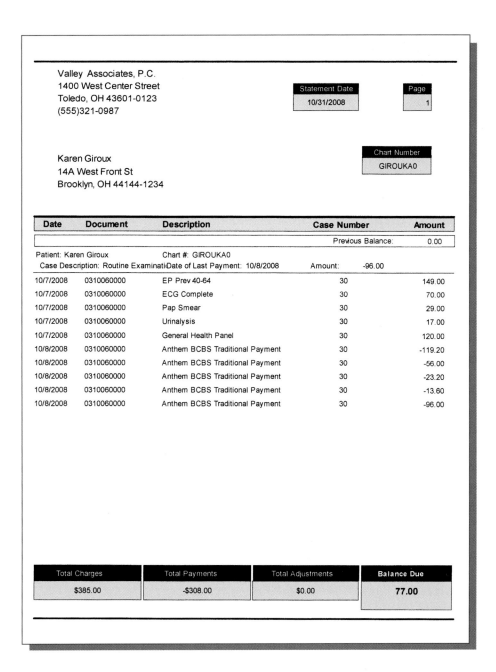

Date	Document	Description	Case Number	Amount
			Previous Balance:	0.00

Valley Associates, P.C.
1400 West Center Street
Toledo, OH 43601-0123
(555)321-0987

Statement Date
10/31/2008

Page
1

Karen Giroux
14A West Front St
Brooklyn, OH 44144-1234

Chart Number
GIROUKA0

Patient: Karen Giroux   Chart #: GIROUKA0
Case Description: Routine Examinati Date of Last Payment: 10/8/2008   Amount: -96.00

Date	Document	Description	Case Number	Amount
10/7/2008	0310060000	EP Prev 40-64	30	149.00
10/7/2008	0310060000	ECG Complete	30	70.00
10/7/2008	0310060000	Pap Smear	30	29.00
10/7/2008	0310060000	Urinalysis	30	17.00
10/7/2008	0310060000	General Health Panel	30	120.00
10/8/2008	0310060000	Anthem BCBS Traditional Payment	30	-119.20
10/8/2008	0310060000	Anthem BCBS Traditional Payment	30	-56.00
10/8/2008	0310060000	Anthem BCBS Traditional Payment	30	-23.20
10/8/2008	0310060000	Anthem BCBS Traditional Payment	30	-13.60
10/8/2008	0310060000	Anthem BCBS Traditional Payment	30	-96.00

Total Charges	Total Payments	Total Adjustments	Balance Due
$385.00	-$308.00	$0.00	77.00

Practice Management Reports and Aging Analysis

The billing program is also used to produce reports about practice finances. Reports that may be generated include

- Claim turnaround times from the largest payers
- The amounts of payments that are currently outstanding (the accounts receivable)
- The average amount billed on each day the office is open in a specified period
- The amount of billing for each physician in the practice, including each physician's no-show rate (patients who did not appear for their appointments)
- The frequency of procedure codes reported by each physician in the practice
- The number and type of errors

Especially important to medical insurance specialists are aging reports. These reports show the age, or how long after the date of the invoice, expected payments from payers and patients are received. As mentioned earlier, insurance aging reports show how long a payer has taken to respond to each claim. For example, in MediSoft, reports show primary, secondary, and tertiary aging. How long each payer takes to pay bills can be compared with the terms of its contract. For example, a PPO with which the practice has a contract might routinely be ten days later than the agreed-to claim turnaround time. The practice manager might review the situation with the payer's customer service manager and ask the payer to adhere to its guidelines.

Collections

Collections involve finding the correct balance between two important goals: ensuring cash flow and ensuring patient satisfaction. Most patients pay their bills on time. However, every practice has some patients who do not pay their bills when they receive their monthly statements. Patients' reasons for not paying range from forgetfulness or inability to pay to dissatisfaction with the services or charges. Medical insurance specialists must take action to resolve problems and collect payments. Note, though, that the collection process really begins with effective communications with patients about their responsibility to pay for services. When patients understand the charges and agree to pay them in advance, collecting the payments is not usually problematic.

Practice Financial Policy

So that patients understand their financial responsibilities, the practice should have and share a financial policy. The policy should tell patients how the practice will handle the following.

- Collecting copayments and past-due balances
- Setting up financial arrangements for unpaid balances
- Charity care or use of a sliding scale for patients with low incomes
- Payments for services not covered by insurance
- Collecting prepayment for services
- Accepting cash, checks, money orders, and credit cards
- Special circumstances for automobile accidents and nonassigned insurance

Many experts recommend asking patients to sign a copy of the financial policy and giving them a copy, keeping the original in the medical record.

Governing Collections

Collections from payers are considered business collections. Collections from patients, however, are consumer collections and are regulated by federal and state law. The Fair Debt Collection Practices Act of 1977 and the Telephone Consumer Protection Act of 1991 regulate debt collections, forbidding unfair practices. General guidelines include the following.

- Do not call a patient before 8 A.M. or after 9 P.M.
- Do not make threats or use profane language.
- Do not discuss the patient's debt with anyone except the person who is responsible for payment. If the patient has a lawyer, discuss the problem only with the lawyer, unless the lawyer gives permission to talk with the patient.
- Do not use any form of deception or violence to collect a debt. For example, do not impersonate a law officer to try to force a patient to pay.

If the practice's printed or displayed payment policy covers adding finance charges on late accounts, it is acceptable to do so. The amount of the finance charge must comply with federal and state law.

Collection Process and Methods

Medical insurance specialists are often responsible for handling, or at least organizing, the collection effort. Collection begins with the **patient aging report**, which shows which patients' payments are overdue (see Figure 9.4). Aging begins on the date of the bill. For each account, an aging report shows the name of the patient, the last payment, and the amount of charges in each of these categories:

- *Current:* Up to thirty days
- *Past:* thirty-one to sixty days
- *Past:* sixty-one to ninety days
- *Past:* Over ninety-one days

For example, Figure 9.4 shows that charges totaling $204.60 are thirty-one to sixty days past due.

Each practice sets its own procedures for the collection process. Large bills have priority over smaller ones. Usually, an automatic reminder notice and a second statement are mailed when a bill has not been paid thirty days after it was issued. Some practices phone a patient with a thirty-day overdue account. If the bill is not then paid, a series of collection letters is generated at intervals, each more stringent in its tone and more direct in its approach. Following is an example of one practice's collection time line; different approaches are used in other practices.

30 days	Bill patient
45 days	Call patient regarding bill
60 days	Letter 1
75 days	Letter 2 and call
80 days	Letter 3
90 days	Turn over to collections

Valley Associates, P.C.
Patient Aging
As of November 30, 2008

Chart	Name	Birthdate	Current 0 - 30	Past 31 - 60	Past 61 - 90	Past 91 ---->	Total Balance
CARUTRO0 Robin Caruthers		3/29/1979		46.00			46.00
Last Pmt: -20.00 On: 10/6/2008		(555)629-0222					
ESTEPWI0 Wilma Estephan		3/14/1940		5.60			5.60
Last Pmt: -22.40 On: 10/8/2008		(555)683-5272					
GIROUKA0 Karen Giroux		3/15/1945		77.00			77.00
Last Pmt: -96.00 On: 10/8/2008		(555)683-5364					
PEREZCA0 Carmen Perez		5/15/1934			62.00		62.00
Last Pmt: -20.00 On: 10/1/2008		(555)692-3314					
PORCEJE0 Jennifer Porcelli		7/5/1970		76.00			76.00
Last Pmt: -15.00 On: 10/13/2008		(555)709-0388					
WILLIWA0 Walter Williams		9/4/1936			116.00		116.00
Last Pmt: -15.00 On: 10/1/2008		(555)936-0216					
Report Aging Totals			$0.00	$204.60	$178.00	$0.00	382.60
Percent of Aging Total			0.0 %	53.5 %	46.5 %	0.0 %	100.00 %

Figure 9.4 Example of Patient Aging Report

Collection Calls and Letters

Telephone calls to patients often result in questions regarding insurance filing, what the insurance carrier allowed, and whether secondary insurance was filed. All this information should be gathered before making a call. Examples of a series of collection letters appear in Figure 9.5, parts a, b, and c.

Collection Agencies

After a number of collection attempts that do not produce results, some practices use outside collection agencies to pursue large unpaid bills. The agency that is selected should have a reputation for fair and ethical handling of collections. When a patient's account is referred to an agency for collection, the medical insurance specialist no longer contacts the patient or sends statements. If a payment is received from a patient while the account is with the agency, the agency is notified. Collection agencies are often paid on the basis of the amount of money they collect, so they must be told about collected amounts.

Credit Arrangements

For large bills or special situations, some practices may elect to extend credit to patients. When credit agreements are made, patients and the practice agree to divide the bill over a period of months. Patients agree to make monthly payments. If no finance charges are applied to unpaid balances, this type of arrangement is between the practice and the patient, and no legal regulations apply. If, however, the practice adds finance charges and the payments are to be made in more than four installments, the arrangement is subject to the Truth in Lending Act, which is part of the Consumer Credit Protection Act. In this case, the practice notifies the patient in writing about the total amount, the

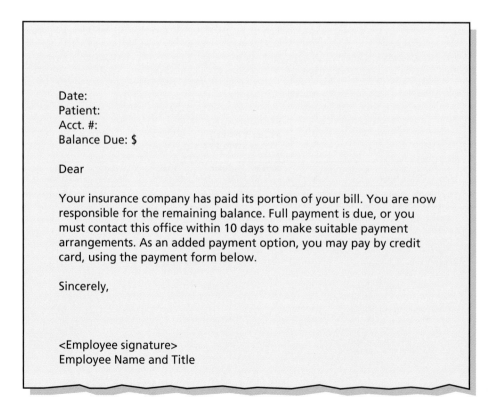

Date:
Patient:
Acct. #:
Balance Due: $

Dear

Your insurance company has paid its portion of your bill. You are now responsible for the remaining balance. Full payment is due, or you must contact this office within 10 days to make suitable payment arrangements. As an added payment option, you may pay by credit card, using the payment form below.

Sincerely,

<Employee signature>
Employee Name and Title

Figure 9.5 Samples of Collection Letters (a) First Letter

Date:
Patient:
Acct. #:
Balance Due: $

Dear

This is a reminder that your account is overdue. If there are any
problems we should know about, please telephone or stop in at the
office. A statement is attached showing your past account activity.

Your prompt payment is requested.

Sincerely,

<Employee signature>
Employee Name and Title

Figure 9.5 (b) Second Letter

Date:
Patient:
Acct. #:
Balance Due: $

Dear

Your account is seriously past due and has been placed with our
in-house collection department. Immediate payment is needed to keep
an unfavorable credit rating from being reported on this account. If you
are unable to pay in full, please call to make acceptable arrangements
for payment. Failure to respond to this notice within 10 days will
precipitate further collection actions.

Sincerely,

<Employee signature>
Employee Name and Title

Figure 9.5 (c) Third Letter

finance charges (stated as a percentage), when each payment is due and the amounts, and the date the last payment is due. Both the practice manager and the patient must sign this agreement.

Writing Off Uncollectible Accounts

When the practice's collection process has been followed and no payment has resulted, the practice has a policy on bills it does not expect to collect. Usually, if all collection attempts have been exhausted and it would cost more to continue than the amount owed, the process is ended. In this case, the amount is called an **uncollectible account** or bad debt and is written off the practice's expected accounts receivable.

Record Retention

Patients' medical records and financial records are kept according to the practice's policy. The practice manager or providers set this policy after reviewing the state regulations that apply. Any federal laws, such as HIPAA regulations, are also taken into account.

The practice's policy about keeping records is summarized in a **retention schedule**, a list of the items from a record that are retained and for how long. The retention schedule usually also covers the method for retention. For example, a policy might state that all established patients' records are stored in the practice's files for three years, and then microfilmed and removed to another storage location for another four years.

The retention schedule that is established must protect both the provider and the patient. Continuity of care is the first concern: the record must be available for anyone who is caring for the patient, within or outside of the practice. Also, the records must be kept in case of a legal proceeding, For example, the provider might be asked to justify the level and nature of treatment when a claim is investigated or challenged (see Chapter 6), requiring access to documentation.

The American Health Information Management Association (AHIMA) Practice Brief on the retention of health information states:

> Each health care provider should develop a retention schedule for patient health information that meets the needs of its patients, physicians, researchers, and other legitimate users, and complies with legal, regulatory, and accreditation requirements. The retention schedule should include guidelines that specify what information should be kept, the time period for which it should be kept, and the storage medium (paper, microfilm, optical disk, magnetic tape, or other).

Although state guidelines cover medical information about patients, most do not specifically cover financial records. In terms of retention, the patient's financial records are generally considered saved according to federal business records retention requirements. Under HIPAA, covered entities must keep records of HIPAA compliance for six years. For example, patients have the right to request an accounting of the disclosures that have been made of their protected health information (see Figure 9.6). In general, the storage method chosen and the means of destroying the records when the retention period ends must strictly adhere to the same confidentiality requirements as patient medical records.

PATIENT REQUEST FOR ACCOUNTING OF DISCLOSURES

Patient Name

Patient Address

Medical Record #   Date of Birth

Name & Address of Requestor if not patient

"Please consider this a request for an accounting of all disclosures for the time frames indicated below (Maximum time frame that can be requested is six years prior to the date of the request, but not before April 14, 2003). I understand that there is a fee for this accounting and wish to proceed. I understand that the accounting will be provided to me within sixty days unless I am notified in writing that an extension of up to thirty days is necessary."

Patient or Requestor to Complete:			Practice to Complete:		
From Date(s):	To Date(s):	Purpose of Disclosure:	Date Request In	Date Information to Patient	Fee

Date:	Signature of Patient or Legal Representative:
Date:	Signature of Patient or Legal Representative:

Figure 9.6 Example of Patient Request for Accounting of Disclosures Form

Thinking It Through—9.4

Based on the patient account information in Figure 9.4 on page 315:

1. What was the last payment made by Carmen Perez? _____

2. For Walter Williams, what amount has been due for more than sixty days? _____

Review

Chapter Summary

1. Payers first perform initial processing checks on claims, rejecting those with missing or clearly incorrect information. During the adjudication process, claims are processed through the payer's automated medical edits; a manual review is done if required; and the payer decides whether to pay, deny, or reduce the claim.

2. Automated edits check for (a) patient eligibility for benefits, (b) time limits for filing claims, (c) preauthorization and referral requirements, (d) duplicate dates of service, (e) noncovered services, (f) the use of valid codes, (g) unbundling of bundled codes, (h) confirmation that services were appropriate and necessary, (i) utilization review, and (j) concurrent care.

3. Medical insurance specialists monitor claims by reviewing the insurance aging report and follow up at properly timed intervals based on the payer's promised turnaround time. The HIPAA 276/277 Heath Care Claim Status Inquiry/Response is used to track overdue claims.

4. The HIPAA 835 Health Care Payment and Remittance Advice is the standard transaction payers use to transmit adjudication details and payments to providers. When a payer's remittance advice (RA) is received, the medical insurance specialist checks each service and payment against the corresponding claim. The claim control number reported on the 835 is used to match up claims sent and payments received. Claims that are unpaid, downcoded, or denied inappropriately may be resubmitted or appealed. Payments, unless electronically transferred to the provider's bank account, are deposited.

5. Filing an appeal may result in payment of a denied or reduced claim. Postpayment audits are usually used to gather information about treatment outcomes, but they may also be used to find overpayments, which must be refunded to the payer. Refunds to patients may also be required.

6. Accounts receivable, made up of money owed to the practice by third-party payers and patients, must be collected on a timely basis for adequate cash flow to cover expenses. Medical insurance specialists maintain patient accounts, generate patient invoices, and produce patient aging reports. They may also play a role in collections.

7. A retention schedule provides guidelines on the items in the patient medical record that must be retained and on the length of time and method for retention. Patients' continuity of care is the first concern. Also, the provider must be able to justify the level and nature of treatment when a claim is investigated or challenged.

Key Terms

accounts receivable (A/R) *page 310*
adjustment *page 313*
appeal *page 305*
auto-posting *page 305*
claim adjustment reason codes *page 305*
claimant *page 309*
claim turnaround time *page 300*
concurrent care *page 298*

day sheet *page 311*
determination *page 300*
electronic funds transfer (EFT) *page 308*
insurance aging report *page 300*
medical necessity denial *page 300*
medical review program *page 297*
patient aging report *page 315*
patient statement *page 311*

preexisting condition *page 297*
retention schedule *page 318*
uncollectible account *page 318*
utilization review *page 298*
waiting period *page 297*
276 *page 301*
277 *page 301*
835 *page 303*

Review Questions

Match the key terms in the left column with the definitions in the right column.

A. medical necessity denial

B. preexisting condition

C. retention schedule

D. uncollectible accounts

E. 276/277

F. waiting period

G. utilization review

H. electronic funds transfer

I. concurrent care

J. determination

_____ 1. The time that the insured must wait from the date of enrollment to the date insurance coverage is effective

_____ 2. A review to determine the appropriateness of health care services delivered to a member of a plan

_____ 3. Medical situation in which a patient receives extensive independent care from two or more attending physicians on the same date of service

_____ 4. A payer's refusal to pay for a reported procedure that does not meet its medical necessity criteria

_____ 5. The HIPAA standard transaction used to follow up on delayed reimbursement

_____ 6. A practice's policy that governs the information from patients' medical records that is to be stored, for how long it is to be retained, and the storage medium to be used

_____ 7. A payer's decision regarding payment of a claim

_____ 8. A banking service for directly transmitting funds from one bank to another

_____ 9. Money that cannot be collected from the practice's payers or patients

_____ 10. An illness or disorder that existed before the insured's medical insurance contract went into effect

Decide whether each statement is true or false, and write T for true or F for false.

_____ 1. A claim may be rejected by a payer because the patient has not paid the premium for the reported date of service.

_____ 2. The medical review program is created by the provider's practice manager to adjudicate claims.

_____ 3. A payer's claims examiners are trained medical professionals.

_____ 4. If a patient's medical record clearly documents a high level of evaluation and management service, the associated procedure code is not likely to be reduced by the payer.

_____ 5. The claim turnaround time should be specified in the payer's manual.

_____ 6. The insurance aging report shows when patients received their statements.

_____ 7. The EFT summarizes the results of the payer's adjudication process.

_____ 8. An appeal can be filed if the provider disagrees with the payer's determination.

_____ 9. The RA lists the patient's liability, which is subtracted from the allowed charge to calculate the amount the provider is paid.

_____ 10. The correct procedure for writing off the part of a fee that a payer does not allow is to delete the billed charge in the patient billing system and enter the allowed charge.

Write the letter of the choice that best completes the statement or answers the question.

_____ 1. A payer's initial processing of a claim screens for
   A. utilization guidelines
   B. medical edits
   C. basic errors in claim data or missing information
   D. claims attachments

_____ 2. Some automated edits are for
   A. patient eligibility, duplicate claims, and noncovered services
   B. valid identification numbers, missing charges, and provider status
   C. medical necessity reduction denial
   D. documentation, utilization, and in-network status

_____ 3. A claim may be downcoded because
   A. the claim does not list a charge for every procedure code
   B. the claim is for noncovered services
   C. the documentation does not justify the level of service
   D. the procedure code applies to a patient of the other gender

_____ 4. Payers should comply with the stated
   A. insurance aging report
   B. claim turnaround time
   C. remittance advice
   D. retention schedule

_____ 5. The person filing an appeal is called
   A. the guarantor
   B. the claims examiner
   C. the medical director
   D. the claimant

_____ 6. Appeals must always be filed
   A. within a specified time
   B. by the provider for the patient
   C. by patients on behalf of patients
   D. in writing

_____ 7. If a postpayment audit determines that a paid claim should have been denied or reduced
   A. the provider is subject to civil penalties
   B. the provider must refund the incorrect payment
   C. the provider bills the patient for the denied amount
   D. none of the above

_____ 8. The day sheet produced by the patient billing system shows
   A. what each patient owes the practice as of that date
   B. what each payer owes the practice as of that date
   C. the payments and charges that occurred on that date
   D. the charges for each physician in the practice on that date

_____ 9. The patient aging report is used to
   A. enter payments in the patient billing system
   B. enter write-offs to patient's accounts
   C. track overdue claims from payers
   D. collect overdue accounts from patients

_____ 10. The HIPAA standard transaction that is used to inquire about the status of a claim is
   A. 837
   B. 835
   C. 276
   D. 277

Provide answers to the following questions:

1. List the ten areas checked during an automated medical edit.

2. Name three possible results of the payer's adjudication process.

Applying Your Knowledge

The following data elements were submitted to a third-party payer. Using the ICD-9-CM, CPT, and the place of service codes in Appendix B, audit the information in each case and advise the payer about the correct action.

Case 9.1

Dx 783.2
CPT 80048
POS 60

Case 9.2

Dx 518.83
CPT 99241–22

Case 9.3

Dx 662.30
CPT 54500

Computer Exploration

Internet Activity

1. The American Medical Association publishes *American Medical News,* weekly coverage of issues in which the organization is interested. Point your Web browser at the AMA's Web site:
    http://www.ama-assn.org
    and click *Journals and American Medical News*
    Click *American Medical News* on the list that appears, and research recent articles related to medical billing and insurance under the category *Medical Markets.*
2. The American Health Lawyers Web site contains information about legal matters in health care. Point your Web browser at
    http://www.healthlawyers.org
    and click *Today in Health Law*
    Report on a topic related to medical billing and insurance.

9.1 Create Claims in MediSoft

Insurance claims can be created in MediSoft on a daily, weekly, or any other timely basis. Claim creation begins with the entry of patient and transaction data, and proceeds to the actual transmission of electronic claims or printing of paper claims.

1. Select Claim Management on the Activities menu. The Claim Management dialog box is displayed.

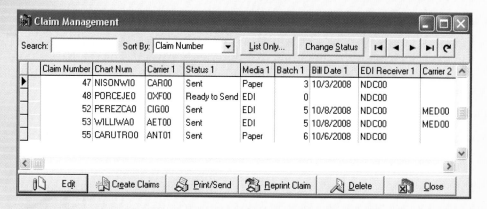

2. Click the Create Claims button. The Create Claims dialog box appears. This dialog box provides a number of options for creating claims. If these boxes were left totally blank and the Create button clicked, the program would create claims for all transactions that have not already been placed on a claim.

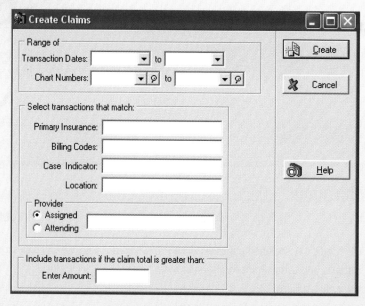

3. If you wanted to create claims for transactions on a given day, you would enter that date in the Transaction Dates boxes. If all other boxes were left blank, the program would create claims for all transactions on that date that were not already placed on a claim.

4. Similarly, the other boxes provide options for further filtering of claims. Claims can be created for specific patient(s), primary insurance carriers, billing codes, case indicators, locations, assigned and/or attending provider, or dollar amounts greater than a specified amount. If you were actually creating claims, once the Create Claims dialog box options were selected, you would click the Create button. For now, click the Cancel button to exit this dialog box.

5. Click the Close button to exit the Claim Management dialog box.

9.2 Examine Claims Already Created in MediSoft

1. Select Claim Management on the Activities menu. The Claim Management dialog box is displayed.
2. This dialog box lists all claims that have already been created in MediSoft. In this sample database, five claims have been created.
3. Click the claim for Walter Williams, chart number WILLIWA0. (*Note:* The claim numbers displayed on your screen may differ from those shown in the examples in this text. MediSoft assigns numbers to insurance claims sequentially. Therefore, depending on when and if you carried out the claim creation exercise in the Appendix, your claim numbers will vary. This is inconsequential as the numbers do not affect the claims in any way.)

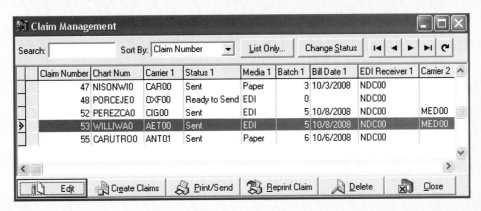

4. Click the Edit button. The Claim dialog box is displayed. This box contains five tabs that list detailed information about the claim.

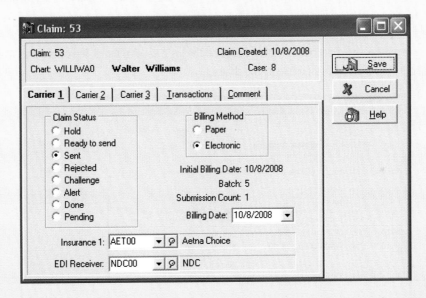

5. The Carrier 1 tab displays information about the claim and the primary insurance carrier, in this case, Aetna Choice. The Claim Status is listed as Sent. The Billing Method is Electronic. The Billing Date is 10/8/2008.

6. Click the Carrier 2 tab. This tab displays information about the claim and the secondary insurance carrier, Medicare Nationwide.

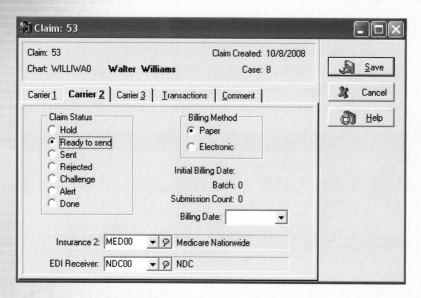

7. Even though Aetna Choice will cover Walter Williams' claim in full, a claim is also created for the secondary insurance carrier for their records. In MediSoft, secondary claims are automatically set up as paper claims because, in general, only primary claims may be sent electronically. In this case, the claim status is "Ready to send." Once a remittance advice is received from the primary insurance carrier, the secondary claim is usually sent along with a copy of the RA.

8. Click the Transactions tab. This tab lists all the transactions that have been placed on this particular claim. Notice that the first two boxes are checked in the Ins 1 Resp and the Ins 2 Resp columns, indicating that Walter Williams has two policies that could be responsible for the charges.

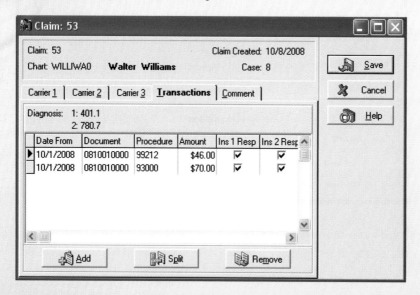

9. Click the Cancel button to Exit the Claim dialog box.
10. Click the Close button to close the Claim Management dialog box.

Computer Exploration

9.3 View an Insurance Aging Report

An insurance aging report is used to track claims filed with insurance carriers. The report shows how long a payer has taken to respond to each claim. In MediSoft, an insurance aging report shows claims that have been sent fewer than 30 days ago, as well as 30–60, 60–90, 90–120, and past 120 days ago. This information is used to follow up on overdue payments from insurance carriers. Reports can be generated for primary, secondary, or tertiary insurance carriers.

1. Open the Reports menu, and click Aging Reports. MediSoft displays a submenu for generating a number of aging reports.

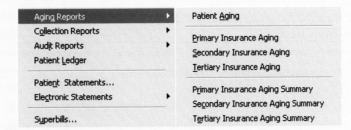

2. Click Primary Insurance Aging.
3. The Print Report Where? dialog box is displayed. All reports in MediSoft can be previewed on the screen, printed, or exported to a file. Select the option to preview the report on-screen, and then click the Start button.
4. The Primary Insurance Aging: Data Selection Questions dialog box appears. All records will be included if the range boxes are left blank. To narrow the results of the report, a range of insurance carriers, billing dates, and/or attending providers can be specified. In this case, change the date in the second Initial Billing Date range box to 11/30/2008, and leave the other boxes blank to include all records.

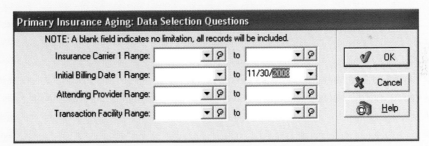

Computer Exploration

5. Click the OK button. A Primary Insurance Aging report appears in the Preview Report window. Use the scroll bars to read the full report. The report shows three unpaid claims from three different insurance carriers that fall in the 31–60 days column.

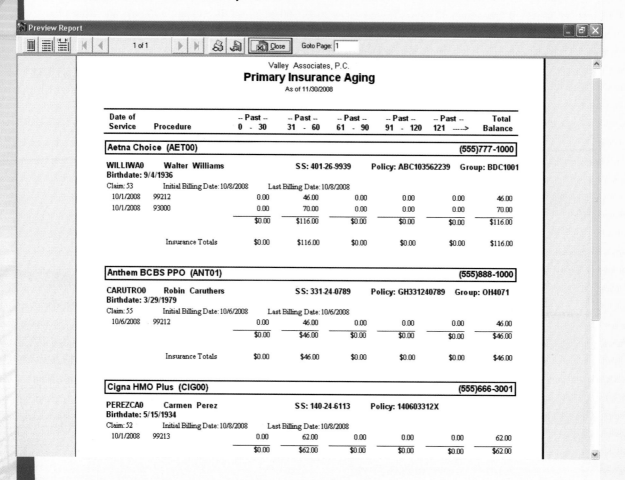

6. The printer icon at the top of the Preview Report window can be used to print the report from the Preview Report window. For now, click the Close button to close the report and return to the main MediSoft window.

Part 4 Health Care Payers

Objectives

After studying this chapter, you should be able to:

1. Identify the major types of private payers.

2. List the five main parts of participation contracts and describe their purpose.

3. Discuss the billing and reimbursement information typically summarized on a plan data form.

4. List the five steps used to ensure that private payer claims are correctly prepared.

5. Discuss the importance of verifying enrollees' eligibility for services and of submitting correct encounter information for capitated services.

Introduction

Patients of medical practices have a variety of health plans. Many are covered by their employers' group insurance. Each plan has a schedule of benefits, rules of coverage, and payment requirements. Medical insurance specialists must know how to get the information they need to answer questions from patients, payers, and staff members of their medical practice, and how to submit accurate, timely health care claims. These tasks require organizing each plan's basic benefit and payment information so that it is easily accessed when preparing claims for patients.

Experienced medical insurance specialists may also be asked to help decide whether entering into various managed care participation contracts is in the practice's financial interest. The provisions of the payers' contracts, allowed fees, and control of patient services need to be reviewed before these decisions are made.

Private Payers

According to the Employee Benefit Research Institute (cited in *Modern Physician*, 12/1/2003), over 60 percent of Americans have medical insurance coverage through their employers. The human resources departments of their companies select a number of health plans for employees to choose among. Some large firms offer as many as 150 different versions of plans (often referred to as insurance "products") from competing third-party payers. The largest employer-sponsored health program in the United States is the **Federal Employees Health Benefits** program **(FEHB)**, which covers more than 8 million federal employees, retirees, and their families through over three hundred health plans from a number of carriers. FEHB is administered by the federal government's Office of Personnel Management (OPM), which receives and deposits premiums and remits payments to the carriers. Each carrier is responsible for furnishing identification cards and benefits brochures to enrollees, adjudicating claims, and maintaining records.

For most employer-sponsored plans, the payer is an insurance company's health care plan or a managed care organization (MCO). Many payers offer a complete range of plan types with various costs and benefits. They often have many versions of managed care plans—offering plans with a range of deductibles and copayments—as well as indemnity plans. For example, Figure 10.1 on page 332 shows the range of group medical plans and riders offered by a major company. The Blue Cross and Blue Shield Association, a private-sector payer with multiple group and individual plan choices, is also discussed below.

Employer-Sponsored Plan Administration

During specified periods called **open enrollment periods**, employees may choose the plan they prefer for the coming benefit period. Employees selecting from among the employer's plans may add **riders** to their policies for additional charges. Riders are also referred to as *options*. For example, a rider for coverage of vision services (usually covering one complete ophthalmological examination and one pair of prescription lenses per year) may be purchased.

Employers negotiate with third-party payers to create customized plans for their employees. To control costs, they may **carve out** parts of a plan—that is, change a plan's standard coverage or providers. For example, an employer may choose to

- Omit a specific benefit that is covered under the standard plan, such as coverage of prescription drugs

Billing Tip

Private Payers
Private payers do not necessarily operate under the same regulations as government-sponsored programs. Each payer's rules and interpretations may vary. The definitions of basic terms (for example, the age range for "neonate") differ, as do preauthorization requirements. Medical insurance specialists must research each payer's rules for correct billing and reimbursement.

	Maximum Provider Choice	⟷		Maximum Control of Cost and Quality
	Indemnity	In Network or Out of Network		In Network Only
	Managed Indemnity	**PPO/Open Access**	**Point-of-Service**	**HMO/Exclusive Provider**
Network	None; use any provider	220,000 physicians 4,300 hospitals	150,000 physicians 2,000 hospitals	150,000 physicians 2,000 hospitals
Care Managed by Primary Care Physicians (PCP)	No	No	Yes: Open access OB/GYN, behavioral, vision	Yes: Open access OB/GYN, behavioral, vision
Access to Providers	May use any provider	Use any PPO network provider; may use out-of-network providers at a higher cost	Use network providers; may use out-of-network providers at higher cost	Must use network providers
Provider Compensation	Fee-for-service, reasonable and customary rate	**In Network:** Discounted fee for service **Out of Network:** Fee-for-service, reasonable and customary rate	**In Network:** Capitation and discounted fee-for-service **Out of Network:** Fee-for-service, reasonable and customary rate	Capitation and discounted fee-for-service
Options	**Prescription Drug Coverage** **Behavioral Care** **Dental Care** **Vision Care** **Medicare HMO** **Life and Disability** **Expectant Mother**			

Figure 10.1 Medical Group Plans Offered by Payer

- Use a different network of providers for a certain type of care, such as negotiating with a local practice network for behavioral health coverage rather than using the standard plan physicians

In these situations, the payer for some services under an employer's plan may be different than for the standard plan. For example, many employers contract with a **pharmacy benefit manager** (PBM) to operate their prescription drug benefits. Because they represent a large group of buyers, PBMs can negotiate favorable prices with pharmaceutical companies for employers' plans.

Employer-Sponsored Plan Types

Employers offer a range of managed care plans. Some also offer indemnity plans. Some firms offer consumer-driven plans, and increasingly flexible savings plans are offered in conjunction with high-deductible indemnity plans.

TABLE 10.1	Comparison of Managed Care Health Plan Structures		
Plan Type	**Patient Base**	**Provider Payment Method**	**Plan Employment of Physicians**
Indemnity	All patients	Fee for service	No
Health Maintenance Organization (HMO): Staff HMO	Only HMO patients	By employment contract	Yes
Group HMO	HMO or nonHMO	By employment contract or capitation	Yes or No
Independent Practice Association (IPA)	HMO or nonHMO	PCP: Capitation Specialist: Fee for service	No
Point-of-Service (POS)	HMO or nonHMO	By contract, but specialist is fee for service	No
Preferred Provider Organization (PPO)	Managed care and nonmanaged care	By contract	No

Managed care plans   Preferred provider organizations (PPOs) are the most popular choice, followed by health maintenance organizations (HMOs), especially the point-of-service (POS) variety. The fewest number of employees choose indemnity plans, usually because such plans cost more. Table 10.1 reviews the basic features and differences among these types of plans (also see Chapter 1).

PPOs charge an annual premium and a copayment; they usually also require an annual deductible. Most do not require payment of coinsurance when the patient uses a preferred (in-network) provider, but a large coinsurance (30 to 50 percent) is due from patients who use out-of-network providers. The majority of the HMO enrollees choose the POS type, in which patients can see either in-network or out-of-network providers. Under the POS model, patients using out-of-network providers must submit a claim, receive only 50 to 80 percent reimbursement of the costs, and pay deductibles and copayments. Both PPOs and HMOs usually cover preventive medical services.

Indemnity plans   Traditional indemnity plans require premium, deductible, and coinsurance payments. They typically cover 70 to 80 percent of costs for covered benefits after the deductible is met. Some plans are structured with a high deductible, such as $5,000 to $10,000, in order to offer policyholders a relatively less expensive premium.

Increasingly, traditional plans incorporate managed care features, as payers compete for employers' contracts and try to control costs. For example, many indemnity plans have a number of utilization requirements, and many now offer some preventive services benefits.

Consumer-driven health plans   Consumer-driven (consumer-directed) health plans have higher copayments or deductibles than PPOs. They are designed to require patients to assume a greater responsibility for managing their health care by choosing from a variety of plan designs. In many plans, employers provide a set amount of money each year for employees to use for any health service they choose. If they empty the accounts, employees must cover a deductible themselves; if money is left in the account, it rolls over to help cover the next year's health expenses. Consumer-driven plans often feature a "tiered" structure, such as three levels of prescription-drug choices.

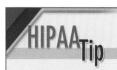

Flexible savings (spending) accounts and cafeteria plans   Some companies offer flexible savings accounts (FSA) or other flexible benefits plans (called cafeteria plans or Section 125 plans) that augment employees' other health insurance coverage. These plans permit employees to put pretax dollars from their salaries in an account that can be used to pay for certain medical and dependent care expenses. The expenses that can be paid include annual premiums, medical expenses that are not covered under the regular insurance plan (such as routine physical examinations and eyeglasses), and child care. The employee files the claim with the plan. Medical practices may supply documentation to the patient for this purpose.

Self-Insured Health Plans

Many large employers, such as automotive companies and airlines, cover the costs of their employees' health plans themselves rather than buying insurance from private payers. Such self-insured health plans (versus "fully insured plans" that pay premiums to the payer) are regulated by the federal **Employee Retirement Income Security Act of 1974 (ERISA)** rather than by state laws. However, state regulations, where they exist, may govern some aspects of benefits and participation. The trend is for state-mandated laws that protect consumers' access to health care.

Most self-insured health plans contract with third–party claims administrators (TPAs), which are outside vendors, to handle their administrative services such as collecting premiums, keeping lists of members up to date, and processing and paying insurance claims.

Blue Cross and Blue Shield

The **Blue Cross and Blue Shield Association (BCBS)**, founded in the 1930s to provide low-cost medical insurance, is a national organization of forty-two independent companies called Member Plans that insure nearly 89 million people. About 50 percent of these plan subscribers (policyholders) join PPOs; 23 percent are in indemnity plans; 19 percent in HMOs; and 8 percent are in point-of-service plans. BCBS has both for-profit and nonprofit companies that offer health plans to individuals, small and large employer groups, senior citizens, federal government employees, and others. In addition to major medical and hospital insurance, the "Blues" also have freestanding plans for dental, vision, mental health, prescription, and hearing coverage.

Subscriber Identification Card

Blue Cross and Blue Shield subscriber identification cards are used to determine the type of plan, since BCBS offers local and national programs through its many individual plans (see Figure 10.2a and b.) In addition to the subscriber's name, most BCBS cards list the following information:

Plan name

Type of plan

Subscriber identification number (usually the subscriber's Social Security number with a three-letter prefix)

Effective date of coverage

BCBS plan codes and coverage codes

Participation in reciprocity plan with other BCBS plans

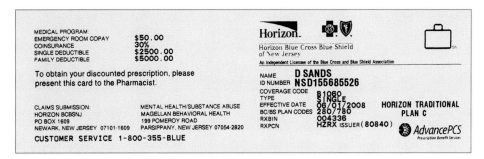

Front

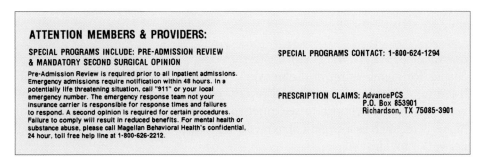

Figure 10.2 Blue Cross and Blue Shield Subscriber Card (a) Front, (b) Back

Copayments, coinsurance, and deductible amounts

Information about additional coverage, such as prescription medication or mental health care

Information about preauthorization requirements

Claims submission address

Contact phone numbers

Types of Plans

A fee-for-service BCBS plan has an individual and family deductible and a coinsurance payment. Individual annual deductibles may range from as little as $100 to $2,500 or more. The family deductible is usually twice the amount of the individual deductible. Once the deductible has been met, the plan pays a percentage of the charges, usually 70, 80, or 90 percent, until an annual maximum out-of-pocket cap has been reached. After that, the plan pays 100 percent of approved charges until the end of the benefit year. At the beginning of the new benefit year, the out-of-pocket caps resets, and 100 percent reimbursement does not occur until the out-of-pocket maximum for the new year has been met. Once the cap has been met, charges by nonparticipating providers are paid at 100 percent of the allowed amount. If the charges exceed the allowed amount, the patient must pay the balance to the provider, even though the annual cap has been met.

BCBS plans also offer many types of managed care programs, including HMOs, PPOs, POSs, and others. In an HMO, a patient must choose a primary care physician who is in the BCBS network. The POS plan offers greater choice to the patient. Members of a POS plan may receive treatment from a provider in the network, or they may choose to see a provider outside the network and pay a higher fee. Depending on the particular plan, the patient may or may not have a primary care provider. In a PPO, physicians and other health care

A. Given the many different insurance plans that medical insurance specialists work with, what do you think are the most important items of information that should be available about a plan?

B. Some practices create their own comprehensive office manuals that collate information about the plans their patients have, while other practices rely solely on payers' provider manuals. What are the pros and cons of each approach?

providers sign a contract with BCBS agreeing to accept reduced fees in exchange for membership in the network. As a network member, providers are listed in a provider directory and receive referrals from other network members. Patients can choose to see a network or a nonnetwork provider, paying higher fees, such as a larger copayment, when receiving treatment from a nonnetwork provider.

BlueCard Program

The **BlueCard** program is a nationwide program that makes it easy for patients to receive treatment when outside their local service area, and also makes it easy for providers to receive payment when treating patients enrolled in plans outside the provider's service area. The program links participating providers and independent BCBS plans throughout the nation with a single electronic claim processing and reimbursement system.

When a subscriber requires medical care while traveling outside of the service area, he or she presents the subscriber ID card to a BCBS participating providers. The provider verifies the subscriber's membership and benefit coverage by calling the BlueCard eligibility number. After providing treatment, the provider submits the claim to the local BCBS plan in his or her service area, which is referred to as the **host plan**. The host plan sends the claim via modem to the patient's **home plan**—the plan in effect when the patient is at home—which processes the claim and sends it back to the host plan. The host plan pays the provider according to local payment methods, and the home plan sends the remittance advice. For example, if a subscriber from New Jersey requires treatment while traveling in Delaware, the provider in Delaware can treat the patient, file the claim, and collect payment from the Delaware plan.

Participation Contracts

Providers, like employers and employees, must evaluate participation in managed care products. They judge which plans to join based on the types of patients they serve and the financial arrangements that are offered to them. Because managed care organizations are the predominant health care delivery systems, most medical practices have a number of contracts with plans in their area. Figure 10.3 shows the notice of participation posted in an orthopedic specialty. Nearly every practice has at least one participation contract, and many have multiple agreements.

Welcome to Newton Major Orthopedic Associates, P.C.

In order to make your visit as pleasant as possible, we have compiled a list of the most commonly asked questions regarding insurance and billing in this office.

With which insurance plans does NMOA participate?

Aetna/US Healthcare Plans
CIGNA
Blue Choice PPO: POS, PPO, Prestige, Select
Focus Workers Compensation PPO
Health Care Value Management, Inc.
Health Choice
Health Direct
Kaiser Permanente
Medicare

Medicaid
MedSpan
MD Health Plan
Oxford Health Plan
Physician Health Services
Prudential Healthcare
POS Plan
Wellcare

What can I expect if NMOA participates with my insurance?

We will file a claim with your insurance company for any charges. Your insurance may require you to pay a copay at the time of services. You are responsible for any deductibles and non-covered services. You may need to obtain a referral from your primary care physician. Failure to obtain a referral may result in rescheduling of your appointment until you can obtain one.

What can I expect if NMOA does not participate with my insurance?

Payment is expected at the time of service. You will receive a statement within two weeks. Use it to file a claim. As a courtesy, NMOA will submit any surgery claims to your insurance carrier, but you are responsible for payment.

Figure 10.3 Example of Practice Participation List

Contract Provisions

When the practice evaluates a managed care organization, an experienced medical insurance specialist may be asked to join the evaluation team, which may be led by the practice manager or by a committee of physicians. Usually, an attorney is also involved in the evaluation process. The managed care organization's business history, National Committee for Quality Assurance (NCQA) accreditation, and licensure status are reviewed. Another factor is whether the MCO offers multiple products—ideally, HMO, PPO, POS, and fee-for-service options.

A major question the team must answer is whether the plan is a good financial opportunity. All plans **reprice** physicians' usual fees, resulting in lower revenue for each procedure. Some plans pay fees that are very low, and even gaining many more patients who have this plan may not make joining the plan

Customer service representatives, claims examiners, and provider relations representatives are employed by payers such as insurance companies and managed care organizations and by third-party administrators.

Customer service representatives handle written, e-mail, and telephone inquires from providers and from policyholders about referrals, billing requirements, claims submission, preauthorization for procedures, precertification for hospital admissions, coverage issues, eligibility for benefits, copayment requirements, and balance billing. They receive training about the various health plans that are offered by the payer, and they must be familiar with the organization of their company so that they can correctly direct inquiries. These entry-level positions require skill in oral communications—such as excellent telephone techniques—as well as written communications, research abilities, and problem solving. Employers also require computer literacy and, often, previous customer service employment.

Claims examiners (also called claims analysts) work with the payer's computer system to process claims. They are trained to apply the payer's rules for determining medically necessary procedures and for bundling or global period coverage. They contact providers for information needed to complete claims, review and check claims attachments, and make a determination to pay, deny, or partially pay the claim. If the claims examiner decides to not pay the claim in full, the appropriate computer entries are selected so that an explanation of the reason for denial or reduced payment is sent out. The position of claims examiner usually requires a high school diploma, experience with claims processing and coding procedures, medical terminology, good oral and written communications skills, and data-entry skills.

Provider relations representatives speak for an entity to its network of physicians. Many hospitals employ these representatives to enroll physicians in their network and to monitor their status. Third-party payers, especially managed care organizations, have provider relations representatives to work with the physicians whom they employ or place under contract. Representatives process the documents needed to enroll physicians in the network, maintain the current list of providers for beneficiaries, and handle questions from providers about policies and procedures. Most representatives have high school diplomas as well as associate degrees or equivalent experience in the health care field. This job requires good written and oral communication skills as well as computer literacy skills.

profitable. Usually, the evaluation team checks the maximum fees the plan pays for the services that the practice's providers most often perform. If the participating provider fee schedule reduces payment for these services too much, the evaluation team may decide not to join, even though participation would bring more patients.

Other aspects of the plan, such as the plan's medical necessity guidelines, may cause the practice to decide against participating. Some physicians do not accept certain plans because, in their view, complying with the plans' health care protocols will limit their professional medical judgment in treating patients.

The following are the main parts of participation contracts:

- Introductory section (often called "recitals" and "definitions")
- Contract purpose and covered medical services

- Physician's responsibilities
- Managed care plan obligations
- Compensation and billing guidelines

Introductory Section

The introductory section is important because it lists the names of the contracting parties and defines the terms used in the contract. Often, the contract mentions that the provider's manual is part of the agreement and is to be referred to for specific points. The section also states the ways the plan may use participating physicians' names. Some plans wish to provide lists of participating physicians to plan members. Other plans, however, want to use the providers' names in newspaper, radio, or television advertisements.

This section also indicates specifically who the payer is. For example, "First Health Plan, a Federally Qualified Health Maintenance Organization," or "Golden Gate Insurance Company, a stock company." Payer information must be noted so that claims are sent to the correct organization. For example, although a self-insured health plan may create the plan, a third-party administrator (TPA) may be responsible for processing and paying claims.

Contract Purpose and Covered Medical Services

These provisions state the type of plan and the medical services that patients are provided under it. In addition to office visits and preventive medical services, which are usual, obstetrician-gynecologist, behavioral health, physical and occupational therapy, emergency and urgent care, and diagnostic laboratory services may be covered.

Under a capitation plan, the exact covered services (the list of CPTs) included in the cap rate should appear (see Chapter 7). For example, when a provider gives a patient a MMR (measles, mumps, and rubella virus) vaccine, two fees are involved: one for giving the injection (called the administration of the immunization) and a second for the dosage of the vaccine itself. Under a capitated primary care contract, the covered medical services provisions state whether both the fee for injecting vaccines and the cost of injectable materials are included in the cap rate, or just the immunization administration.

Physician's Responsibilities

The physician's responsibilities under the plan include the following:

- *Services:* The contract stipulates the services that the provider must offer to plan members.
- *Acceptance of plan members:* The contact states whether providers must see all plan members who wish to use their services or some percentage or specific number of members. For example, capitated plans often require primary care physicians to accept at least a certain number of patients who are enrolled in the plan. If treating this number of patients means that the plan's enrollees will make up a large part of the practice, providers must evaluate whether the plan's payment structure is high enough.
- *Referrals:* This part of the contract states whether providers must refer only to other participating providers. It also covers the conditions under which the referral rules do not apply, such as in an emergency.
- *Preauthorizations:* If the provider is responsible for securing preauthorizations for the patient, as is the case in most HMOs, this is stated.

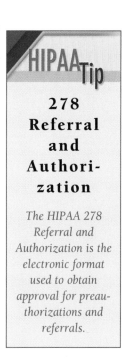

HIPAATip

278 Referral and Authorization

The HIPAA 278 Referral and Authorization is the electronic format used to obtain approval for preauthorizations and referrals.

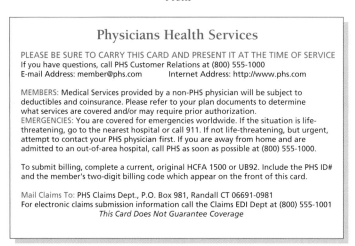

Front

Physicians Health Services

PLEASE BE SURE TO CARRY THIS CARD AND PRESENT IT AT THE TIME OF SERVICE
If you have questions, call PHS Customer Relations at (800) 555-1000
E-mail Address: member@phs.com   Internet Address: http://www.phs.com

MEMBERS: Medical Services provided by a non-PHS physician will be subject to
deductibles and coinsurance. Please refer to your plan documents to determine
what services are covered and/or may require prior authorization.
EMERGENCIES: You are covered for emergencies worldwide. If the situation is life-
threatening, go to the nearest hospital or call 911. If not life-threatening, but urgent,
attempt to contact your PHS physician first. If you are away from home and are
admitted to an out-of-area hospital, call PHS as soon as possible at (800) 555-1000.

To submit billing, complete a current, original HCFA 1500 or UB92. Include the PHS ID#
and the member's two-digit billing code which appear on the front of this card.

Mail Claims To: PHS Claims Dept., P.O. Box 981, Randall CT 06691-0981
For electronic claims submission information call the Claims EDI Dept at (800) 555-1001
This Card Does Not Guarantee Coverage

Back

Figure 10.4 Example of an Insurance Card for a POS Plan

- *Other provisions:* Providers' credentials, health plan protocols, HIPAA Privacy policies, record retention, and other guidelines from the payer's medical review program are covered.

Managed Care Plan Obligations

Managed care plan obligations include the following:

- *Identification of enrolled patients:* The plan's method of identifying enrolled patients should be specified. Usually, this is with an identification card like the one shown in Figure 10.4. In this example, the provider network, the schedule of benefits, the office visit copayment, the name of the policyholder, the group, the type of contract, the patient's identification number, and the patient's dependents are listed.
- *Payments:* Paying the physician for services according to the claim turnaround time that is specified in the contract.
- *Other compensation:* This indicates whether any incentives, bonuses, and withholds apply (see Chapter 7).
- *Protection against loss:* If the provider is assuming financial risk for the cost of care, as happens under capitation, the contract should have a **stop-loss provision.** This clause limits the provider's care-related expenditures if there

is an unexpectedly high use of services. For example, a cap rate might be based on an equal number of each level of E/M service. If every patient encounter during one month required comprehensive histories and examinations with complex medical decision making, or if one patient required multiple visits, pushing the encounter cost far beyond expectations, the cap rate would not adequately pay for the services that were provided. Stop-loss provisions state a dollar amount over which the provider is not responsible, to protect providers from the full financial impact of their risk.

Under plans in which providers must refer only to other participating providers, the providers' compliance is evaluated by the plan, and incentives or bonuses may be tied to how well a provider observes the referral rules. For this reason, a stated obligation of the plan should be to provide and regularly update the list of participating providers, so that providers are sure they are referring their patients correctly.

HIPAA Tip

Withdrawing from a Contract

Most participation contracts require physicians to notify patients if they withdraw from their managed care organization.

Compensation and Billing Guidelines

The compensation and billing guidelines cover fees, billing requirements, claim filing deadlines, patients' financial responsibilities, and balance-billing rules. The rules for collecting patients' payments—whether at time of service or after adjudication—are listed. The guidelines also cover coordination of benefits (COB) when another plan is primary. The billing guidelines may be printed in the contract; usually, though, the contract states that the guidelines appear in the plan's provider's manual.

Billing and Reimbursement Information

Many aspects of participation contracts affect the billing and reimbursement process. When the practice decides to participate in a plan, the medical insurance specialist analyzes the contract and the plan's manual. Information about the plan is organized for ease of use. (Some offices use a form such as that shown in Figure 10.5 on page 342.) The following types of information are summarized:

Basic Payer Information

- Plan type—either HMO, POS, PPO, FFS (fee-for-service), or other
- Plan name
- Payer contact information—where claims are to be sent, and a contact for queries and follow-up
- Covered services—which physician services, preventive services, and prescription drugs (formulary) are covered

Information Regarding Patient Services

- Eligibility verification contact—the person to contact to verify patients' eligibility for services
- Referral, preauthorization, and precertification requirements

Billing Information

- Type of claims (HIPAA 837 only, or paper as well)
- Payer turnaround time (number of turnaround days for claims processing and payment)

Patient Financial Responsibilities

- Copayment requirements (the same for each encounter, for example, or varied according to the type of service)

PLAN TYPE: HMO   POS   PPO   FFS   Other

PLAN NAME:

Send claims to:
Address:
Phone no.:   Fax no.:
Contact person: E-mail address:

Coverage provided for:
Physician services:
Preventive services:
Formulary:

Patient eligibility:
Phone no.:   Fax no.:
Contact person: E-mail address:

Preauthorization required
For: YES   NO
Referrals
Lab services
Emergency/urgent care
Other:
Precertification required
For:
Elective admissions
Outpatient surgeries
Other:

Billing information
EC?   Paper w/attachments?   Payment due:
Format?   Other   30____60____Other____

Patient responsibilities
Copayment(s) for:
Deductible: Status:
Coinsurance:

Balance billing?
Withholds?

Figure 10.5 **Plan Data Form**

- Other required payments, such as deductibles and coinsurance
- Balance billing or withholds

When the practice participates in a plan, the medical insurance specialist should also have access to other detailed information that affects billing. For example:

- The code edits that are programmed, such as "CPT 99215 is paid only once every six months"

- The global follow-up times for major and minor surgical procedures
- The policies for multiple procedure reimbursement (some payers fully reimburse multiple procedures performed on the same date of service; others pay fully for only the first service, and pay the rest at a reduced percentage)
- The procedures to be followed by the practice to verify patient enrollment and coverage
- Documentation requirements (for example, some contracts cover prolonged services—CPT 99354–99357—only with specific documentation)
- How to appeal a denied or a downcoded claim

Copayment Requirements and Calculations

Payers vary as to the copayment(s) required. Some plans require a copayment only when an E/M service is provided, and others require it when the patient visits an office for any procedure or service. Copayment amounts may also vary according to the service performed. Some plans have different copayment amounts for office visits, emergency room visits, ambulance services, and preventive services. When two services, such as an E/M service and a billable procedure, are performed on the same date of service, either one or two copayments may be required.

Another variable in collecting copayments involves primary or secondary plans. Medical insurance specialists should verify whether a copayment is to be collected under the secondary plan. Usually it is not, unless the primary plan does not cover the service or if the member is satisfying a deductible for the primary plan.

The payer's rules about copayment calculations also need to be understood. Plans have two different ways of handling copayments that are collected from patients at the time of service. Most plans require the patient's copayment to be subtracted from the amount due to the provider from the payer. This treats the copayment like a deductible or coinsurance payment. The contract (or provider's manual) states the policy in terms such as "All member copayments, deductibles, and coinsurance apply." (The word *apply* here means that they should be taken into account when the payer calculates the balance due to the provider.)

Some plans, though, permit the provider to keep the patient's copayment without deducting it from the fee. In this case, usually the plan pays a lower fee for the service, so often the provider collects the same amount in both situations. Either way is acceptable and is a matter of contract wording. The rules must be clear to the medical insurance specialist for correct calculations of the expected payment from the payer.

The following examples show how the two different ways of handling copayments affect the calculation of the amount due to the provider. In the first example, the patient's copayment is subtracted from the allowed fee for the visit.

The plan: a PPO that pays 75 percent of the provider's usual charge; a $5 copayment is due, and copayment is applied toward provider payment

Provider usual charge	$50.00
Payer allowed fee ($50 × 75 percent)	37.50
Patient copay subtracted	−5.00
Payer pays	32.50
Provider collects a total of	$37.50

In the following example, the plan's rule is that the patient's copayment is not subtracted from the amount due from the payer to the provider. However, notice that the plan pays 65 percent, not 75 percent, of the provider's usual fee, so the provider receives the same amount as in the example above:

Billing Tip

Increasing Reimbursed Services
When the practice has a participation contract, medical insurance specialists should keep a record of services that were not paid over a year's billing period. This record provides a basis for negotiating with the payer to revise the contract in order to reimburse more services.

Billing Tip

Collecting Copays
Patients should be told that the practice is obligated to follow payer copayment guidelines. The practice must report medical services properly, and the patient is responsible according to the rules.

Billing Tip

Consult Versus Referral
Managed care plans may have forms that interchange or misuse the terms refer *and* consult. A consultation occurs when a physician, at the request of the patient's attending physician, examines the patient and reports an opinion to the requestor. Under a referral, care (a portion or all) is transferred to another physician. However, a plan's referral form may in fact be the correct one to use when consultation is required. This usage should be clarified with the plan's provider support representative.

The plan: a PPO that pays 65 percent of the provider's usual charge; copayment is not subtracted from the fee

Provider usual charge	$50.00
Payer allowed fee ($50 × 65 percent)	32.50
Copay not subtracted	5.00
Provider collects a total of	$37.50

Surgical Procedures

Most managed care plans have rules for approving emergency surgical procedures and elective surgery. Emergency surgery must usually be approved within a specified period, such as forty-eight hours, after admission was required. **Elective surgery** is a procedure that can be scheduled ahead of time, but which may be medically necessary. It usually requires **precertification**—generally defined by plans as preauthorization for hospital-based services and outpatient surgeries—during a specified period, such as at least twenty-four hours, before the service is performed. The precertification requirement is usually shown on the patient's insurance card (see Figure 10.6). The practice must send a

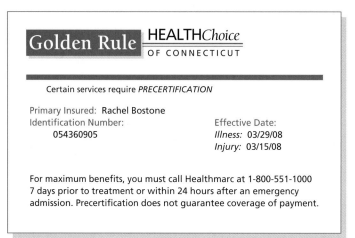

Front

Back

Figure 10.6 Example of an Insurance Card Showing Precertification Requirement

completed precertification form for review in advance of the admission. Figure 10.7 shows an example of a precertification form.

Some elective surgical procedures are done on an inpatient basis, so the patient is admitted to the hospital; others are done on an outpatient basis. The following are common outpatient surgeries:

- Abdominal hernia
- Bunionectomy
- Carpal tunnel
- Destruction of cutaneous vascular proliferative lesions
- Knee arthroscopy
- Otoplasty
- Sclerotherapy

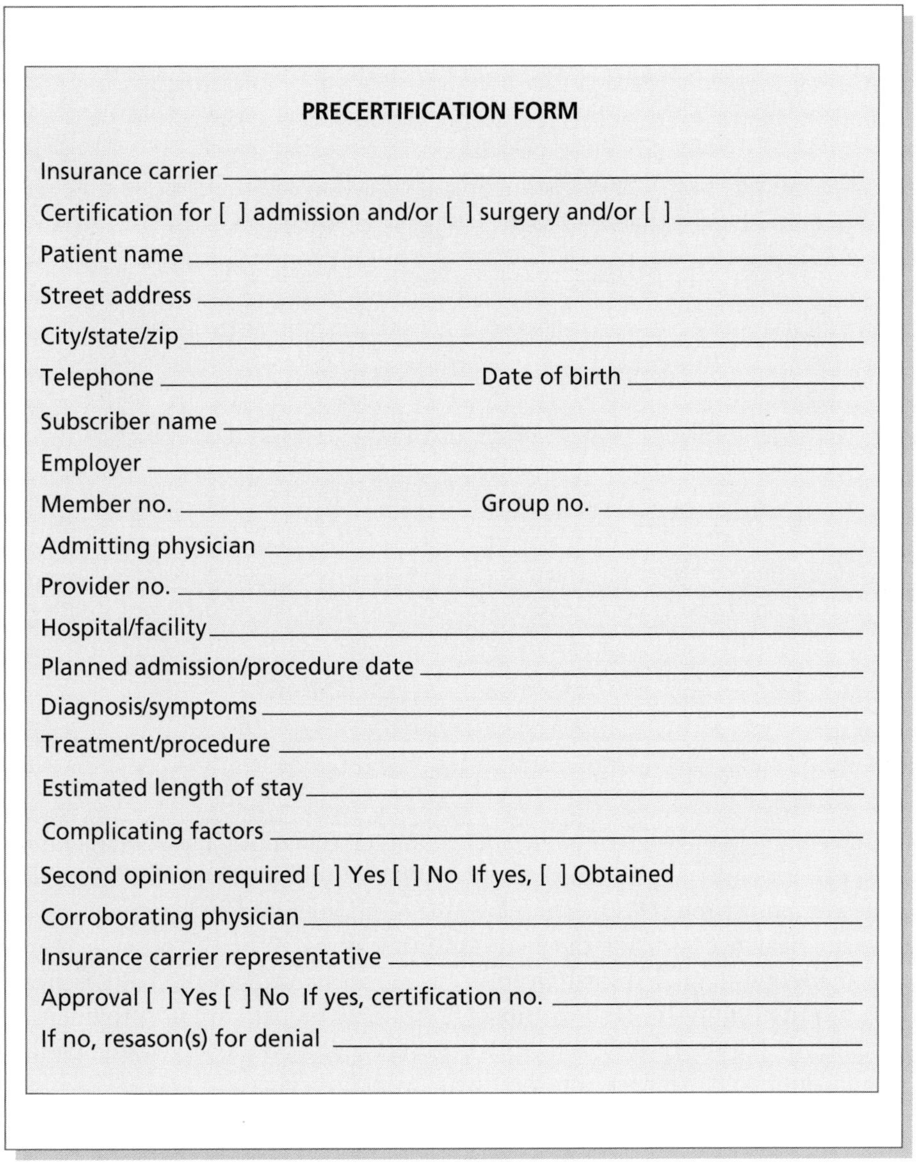

PRECERTIFICATION FORM

Insurance carrier _____

Certification for [ ] admission and/or [ ] surgery and/or [ ] _____

Patient name _____

Street address _____

City/state/zip _____

Telephone _____ Date of birth _____

Subscriber name _____

Employer _____

Member no. _____ Group no. _____

Admitting physician _____

Provider no. _____

Hospital/facility_____

Planned admission/procedure date _____

Diagnosis/symptoms _____

Treatment/procedure _____

Estimated length of stay_____

Complicating factors _____

Second opinion required [ ] Yes [ ] No If yes, [ ] Obtained

Corroborating physician _____

Insurance carrier representative _____

Approval [ ] Yes [ ] No If yes, certification no. _____

If no, resason(s) for denial _____

Figure 10.7 Precertification Form for Hospital Admission or Surgery

In what section of a PPO participation contract is each of the following phrases located?

A. Physician has accurately completed the Participating Physician Credentialing Application that accompanies this agreement and has been accepted by the Plan. Physician shall promptly notify Plan of any change in this information, including any change in its principal place of business, within seven days of such change.

_____

B. "Members" means enrollees or enrolled dependents covered by a Plan benefit agreement.

_____

C. Physician agrees to accept the Plan fee schedule or physician's billed charges, whichever is less, as payment in full for all medical services provided to members.

_____

D. Physician agrees to allow review and duplication of any data free of charge and other records maintained on members which relate to this agreement.

_____

E. Plan agrees to provide current identification cards for members.

_____

F. Plan shall deduct any copayments and deductible amounts required by the Plan benefit agreement from the allowed payment due Physician under this agreement.

_____

G. Plan intends, by entering into this agreement, to make available quality health care to Plan members by contracting with Physician. Physician intends to provide such care in a cost-effective manner.

_____

For a major course of treatment, such as surgery, chemotherapy, and radiation for a patient with cancer, many private payers use the services of a **utilization review organization (URO)**. These organizations are hired by the payer to evaluate medical necessity of the planned procedures. When a provider (or a patient) requests precertification for such a treatment plan, the URO issues a report of its findings. As shown in Figure 10.8, the patient and provider are both notified of the results. If the planned services are not covered, the patient should agree to pay for them before the treatment begins.

```
Case number:    G631000
Procedure:      Axillary node dissection

Dear Patient:

As you may know, ABC is a utilization review company that contracts
with insurance companies, managed care organizations, and self-
insured groups to review the health care services provided to people
covered under their medical plans and to make recommendations
regarding the medical necessity and efficiency of these health care
services. ABC is not an insurer, and does not make eligibility, benefit,
or coverage decisions.

We have received information about the procedure scheduled for
08/12/2001 at Downtown Hospital. Based on review of this information,
we find this outpatient procedure to be medically necessary and
efficient.

If the treatment plan is changed, or if admission to the hospital is
necessary, please contact your insurance company immediately.

ABC's recommendation is not a decision regarding payment of a
particular claim. Your medical plan payer is responsible for making
final payment and eligibility decisions. Any questions about a claim,
deductible, or copayment should be directed to your medical plan.

Sincerely,


ABC Reviewer
Medical Care Coordinator


cc:   George Ballister, M.D.
      Downtown Hospital
```

Figure 10.8 Example of Letter from Utilization Company

Private Payer Claim Management

This section covers the steps to follow to create correct claims for all fee-based
services, whether the patient is in a managed care or a traditional plan.

Step 1: Identify the Plan and the Payer

Since there are more than six thousand insurance companies and many move,
go out of business, or merge with other companies each year, verifying current
information on each patient's plan's address, phone numbers, and claim submission requirements is vital. Resources such as directories of insurance carriers and Web sites should be used to locate contact information.

Billing Tip

Nonparticipation
If the provider is not a
participant, patients are
notified about their responsibility for payment and the
practice's policy for collecting it in advance
of services.

The HIPAA 270/271 Eligibility for a Health Plan transaction (the inquiry from the provider and the response from the payer) is the electronic format used to verify benefits.

TABLE 10.2	Determining Primary Coverage

- If the patient has only one policy, it is primary.
- If the patient has coverage under two plans, the plan that has been in effect for the patient for the longest period of time is primary. However, if an active employee has a plan with the present employer and is still covered by a former employer's plan as a retiree or a laid-off employee, the current employer's plan is primary.
- If the patient is also covered as a dependent under another insurance policy, the patient's plan is primary.
- If an employed patient has coverage under the employer's plan and additional coverage under a government-sponsored plan, the employer's plan is primary. For example, if a patient is enrolled in a PPO through employment and is also on Medicare, the PPO is primary.
- If a retired patient is covered by a spouse's employer's plan, and the spouse is still employed, the spouse's plan is primary, even if the retired person has Medicare.
- If the patient is a dependent child covered by both parents' plans, and the parents are not separated or divorced (or if the parents have joint custody of the child), the primary plan is determined by the birthday rule (see page 84).
- If two or more plans cover dependent children of separated or divorced parents who do not have joint custody of their children, the children's primary plan is determined in this order:
  —The plan of the custodial parent
  —The plan of the spouse of the custodial parent (if the parent has remarried)
  —The plan of the parent without custody

The initial information about the patient's plan is taken from the patient's information form (PIF). Changes in insurance coverage are reported by patients when they update the data on the patient information form (see Chapter 3).

Step 2: Verify Patient Eligibility Under the Primary Insurance

This step has two parts. First, the primary insurance plan is determined; and second, eligibility under that insurance plan is verified. Table 10.2 lists the points that must be reviewed in order to determine a patient's primary insurance plan.

The second step is to verify patients' eligibility for benefits under the primary plan. Eligibility under employer-sponsored plans may be affected by a number of factors:

- Coverage may end on the last day of the month in which the employee's active full-time service ends, such as for disability, layoff, or termination.
- The employee may no longer qualify as a member of the group. For example, some companies do not provide benefits for part time employees. If a full-time employee changes to part-time employment, the coverage ends.
- The employee has not met required premium payments.
- An eligible dependent's coverage may end on the last day of the month in which the dependent status ends, such as reaching the age limit stated in the policy.

After photocopying the front and the back of insurance cards for new patients and for established patients whose insurance has changed, the medical insurance specialist contacts the payer to double-check that the patient is eligible for services. Depending on the type of practice, eligibility for the following benefits may be specifically verified:

- Office visits
- Lab coverage
- Diagnostic X-rays
- PAP smear coverage

- Coverage of psychiatric visits, including the number of visits covered and the coinsurance for each
- Physical or occupational therapy
- Durable medical equipment (DME)
- Foot care

If the provider is a primary care physician and the plan requires registration of a PCP, the insurance card often lists the correct provider's name.

Step 3: Check Patient's Additional Insurance Coverage

Secondary insurance is another insurance policy under which the patient is a beneficiary. Supplemental insurance is a "fill-the-gap" insurance plan that covers parts of expenses, such as coinsurance, that the policyholder must otherwise pay. Under coordination of benefits provisions, if the patient has signed an assignment of benefits statement, the provider is responsible for reporting any additional insurance coverage to the primary payer. Medical insurance specialists review the PIF to determine whether the patient has secondary or supplemental coverage that should be reported on the primary payer's claim.

A secondary claim is reported to a second payer after the remittance advice (RA) is received on the primary claim. Supplemental insurance held with the same payer can be reported on a single claim. Claims for supplemental insurance held with other than the primary payer are also reported after the primary payer's RA is received.

Step 4: Conduct an Internal Review of Claims Before Submission

The best way to reduce the possibility that claims will be rejected or downcoded due to compliance errors is the internal claim audit (see Chapter 6). During this review, a staff member other than the person who prepared the claim checks a number of important points on the claim:

- Are the diagnosis and procedure codes logically related and supported by the documentation?
- Were the payer's code edits and other coding rules observed? To research this question, medical insurance specialists may need to review the payer's coverage bulletins. Many payers provide these on their Web sites as well as in printed form. For example, Figure 10.9 on page 350 illustrates a payer's rules for billing echocardiographs. These bulletins should be organized so that the necessary billing information is easy to research.
- Were the payer's requirements for referrals, preauthorization, and precertification followed?

The plan's claim submission guidelines are also followed. The medical insurance specialist may contact the payer representative to clarify the procedure for claim attachments or other points.

Step 5: Monitor and Follow-up on Claims

The medical insurance specialist follows-up on primary insurance claims to be sure that they are being processed by the payer. Missing or incorrect information is supplied as requested. Then, the payer's promised payment date is used to follow-up on late claims.

When RAs arrive, they should be promptly processed. The expected payments are closely checked, and procedure codes are matched up. Secondary insurance claims are completed and transmitted if appropriate.

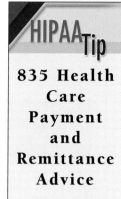

HIPAA Tip

835 Health Care Payment and Remittance Advice

The HIPAA RA is the 835 Health Care Payment and Remittance Advice transaction.

Billing Tip

Verifying Payments per Contracted Fee Schedule Medical insurance specialists should verify that payers' payments are correct according to the fee schedules in their contracts. This double-check is particularly important if remittance advices are autoposted. Most billing programs are able to track contracted rates, and some RAs should be manually posted as an audit to uncover any payment problems.

PRIMARY CARE PHYSICIAN REFERRAL LOG

Physician name: _____

Patient name	Date referred	Patient identification number	Telephone contact name	Referred-to specialist name	Referred-to specialist NPI	Referral notes &/or limitations

Figure 10.9 Example of Payer Coverage Policy Bulletin

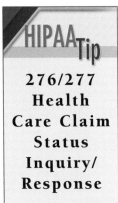

Communications with Payers

Good communication between payers and the medical insurance staff is essential for effective contract and claim management. As claims are processed, questions and requests for information go back and forth between the practice staff and the payer's claims processing group. When claims are long overdue or there are repeated difficulties, however, these problems are the responsibility of the payer's provider representatives. To avoid major problems, many practices routinely meet with major payers' representatives. These meetings address the practice's specific problems and questions, which should be organized in advance, and update the practice on new regulations or changes. A meeting should also be held when a new participation contract is signed to discuss the payer's major guidelines, fee schedule, and medical record documentation requirements.

If RAs indicate a discrepancy between the provider's manual and code edits that are applied, or if code edits are undocumented by the payer, a written request to the payer for an explanation of their policies in writing should be sent.

Capitation Management

Most multispecialty practices have over five capitated contracts, and specialists usually have about three of these agreements. When the practice participates in a capitated contract, careful attention must be paid to patient eligibility, referral requirements, encounter reports, claim write-offs, and billing procedures.

Patient Eligibility

Under most capitated agreements with primary care physicians, providers receive monthly payments that cover the patients who chose them as their PCPs for that month. The typical payment for global services is around $150. The **monthly enrollment list** that is sent with the payment should list the current names. This list, also called a "provider patient listing," contains patients' names, identification numbers, dates of birth, type of plan or program, and effective date of registration to the PCP.

At times, however, the list does not contain members who should be listed, or a disenrolled member's name has not been removed. To be sure that the patient is eligible for services, the medical insurance specialist, after following the normal step of photocopying the patient's insurance card, also contacts the payer to double-check.

Referral Requirements

HMOs may require PCPs to refer patients to an in-network provider or get authorization from the plan to refer to an out-of-network provider. Patients who self-refer to nonparticipating providers may be balance-billed for those services. Both PCPs and specialists may be required to keep logs of referral activities.

Encounter Reports and Claim Write-offs

Most HMOs require capitated providers to submit encounter reports for patient encounters. Some do not require regular procedural coding and charges on the reports. Instead of using different codes for established or new patients and five levels of visits, the payer's form may just list "office visit" to be checked off. Some plans require the use of a regular claim with CPT procedural coding.

The medical billing program is set up to write off capitated accounts. If this is not done, the program's reports double-count the revenue for patient encounters—once, at the beginning of the month when the capitated payment is entered for the patient, and then again when a claim is created for a patient who has had an encounter during the period. To fix this, the regular charges that appear on encounter reports or claims are written off. Only the capitated payment remains on the patient's account.

Billing for Excluded Services

Under a capitated contract, providers charge for services not covered by the cap rate. Medical insurance specialists need to organize this information for billing. For example, a special encounter form for the capitated plan might list the CPTs covered under the cap rate and then list the CPTs that can be billed. The plan's data form should indicate the plan's payment method for these additional services, such as discounted fee-for-service.

Thinking It Through—10.3

What procedures would you suggest to ensure that providers are paid according to the payer's guidelines?

Billing Tip

Payment for New Procedures
Payment for new procedures may be announced by a payer, such as under a Medicare directive (see Chapter 11). If the practice performs this procedure, it should send a letter to the other major payers explaining that this procedure will be reported for payment in the future, and requesting their allowed charge and any other regulations for payment. New procedures often require greater documentation, for instance.

Private Payer Claim Completion

Private payer claims are completed using either the HIPAA 837 claim or the CMS-1500 paper claim. The 837 is used for most private payer primary and secondary claims. Chapter 8 covers these claims in detail. Claim preparation tips are presented here.

Medical insurance specialists should be aware of the following items that may be required for correct claims to private payers:

- *Taxonomy codes:* The participation contract may state that certain specialties receive a higher rate for various procedures. For example, if a pediatrician is board-certified in pediatric cardiology, the correct taxonomy code—either for pediatrician or for pediatric cardiology—would be reported with the associated service.
- *Identifying numbers:* Many private payers require the claim to contain the providers' identifying numbers. BCBS plans usually require the Blue Provider Number.
- *Contract information:* The participation contract may require these additional data elements: a contract type code, contract amount, contract percent, contract code, discount percent, or contract version identifier.

A major problem with generating clean private payer claims is that reimbursement is based on contracts, and the terms and payment policies are not always clear. However, the trend is for managed care organizations, in particular, to improve providers' understanding of what meets the payers' definition of medical necessity.

A major example of this trend is the Web-based tool that one BCBS plan offers. It lets physician practices access information on specific code-editing policies and the clinical reasons for them. The tool contains a list of procedures the payer covers, the costs for those procedures, and whether the procedures have to be performed separately or can be combined in a single office visit or operation. The tool is designed to reduce the time spent on claim inquiries and to increase timely and accurate payments.

Review

Chapter Summary

1. The major types of private payers are commercial payers such as managed care organizations, insurance carriers such as Blue Cross and Blue Shield (BCBS) plans, self-insured health plans, and third-party claims administrators.

2. Participation contracts have five main parts. The introductory section provides the names of the parties to the agreement, contract definitions, and the payer. The contract purpose and covered medical services section lists the type and purpose of the plan and the medical services it covers for its enrollees. The third section covers the physician's responsibilities as a participating provider. The fourth section covers the plan's responsibilities toward the participating provider. The fifth section lists the compensation and billing guidelines, such as fees, billing rules, filing deadlines, patients' financial responsibilities, and coordination of benefits.

3. The following types of information are typically summarized on a plan data form: payer information (plan name and type, payer contact information, covered service groups), patient information regarding services (eligibility verification contact; referral, preauthorization, and precertification requirements), billing information (format for claims, payer turnaround time), and patient financial responsibilities (copayment requirements; other required payments, such as deductibles and coinsurance).

4. Five steps are followed to ensure that correct claims are prepared: (a) identify the plan and the payer, (b) verify patient eligibility under the primary insurance, (c) check patient's secondary coverage, (d) conduct an internal review of claims before submission, and (e) monitor and follow-up on claims.

5. Under capitated contracts, medical insurance specialists verify patient eligibility with the plan, because enrollment data are not always up to date. Encounter information, whether it contains complete coding or just diagnostic coding, must accurately reflect the necessity for the provider's services.

Key Terms

Review Questions

Match the key terms in the left column with the definitions in the right column.

A. monthly enrollment list

B. precertification

C. rider

D. subscriber

E. carve out

F. utilization review company

G. Employee Retirement Income Security Act of 1974

H. home plan

I. stop-loss provision

J. elective surgery

_____ 1. Payer preauthorization for elective hospital-based services and outpatient surgeries

_____ 2. Individual insured by a BCBS plan

_____ 3. A federal law that provides incentives and protection against litigation for companies that set up employee health and pension plans

_____ 4. A part of a standard health plan that is changed under a negotiated employer-sponsored plan

_____ 5. Document of eligible members of a capitated plan registered with a particular PCP for a monthly period

_____ 6. Document that modifies an insurance contract

_____ 7. Surgical procedure that can be scheduled in advance

_____ 8. In a BlueCard program, the provider's local BCBS plan

_____ 9. A company hired by a payer to evaluate the appropriateness and medical necessity of hospital-based health care services

_____ 10. Contractual guarantee against a participating provider's financial loss due to an unusually large demand for high-cost services

Decide whether each statement is true or false, and then write T for true or F for false.

_____ 1. Preferred provider organizations are the most popular type of managed care plan.

_____ 2. A carve out may be used to omit a specific plan benefit that is usually covered.

_____ 3. Self-insured health plans are required by ERISA to use pharmacy benefit managers.

_____ 4. The introductory section of a participation contract specifies the payer.

_____ 5. Stop-loss provisions protect the plan from the financial impact of an unusually high number of expensive claims.

_____ 6. If the participation contract states that copayments apply, the payer subtracts the patient's copayment from the provider's reimbursement.

_____ 7. Elective surgery is not reimbursed because it is not medically necessary.

_____ 8. Encounter reports for capitated services contain diagnosis codes.

_____ 9. The employer's plan is secondary if the patient has Medicare coverage.

_____ 10. Secondary claims are submitted at the same time as primary claims.

Write the letter of the choice that best completes the statement or answers the question.

_____ 1. The largest employer-sponsored health program in the United States is
A. Medicare
B. Medicaid
C. Federal Employees Health Benefits program
D. workers' compensation

_____ 2. In employer-sponsored health plans, employees may choose their plan during the
   A. carve out   C. contract period
   B. open enrollment period   D. birthday rule period

_____ 3. If a patient has secondary insurance under a spouse's plan, what information is needed before transmitting a claim to the secondary plan?
   A. RA data   C. PPO data
   B. 271 data   D. none of the above

_____ 4. Self-insured health plans are regulated by
   A. PHI   C. FEHB
   B. PPO   D. ERISA

_____ 5. Blue Cross and Blue Shield plans offer
   A. all major types of health plans
   B. only indemnity plans
   C. only PPOs
   D. only HMOs

_____ 6. Elective surgery usually requires
   A. a deductible   C. a referral
   B. precertification   D. none of the above

_____ 7. Which of the following appears only on secondary claims?
   A. primary insurance group policy number
   B. primary insurance employer name
   C. primary plan name
   D. primary payer payment

_____ 8. Under an HMO plan, the physician practice receives
   A. an encounter report   C. a monthly enrollment list
   B. precertification for services D. a secondary insurance identification number

_____ 9. What document is researched to uncover rules for private payers' copayments?
   A. ERISA   C. HIPAA Security Rule
   B. participation contract   D. none of the above

_____ 10. What code that may be reported on a health care claim describes the specialty of the provider?
   A. CPT   C. secondary identifier
   B. ICD   D. taxonomy

Provide answers to the following questions in the spaces provided.

   1. List the five main parts of participation contracts.

   2. What five steps should be followed to effectively manage fee-for-service claims?

Applying your Knowledge

Case 10.1

Determine the primary plan:

A. George Rangley enrolled in the ACR plan in 2005 and in the New York Health plan in 2004.

George's primary plan:_____

B. Mary is the child of Gloria and Craig Bivilaque, who are divorced. Mary is a dependent under both Craig's and Gloria's plans. Gloria has custody of Mary.

Mary's primary plan:_____

C. Karen Kaplan's date of birth is 10/11/1970; her husband Carl was born on 12/8/1971. Their child Ralph was born on 4/15/2000. Ralph is a dependent under both Karen's and Carl's plans.

Ralph's primary plan:_____

D. Belle Estaphan has medical insurance from Internet Services, from which she retired last year. She is on Medicare, but is also covered under her husband Bernard's plan from Orion International, where he works.

Belle's primary plan:_____

E. Jim Larenges is covered under his spouse's plan and also has medical insurance through his employer.

Jim's primary plan:_____

Case 10.2

Based on the following notes, fill out the precertification form for Betty Sinowitcz.

Encounter Data: 5/4/2006

Patient: Elizabeth R. Sinowitcz

Date of Birth: 8/2/1937

Address: 45 Maple Hill Road, Apt. 12-B, Rangeley, MN 55555

Home Telephone: 555–123–9887

Employer: Argon Electric Company, 238 Industry Way, Rangeley, MN 55554

Work Telephone: 555–124–8754

Betty is on Medicare. She also has insurance coverage through Argon Electric in the Horizon PPO. Her insurance card shows her member number as 65-PO; no group number is shown.

Betty was referred to Dr. Hank R. Ferrara, a Horizon-participating ophthalmologist (PIN 349–00–G), for evaluation of her blurred and dimmed vision. After conducting an examination and taking the necessary history, Dr. Ferrara diagnoses the patient's condition as a cataract of the left eye that is close to mature (ICD 366.10). Dr. Ferrara decides to schedule Betty for lens extraction; the procedure is ambulatory care surgery with same-day admission and discharge. The procedure will be done at Mischogie Hospital's Outpatient Clinic on 5/10. Horizon PPO requires precertification for this procedure (CPT 66984).

Case 10.3

Jan Wommelsdorf, of Fargo, North Dakota, was on vacation in Portland, Oregon, when she became ill. She has BCBS BlueCard insurance, so she telephoned the BlueCard toll-free number to find a provider near her in Seattle. She was examined by Dr. Vijay Sundaram and provided with a special diet to follow until she returns home and visits her regular physician.

A. Who submits the claim, Jan Wommelsdorf or Dr. Sundaram?

B. Is the claim submitted to Jan's local BCBS plan in North Dakota or to Dr. Sundaram's local plan in Washington?

Computer Exploration

Internet Activity

1. FEHB beneficiaries have an annual open enrollment season, during which they can decide whether to remain in their current health plan or switch to a different plan. Point your Web browser at
   http://www.opm.gov and explore *Employment and Benefits.* Investigate the options under FEHB and their FSA plans.

2. Explore the Web site for the national Blue Cross and Blue Shield Association at
   http://www.bluecares.com
   Enter your Zip code, and look up information about the Blue Cross and Blue Shield affiliate for the state in which you live. What types of plans are offered?

3. Go to the Web site for Anthem Blue Cross and Blue Shield at
   http://www.anthem.com
   Click the link to find out more about their insurance products and services. Pick two of the states on the list, and note the products and services offered.

4. Private payers provide valuable information on their Web sites, such as coverage bulletins, available plans, and benefits. Point your Web browser at the site of a major carrier and explore its health plan information. Two suggestions are:
   http://www.cigna.com
   and
   http://www.aetna.com

NDCMediSoft Exploration

10.1 Review Insurance Carrier Entries in MediSoft

Information about insurance carriers is entered in MediSoft when the program is set up and is modified as necessary.

1. To access the Insurance Carrier List dialog box, select Insurance Carriers on the Lists menu. The Insurance Carrier dialog box is displayed.

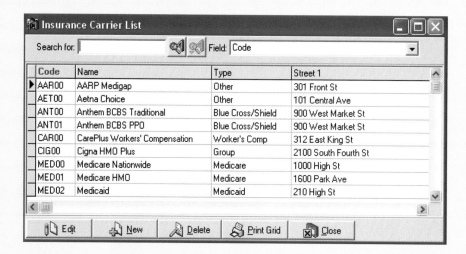

2. The Insurance Carrier List dialog box contains a list of all insurance carriers that have been entered in the MediSoft program. Look closely at the window. Notice that the carriers are listed by Code. This Code is a unique identifier assigned to each insurance carrier. It is typically the first three letters of the carrier's name, followed by a two-digit number. For example, notice that Anthem BCBS Traditional is assigned a Code of ANT00 and that Anthem BCBS PPO is assigned ANT01.

3. Highlight Aetna Choice, and click the Edit button. This action displays the information for the Aetna Choice insurance plan. Notice that the Code is AET00.

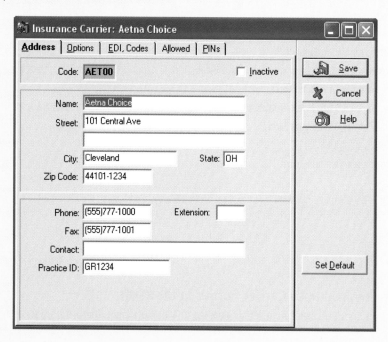

4. The Insurance Carrier dialog box contains five tabs: Address; Options; EMC, Codes; Allowed; and PINs. The Address tab lists standard address, phone, and fax information as well as a contact person at the company (optional) and the practice's ID number, if one has been assigned. The practice ID is a number given to the practice by the insurance carrier.

Computer Exploration

5. Click the Options tab. The top section of the Options tab lists the plan name, the type of plan, the plan ID (a HIPAA-compliant field created in anticipation of the use of a national plan identifier), an alternate carrier ID field (an open field for use by external programs), and whether to delay secondary billing until an RA has been received from the primary carrier. If the Delay Secondary Billing box is checked, a claim will not be printed for this carrier until a payment or adjustment entry has been made for the primary carrier.

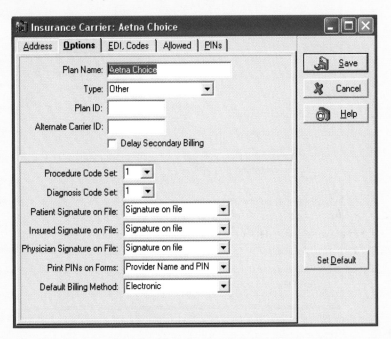

6. The lower half of the Options tab indicates which procedure and diagnosis code sets are to be used with this carrier. (Remember, up to two alternate codes can be entered for each procedure and diagnosis code.)

The selection in the three Signature on File fields determines what is entered in form locators 12, 13, and 31 of the HCFA-1500. This selection does not determine the content of the form locaters, but how the content is displayed. Options include to print "Signature on file," leave the form locator blank, or to print a name. This selection varies from one insurance carrier to another.

The Default Billing Method is set to paper or electronic, depending on the decision of the practice and the carrier's requirements. In the Valley Associates, P.C., sample database, the default billing method is currently set to electronic for all of the carriers.

7. Click the EMC, Codes tab. The fields in the top half of the tab refer to specific entries regarding the electronic claims receiver. In this case, the receiver is NDCOO, which is National Data Corporation, an electronic claims clearinghouse. The other fields are completed based on information provided by the electronic claims receiver.

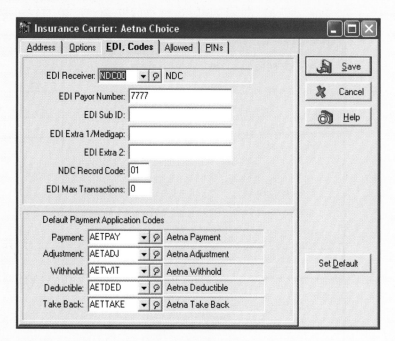

8. The lower section of the tab determines which payment, adjustment, withhold, and deductible codes are used when transactions are entered for this carrier. These codes are set up in the Procedure/Payment/Adjustment List dialog box, accessed by choosing Procedure/Payment/Adjustment Codes on the Lists menu.

9. Click the Allowed tab. This tab contains a column to enter the carrier's allowed amount for each procedure code in the database. In the sample database, an allowed entry for code 10120 has been entered. In an actual medical practice database, all the fields in the Allowed column would contain entries.

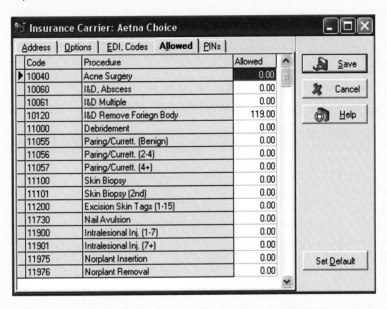

10. Click the PINs tab. The PINs tab is used to list the carrier's PINs and Group IDs for each physician in the medical group. This information is required at different points in a claim, depending on the type of carrier and the circumstances of the claim.

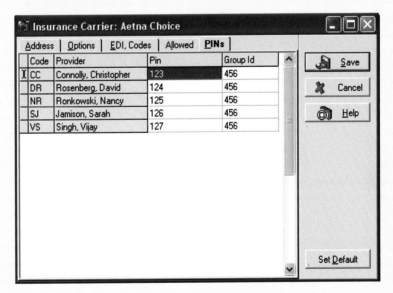

11. Click the Cancel button to close the Insurance Carrier dialog box.
12. Click the Close button to close the Insurance Carrier List dialog box.

Computer Exploration

10.2 Printing Primary and Secondary Claims

Whether an insurance claim is transmitted or printed as a primary or a secondary claim is determined by what is entered in the patient's Case folder.

1. Select Patients/Guarantors and Cases on the Lists menu. The Patient List dialog box appears.
2. Enter "L" in the Search For box to select Nancy Lankhaar's information.
3. Click Rash under Case Description on the right side of the dialog box to highlight her case.
4. Click the Edit Case button. The Case folder is displayed.
5. The Policy 1 tab contains information about the primary insurance carrier. Click the Policy 1 tab. Notice that the primary insurance carrier is Medicare Nationwide. This carrier will be billed first.

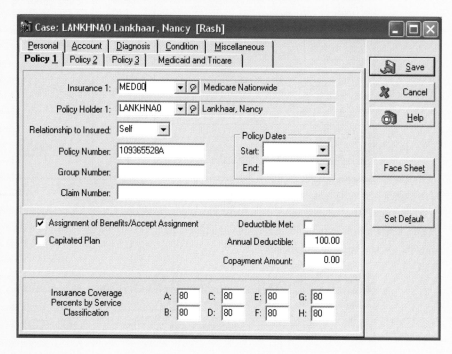

6. Click the Policy 2 tab. This tab lists information about the secondary insurance carrier. In this case, the secondary policy is AARP Medigap.

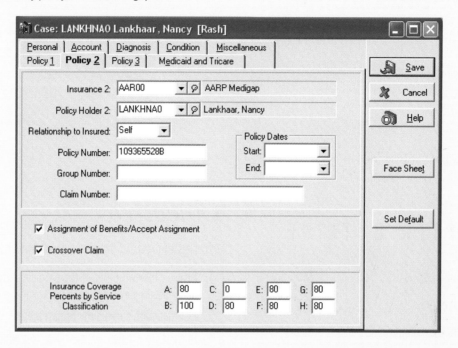

7. Notice that the Crossover Claim box is checked. When this box is checked, it indicates that no secondary claim needs to be filed by the practice, because the primary carrier forwards the claim directly to the secondary carrier. Medicare provides this service for many secondary carriers.

   If the Crossover Claim box is not checked, the practice would file a claim with the secondary carrier when an RA is received from the primary carrier.

8. Click the Cancel button to close the Case folder.

9. Click the Close button to close the Patient List dialog box.

Medicare

Objectives

After studying this chapter, you should be able to:

1. Discuss the two parts of the Medicare program and briefly describe the coverage each part provides to beneficiaries.

2. List Medicare's eligibility requirements.

3. Discuss the types of services excluded from Medicare coverage.

4. Compare participating and nonparticipating providers' methods of reimbursement.

5. Discuss the two major types of Medicare Part B plans available to beneficiaries.

6. Discuss Medigap insurance and explain the coverage it offers.

7. List several situations in which Medicare is the secondary payer on a claim.

8. Prepare correct Medicare primary and secondary claims.

Introduction

Medicare is a federal medical insurance program established in 1965 under Title XVIII of the Social Security Act. The first benefits were paid in January 1966. In 2000, 41.9 million people received estimated benefits of $230.8 billion. The Medicare program is managed by the Centers for Medicare and Medicaid Services (CMS). It is arguably the most complex health insurance program, with numerous rules and regulations that must be followed for claims to be paid. To complicate matters, these rules change frequently, and keeping up with the changes is a challenge for most providers and medical information specialists.

The federal government does not pay Medicare claims directly; instead, it contracts with insurance organizations to process its claims. Insurance companies that process claims sent by hospitals, skilled nursing facilities, intermediate care facilities, long-term care facilities, and home health care agencies are known as **fiscal intermediaries**. Insurance companies that process claims sent by physicians, providers, and suppliers are referred to as carriers. The flow of claims from the provider to the carrier and back is illustrated in Figure 11.1.

Medicare Program

The Medicare program has two parts that cover different types of services. To receive benefits under either part of the Medicare program, individuals must meet certain eligibility requirements.

Medicare Part A pays for inpatient hospital care, skilled nursing facility care, home health care, respite care, and hospice care. Anyone who receives Social Security benefits is automatically enrolled in Part A. No premiums are required of beneficiaries because the program is partially funded by payroll taxes collected from individuals, employers, and the federal government. Individuals

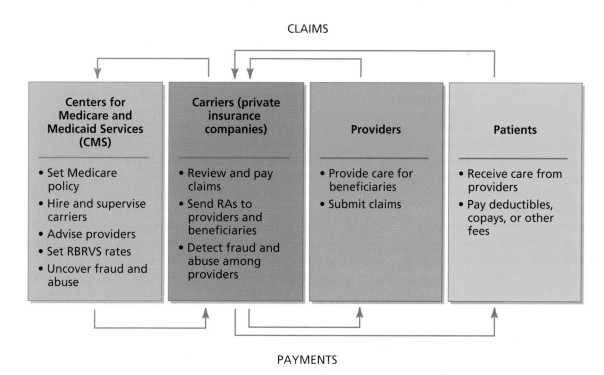

Figure 11.1 The Medicare Claims Process

TABLE 11.1	Medicare Part A Coverage

A semiprivate bed in a hospital (up to 90 hospital days for each 90-day benefit period) and inpatient services. Benefit periods begin the first day a Medicare patient is given inpatient hospital services and end when the patient has been out of a hospital or skilled nursing facility for 60 consecutive days.

A semiprivate bed in a skilled nursing facility.

Care in a psychiatric hospital (up to 190 days in a lifetime).

Hospice care and respite care when a terminally ill patient is admitted to a hospice.

Nursing home care (if the patient spent at least 3 days in a benefit period as an inpatient).

Transplants for heart, lung, kidney, pancreas, intestine, bone marrow, cornea, and liver—under certain conditions and when performed at Medicare-certified facilities.

Home health services for patients confined to their homes because of an illness or injury. Services covered include intermittent nursing care and physical, occupational, or speech therapy; part-time services of home health aides, medical supplies, and equipment (no drugs). These patients are generally confined to their homes by injury or illness.

TABLE 11.2	Medicare Part B Coverage

Physician services including surgery, consultations, home, office, and institutional services and supplies incidental to physician services; drugs and biologicals that cannot be self-administered; physical therapy; speech pathology; blood and blood transfusions; physician interpretation of Pap smears.

Outpatient hospital services, including diagnostic services; physical, occupational, or speech therapy; mental health services; hospital services provided in connection with a physician's services; ambulatory surgery; and emergency hospital services.

Diagnostic X-ray and laboratory tests and other diagnostic tests.

X-ray, radium, and radioactive isotope therapy.

Durable medical equipment such as oxygen, hospital beds, and other equipment.

Artificial devices that replace all or part of an internal body organ; ostomy bags and supplies; one pair of glasses or contact lenses after cataract surgery (if an intraocular lens has been inserted).

Braces, artificial limbs, and artificial eyes.

Rural and community health clinic services performed by licensed nurses and physician's assistants, plus similar services provided to homebound patients in certain areas.

Certified registered nurse anesthetist (CRNA), nurse midwife, and physician's assistant services.

Psychologist and social worker services (in connection with a physician's service).

Chiropractic services (subject to limits).

Ambulance service (when the patient's condition rules out other means of transportation).

Home dialysis supplies and equipment, self-care home dialysis support services, and institutional dialysis services and supplies.

Medical nutrition therapy services for people who have diabetes or kidney disease.

Certain preventive services for qualified individuals, including bone mass measurements, colorectal cancer screening, certain diabetes services and supplies, glaucoma screening, mammogram screening, Pap test and pelvic examination, prostate cancer screening, and shots.

age sixty-five or older who are not eligible for Social Security benefits may enroll in Part A, but they must pay premiums for the coverage. Details of Part A coverage are provided in Table 11.1.

Medicare Part B helps pay for a wide range of procedures and supplies. For example, it covers physician services, outpatient hospital services, diagnostic tests, clinical laboratory services, and outpatient physical and speech therapy, as long as these services are considered medically necessary (see Table 11.2 for coverage details). Individuals entitled to Part A benefits are automatically qualified to enroll in Part B. U.S. citizens and permanent residents over the age of sixty-five are also eligible.

Part B is a voluntary program; eligible persons may or may not take part in it. Those desiring Part B coverage must enroll; coverage is not automatic. Unlike Part A, Part B coverage is not premium-free; in 2004, it cost $66.60 per month. The plan is funded by beneficiary premiums and by the federal government.

Eligibility Requirements

To qualify for Medicare benefits, individuals must meet Medicare's eligibility requirements under one of its six beneficiary categories:

1. *Individuals 65 or older:* Persons age sixty-five or older who have paid FICA taxes or Railroad Retirement taxes for at least forty calendar quarters.
2. *Disabled adults:* Individuals who have been receiving Social Security disability benefits or Railroad Retirement Board disability benefits for more than two years. Coverage begins five months after the two years of entitlement.
3. *Individuals disabled before age eighteen:* Individuals under eighteen who meet the disability criteria of the Social Security Act.
4. *Spouses of entitled individuals:* Spouses of deceased, disabled, or retired individuals who were or still are entitled to Medicare benefits.
5. *Retired federal employees enrolled in the Civil Service Retirement System (CSRS):* Retired CSRS employees and their spouses.
6. *Individuals with end-stage renal disease (ESRD):* Individuals of any age who receive dialysis or a renal transplant for ESRD. Coverage typically begins on the first day of the month following the start of dialysis treatments. In the case of a transplant, entitlement begins the month the individual is hospitalized for the transplant (the transplant must be completed within two months). The donor is covered for services related to the donation of the organ only.

Health Insurance Card

Each Medicare enrollee receives a health insurance card (HIC) (see Figure 11.2). This card lists the beneficiary's name, sex, effective dates for Part A and Part B coverage, and Medicare number. The Medicare number is assigned by the Centers for Medicare and Medicaid Services and usually consists of the Social Security number followed by a numeric or alphanumeric suffix.

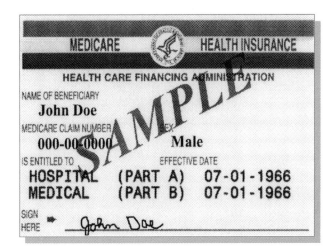

Figure 11.2 Medicare Health Insurance Card (HIC)

Billing Tip

Premiums Rising
The monthly Medicare premium started at $3 in 1966, climbed gradually to $7.20 in 1976, and reached $50 in 2001. The 2004 premium is 33 percent higher than in 2001. It is also increasing for people with incomes greater than $80,000 a year; roughly tripling for people with incomes over $200,000.

Excluded Services and Not Medically Necessary Services

What Medicare covers is determined by federal legislation, rather than by medical practice. For this reason, Medicare does not provide coverage for certain services and procedures. Claims may be denied because the service provided is excluded by Medicare, or because the service was not reasonable and necessary for the specific patient.

Excluded services are services that are not covered under any circumstances, such as routine physical examinations and cosmetic surgery. The services that are excluded change from year to year. For example, in 2003, these services were excluded

- Routine preventive physical examinations, including X-rays and laboratory tests, *except* screening mammograms, physician interpretation of Pap smears, bone mass measurements, and screening for prostate cancer, colorectal cancer, and glaucoma
- Immunizations, with the exception of influenza, hepatitis B, and pneumococcal vaccines
- Routine dental examinations
- Routine medical appliances
- Specific foot care procedures, including most instances of treatment or surgery for subluxation of the foot, supportive shoes, treatment of flat foot, and routine foot care
- Examinations for the prescription of hearing aids or actual hearing aid devices
- Examinations for the prescription of eyeglasses or contact lenses or actual eyeglasses or contact lenses (unless an underlying disease is the cause)
- Services provided by a nonphysician in a hospital inpatient setting that were not ordered or provided by an employee under contract with the hospital
- Services provided as a result of a noncovered procedure, such as laboratory tests ordered in conjunction with a noncovered surgical procedure
- Most custodial services, including daily administration of medication, routine care of a catheter, and routine administration of oxygen therapy
- Long-term care, for example, most nursing home care
- Cosmetic surgery
- Acupuncture
- Health care received while traveling outside the United States

Other services that are not covered are classified as not medically necessary under Medicare guidelines. These services are not covered by Medicare unless certain conditions are met, such as particular diagnoses. For example, a vitamin B_{12} injection is a covered service only for patients with certain diagnoses, such as pernicious anemia. If the patient does not have one of the specified diagnoses, the B_{12} injection is categorized as not reasonable and necessary. The Medicare code edits under Medicare National Correct Coding Initiative (NCCI; see Chapter 6) will deny the claim.

To be considered medically necessary, a treatment must be

- Appropriate for the symptoms or diagnoses of the illness or injury
- Not an elective procedure
- Not an experimental or investigational procedure
- An essential treatment; not performed for the patient's convenience
- Delivered at the most appropriate level that can safely and effectively be administered to the patient

Several common categories of medical necessity denials include

- *The diagnosis does not match the service:* In this case, *match* means that the diagnosis does not justify the procedures performed. In some instances, the denial is the result of a clerical error—for example, a fifth digit was dropped from an ICD-9-CM code. In these instances, many times the claim can be corrected and will eventually be paid. In other situations, the diagnosis is not specific enough to justify the treatment.
- *Too many services in a brief period of time:* Examples include more than one office visit in a day, or too many visits for treatment of a minor problem.
- *Level of service denials:* Claims in this category are either denied or downcoded (coded at a lower level) because the services provided were in excess of those required to adequately diagnose and/or treat the problem. Level of service denials typically occur on claims for office visits. Rather than deny the claim, the payer will downcode the procedure—for example, change a CPT E/M code from 99214 to 99212.

The CMS Web site contains a Medicare Coverage home page (http://www.cms.hhs.gov/coverage/default2.asp) that informs the public about coverage issues and about how coverage decisions are made. The page contains links to the coverage database and to issues about how national coverage is determined. The site is designed to make the ongoing policymaking process for Medicare coverage more visible and understandable.

Billing Tip

CMS Manual System On Line
CMS has created the CMS Manual System to transition from a paper-based to a Web-based manual system. Located at http://cms.hhs.gov/manuals/, this site contains all program manuals as well as revisions, business requirements, and one-time notifications.

Medicare Participation

Annually, physicians choose whether they want to participate in the Medicare program. Participating physicians agree to accept assignment for all Medicare claims and to accept Medicare's allowed charge as payment in full for services. They also agree to submit claims on behalf of the patient at no charge and to receive payment directly from Medicare on the patient's behalf. Participants are responsible for knowing the rules and regulations of the program as they affect their patients.

To ensure that only qualified providers are enrolled in Medicare, CMS requires all participating providers to complete form CMS 855, the Medicare Provider/Supplier Enrollment Application. It contains data about education and credentials, as appropriate to the type of provider or supplier. Providers must attest to the accuracy of the information reported every three years.

Incentives

Medicare carriers offer incentives to physicians to encourage participation. For example:

- Medicare Physician Fee Schedule (MPFS) amounts are 5 percent higher than for nonparticipating (nonPAR) providers.
- Participating providers do not have to forward claims for beneficiaries who also have supplemental insurance coverage and who assign their supplemental insurance payments to the participating provider. The Medicare carrier automatically forwards the claim to the supplemental carrier, and payments are made directly to the provider from both the primary and secondary payers, with no extra administrative work on the provider's end.
- Participating providers are listed in the carrier's online directory of Medicare-participating providers and receive referrals in some circumstances.

Billing Tip

MPFS On Line
CMS provides free information on the services covered by the Medicare Physician Fee Schedule (MPFS) at http://cms.hhs.gov/ physicians/default .asp. Listed are more than 10,000 physician services, the associated RVUs, and various Medicare payment policies.

Payments

Physicians who participate agree to accept the charge amounts listed in the Medicare Physician Fee Schedule (MPFS) as payment in full for all covered services. MPFS was developed from the resource-based relative value scale (RBRVS) system (see Chapter 7) using three cost factor components: (1) the work relative value unit (RVU)—the time required for the physician to complete the service and the difficulty of the work; (2) the practice RVU—the overhead costs of running the practice; and (3) the malpractice RVU—the cost of liability or malpractice insurance. Each component is multiplied by a geographic practice cost index (GPCI) that takes into account local variations when establishing a price for a service. On average, the Medicare payment rate is about 20 percent lower than average private payer rates.

Notice of Exclusions from Medicare Benefits

Participating providers may bill patients for services that are not covered by the Medicare program, such as routine physicals and many screening tests. Although it is not required, it is a good policy to give patients written notification that Medicare will not pay for a service before providing it, so that patients understand their financial responsibility to pay for the service. The CMS form entitled **Notice of Exclusions from Medicare Benefits (NEMB)** is available for this purpose (see Figure 11.3). NEMBs are used on an entirely voluntary basis by providers. Their purpose is to advise beneficiaries, before services that are not Medicare benefits are furnished, that Medicare will not pay for them, and to provide beneficiaries with an estimate of how much they may have to pay. Providers may also choose to design their own NEMBs based on the services they offer.

Advance Beneficiary Notice

Participating physicians also agree to not bill patients for services that Medicare declares not reasonable and necessary, unless the patients were informed ahead of time in writing and agreed to pay for the services. For this reason, if a provider has reason to believe that a procedure will not be covered by Medicare because it is deemed not reasonable and necessary, the provider must notify the patient before the treatment using a standard **advance beneficiary notice (ABN)** from CMS (see Figure 11.4 on page 372). The ABN form is designed to

- Identify the service or item that Medicare is unlikely to pay for
- State the reason Medicare is unlikely to pay

NOTICE OF EXCLUSIONS FROM MEDICARE BENEFITS (NEMB)
There are items and services for which Medicare will not pay.

- Medicare does **not** pay for all of your health care costs. Medicare only pays for covered benefits. **Some items and services are not Medicare benefits and Medicare will not pay for them.**
- When you receive an item or service that is not a Medicare benefit, **you are responsible to pay for it,** personally or through any other insurance that you may have.

  The purpose of this notice is to help you make an informed choice about whether or not you want to receive these items or services, knowing that you will have to pay for them yourself. **Before you make a decision, you should read this entire notice carefully.**

  Ask us to explain, if you don't understand why Medicare won't pay.

  Ask us how much these items or services will cost you (**Estimated Cost: $_____**).

Medicare will not pay for: _____
_____ ;

❑   **1. Because it does not meet the definition of any Medicare benefit.**

❑   **2. Because of the following exclusion * from Medicare benefits:**

❑ Personal comfort items.	❑ Routine physicals and most tests for screening.
❑ Most shots (vaccinations).	❑ Routine eye care, eyeglasses and examinations.
❑ Hearing aids and hearing examinations.	❑ Cosmetic surgery.
❑ Most outpatient prescription drugs.	❑ Dental care and dentures (in most cases).
❑ Orthopedic shoes and foot supports (orthotics).	❑ Routine foot care and flat foot care.
❑ Health care received outside of the USA.	❑ Services by immediate relatives.
❑ Services required as a result of war.	❑ Services under a physician's private contract.

❑ Services paid for by a governmental entity that is not Medicare.

❑ Services for which the patient has no legal obligation to pay.

❑ Home health services furnished under a plan of care, if the agency does not submit the claim.

❑ Items and services excluded under the Assisted Suicide Funding Restriction Act of 1997.

❑ Items or services furnished in a competitive acquisition area by any entity that does not have a contract with the Department of Health and Human Services (except in a case of urgent need).

❑ Physicians' services performed by a physician assistant, midwife, psychologist, or nurse anesthetist, when furnished to an inpatient, unless they are furnished under arrangements by the hospital.

❑ Items and services furnished to an individual who is a resident of a skilled nursing facility (a SNF) or of a part of a facility that includes a SNF, unless they are furnished under arrangements by the SNF.

❑ Services of an assistant at surgery without prior approval from the peer review organization.

❑ Outpatient occupational and physical therapy services furnished incident to a physician's services.

*   **This is only a general summary of exclusions from Medicare benefits. It is not a legal document. The official Medicare program provisions are contained in relevant laws, regulations, and rulings.**

Figure 11.3 Notice of Exclusions from Medicare Benefits (NEMB)

- Estimate how much the service or item will cost the beneficiary if Medicare does not pay

The ABN for general use is referred to as form CMS-R-131-G. Variations of the form for laboratory use (CMS-R-131-L) and home health care (CMS-R-296) are also available.

ABNs are not required for excluded services; they are to be used only for services that may not be deemed reasonable and necessary by Medicare. As with a NEMB, the purpose of the ABN is to help the patient or beneficiary make an informed decision about services he or she might have to pay for out-of-pocket. In addition, if the provider could have been expected to know that a service would not be covered, and performed the service without informing the patient, the provider may be liable for the charges.

Modifiers for ABNs

Modifiers are attached to procedure codes when reporting a noncovered Medicare service on health care claims. There are three choices of modifiers:

- *GZ*—an item or service expected to be denied as not reasonable and necessary. This might be used, for example, for a noncovered screening test, or a service reported with a noncovered ICD-9 code, or a service provided within frequency limits. Use the –GZ modifier only if the item or service is expected to be denied but the physician's office does *not* have a signed ABN. This might occur in an emergency care situation, or a patient might not be available to sign the document before a specimen is tested. The patient cannot be billed for the service if Medicare does not pay.

- *GA*—a waiver of liability statement is on file. This modifier also applies when services are expected to be denied as not reasonable and necessary.

Figure 11.4 Advance Beneficiary Notice (ABN)

However, it indicates that there is a signed ABN on file in the physician's office. If the claim is not paid by Medicare, the patient is responsible for payment of the charges.

- *GY*—an item or service that is statutorily excluded or does not meet the definition of a Medicare benefit. This would be used for services *never* covered by Medicare, such as routine physicals or cosmetic surgeries. It indicates that an ABN is not required. The claim will be denied by Medicare, and the patient is responsible for payment of the charges.

Nonparticipating Providers

Nonparticipating physicians decide whether to accept assignment on a claim-by-claim basis.

Payment Under Acceptance of Assignment

Providers who elect not to participate in the Medicare program but who accept assignment on a claim are paid 5 percent less for their services than PAR providers. For example, if the Medicare-allowed amount for a service is $100, the PAR provider receives $80 (80 percent of $100), and the nonPAR provider receives $76 ($80 minus 5 percent).

Nonparticipating providers must also provide a surgical financial disclosure—advance written notification—when performing elective surgery that has a $500 or greater charge. The form must contain specific wording and must include an estimated charge for the procedure (see Figure 11.5 for an example).

Like participating providers, nonPAR providers may bill patients for services that are excluded from coverage in the Medicare program. Therefore, it is good practice to provide patients with an NEMB notifying them that Medicare will not pay for a service before providing the service.

Dear (Patient's name):

I do not plan to accept assignment for your surgery. The law requires that where assignment is not taken and the charge is $500 or more, the following information must be provided prior to surgery. These estimates assume that you have already met the $100 annual Medicare Part B deductible.

Type of Surgery

_____

Estimated charge for surgery $_____

Estimated Medicare payment $_____

Your estimated out-of-pocket expense $_____

_____   _____
Patient signature   Date

Figure 11.5 Advance Notice for Elective Surgery Form

Payment for Unassigned Claims: The Limiting Charge

NonPAR providers who do not accept assignment are subject to Medicare's charge limits. The Medicare Comprehensive Limiting Charge Compliance Program (CLCCP) was created to prevent nonparticipating physicians from collecting the balance from Medicare patients. Physicians may not charge a Medicare patient more than 115 percent of the amount listed in the Medicare nonparticipating fee schedule. This amount—115 percent of the fee listed in the nonPAR MFS—is called the **limiting charge**. Medicare issues bulletins to physicians that list fees and limiting charges.

The limiting charge does not apply to immunizations, supplies, or ambulance service. Physicians who collect amounts in excess of the limiting charge are subject to financial penalties and may be excluded from the Medicare program for a specific time period.

For a nonassigned claim, the provider can collect the full payment from the patient at the time of the visit. The claim is then submitted to Medicare. If approved, Medicare will pay 80 percent of the allowed amount on the nonPAR fee schedule—not the limiting amount. Medicare sends this payment directly to the patient, since the physician has already been paid.

A participating provider may also be part of a clinic or group that does not participate. In this case, the beneficiary may be charged more if the visit takes place at the clinic or group location than if it takes place at the provider's private office.

The following example illustrates the different fee structures for PARs, nonPARs who accept assignment, and nonPARs who do not accept assignment.

Participating Provider

Physician's standard fee	$120.00
Medicare fee	$ 60.00
Medicare pays 80% ($60.00 × 80%)	$ 48.00
Patient or supplemental plan pays 20% ($60.00 × 20%)	$ 12.00
Provider adjustment (write-off) ($120.00 − $60.00)	$ 60.00

Nonparticipating Provider (Accepts Assignment)

Physician's standard fee	$120.00
Medicare nonPAR fee	$ 57.00
Medicare pays 80% ($57.00 × 80%)	$ 45.60
Patient or supplemental plan pays 20% ($57.00 × 20%)	$ 11.40
Provider adjustment (write-off) ($120.00 − $57.00)	$ 63.00

Nonparticipating Provider (Does Not Accept Assignment)

Physician's standard fee	$120.00
Medicare nonPAR fee	$ 57.00
Limiting Charge (115% × $57.00)	$ 65.55
Patient billed	$ 65.55
Medicare pays patient (80% × $57.00)	$ 45.60
Total provider can collect	$ 65.55
Patient out-of-pocket expense ($65.55 − $45.60)	$ 19.95

- Medicare Managed Care Plans
- Medicare Preferred Provider Organization Plans (PPOs)
- Medicare Private Fee-for-Service Plans
- Health Savings Accounts

Medicare Managed Care Plans

Many Medicare beneficiaries are enrolled in managed care programs. In 2002, approximately 5 million beneficiaries were enrolled in Medicare HMOs, while approximately 35 million were enrolled in traditional fee-for-service plans. Most managed care plans charge a monthly premium and a small copayment for each office visit, but not a deductible.

Like private payer managed care plans, Medicare managed care plans often restrict the delivery of services to a specific network of physicians, hospitals, and facilities. Some plans offer the option of receiving services from providers outside the network for a higher fee. On the other hand, they offer coverage for services not reimbursed in a traditional fee-for-service plan, such as additional days in the hospital.

To maintain uniform coverage within a geographic area, CMS requires managed care plans to provide all of the Medicare benefits available in the service area. Beyond that restriction, plans are free to offer coverage for additional services not covered under fee-for-service plans, such as prescription drugs, preventive care (including physical examinations and inoculations), eyeglasses and hearing aids, dental care, care for treatment received while traveling overseas, and so on.

Participants in managed care plans are generally required to select a primary care provider from within the network. The PCP provides treatment and manages the patient's medical care through referrals. Some plans require the patient to receive treatment within the plan's network. If a patient goes out of the network for services, the plan will not pay; the patient must pay the entire bill. This restriction does not apply to emergency treatment (which may be provided anywhere in the United States) and **urgently needed care** (care provided while temporarily outside the plan's network area).

Other plans, called point-of-service (POS), permit a patient to receive some services from outside the network, for which the plan will pay a percentage of the fee rather than the entire bill. The patient is responsible for the balance of the charges, usually at least 20 percent. Under yet another option, patients may also see health care providers within or outside of the plan's network; charges for services received within the network are subject to a small copayment, and those outside the network are handled like other fee-for-service Medicare claims—in other words, they are not paid by the managed care plan, but are covered under regular Medicare, subject to the deductible and coinsurance. These also offer extra coverage for such services as preventive care and prescription drugs at an additional cost.

Managed care plans offer beneficiaries a number of advantages:

- Low copayment when receiving treatment
- Minimal paperwork
- Coverage for additional services
- No need for a supplemental Medigap policy (see below)

Disadvantages of Medicare managed care plans include the following:

- Physician choices limited to those in the particular plan
- Typically need to obtain prior approval from the primary care physician before seeing a specialist, undergoing elective surgery, and receiving other services

1. Does a participating provider in a traditional fee-for-service plan always get paid more for a service than a nonparticipating provider who does not accept assignment?

2. Does a patient in a traditional fee-for-service plan always pay higher fees when services are provided by a nonparticipating provider who does not accept assignment?

Preferred Provider Organization (PPO)

In the Medicare Preferred Provider Organization Plan (PPO), patients are given a financial incentive to use doctors within a network, but they may choose to go outside the network. Visits outside the network incur additional costs, which may include a higher copayment or higher coinsurance. A PPO contracts with a certain group of providers to offer health care services to patients. Unlike HMOs, many PPOs do not require patients to select a PCP.

Private Fee-for-Service (PFFS)

Under a private fee-for-service plan, patients receive services from the provider or facility of their choosing, as long as Medicare has approved the provider or facility. The plan is operated by a private insurance company that contracts with Medicare to provide services to beneficiaries. The plan sets its own rates for services, and physicians are allowed to bill patients the amount of the charge not covered by the plan, as long as it does not exceed 15 percent. A copayment may or may not be required. Under a private fee-for-service plan, patients may pay rates that are higher or lower than the rates on the Medicare Fee Schedule, but they cannot be charged for balance billing.

Health Savings Accounts

The Medicare Modernization Act creates a new plan for Medicare called a **Health Savings Account.** Similar to private medical savings accounts, this plan combines a high-deductible fee-for-service plan with a tax-exempt trust to pay for qualified medical expenses. The deductible must be at least $1,000 a year for individuals and $2,000 for couples.

Compliance Guideline

Medigap plans can legally be sold only to people covered by the Medicare fee-for-service plan (Original Medicare Plan). Patients covered by a Medicare managed care plan or by Medicaid (see Chapter 12) do not need Medigap policies.

Medigap and Supplemental Insurance

Individuals enrolled in Medicare Part B Original Medicare Plan often have additional insurance, either in the form of Medigap insurance they purchase or a supplemental insurance plan provided by a former employer. These plans frequently reimburse the patient's Part B deductible and additional procedures that Medicare does not cover. If Medicare does not pay a claim, Medigap and supplemental carriers are not required to pay the claim either.

Medigap Insurance

Medigap is private insurance that beneficiaries may purchase to fill in some of the gaps—unpaid amounts—in Medicare coverage. These gaps include the annual deductible, any coinsurance that is required, and payment for some noncovered services, such as prescription drugs and at-home recovery. Even though private insurance carriers offer Medigap plans, coverage and standards are regulated by federal and state law.

In exchange for Medigap coverage, the policyholder pays a monthly premium. A number of different options are available. These choices are labeled A through J. Monthly premiums vary widely across the different plan levels, as well as within a single plan level, depending on the insurance company selected. While coverage varies from policy to policy, a set of core benefits is common to all Medigap plans:

- Part A daily coinsurance amount for days 61 to 90 of hospitalization
- Part A daily coinsurance amount for each of Medicare's 60 lifetime inpatient hospital days
- 100 percent of covered hospital charges for 365 additional days after all Medicare hospital benefits have been used
- Part B coinsurance amount (usually 20 percent of approved charges) after the deductible ($100)
- First three pints of blood per calendar year

Plans B through J also pay the Part A hospital deductible for each hospitalization. See Figure 11.7 for a complete listing of Medigap plans and the coverage they provide.

When a patient with Medigap coverage is treated by a participating provider, Medicare automatically forwards claim information to the Medigap payer, including the amount Medicare approved and paid for the procedures. Once the Medigap carrier adjudicates the claim, the provider is paid directly, eliminating the need for a separate Medigap claim. The beneficiary receives copies of the Medicare Summary Notices that explain the charges paid and due.

A	B	C	D	E	F	G	H	I	J*
Basic Benefit	Basic Benefit	Basic Benefit	Basic Benefit	Basic Benefit	Basic Benefit	Basic Benefit	Basic Benefit	Basic Benefit	Basic Benefit
		Skilled Nursing Coinsurance	Skilled Nursing Coinsurance	Skilled Nursing Coinsurance	Skilled Nursing Coinsurance	Skilled Nursing Coinsurance	Skilled Nursing Coinsurance	Skilled Nursing Coinsurance	Skilled Nursing Coinsurance
	Part A Deductible	Part A Deductible	Part A Deductible	Part A Deductible	Part A Deductible	Part A Deductible	Part A Deductible	Part A Deductible	Part A Deductible
		Part B Deductible			Part B Deductible				Part B Deductible
					Part Excess (100%)	Part Excess (80%)		Part Excess (100%)	Part Excess (100%)
		Foreign Travel Emergency	Foreign Travel Emergency	Foreign Travel Emergency	Foreign Travel Emergency	Foreign Travel Emergency	Foreign Travel Emergency	Foreign Travel Emergency	Foreign Travel Emergency
			At-Home Recovery			At-Home Recovery		At-Home Recovery	At-Home Recovery
							Basic Drug Benefit (50%) ($3,000 Limit)	Basic Drug Benefit (50%) ($3,000 Limit)	Extended Drug Benefit ($3,000 Limit)
				Preventive Care ($120 Limit)					Preventive Care ($120 Limit)

*High-deductible plans available.

Figure 11.7 Medigap Coverage, Plans A-J

Supplemental Insurance

Supplemental insurance is a plan an individual may be able to purchase when retiring from a company. A supplemental plan is designed to provide additional coverage for an individual receiving benefits under Medicare Part B. Supplemental policies provide benefits similar to those offered in the employer's standard group health plan. CMS does not regulate the supplemental plan's coverage, in contrast to what it does with Medigap insurance.

Medicare as the Secondary Payer

In certain situations, Medicare pays benefits on a claim only after another insurance carrier—the primary carrier—has processed the claim. The medical insurance specialist is responsible for knowing when Medicare is the secondary payer and, in those cases, submitting claims to the primary payer first. A form such as that shown in Figure 11.8 is used to gather and validate information about Medicare patients' primary plans.

Plans Primary to Medicare

Over Age Sixty-Five and Employed

When an individual is employed and receives coverage through the employer's group health plan, Medicare is the secondary payer. Medicare is also secondary when an individual over age sixty-five receives coverage through a spouse's employer (the spouse does not have to be sixty-five or older). On the other hand, Medicare is the primary carrier for

- Individuals who are working for an employer with twenty employees or fewer
- Individuals who are covered by another policy that is not a group policy
- Individuals who are enrolled in Part B, but not Part A, of the Medicare program
- Individuals who must pay premiums to receive Part A coverage
- Individuals who are retired and receiving coverage under a group policy from a previous employer

Disabled

If an individual under age sixty-five is disabled and receives coverage through an employer group health plan (which may be held by the individual, a spouse, or another family member), Medicare is the secondary payer. If the individual or family member is not actively employed, Medicare is the primary payer. Medicare is also the primary payer for

- Individuals and family members who are retired and receiving coverage under a group policy from a previous employer.
- Individuals and family members who are working for an employer with a hundred employees or fewer.
- Individuals and family members receiving coverage under the **Consolidated Omnibus Budget Reconciliation Act (COBRA)**. COBRA requires employers to allow employees, their spouses, and their dependents to continue group health insurance coverage for a minimum of eighteen months after their employment with the company ends. Premiums are paid by the employee without any contribution from the employer.
- Individuals who are covered by another policy that is not a group policy.

Patient's Name _____   Medicare # _____

▪ Medicare Secondary Payer Screening Questionnaire

1. Are you covered by the Veterans Administration, the Black Lung   ( ) Yes   ( ) No
   Program, or Workers Compensation? If so which one? -
   _____

2. Is this illness or injury due to any type of accident?   ( ) Yes   ( ) No

3. Are you age 65 or older?   ( ) Yes   ( ) No

   a. Are you currently employed?   ( ) Yes   ( ) No

   b. Is your spouse currently employed?   ( ) Yes   ( ) No

4. Are you age 65 or under?   ( ) Yes   ( ) No

   a. Are you covered by any employer Group Health Plan?   ( ) Yes   ( ) No

   b. Or another large Group Health Plan?   ( ) Yes   ( ) No

▪ Authorization Statement and Payment Agreement

I declare under penalty of perjury that I do not have another primary insurance carrier to pay for medical care rendered to me by _____, and that all information with regard to residence, employment, and income is correct to the best of my knowledge.

I request that payment of authorized Medicare Benefits be made to this health center for any services furnished to me by its physicians or suppliers.

I understand that my signature requests that payment be made and that it authorizes release of medical information necessary to pay the claim(s). If a secondary insurance carrier is involved my signature also authorizes releasing information to the insurer or agency shown.

In Medicare assigned cases, the physician or supplier agrees to accept the charge determined by the Medicare Carrier as full charge, and the patient is responsible only for the deductible (Excluding UGS/Medicare) coinsurance and noncovered services. Coinsurance and deductible are based upon charge determined by the Medicare carrier.

_____   _____
Signature of Patient or Authorized Representative   Date

_____   _____
Witnessed by   Date

Figure 11.8 Medicare Secondary Payer Screening Questionnaire

End-Stage Renal Disease (ESRD)

During a coordination-of-benefits period (currently thirty months), Medicare is the secondary payer for individuals who receive coverage through an employer-sponsored group health plan and who fail to apply for ESRD-based Medicare coverage. The coordination-of-benefits period begins the first month the individual is eligible for or entitled to Part A benefits based on an ESRD diagnosis. This rule is in effect regardless of whether the individual is employed or retired.

Workers' Compensation

If an individual receives treatment for a job-related injury or illness, Medicare coverage is secondary to workers' compensation coverage (see Chapter 14). Included in this category is the Federal Black Lung Program, a government program that provides insurance coverage for coal miners. When an individual

Ron Polonsky is a seventy-one-year-old retired distribution manager. He and his wife, Sandra, live in Lincoln, Nebraska. Sandra is fifty-seven and employed as a high-school science teacher. She has family coverage through a group health insurance plan offered by the state of Nebraska. Ron is covered as a dependent on her plan. The Medicare Part B carrier for Nebraska is Blue Cross and Blue Shield of Kansas.

Which carrier is Ron's primary insurance carrier? Why?

Compliance Guideline

Patient Coinsurance When Medicare Is Secondary
Medicare patients should not be charged for the primary insurance coinsurance until the RA is received and examined, because the patient is entitled to have Medicare pay these charges. If the patient has not met the annual Part B deductible, then the patient would be responsible for the coinsurance, and that amount is applied toward the deductible.

suffers from a lung disorder caused by working in a mine, Medicare is secondary to the Black Lung coverage. If the procedure or diagnosis is not for a mining-related lung condition, Medicare is the primary payer.

Automobile, No-Fault, and Liability Insurance

Medicare is always the secondary payer when treatment is for an accident-related claim, whether automobile, no-fault (injuries that occur on private property, regardless of who is at fault), or liability (injuries that occur on private property when a party is held responsible).

Veterans' Benefits

If a veteran is entitled to Medicare benefits, he or she may choose whether to receive coverage through Medicare or through the Department of Veterans Affairs.

Calculating Medicare Payments as the Secondary Payer

The physician office must file a Medicare claim when it is the secondary payer. To do so, the medical insurance specialist must know how to credit the patient's deductible and whether the patient's primary insurance coinsurance is covered by Medicare.

Three formulas are used to calculate how much of the coinsurance will be paid. Of the three amounts, Medicare will pay the lowest. The formulas use Medicare's allowable charge, the primary insurer's allowable charge, and the actual amount paid by the primary payer. Medicare, as secondary, pays 100 percent of most coinsurance payments if the patient's Part B deductible has been paid.

The three formulas are:

1. Primary payer's allowed charge minus payment made on claim
2. What Medicare would pay (80 percent of Medicare allowed charge)
3. Higher allowed charge (either primary payer or Medicare) minus payment made on the claim

Example: A patient's visit charge is $100 and the primary payer pays $80, with a $20 patient coinsurance. Medicare allows $80 for the service. The patient has met the Part B deductible. The calculations using the three formulas result in amounts of (1) $100 – $80 = $20, (2) $80 × 80 percent = $64, and (3) $100 – $80 = $20. Medicare will pay $20, since this is the lowest dollar amount from the three calculations.

To file a Medicare secondary payer claim, the amount the primary insurer paid is reported on the Medicare claim. The secondary claim should be sent to

Medicare even when there is a zero balance, so that the patient receives the correct credits toward the Part B annual deductible. Sending zero balance claims to Medicare should be done for all claims, even if the patient's Part B deductible has been met for the year, for compliance with Medicare rules.

Claim Preparation and Transmittal

Under HIPAA, electronic billing complying with the Transactions and Code Sets standards is mandatory for almost all Medicare providers. Electronic filing offers many advantages:

- Claims are acknowledged by the payer when they are received.
- Claim status and eligibility information is returned within twenty-four hours.
- Electronic remittance notices, rather than paper remittance notices, are sent.
- Payment is faster with electronic claims, which can be paid after thirteen days (paper claims took at least twenty-seven days to be paid).
- Payments can be deposited directly in the provider's bank account using electronic funds transfer (EFT).
- Technical support for electronic billing is available on line and is updated regularly.

Filing Medicare claims can be complex. A medical insurance specialist must be familiar with the rules and regulations for the practice's Medicare carrier, since filing rules vary somewhat from payer to payer. The following topics are common to most Medicare carriers.

HCPCS Coding and NCCI Edits

Medicare requires the Healthcare Common Procedure Coding System (HCPCS) for coding services provided to Medicare patients. (See Chapter 5 for more information on HCPCS coding.) Medicare's National Correct Coding Initiative (NCCI) is a list of CPT code combinations that, if used, would cause a claim to be rejected. The NCCI is explained in Chapter 6. The list is updated on a quarterly basis and must be followed closely. Many practices use a software tool to check Medicare claims against the NCCI before transmitting them.

Local Coverage Determinations

Local Coverage Determinations (LCDs) are notices sent to physicians on a regular basis. Previously called Local Medicare Review Policies (LMRPs), an LCD contains detailed and updated information about the coding and medical necessity of a specific service, including

- A description of the service
- A list of indications (instances in which the service is deemed medically necessary)
- The appropriate HCPCS code
- The appropriate ICD-9-CM code
- A bibliography containing recent clinical articles to support the Medicare policy

Medicare Prepayment Requests

Medicare prepayment documentation requests, also called development letters, may be sent by the Medicare carrier to physicians after claims are transmitted.

HIPAA Tip

Small Provider Exemption

Only a "small provider of services"—a physician with fewer than 10 full-time equivalent employees—is exempt from the requirement to file HIPAA-compliant claims.

Billing Tip

LCDs On Line
CMS has a Web site at http://www.cms.hhs.gov/mcd which is updated monthly and contains the complete LCD database. As LCDs provide the most current, detailed information, correct coding and billing require knowledge of the material they contain.

Billing Tip

Preventive Services
Because Medicare pays for some preventive services but not most annual physical exams, practices subtract the cost of the covered services from the exam cost when preparing a claim for a physician's services for the patient on the same date. For example, the cost of a pelvic exam and Pap collection would be subtracted from the preventive service fee for a woman's routine physical.

The letters request more information to establish the medical necessity of the billed procedures. They are often sent when modifiers –22, –52, –53, –62, or –78 have been reported. They are also common when unlisted procedure codes or high-level evaluation and management codes are used, and for procedures when a local medical review policy has not been determined. A response from the provider must be made within 45 days.

NPIs

With the adoption of the National Provider Identifier (NPI) system (see Chapter 8), the National Physician Identification Number (NPI) is reported for a physician.

Prior Authorization; CLIA

Some surgical procedures require preauthorization from qualified independent contractors (QICs), formerly known as Peer Review Organizations (PROs). A **qualified independent contractor** is a state-based group of physicians who are paid by the government to review aspects of the Medicare program, including the quality and appropriateness of services provided and fees charged.

Claims that include lab services performed on-site must report the lab's ten-digit **Clinical Laboratory Improvement Amendments (CLIA)** certification number. All lab services for Medicare and Medicaid patients must be performed by CLIA-certified providers.

Global Surgical Package

Under Medicare regulations, a physician cannot bill separately for each visit or procedure connected with a bundled surgical procedure (unbundling). Instead, a charge for a global surgical package includes services provided by the physician for a certain period of time; which varies depending on the specific procedure. A simple surgery may have a coverage period of only the day of surgery. A complicated procedure may have a coverage period of one day of preoperative and ninety days of postoperative care.

Some of the services that are part of a global surgical package are

- *Preoperative office visits:* The day before surgery for major procedures and the day of surgery for minor procedures
- *Intraoperative services:* Procedures that are part of the surgery procedure itself
- *Postoperative visits:* Visits after the surgery to monitor recovery from the procedure
- *Postsurgical pain management:* Procedures after the surgery to minimize the pain the patient experiences
- *Postsurgical complications:* Treatment for complications that arise after surgery that do not necessitate further surgery
- *Supplies:* Supplies used during the procedure
- *Miscellaneous:* Miscellaneous services, such as removal of sutures, tubes, and catheters

Some of the services that are not part of a global surgical package are

- Office visits before the need for surgery was established, even if the visit was for symptoms that led to the decision for surgery
- Office visits that are not directly related to the surgical diagnosis

- Diagnostic tests and procedures
- Services of other physicians, unless an agreement of transfer is in place
- Surgery for complications that occur after the original procedure and require a return to the operating room

Incident-to Billing

Medicare pays for services and supplies that are furnished incident to a physician's services are commonly included in bills, and for which payment is not made under a separate benefit category. Incident-to services and supplies are those performed or provided by medical staff other than the physician under the physician's supervision. The deciding factor for billing is the direct physical supervision by the physician. Specific rules concerning which Medicare identifier numbers and fees to use must be researched before incident-to claims are submitted.

Roster Billing

Roster billing is a simplified process that allows providers to submit a single claim form with the names, health insurance claim numbers, dates of birth, sex, dates of service, and signatures for Medicare patients who received vaccinations for influenza and pneumococcal vaccines covered by Medicare. These claims do not have to be sent electronically.

Use of Outside Billing Services and Clearinghouses

Many physician practices contract with an outside billing service or clearinghouse to submit claims to Medicare. Such business associates may provide coding, data entry, and claim preparation/transmission services. Medicare must approve the billing arrangements in advance. The service is required to have written compliance policies that ensure coding and billing are based on correct, complete medical documentation.

To safeguard against fraud, all payments are made in the name of the provider and transmitted to the pay-to provider. Providers are also required to review their monthly remittance advices when a billing service is used and to notify CMS if they believe false claims have been generated. CMS's PECOS (Provider Enrollment, Chain, and Ownership System) records data about the billing service or clearinghouse providers use.

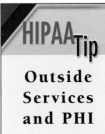

HIPAATip

Outside Services and PHI

Outside vendors must warrant that they will protect PHI according to the practice's Notice of Privacy Practices. Security Rule measures must also be in place to protect shared medical charts and billing data.

Preparing Medicare Claims

Medicare receives about a billion requests for payment each year. Electronic submission is required just for initial Medicare claims transmitted to Medicare carriers. Other transactions, such as changes, adjustments, or appeals to the initial claim, are not required to be electronic. Claims are processed by the Medicare multicarrier system (MCS).

Medicare Required Data Elements on the HIPAA 837 Claim

In addition to the standard data elements that are required on HIPAA claims (see Chapter 8), medical insurance specialists should be alert for the following elements.

Medicare Assignment Code

This information indicates whether the provider accepts Medicare assignment. The choices are as follows:

Code	Definition
A	Assigned
B	Assignment accepted on clinical lab services only
C	Not assigned
P	Patient refuses to assign benefits

Insurance Type Code

This code is required for a claim being sent to Medicare when Medicare is not the primary payer. Choices include:

Code	Definition
AP	Auto Insurance Policy
C1	Commercial
CP	Medicare Conditionally Primary
GP	Group Policy
HM	Health Maintenance Organization (HMO)
IP	Individual Policy
LD	Long-Term Policy
LT	Litigation
MB	Medicare Part B
MC	Medicaid
MI	Medigap Part B
MP	Medicare Primary
OT	Other
PP	Personal Payment (Cash - No Insurance)
SP	Supplemental Policy

Assumed Care Date/Relinquished Care Date

This information is required when providers share post-operative care; the date a provider assumed or gave up care is reported.

CLIA Number

The CLIA Number is reported on claims that bill for any laboratory performing tests covered by the CLIA Act.

CMS-1500 Claim Completion

When the CMS-1500 paper claim is required, follow the guidelines on pages 387–388.

Billing Tip

Invalid or Missing ICD-9-CM Codes Cause Rejections
If the claim contains an invalid diagnosis code, or the ICD-9-CM code is missing, it will be returned as unprocessable by the Medicare multi-carrier system. Practices may also be subject to a $100 fine for each violation of the HIPAA standard.

Medicare CMS-1500 Claim Completion

Form Locator	Data
1	Select Medicare; if the patient has other primary insurance and Medicare is the secondary payer (MSP), select Medicare along with the Group Health Plan or Other box.
1A	ID number from the patient's Medicare Health Insurance Card.
2	Patient's name as it appears on the insurance card.
3	Date of birth (eight-digit format); gender.
4	For MSP Insured's name or if the insured is the patient, enter "Same."
5	Patient's address.
6	Patient's relationship to the insured: self, spouse, child, or other.
7	Insured's address or "Same."
8	Patient's marital status and patient's employment status: employed, full-time student, or part-time student.
9	Form locators 9-9D refer to Medigap insurance policies. Form locator 9 is completed when a Medicare patient agrees to assign benefits of a Medigap policy to a Medicare participating provider. If the policyholder of the Medigap coverage is not the patient, enter the insured's name. If a Medicare patient has a secondary insurance plan that is not Medigap, form locator 9 should be left blank. Medicare forwards claims for these policies directly to the secondary carriers, as long as the carrier has a contract with Medicare. If the supplemental carrier does not have a contract with Medicare, the patient is responsible for submitting the claim to the supplemental carrier once a MSN is received.
9A	"Medigap," "Mgap," or "MG" followed by the policy number.
9B	Medigap policyholder's date of birth.
9C	Claims processing address for the Medigap insurer, which is usually found on the enrollee's Medigap identification card.
9D	Medigap insurance plan name or the Medigap insurer's identifier.
10a–10c	Form locators 10a-10d are used to indicate whether the patient's condition is the result of a work injury, an automobile accident, or another type of accident. If the services provided are related to one of these occurrences, indicate this by selecting Yes or No in the appropriate box. If the services are related to an automobile accident, enter the two-character postal code for the state where the accident occurred. *Other* refers to injuries or conditions that can be reported to a liability insurance carrier or no-fault insurance program. If any of the Yes form locators are selected, other insurance coverage (such as workers' compensation) may be primary to Medicare. Identify the primary insurance carrier in form locator 11.
11	Form locator 11 indicates whether the patient has any insurance primary to Medicare. If there is no plan primary to Medicare, enter "None." If there is coverage primary to Medicare, the insured's policy identification number is entered, and form locators 11a-11c must also be completed.
11a	Policyholder's date of birth and sex if they differ from the information in form locator 3.
11b	If the policy is obtained through an employer or a school, enter the name in form locator 11b. Otherwise, leave form locator 11b blank. If the patient's employment status has changed—for example, if the patient has retired—enter "Retired" followed by the retirement date.
11c	Name of the primary carrier.
12	Signature on file.
13	Blank if the patient's only insurance coverage is through Medicare. If the patient has additional coverage through another insurance plan, such as a Medigap plan, form locator 13 must contain a signature to authorize payment from the additional plan directly to the provider.
14	Date that symptoms first began. For pregnancy, enter the date of the patient's last menstrual period (LMP). If a Medicare patient is receiving chiropractic services, enter the date that this course of treatment began. The X-ray date should be entered in form locator 19.

Medicare CMS-1500 Claim Completion—*continued*

Form Locator	Data
15	Blank.
16	Completed only if the patient's illness or injury is a result of his or her employment; enter the dates the patient has been unable to work.
17	Referring (ordering) physician's name.
17a	NPI of the referring or ordering physician.
18	Admission and discharge dates of hospitalization.
19	Varying information, depending on the nature of the claim.
20	If diagnostic tests subject to purchase price limitations were completed, the Yes box should be selected and the dollar amount of the charge listed under Charges. Yes indicates that the tests were not performed in the provider's office. If Yes is selected, form locator 32 must also be completed. If no outside lab work was purchased, No is selected.
21	ICD-9 code(s).
22	Blank.
23	Prior Authorization Number or CLIA number.
24A	Dates that a procedure, service, or supply was provided. If the same service is provided multiple times, list the To and From dates once and indicate the number of days or units in form locator 24G.
24B	Place of service (POS) code.
24C	Blank.
24D	HCPCS code and up to three modifiers for each.
24E	Diagnosis Code key.
24F	Charges for each service.
24G	Number of days or units.
24H	Blank.
24I	Blank.
24J	Blank.
24K	NPI of the provider if a member of a group practice.
25	Physician or supplier's NPI.
26	Patient account number used by the practice; not required by Medicare.
27	If the physician accepts assignment, the Yes box is selected. If the patient is also covered by a Medigap plan and the patient has authorized payment directly to the provider, the provider must also be a Medicare participating physician and must accept assignment.
28	Total charges.
29	Amount of the patient payment (coinsurance or deductible) that is applied to the services listed on this claim; if no payment was made, enter "None" or "$0.00." If there is also payment from another insurance carrier, a copy of the RA or claim denial should be forwarded.
30	Blank.
31	Signature on file.
32	If the facility and address where services were performed is the same as the one listed in form locator 33, enter "Same." If services were provided at a location other than the office or home, such as a hospital, clinic, laboratory, or other facility, enter the name and address of the facility.
33	If the providing physician is not a member of a group practice, enter the NPI; if the physician is part of a group, enter the practice's NPI for the providing physician.

MSP Claims

The Medicare Coordination of Benefits (COB) program is set up to identify the health benefits available to a Medicare beneficiary so that mistaken payment of Medicare benefits can be prevented. Any inquiries regarding Medicare as second payer situations are directed to the COB. The COB database provides full and up-to-date information on a beneficiary's eligibility for benefits and the availability of other health insurance that is primary to Medicare.

Under HIPAA rules, if Medicare is the secondary payer to one primary payer, the claim must be submitted using the HIPAA 837 transaction. For these claims, the 837 must report the primary payer paid amount for the claim or for a particular service line (procedure). The primary payer allowed amount must be reported in the Allow Amount field. Claims where more than one plan is responsible for payment prior to Medicare, however, should be submitted using the CMS-1500 claim form. The other payers' RAs must be attached when this claim is sent to Medicare for processing.

HIPAATip

The Medicare Modernization Act includes new guidelines for first-level appeals

Part B Appeals

Patients' MSNs contain a statement informing beneficiaries that they have a right to request an itemized statement from the provider. A provider who does not comply with the patient's request within thirty days may be fined $100 per outstanding request. Beneficiaries have the right to examine the itemized statement and request review of questionable or unclear charges. The provider is required to work with the enrollee to explain any discrepancies.

Providers receive a **Medicare Remittance Notice (MRN)** from payers that summarizes a batch of claims, rather than a separate MSN for each claim. Providers also have a right to appeal a claim decision when they do not agree with the carrier's determination. If a claim is denied for medical necessity reasons, the Freedom of Information Act allows the physician to request a copy of the specific policy that led to the decision to reject the claim. If a Local Coverage Determination (LCD) was used in reviewing the claim, carriers must cite this in their denial notice to help providers decide if they want to appeal the denial. The appeals process varies from carrier to carrier, but a typical appeals process is outlined below. A form used for the process is shown in Figure 11.9.

The first step in the appeals process is to request a review of the claim. This review usually takes place over the telephone, and must be requested within 120 days of the date of the MRN. If the review does not lead to a satisfactory resolution, a written review may be requested.

The next step after a written review is a hearing request. This request must be made within six months of the review decision notification, and it may be used only when the amount in question is greater than $100. The hearing decision must be rendered within 120 days. There are three different types of hearings:

1. *Telephone:* Supporting information is submitted in advance, and a telephone call is arranged between a hearing officer and the appealing party.
2. *In person:* An in-person meeting takes place with the hearing officer and the appealing party.
3. *On the record:* Supporting information is submitted in advance, after which a hearing officer reviews the case.

Request For Review of a Medicare Part B Claim

NOTICE - Anyone who misrepresents or falsifies essential information requested
by this form may upon conviction be subject to fine and imprisonment under Federal Law.

Print legibly and complete all information. Only *one form* may be used *per* Medicare patient.

1. Carrier's Name and Address   Medicare B Review Department
                                           P. O. Box C1016
                                           Meriden, CT 06454

2. Name of Patient   **3.Medicare Health Insurance Claim Number**
                                           (9 digits followed by an alpha/numeric suffix)

4. I do not agree with the determination you made on ICN
    (1 form per patient)

5. The reason(s) I disagree with the determination is/are: (Please check those that apply)
____ Service/Claim underpaid/reduced ____   Service/Claim overpaid
____ Duplicate   ____   Service(s) overutilized and/or not medically necessary
____ OTHER: (Please be specific)

_____
_____
_____
_____

6. For services in question, please provide:
Date(s) of Service: Quantity Billed: Modifier: Procedure Code:
_____ _____   _____   _____   _____
_____ _____   _____   _____   _____
_____ _____   _____   _____   _____
_____ _____   _____   _____   _____

7. Additional information to consider including specific diagnosis, illness and/or condition:
_____
_____
_____
_____
_____

8. Attachments to consider: (Please check all that apply)
____   Medical Records   ____   Copy of Claim
____   Ambulance Run Sheet   ____   Certificate of Medical Necessity
____   Office Records/Progress Notes
____   OTHER: (Please be specific)

_____
_____
_____

9. Signature of Claimant or Representative:
(Print) _____   Telephone Number:
                                               _____
(Written) _____

**If you are providing a cover letter or attachments for multiple review cases;
you must have a separate copy for each review form submitted.**

Figure 11.9 Request for Review of a Medicare Part B Claim

If the hearing does not resolve the matter, there are additional appeal levels, including:

- *Administrative law judge (ALJ):* If the amount in dispute is greater than $100, the matter may go before an administrative law judge.
- *Office of Hearing and Appeals:* If the administrative law judge fails to render a satisfactory decision, the case may be brought to the Social Security Administration's Appeals Council of the Office of Hearing and Appeals.
- *United States District Court:* Finally, the appeal may be taken to the U.S. District Court for review if the amount in dispute is at least $1,000.

Medicare beneficiaries also have the right to challenge the policy that underlies a denied claim. These challenges of local coverage determinations are initially reviewed by an administrative law judge. Appeals of national coverage determinations and of ALJ decisions are reviewed by the HHS appeals board, and their decisions could be appealed to federal court.

Audits, Fraud, and Abuse

Many providers think that fraud and abuse apply only to unscrupulous agents who deliberately try to swindle money from the Medicare system. While some intentional violations do occur, so do many unintentional abuses. These are often committed in practices that are either not aware of proper Medicare procedures or are aware of the regulations but do not make a consistent effort to comply with them.

Despite the government's efforts to detect fraudulent activities, fraud and abuse cost the Medicare program millions of dollars every year. Some examples of fraudulent activities include billing for services or supplies that were not provided, altering claims to receive higher payments, and coding routine services that would normally not be covered as more complex services eligible for coverage. Abuse includes seeking payment for services that do not meet professional standards and submitting claims for services or supplies that exceed normal quantities. (This topic is covered in more detail in Chapter 6.)

Medicare Audits

Medicare carriers conduct four types of routine audits. Medical insurance specialists are often assigned to respond to these requests from the Medicare carrier.

1. *One chart audit:* The Medicare carrier sends a request to the practice for one medical record—usually for an E/M service—on one date of service.
2. *Electronic claims submission:* Medicare carriers conduct this prepayment audit to confirm that reported services in fact were performed. The documentation is reviewed to make sure the patients were seen; other aspects of completeness and compliance of the documentation are not examined.
3. *Focused medical review:* The Medicare carrier asks for a small number of records with complete documentation for a specified date of service.
4. *Comprehensive medical review:* Providers whose medical records raise questions are subject to a comprehensive medical review. The Medicare carrier asks for at least fifteen records over a six-month period, and checks all details.

When a series of requests leads to a comprehensive medical review, the matter is especially serious. When this level of audit is requested by Medicare, medical insurance specialists should

- Notify the compliance officer
- Send the complete documentation available for each medical record, including all notes, correspondence, and test results
- Keep copies of everything that has been sent

The Medicare carrier notifies the practice of the audit's results, listing whether each charge on the audited claims was accepted, denied, or downcoded. If payments were previously received from Medicare for charges that are now denied or reduced, the resulting overpayments must be reimbursed to the Medicare program. Providers may also wish to appeal decisions (see Chapter 9).

If warranted by the suggestion of fraudulent patterns, Medicare may refer the case to the Office of the Inspector General (OIG) for fraud and abuse investigation. OIG attorneys must follow certain procedures before they allege that a physician has violated the False Claims Act. The guidelines require the government employee to examine the applicable laws and the published interpretations of the laws, and then to

Because it is critical for medical practices to comply with the rules and regulations of the Centers for Medicare and Medicaid Services (CMS) in coding and reporting Medicare claims, many practices appoint or hire a Medicare compliance specialist. Usually a member of the billing department, the Medicare compliance specialist performs or reviews all of the Medicare claims that are transmitted by the practice.

The Medicare compliance specialist is responsible for knowing the current rules regarding Medicare bundling and global periods based on the CCI edits, local carrier rules for payment of procedures versus durable medical equipment (DME) and other supplies, the current Medicare Fee Schedule, the services for which patients may or may not be billed, overpayment procedures, and other Medicare rules issued by CMS and by the local Medicare carrier. Medicare specialists train the physicians and other professional medical staff in the current rules, and are involved when an appeal is filed. They are also responsible for conducting internal audits to ensure compliance and for contributing to the practice's compliance plan. If an external audit occurs, the Medicare specialist is involved with presenting the documentation to explain the billing practices and show how they comply with regulations.

Medicare compliance specialists are often appointed from the current billing staff, or a new staff member may be hired. Some practices choose to use a compliance consultant to audit the practice's billing and reporting procedures for conformity to current regulations.

- Verify the data and other evidence that have been received in the case
- Investigate the provider
- Assess the provider's possible knowledge of committing a violation, including (1) whether the provider was ever notified of a problem, (2) how clear the rule or policy is, (3) how pervasive or large the alleged false claims are, (4) whether the provider has been audited before and, if so, what efforts were made to fix the problem, (5) whether the provider has asked for guidance about the issue in question, such as by the advisory opinion process, and (6) whether the provider has a compliance plan.

After this information is examined, the OIG then decides whether to charge the provider with fraud and refer the case for prosecution by the Department of Justice (DOJ).

Fraud Detection and Investigation

Medicare and the OIG have undertaken a number of steps to detect fraud and abuse, from increased efforts to detect and pursue violators to rewards offered to beneficiaries and employees who provide information about suspected fraudulent practices. The Medicare fraud hotline receives thousands of calls from the public every year, leading to the recovery of millions of dollars. Medicare receives leads from a variety of sources, including carriers, beneficiaries, employees in providers' offices, and federal agencies such as the Social Security Administration and state Medicaid offices. The majority of leads come from carriers, beneficiaries, and former employees of carriers.

Quality Improvement Organizations (QIOs)

Quality improvement organizations regularly review various components of the Medicare program, such as hospital admissions and discharges, procedures performed, documentation, and charges outside the standard range. QIOs are responsible for assuring that

- Services meet professional standards for quality in health care delivery
- Services are provided only when deemed medically necessary and are delivered in an economical manner
- Medical necessity and quality of services delivered are well documented

A provider suspected of fraudulent activities is referred to the QIO for review. If the QIO discovers sufficient irregularities, a meeting is set up between the provider and members of the QIO. Following the meeting, the QIO delivers a recommendation to the OIG, which determines whether penalties are appropriate.

Carriers

Since carriers process all Medicare Part B claims, they are in a unique position to uncover suspected abuse. Recognizing this, Medicare regulations require each carrier to set up two departments to identify and investigate possible fraud. The Medical Review Unit (MR) is responsible for analyzing claims data and watching for patterns of irregularities, including conducting a postpayment review. MR personnel develop standard patterns for each provider and compare current activity against the normal pattern. When an irregularity is detected, the MR contacts the provider to request an end to the suspicious practice. If the provider does not cease, the case may be referred to the Fraud Unit. The Fraud Unit is responsible for uncovering and deterring fraud and abuse. When the MR refers a case, the Fraud Unit investigates and, if appropriate, sends the case to the OIG's regional office.

Providers or suppliers found guilty of fraud or abuse are subject to monetary penalties and other sanctions, such as having payments withheld or assignment privileges revoked, and exclusion from the Medicare program.

Chapter Summary

1. Medicare Part A provides coverage for care in hospitals and skilled nursing facilities, home health care, and hospice care. Part B provides coverage for physician services, diagnostic X-rays and laboratory tests, some preventive care examinations and tests, outpatient hospital visits, durable medical equipment, and other nonhospital services.

2. Individuals eligible for Medicare are in one of six categories: (a) age sixty-five or older; (b) disabled adults; (c) disabled before age eighteen; (d) spouses of deceased, disabled, or retired employees; (e) retired federal employees enrolled in the Civil Service Retirement System (CSRS); or (f) individuals of any age diagnosed with end-stage renal disease (ESRD).

3. Medicare does not cover most routine and custodial care, examinations for eyeglasses or hearing aids, some foot care procedures, services not ordered by a physician, cosmetic surgery, health care received while traveling outside the United States, and procedures deemed not reasonable and medically necessary.

4. Participating providers agree to accept assignment for all Medicare claims and to accept Medicare's fee as payment in full for services. Nonparticipating providers choose whether to accept assignment on a claim-by-claim basis. NonPAR providers bill 5 percent less than PAR providers on assigned claims; on unassigned claims, nonPAR providers are subject to Medicare's limiting charges.

5. Medicare beneficiaries can choose from (a) a fee-for-service plan referred to as the Original Medicare Plan that provides maximum freedom of choice when selecting a provider or specialist or (b) Medicare Advantage, a group of plans including managed care plans that offer additional services but restricts beneficiaries to a network of providers, a preferred provider organization (PPO) plan, private fee-for-service, and health medical savings accounts.

6. Medigap insurance pays for services that are not covered by Medicare. Coverage varies with specific Medigap plans, but all provide coverage for patient deductibles and coinsurance. Some also cover excluded services such as prescription drugs and limited preventive care.

7. Medicare is the secondary payer when (a) the patient is covered by an employer group health insurance plan or is covered through an employed spouse's plan; (b) the patient is disabled, under age sixty-five, and covered by an employee group health plan; (c) the patient is diagnosed with ESRD but is covered by an employer-sponsored group health plan; (d) the services are covered by workers' compensation insurance; (e) the services are for injuries in an automobile accident; and (f) the patient is a veteran who chooses to receive services through the Department of Veterans Affairs.

Key Terms

advance beneficiary notice (ABN) *page 370*

Clinical Laboratory Improvement Amendments (CLIA) *page 384*

Consolidated Omnibus Budget Reconciliation Act (COBRA) *page 380*

fiscal intermediary *page 365*

Health Savings Account *page 378*

limiting charge *page 374*

Local Coverage Determination (LCD) *page 383*

Medicare Advantage *page 376*

Medicare Modernization Act *page 375*

Medicare Part A *page 365*

Medicare Part B *page 366*

Medicare Remittance Notice (MRN) *page 389*

Medicare Summary Notice (MSN) *page 375*

Medigap *page 378*

Notice of Exclusions from Medicare Benefits (NEMB) *page 370*

Original Medicare Plan *page 375*

quality improvement organizations (QIO) *page 384*

roster billing *page 385*

supplemental insurance *page 380*

urgently needed care *page 377*

Review Questions

Match the key terms in the left column with the definitions in the right column.

A. Advance Beneficiary Notice (ABN)

B. Health Savings Account

C. Medicare Advantage

D. supplemental insurance

E. limiting charge

F. fiscal intermediary

G. Notice of Exclusions from Medicare Benefits (NEMB)

H. quality improvement organizations (QIOs)

I. urgently needed care

J. Medicare Summary Notice (MSN)

_____ 1. A carrier or payer that has a contract with Medicare to process insurance claims on behalf of Medicare

_____ 2. A group of insurance plans offered under Medicare Part B, intended to provide beneficiaries with a wider selection of plans

_____ 3. Nonparticipating physicians cannot charge more than this amount on unassigned claims (115 percent of the Medicare Fee Schedule)

_____ 4. A form given to patients when the physician practice thinks that a service to be provided will not be considered medically necessary or reasonable by Medicare

_____ 5. Emergency treatment needed by a managed care patient while traveling outside the plan's network area

_____ 6. A form that advises beneficiaries, before services that are not Medicare benefits are furnished, that Medicare will not pay for them, and provides an estimate of how much they may have to pay

_____ 7. A document furnished to Medicare beneficiaries by the Medicare program that lists the services they received and the payments the program made for them

_____ 8. A high-deductible fee-for-service Medicare plan

_____ 9. A type of insurance plan purchased from a former employer that provides coverage in addition to Medicare Part B

_____ 10. A group of physicians paid by the government to review aspects of the Medicare program, including the quality and appropriateness of services provided and fees charged

Decide whether each statement is true or false, and write T for true or F for false.

_____ 1. Fiscal intermediaries are the claims processors for Medicare Part B.

_____ 2. Screening mammograms are excluded services for Medicare Part B.

_____ 3. A procedure is classified as not medically necessary if it is an elective procedure.

_____ 4. Physicians who agree to participate can choose to accept assignment on a claim-by-claim basis.

_____ 5. Participating and nonparticipating providers may bill patients at their standard rates for services excluded from Medicare coverage.

_____ 6. Medicare Advantage plans usually offer coverage for some services that are not covered by the Original Medicare Plan.

_____ 7. All Medigap policies provide coverage for Part B coinsurance.

_____ 8. Medicare is the secondary payer for all beneficiaries over age sixty-five and working.

_____ 9. Local Coverage Determinations (LCDs) are notices sent to physicians about the coding and medical necessity of specific services.

_____ 10. Physicians may contract with outside billing services to provide diagnostic and procedural coding on Medicare claims.

Write the letter choice that best completes the statement or answers the question.

_____ 1. Most cases of fraud and abuse in the Medicare program are reported by
    A. physicians   C. beneficiaries and carriers
    B. OIG Investigators   D. carriers

_____ 2. The Original Medicare Plan requires a premium, a deductible, and
    A. Medigap   C. coinsurance
    B. supplemental insurance   D. HIPAA TCS

_____ 3. Which modifier indicates that a signed ABN is on file?
    A. AB   C. GZ
    B. GA   D. GY

_____ 4. Under Medicare's global surgical package regulations, a physician may bill a patient separately for
    A. supplies used during the surgical procedure
    B. procedures performed after the surgery to minimize pain
    C. diagnostic tests required to determine the need for surgery
    D. the removal of tubes, sutures, or catheters

_____ 5. HIPAA regulations require the Medicare program to comply with
    A. Privacy Rule   C. Transactions and Code Sets standards
    B. Security Rule   D. All of the above

_____ 6. Under Medicare Advantage, a physician billing under a private fee-for-service contract can bill patients for the amount not paid by Medicare, subject to a _____ limit.
    A. 5 percent   C. 15 percent
    B. 10 percent   D. 115 percent

_____ 7. Under the Medicare Part B traditional fee-for-service plan, Medicare pays _____ percent of the charges.
    A. 75   C. 90
    B. 80   D. 100

_____ 8. A code of C for the Medicare Assignment Code indicates that
    A. The claim is assigned   C. The patient refuses to assign benefits
    B. The claim is not assigned   D. None of the above

_____ 9. A Medicare prepayment documentation request is sent by
    A. the physician   C. the primary payer
    B. the Medicare carrier   D. the local coverage policy

Provide answers to the following questions.

1. What is the difference between a Medigap policy and a supplemental policy?

2. Why are there no premium charges for most individuals enrolled in Medicare Part A?

3. What is the difference between excluded services and services that are not reasonable and necessary?

Applying Your Knowledge

The objective of these cases is to correctly complete a claim, applying what you have learned in the chapter to each case situation. Each case consists of two sections. The first section contains information about the patient, the insurance coverage, and the current medical condition. The second section is an encounter form from Valley Associates, P.C.

If you are using NDCMedisoft to complete the cases, read the Guide to NDCMedisoft before beginning. Information from the first section, the patient information form, has already been entered in the program for you. You must enter information from the second section, the encounter form, to complete the claim. If you are gaining experience by completing a paper CMS-1500 claim form, follow the instructions on pages 387–388.

The following provider information, which is also available in the NDCMediSoft database, should be used for the case studies in Chapter 11.

Provider Information

Name:	Christoper M. Connolly, M.D.
Practice Name:	Valley Associates, P.C.
Address:	1400 West Center Street Toledo, OH 43601-0213
Phone:	555-321-0987
Employer ID Number:	16-1234567
Medicare PIN:	AB1234
Assignment:	Accepts
Physician Signature:	On File (1-1-2005)

Case 11.1

From the Patient Information Form:

Name	Donald Martone	*Health Plan*	Medicare Nationwide
Sex	M	*Health Insurance No.*	3124/60239A
Birth Date	06/24/1939	*Copayment Amount*	None
Marital Status	S	*Signature*	On File (1-1-2008)
Employer	(Retired)	*Condition Related to:*	
Address	83 Summit Rd. Cleveland, OH 44101-0123	*Employment*	No
		Auto Accident	No
		Other Accident	No
Telephone:	553-333-0412	*Accept Assignment*	Yes
SSN	312-46-0239	*Physician Signature*	On File (1-1-2005)

Encounter Form on page 398

VALLEY ASSOCIATES, P.C.

Christopher M. Connolly, M.D. - General Practice

555-321-0987

FED I.D. #16-1234567

PATIENT NAME	APPT. DATE/TIME	
Donald Martone	10/06/2008	9:30am

PATIENT NO.	DX
MARTODO0	**1.** 465.9 upper respiratory infection **2.** 786.2 cough **3.** 780.6 fever **4.**

DESCRIPTION	✓	CPT	FEE	DESCRIPTION	✓	CPT	FEE
EXAMINATION				**PROCEDURES**			
New Patient				Diagnostic Anoscopy		46600	
Problem Focused		99201		ECG Complete		93000	
Expanded Problem Focused		99202		I&D, Abscess		10060	
Detailed		99203		Pap Smear		88150	
Comprehensive		99204		Removal of Cerumen		69210	
Comprehensive/Complex		99205		Removal 1 Lesion		17000	
Established Patient				Removal 2-14 Lesions		17003	
Minimum		99211		Removal 15+ Lesions		17004	
Problem Focused	✓	99212	28	Rhythm ECG w/Report		93040	
Expanded Problem Focused		99213		Rhythm ECG w/Tracing		93041	
Detailed		99214		Sigmoidoscopy, diag.		45330	
Comprehensive/Complex		99215					
				LABORATORY			
PREVENTIVE VISIT				Bacteria Culture		87081	
New Patient				Fungal Culture		87101	
Age 12-17		99384		Glucose Finger Stick		82948	
Age 18-39		99385		Lipid Panel		80061	
Age 40-64		99386		Specimen Handling		99000	
Age 65+		99387		Stool/Occult Blood		82270	
Established Patient				Tine Test		85008	
Age 12-17		99394		Tuberculin PPD		85590	
Age 18-39		99395		Urinalysis		81000	
Age 40-64		99396		Venipuncture		36415	
Age 65+		99397					
				INJECTION/IMMUN.			
CONSULTATION: OFFICE/ER				DT Immun		90702	
Requested By:				Hepatitis A Immun		90632	
Problem Focused		99241		Hepatitis B Immun		90746	
Expanded Problem Focused		99242		Influenza Immun		90659	
Detailed		99243		Pneumovax		90732	
Comprehensive		99244					
Comprehensive/Complex		99245		**TOTAL FEES**			

Case 11.2

Name	Wendy Walker	Health Plan	Medicare HMO
Sex	F	Health Insurance No.	321690809A
Birth Date	11/14/1935	Copayment Amount	$10
Marital Status	S	Signature	On File (1-1-2008)
Employer	(Retired)	Condition Related to:	
Address	85 Woodmont Dr.	Employment	No
	Alliance, OH	Auto Accident	No
	44601-1234	Other Accident	No
Telephone:	555-024-1689	Accept Assignment	Yes
SSN	321-69-0809	Physician Signature	On File (1-1-2005)

VALLEY ASSOCIATES, P.C.
Christopher M. Connolly, M.D. - General Practice
555-321-0987
FED I.D. #16-1234567

PATIENT NAME				APPT. DATE/TIME			
Wendy Walker				10/06/2008		10:30am	
PATIENT NO.				**DX**			
WALKEWE0				1. 719.45 pain in hips 2. 719.50 joint stiffness NEC 3. 780.6 fever 4.			

DESCRIPTION	✓	CPT	FEE	DESCRIPTION	✓	CPT	FEE
EXAMINATION				**PROCEDURES**			
New Patient				Diagnostic Anoscopy		46600	
Problem Focused		99201		ECG Complete		93000	
Expanded Problem Focused		99202		I&D, Abscess		10060	
Detailed		99203		Pap Smear		88150	
Comprehensive		99204		Removal of Cerumen		69210	
Comprehensive/Complex		99205		Removal 1 Lesion		17000	
Established Patient				Removal 2-14 Lesions		17003	
Minimum		99211		Removal 15+ Lesions		17004	
Problem Focused		99212		Rhythm ECG w/Report		93040	
Expanded Problem Focused		99213		Rhythm ECG w/Tracing		93041	
Detailed	✓	99214	59	Sigmoidoscopy, diag.		45330	
Comprehensive/Complex		99215					

Case 11.3

Name	Andrea Spinelli	Health Plan	Medicare HMO
Sex	F	Health Insurance No.	701694342A
Birth Date	01/01/1941	Copayment Amount	$10
Marital Status	S	Signature	On File (1-1-2008)
Employer	(Retired)	Condition Related to:	
Address	23 N Brook Ave.	Employment	No
	Sandusky, OH	Auto Accident	No
	44870-8901	Other Accident	No
SSN	701-69-4342	Accept Assignment	No
Telephone	555-402-0396	Physician Signature	On File (1-1-2005)

VALLEY ASSOCIATES, P.C.
Christopher M. Connolly, M.D. - General Practice
555-321-0987
FED I.D. #16-1234567

PATIENT NAME	APPT. DATE/TIME	
Andrea Spinelli	10/09/2008	1:30pm
PATIENT NO.	**DX**	
SPINEAN0	1. 380.4 cerumen in ear 2. 3. 4.	

DESCRIPTION	✓	CPT	FEE	DESCRIPTION	✓	CPT	FEE
EXAMINATION				**PROCEDURES**			
New Patient				Diagnostic Anoscopy		46600	
Problem Focused		99201		ECG Complete		93000	
Expanded Problem Focused		99202		I&D, Abscess		10060	
Detailed		99203		Pap Smear		88150	
Comprehensive		99204		Removal of Cerumen	✓	69210	34.50
Comprehensive/Complex		99205		Removal 1 Lesion		17000	
Established Patient				Removal 2-14 Lesions		17003	
Minimum		99211		Removal 15+ Lesions		17004	
Problem Focused		99212		Rhythm ECG w/Report		93040	
Expanded Problem Focused		99213		Rhythm ECG w/Tracing		93041	
Detailed		99214		Sigmoidoscopy, diag.		45330	
Comprehensive/Complex		99215					

Case 11.4

From the Patient Information Form

Name	Carmen Perez
Sex	M
Birth Date	05/15/1934
Marital Status	M
Employer	(Retired)
Address	225 Potomac Dr
	Shaker Heights, OH
	44118-2345
Telephone	555-692-3314
SSN	140-24-6113

Secondary Insurance Information

Health Plan	Nationwide Medicare
Health Insurance No.	140246113A

Signature	On File (1-1-2008)
Condition Related to:	
Employment	No
Auto Accident	No
Other Accident	No
Accept Assignment	Yes
Physician Signature	On File (1-1-2005)

Primary Insurance Information

Insured	Monica Perez
Pt Relationship to Insured	Spouse
Insured's Date of Birth	03/14/1936
Insured's Employer	Kinko's
SSN	140-60-3312
Insurance Plan	Cigna HMOPlus
Insurance ID No.	140603312X
Copayment Amount	$10

VALLEY ASSOCIATES, P.C.
Christopher M. Connolly, M.D. - General Practice
555-321-0987
FED I.D. #16-1234567

PATIENT NAME	APPT. DATE/TIME
Carmen Perez	10/08/2008 2:00pm

PATIENT NO.	DX
PEREZCA0	**1.** 493 extrinsic asthma **2.** **3.** **4.**

DESCRIPTION	✓	CPT	FEE	DESCRIPTION	✓	CPT	FEE
EXAMINATION				**PROCEDURES**			
New Patient				Diagnostic Anoscopy		46600	
Problem Focused		99201		ECG Complete		93000	
Expanded Problem Focused		99202		I&D, Abscess		10060	
Detailed		99203		Pap Smear		88150	
Comprehensive		99204		Removal of Cerumen		69210	
Comprehensive/Complex		99205		Removal 1 Lesion		17000	
Established Patient				Removal 2-14 Lesions		17003	
Minimum	✓	99211	30	Removal 15+ Lesions		17004	
Problem Focused		99212		Rhythm ECG w/Report		93040	
Expanded Problem Focused		99213		Rhythm ECG w/Tracing		93041	
Detailed		99214		Sigmoidoscopy, diag.		45330	
Comprehensive/Complex		99215					

Case 11.5

Name	Nancy Lankhaar
Sex	F
Birth Date	08/12/1935
Marital Status	S
Employer	(Retired)
Address	44 Crescent Rd Cleveland, OH 44101-3456
Telephone	555-787-3424
SSN	109-36-5528
Health Plan	Nationwide Medicare
Health Insurance No.	109365528A
Signature	On File (1-1-2008)

Secondary Insurance Information

Insured	Same
Insurance Plan	AARP Medigap
Insurance ID No.	109365528B
Condition Related to:	
Employment	No
Auto Accident	No
Other Accident	No
Accept Assignment	Yes
Physician Signature	On File (1-1-2005)

VALLEY ASSOCIATES, P.C.
Christopher M. Connolly, M.D. - General Practice
555-321-0987
FED I.D. #16-1234567

PATIENT NAME				APPT. DATE/TIME			
Nancy Lankhaar				10/07/2008		11:00am	
PATIENT NO.				**DX**			
LANKHNA0				**1.** 782.1 rash on leg **2.** **3.** **4.**			

DESCRIPTION	✓	CPT	FEE	DESCRIPTION	✓	CPT	FEE
EXAMINATION				**PROCEDURES**			
New Patient				Diagnostic Anoscopy		46600	
Problem Focused		99201		ECG Complete		93000	
Expanded Problem Focused		99202		I&D, Abscess		10060	
Detailed		99203		Pap Smear		88150	
Comprehensive		99204		Removal of Cerumen		69210	
Comprehensive/Complex		99205		Removal 1 Lesion		17000	
Established Patient				Removal 2-14 Lesions		17003	
Minimum		99211		Removal 15+ Lesions		17004	
Problem Focused	✓	99212	28	Rhythm ECG w/Report		93040	
Expanded Problem Focused		99213		Rhythm ECG w/Tracing		93041	
Detailed		99214		Sigmoidoscopy, diag.		45330	
Comprehensive/Complex		99215					

Case 11.6

Name	Walter Williams
Sex	M
Birth Date	09/04/1936
Marital Status	M
Employer	(Retired)
Address	17 Mill Road
	Brooklyn, OH
	44144-4567
Telephone	555-936-0216
SSN	401-26-9939

Secondary Insurance Information

Health Plan	Nationwide Medicare
Health Insurance No.	401269939A
Signature	On File
Condition Related to:	
Employment	No

Auto Accident	No
Other Accident	No
Accept Assignment	Yes
Physician Signature	On File (1-1-2005)

Primary Insurance Information

Insured	Vereen Williams
Pt Relationship to Insured	Spouse
Insured's Date of Birth	07/14/1945
Insured's Sex	F
Insured's Address	Same
Insured's Employer	Brooklyn Day Care
SSN	103-56-2239
Insurance Plan	Aetna Choice
Insurance ID No.	ABC103562239
Insurance Group No.	BDC1001
Copayment Amount	$15

VALLEY ASSOCIATES, P.C.
Christopher M. Connolly, M.D. - General Practice
555-321-0987
FED I.D. #16-1234567

PATIENT NAME	APPT. DATE/TIME	
Walter Williams	10/03/2008	9:00am

PATIENT NO.	DX
WILLIWA0	**1.** 401.1 benign essential hypertension
	2. 780.7 fatigue
	3.
	4.

				LABORATORY		
				Bacteria Culture	87081	
				Fungal Culture	87101	
				Glucose Finger Stick	82948	
				Lipid Panel	80061	
				Specimen Handling	99000	
				Stool/Occult Blood	82270	
				Tine Test	85008	
				Tuberculin PPD	85590	
				Urinalysis	81000	
				Venipuncture	✓ 36415	17

Case 11.7

From the Patient Informatin Form

Name	Donna Gaeta
Sex	F
Birth Date	12/02/1937
Marital Status	S
Employer	(Retired)
Address	11 Brigade Hill Road Toledo, OH 43601-5678
Telephone	555-402-0621
SSN	138-46-2400
Health Plan	Nationwide Medicare
Copayment Amount	None
Health Insurance No.	138462400A
Signature	On File (1-1-2008)
Condition Related to:	
Employment	No
Auto Accident	No
Other Accident	No
Accept Assignment	No
Physician Signature	On File (1-1-2005)

VALLEY ASSOCIATES, P.C.
Christopher M. Connolly, M.D. - General Practice
555-321-0987
FED I.D. #16-1234567

PATIENT NAME	APPT. DATE/TIME	
Donna Gaeta	10/07/2008	3:30pm

PATIENT NO.	DX
GAETADO0	**1.** v70.0 routine medical exam **2.** **3.** **4.**

DESCRIPTION	✓	CPT	FEE	DESCRIPTION	✓	CPT	FEE
EXAMINATION				**PROCEDURES**			
New Patient				Diagnostic Anoscopy		46600	
Problem Focused		99201		ECG Complete	✓	93000	29
Expanded Problem Focused		99202		I&D, Abscess		10060	
Detailed		99203		Pap Smear	✓	88150	29
Comprehensive		99204		Removal of Cerumen		69210	
Comprehensive/Complex		99205		Removal 1 Lesion		17000	
Established Patient				Removal 2-14 Lesions		17003	
Minimum		99211		Removal 15+ Lesions		17004	
Problem Focused		99212		Rhythm ECG w/Report		93040	
Expanded Problem Focused		99213		Rhythm ECG w/Tracing		93041	
Detailed		99214		Sigmoidoscopy, diag.		45330	
Comprehensive/Complex		99215					
				LABORATORY			
PREVENTIVE VISIT				Bacteria Culture		87081	
New Patient				Fungal Culture		87101	
Age 12-17		99384		Glucose Finger Stick		82948	
Age 18-39		99385		Lipid Panel		80061	
Age 40-64		99386		Specimen Handling		99000	
Age 65+	✓	99387	142	Stool/Occult Blood		82270	
Established Patient				Tine Test		85008	
Age 12-17		99394		Tuberculin PPD		85590	
Age 18-39		99395		Urinalysis	✓	81000	17
Age 40-64		99396		Venipuncture	✓	36415	17
Age 65+		99397					
				INJECTION/IMMUN.			
CONSULTATION: OFFICE/ER				DT Immun		90702	
Requested By:				Hepatitis A Immun		90632	
Problem Focused		99241		Hepatitis B Immun		90746	
Expanded Problem Focused		99242		Influenza Immun		90659	
Detailed		99243		Pneumovax		90732	
Comprehensive		99244					
Comprehensive/Complex		99245		**TOTAL FEES**			

Case 11.8

From the Patient Information Form

Name	Eric Huang
Sex	M
Birth Date	03/13/1940
Marital Status	M
Employer	(Retired)
Address	1109 Bauer St.
	Shaker Heights, OH
	44118-6789
Telephone	555-639-1787
SSN	302-46-1884
Health Plan	Nationwide Medicare
Copayment Amount	None
Health Insurance No.	302461884A
Signature	On File (1-1-2008)
Condition Related to:	
Employment	No
Auto Accident	No
Other Accident	No
Accept Assignment	Yes
Physician Signature	On File (1-1-2005)

VALLEY ASSOCIATES, P.C.
Christopher M. Connolly, M.D. - General Practice
555-321-0987
FED I.D. #16-1234567

PATIENT NAME	APPT. DATE/TIME
Eric Huang	10/09/2008 9:00am

PATIENT NO.	DX
HUANGER0	**1.** 782.4 jaundice **2.** **3.** **4.**

DESCRIPTION	✓	CPT	FEE	DESCRIPTION	✓	CPT	FEE
EXAMINATION				**PROCEDURES**			
New Patient				Diagnostic Anoscopy		46600	
Problem Focused		99201		ECG Complete		93000	
Expanded Problem Focused		99202		I&D, Abscess		10060	
Detailed		99203		Pap Smear		88150	
Comprehensive		99204		Removal of Cerumen		69210	
Comprehensive/Complex		99205		Removal 1 Lesion		17000	
Established Patient				Removal 2-14 Lesions		17003	
Minimum		99211		Removal 15+ Lesions		17004	
Problem Focused		99212		Rhythm ECG w/Report		93040	
Expanded Problem Focused		99213		Rhythm ECG w/Tracing		93041	
Detailed		99214		Sigmoidoscopy, diag.		45330	
Comprehensive/Complex		99215					
				LABORATORY			
PREVENTIVE VISIT				Bacteria Culture		87081	
New Patient				Fungal Culture		87101	
Age 12-17		99384		Glucose Finger Stick		82948	
Age 18-39		99385		Lipid Panel		80061	
Age 40-64		99386		Specimen Handling		99000	
Age 65+		99387		Stool/Occult Blood		82270	
Established Patient				Tine Test		85008	
Age 12-17		99394		Tuberculin PPD		85590	
Age 18-39		99395		Urinalysis		81000	
Age 40-64		99396		Venipuncture		36415	
Age 65+		99397					
				INJECTION/IMMUN.			
CONSULTATION: OFFICE/ER				DT Immun		90702	
Requested By:				Hepatitis A Immun		90632	
Problem Focused		99241		Hepatitis B Immun		90746	
Expanded Problem Focused		99242		Influenza Immun		90659	
Detailed	✓	99243	97	Pneumovax		90732	
Comprehensive		99244					
Comprehensive/Complex		99245		**TOTAL FEES**			

Case 11.9

From the Patient Information Form

Name	Lakshmi Prasad
Sex	F
Birth Date	08/02/1940
Marital Status	M
Employment Status	Part-time
Employer	Towne Restaurant
Address	38 Mountain Ave. Alliance, OH 44601-5678
Telephone	555-492-3601
SSN	351-42-6798
Health Plan	Nationwide Medicare
Health Insurance No.	351426798A
Copayment Amount	None
Signature	On File (1-1-2008)
Condition Related to:	
Employment	No
Auto Accident	No
Other Accident	No
Accept Assignment	Yes
Physician Signature	On File (1-1-2005)

VALLEY ASSOCIATES, P.C.
Christopher M. Connolly, M.D. - General Practice
555-321-0987
FED I.D. #16-1234567

PATIENT NAME	APPT. DATE/TIME
Lakshmi Prasad	10/09/2008 11:00am

PATIENT NO.	DX
PRASALA0	**1.** v70.0 routine medical exam **2.** **3.** **4.**

DESCRIPTION	✓	CPT	FEE	DESCRIPTION	✓	CPT	FEE
EXAMINATION				**PROCEDURES**			
New Patient				Diagnostic Anoscopy		46600	
Problem Focused		99201		ECG Complete		93000	
Expanded Problem Focused		99202		I&D, Abscess		10060	
Detailed		99203		Pap Smear	✓	88150	29
Comprehensive		99204		Removal of Cerumen		69210	
Comprehensive/Complex		99205		Removal 1 Lesion		17000	
Established Patient				Removal 2-14 Lesions		17003	
Minimum		99211		Removal 15+ Lesions		17004	
Problem Focused		99212		Rhythm ECG w/Report		93040	
Expanded Problem Focused		99213		Rhythm ECG w/Tracing		93041	
Detailed		99214		Sigmoidoscopy, diag.		45330	
Comprehensive/Complex		99215					
				LABORATORY			
PREVENTIVE VISIT				Bacteria Culture		87081	
New Patient				Fungal Culture		87101	
Age 12-17		99384		Glucose Finger Stick		82948	
Age 18-39		99385		Lipid Panel		80061	
Age 40-64		99386		Specimen Handling		99000	
Age 65+		99387		Stool/Occult Blood		82270	
Established Patient				Tine Test		85008	
Age 12-17		99394		Tuberculin PPD		85590	
Age 18-39		99395		Urinalysis		81000	
Age 40-64		99396		Venipuncture		36415	
Age 65+	✓	99397	118				
				INJECTION/IMMUN.			
CONSULTATION: OFFICE/ER				DT Immun		90702	
Requested By:				Hepatitis A Immun		90632	
Problem Focused		99241		Hepatitis B Immun		90746	
Expanded Problem Focused		99242		Influenza Immun	✓	90659	68
Detailed		99243		Pneumovax		90732	
Comprehensive		99244					
Comprehensive/Complex		99245		**TOTAL FEES**			

Case 11.10

From the Patient Information Form

Name	Donald Aiken
Sex	M
Birth Date	04/30/1935
Marital Status	S
Employer	(Retired)
Address	24 Beacon Crest Dr. Sandusky, OH 44870-2345
Telephone	555-602-9947
SSN	138-02-1649
Health Plan	Nationwide Medicare
Health Insurance No.	138021649A
Copayment Amount	None
Signature	On File (1-1-2008)
Condition Related to:	
Employment	No
Auto Accident	No
Other Accident	No
Accept Assignment	Yes
Physician Signature	On File (1-1-2005)

VALLEY ASSOCIATES, P.C.
Christopher M. Connolly, M.D. - General Practice
555-321-0987
FED I.D. #16-1234567

PATIENT NAME	APPT. DATE/TIME	
Donald Aiken	10/10/2008	10:30am

PATIENT NO.	DX
AIKENDO0	**1.** 281.0 pernicious anemia **2.** 782.4 jaundice **3.** **4.**

DESCRIPTION	✓	CPT	FEE	DESCRIPTION	✓	CPT	FEE
EXAMINATION				**PROCEDURES**			
New Patient				Diagnostic Anoscopy		46600	
Problem Focused		99201		ECG Complete		93000	
Expanded Problem Focused		99202		I&D, Abscess		10060	
Detailed	✓	99203	69	Pap Smear		88150	
Comprehensive		99204		Removal of Cerumen		69210	
Comprehensive/Complex		99205		Removal 1 Lesion		17000	
Established Patient				Removal 2-14 Lesions		17003	
Minimum		99211		Removal 15+ Lesions		17004	
Problem Focused		99212		Rhythm ECG w/Report		93040	
Expanded Problem Focused		99213		Rhythm ECG w/Tracing		93041	
Detailed		99214		Sigmoidoscopy, diag.		45330	
Comprehensive/Complex		99215					
				LABORATORY			
PREVENTIVE VISIT				Bacteria Culture		87081	
New Patient				Fungal Culture		87101	
Age 12-17		99384		Glucose Finger Stick		82948	
Age 18-39		99385		Lipid Panel		80061	
Age 40-64		99386		Specimen Handling		99000	
Age 65+		99387		Stool/Occult Blood		82270	
Established Patient				Tine Test		85008	
Age 12-17		99394		Tuberculin PPD		85590	
Age 18-39		99395		Urinalysis		81000	
Age 40-64		99396		Venipuncture	✓	36415	17
Age 65+		99397					
				INJECTION/IMMUN.			
CONSULTATION: OFFICE/ER				DT Immun		90702	
Requested By:				Hepatitis A Immun		90632	
Problem Focused		99241		Hepatitis B Immun		90746	
Expanded Problem Focused		99242		Influenza Immun		90659	
Detailed		99243		Pneumovax		90732	
Comprehensive		99244					
Comprehensive/Complex		99245		**TOTAL FEES**			

Case 11.11

From the Patient Information Form

Name	Joseph Zylerberg
Sex	M
Birth Date	03/14/1935
Marital Status	S
Employer	(Retired)
Address	18 Alpine Dr.
	Alliance, OH
	44601-9012
Telephone	555-692-3417
SSN	201-36-4413
Health Plan	Nationwide Medicare
Health Insurance No.	201364413A
Signature	On File (1-1-2008)

Secondary Insurance Information

Insured	Same
Pt Relationship to Insured	
Insured's Date of Birth	
Insured's Employer	
SSN	
Insurance Plan	Medicaid
Insurance ID No.	201364413C
Insurance Group No.	
Condition Related to:	
Employment	No
Auto Accident	No
Other Accident	No
Accept Assignment	Yes
Physician Signature	On File (1-1-2005)

VALLEY ASSOCIATES, P.C.
Christopher M. Connolly, M.D. - Internal Medicine
555-967-0303
FED I.D. #16-1234567

PATIENT NAME	APPT. DATE/TIME	
Joseph Zylerberg	10/09/2008	4:30pm

PATIENT NO.	DX
ZYLERJO0	**1.** 413.9 angina pectoris **2.** 414.01 atherosclerotic heart disease **3.** **4.**

DESCRIPTION	✓	CPT	FEE	DESCRIPTION	✓	CPT	FEE
EXAMINATION				**PROCEDURES**			
New Patient				Diagnostic Anoscopy		46600	
Problem Focused		99201		ECG Complete	✓	93000	29
Expanded Problem Focused		99202		I&D, Abscess		10060	
Detailed		99203		Pap Smear		88150	
Comprehensive	✓	99204	103	Removal of Cerumen		69210	
Comprehensive/Complex		99205		Removal 1 Lesion		17000	
Established Patient				Removal 2-14 Lesions		17003	
Minimum		99211		Removal 15+ Lesions		17004	
Problem Focused		99212		Rhythm ECG w/Report		93040	
Expanded Problem Focused		99213		Rhythm ECG w/Tracing		93041	
Detailed		99214		Sigmoidoscopy, diag.		45330	
Comprehensive/Complex		99215					
				LABORATORY			
PREVENTIVE VISIT				Bacteria Culture		87081	
New Patient				Fungal Culture		87101	
Age 12-17		99384		Glucose Finger Stick		82948	
Age 18-39		99385		Lipid Panel		80061	
Age 40-64		99386		Specimen Handling		99000	
Age 65+		99387		Stool/Occult Blood		82270	
Established Patient				Tine Test		85008	
Age 12-17		99394		Tuberculin PPD		85590	
Age 18-39		99395		Urinalysis		81000	
Age 40-64		99396		Venipuncture		36415	
Age 65+		99397					
				INJECTION/IMMUN.			
CONSULTATION: OFFICE/ER				DT Immun		90702	
Requested By:				Hepatitis A Immun		90632	
Problem Focused		99241		Hepatitis B Immun		90746	
Expanded Problem Focused		99242		Influenza Immun		90659	
Detailed		99243		Pneumovax		90732	
Comprehensive		99244					
Comprehensive/Complex		99245					
				TOTAL FEES			

Case 11.12

Name	Hector Munoz
Sex	M
Birth Date	10/19/1931
Marital Status	M
Employer	(Retired)
Address	7 John Court
	Toledo, OH
	43601-0123
Telephone	555-326-1742
SSN	301-46-2901
Health Plan	Nationwide Medicare
Health Insurance No.	301462901A
Copayment Amount	None
Signature	On File (1-1-2008)

Secondary Insurance Information

Insured	Same
Insurance Plan	AARP Medigap
Insurance ID No.	301462901B
Condition Related to:	
Employment	No
Auto Accident	No
Other Accident	No
Accept Assignment	Yes
Physician Signature	On File (1-1-2005)

VALLEY ASSOCIATES, P.C.
Christopher M. Connolly, M.D. - General Practice
555-321-0987
FED I.D. #16-1234567

PATIENT NAME	APPT. DATE/TIME	
Hector Munoz	10/10/2008	9:30am
PATIENT NO.	**DX**	
MUNOZHE0	**1.** 682.0 abscess on chin	
	2.	
	3.	
	4.	

DESCRIPTION	✓	CPT	FEE	DESCRIPTION	✓	CPT	FEE
EXAMINATION				**PROCEDURES**			
New Patient				Diagnostic Anoscopy		46600	
Problem Focused		99201		ECG Complete		93000	
Expanded Problem Focused	✓	99202	50	I&D, Abscess	✓	10060	57
Detailed		99203		Pap Smear		88150	
Comprehensive		99204		Removal of Cerumen		69210	
Comprehensive/Complex		99205		Removal 1 Lesion		17000	
Established Patient				Removal 2-14 Lesions		17003	
Minimum		99211		Removal 15+ Lesions		17004	
Problem Focused		99212		Rhythm ECG w/Report		93040	
Expanded Problem Focused		99213		Rhythm ECG w/Tracing		93041	
Detailed		99214		Sigmoidoscopy, diag.		45330	
Comprehensive/Complex		99215					

Computer Exploration

1. Visit the official U.S. government Web site for Medicare: http://www.medicare.gov
   Use the Medicare Personal Plan Finder to help you decide on the right Medicare health plan for a senior family member or friend. Compare benefits, costs, options, and provider quality information.
2. Go to the Centers for Medicare and Medicaid Services (CMS) Web site at: http://www.cms.hhs.gov
   Select the link for the Quarterly Provider Update, which contains quarterly updates on all changes to Medicare's regulations and instructions that affect providers. Click the link for the latest issue's table of contents, and then select the link for Physicians in the list of specific Medicare providers. Read about one Medicare regulation that physicians should know about that is currently undergoing change.
3. Go to the Centers for Medicare and Medicaid Services (CMS) Web site for Medicare at:
   http://www.cms.hhs.gov
   Select the Professionals link (rather than the Consumers link), and then select the Physicians link. Look for information about participating and nonparticipating providers and the Medicare Physician Fee Schedule (MPFS). Read the most recent information on that topic. Under the Contacts topic, look up the Medicare Part B carrier for your state.

NDCMedisoft Activity

11.1 Review MediSoft Entries Specific to Medicare

This activity explores various entries in MediSoft for a patient whose primary insurance carrier is Medicare.

1. Wilma Estephan's primary insurance carrier is Medicare Nationwide, a traditional fee-for-service plan. Open the Lists menu and select Patients/Guarantors and Cases.
2. In the Search For box, key ES to display Wilma Estephan's information in the Patient List dialog box.
3. Click the Edit Patient button to display the Name, Address tab.

4. Note that Wilma Estephan's Social Security Number, displayed at the bottom of the dialog box, is 140-32-4102. Click the Cancel button to close the Patient/Guarantor dialog box and return to the Patient List dialog box.

5. In the right side of the Patient List dialog box, click Wilma Estephan's Hypertension case to select it, and then click the Edit Case button.

6. In the Case dialog box that is displayed, click the Policy 1 tab.

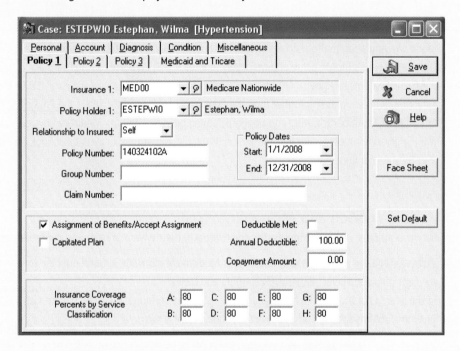

7. The Policy 1 tab shows that Medicare Nationwide is the primary carrier. Note that Wilma Estephan's policy number is 140324102A. This number is the same as her Social Security Number with an A after it. Medicare beneficiaries' policy numbers are comprised of their Social Security Number and a suffix (or in some cases a prefix) that indicates exact details about their benefits. Here the A signifies that she is a retired worker over age 65.

8. The Policy 1 tab also indicates that there is a $100 annual deductible—the standard deductible associated with Part B coverage. The Insurance Coverage Percents by Service Classification boxes at the bottom of the tab indicate that Medicare pays for 80 percent of covered services. The beneficiary is responsible for the remaining 20 percent.

Click the Account tab.

Computer Exploration

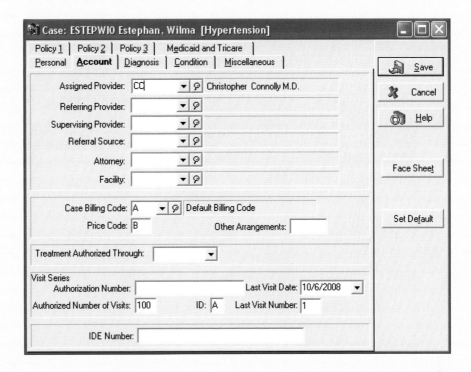

Case: ESTEPWIO Estephan, Wilma [Hypertension]

Policy 1 | Policy 2 | Policy 3 | Medicaid and Tricare
Personal | **Account** | Diagnosis | Condition | Miscellaneous

Assigned Provider: CC ▼ ⌕ Christopher Connolly M.D.
Referring Provider: ▼ ⌕
Supervising Provider: ▼ ⌕
Referral Source: ▼ ⌕
Attorney: ▼ ⌕
Facility: ▼ ⌕

Case Billing Code: A ▼ ⌕ Default Billing Code
Price Code: B   Other Arrangements:

Treatment Authorized Through: ▼

Visit Series
Authorization Number: Last Visit Date: 10/6/2008 ▼
Authorized Number of Visits: 100   ID: A   Last Visit Number: 1

IDE Number:

Save
Cancel
Help
Face Sheet
Set Default

9. In the Account tab, the Price Code box reads B. In the Valley Associates, P.C. sample database, Price Code B represents the Medicare Fee Schedule. Medicare and Medicaid are the only insurance carriers that use Price Code B in this sample database.

10. To see what effect Price Code B has on charge transactions, the Transaction Entry dialog box needs to be opened. Click the Cancel button to close the Case dialog box, and then click the Close button to close the Patient List dialog box.

11. Click Enter Transactions in the Activities menu. Key ES in the Chart box, and press Enter to display Wilma Estephan's transaction information.

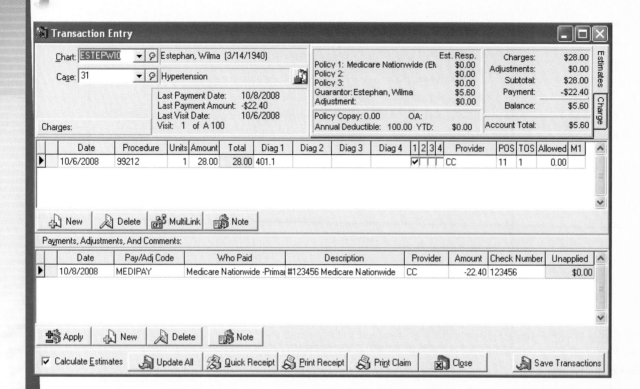

12. Click in the Procedure box under Charges, and then click the small magnifying glass icon to the right of the triangle button to display the Procedure Search Window.

13. Make sure the Field box is set to Code 1, and then key 99212 in the Search For box. This is the code for Wilma Estephan's procedure in the Charges section of the Transaction Entry dialog box.

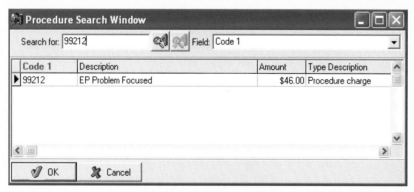

14. MediSoft locates the code in the Procedure Search Window, and displays the code's description (EP Problem Focused) and amount ($46). Click the Cancel button to close the Procedure Search Window.

15. Back in the Transaction Entry dialog box, note that the amount box for the same procedure displays $28. This amount represents the Price Code B amount, as set up in the Procedure/Payment/Adjustment Codes dialog box. The amount in the Procedure Search Window represents the Price Code A amount, the default. For this reason, the Price Code box in the Account tab of the Case dialog box must be set correctly, according to the carrier.

16. Click the Close button to exit the Transaction Entry dialog box.

Medicaid

CHAPTER OUTLINE

Objectives

After studying this chapter, you should be able to:

1. Describe the federal Medicaid eligibility requirements.
2. Discuss the effects of the Welfare Reform Act on Medicaid eligibility.
3. Explain the difference between *categorically needy* and *medically needy*.
4. Describe the income and asset guidelines used by most states to determine eligibility.
5. List the services that Medicaid usually does not cover.
6. List the types of plans that states offer to Medicaid recipients.
7. Discuss the claim filing procedures when a Medicaid recipient has other insurance coverage.
8. Prepare correct Medicaid claims.

Introduction

The Medicaid program was established under Title XIX of the Social Security Act of 1965 to pay for the health care needs of individuals and families with low incomes and few resources. The program is jointly funded by the federal and state governments. The federal government makes payments to states under the **Federal Medicaid Assistance Percentage (FMAP).** The amount of the payment is based on the state's average per capita income in relation to the national income average. The Centers for Medicare and Medicaid Services (CMS) projects that combined federal and state Medicaid expenditures, for more than 42 million eligible persons, will be $310.4 billion in 2004. Of this amount, the federal share is expected to be about 57 percent.

Individuals who apply for Medicaid benefits must meet minimum federal requirements and any additional requirements of the state in which they live. A person eligible in one state may be denied coverage in another state. Coverage also varies, with some states providing coverage for fewer than 40 percent of residents below the poverty level and other states covering as much as 60 percent of the same population. Because of this state-to-state variation, and because Medicaid rules and regulations change frequently, this chapter presents a general overview of the program.

To apply for Medicaid benefits, individuals must call or write their local Income Maintenance office or Department of Social Services and request an application. Once completed, the application is returned to the office, along with proof of income, assets, and any other relevant proof of eligibility. Applications are usually processed in forty-five to sixty days. An applicant who is denied coverage may appeal the decision through a Fair Hearing. Beneficiaries must notify the agency immediately if their income, assets, or living situations change.

Federal Eligibility

Federal guidelines mandate coverage for individuals referred to as **categorically needy**—persons with low incomes and few resources, and certain Medicare beneficiaries with low incomes. The categorically needy typically include families with dependent children who receive some form of cash assistance, individuals eligible to receive Supplemental Security Income (SSI), pregnant women with low incomes, and infants and children who meet low-income requirements.

The federal government requires states to offer benefits to the following groups:

- Persons with low incomes and few resources who receive financial assistance under **Temporary Assistance for Needy Families (TANF)**
- Persons who are eligible for TANF but who do not receive financial assistance
- Persons who receive foster care or adoption assistance under Title IV-E of the Social Security Act
- Children under six years of age who meet TANF requirements or whose family income is below 133 percent of the poverty level
- Persons in some groups who lose cash assistance when their work income or Social Security benefits exceed allowable limits (temporary Medicaid eligibility)

- Pregnant women whose family income is below 133 percent of the poverty level (coverage limited to pregnancy-related medical care)
- Infants born to Medicaid-eligible pregnant women
- Persons who are age sixty-five and over, legally blind, or totally disabled and who receive Supplemental Security Income (SSI)
- Certain low-income Medicare recipients

State Children's Health Insurance Program

From time to time, the federal government enacts legislation that affects the Medicaid program. The **State Children's Health Insurance Program (SCHIP)**, part of the Balanced Budget Act of 1997, offers states the opportunity to develop and implement plans for health insurance coverage for uninsured children. Children served by SCHIP come from low-income families whose incomes are not low enough to qualify for Medicaid. The program covers children up to age nineteen.

The program is funded jointly by the federal government and the states. It provides coverage for many preventive services, physician services, and inpatient and outpatient services. States may meet SCHIP requirements by expanding their current Medicaid program to include uninsured children, by establishing a new program, or by some combination of the two methods. Once each state's plan is approved, the federal government provides matching funds. In recent years, through state waivers, states have been given greater flexibility to expand their insurance coverage to the uninsured. This has resulted in an increased enrollment in Medicaid and SCHIP. In 2003 an estimated 5 million children were covered under SCHIP. Unlike in previous years, legislation introduced in 2003 allowed states to start carrying over a certain amount of unspent SCHIP money from previous years, making more money available to the expanding program.

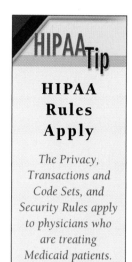

HIPAA Tip

HIPAA Rules Apply

The Privacy, Transactions and Code Sets, and Security Rules apply to physicians who are treating Medicaid patients.

Early and Periodic Screening, Diagnosis, and Treatment

Early and Periodic Screening, Diagnosis, and Treatment (EPSDT) provides health care benefits to children under age twenty-one who are enrolled in Medicaid. States are required by federal law to inform all Medicaid-eligible persons who are under age twenty-one of the availability of EPSDT and immunizations. Patients are not charged a fee for EPSDT services; however, some families do pay a monthly premium.

The EPSDT program emphasizes preventive care. Health screenings (known as well-child checkups) for medical, vision, hearing, and dental are performed at regular intervals. These examinations must include at least the following nine components:

1. A comprehensive health and developmental history, including assessment of both physical and mental health
2. A comprehensive, unclothed physical examination
3. Appropriate immunizations
4. Laboratory tests (including lead blood testing at twelve and twenty-four months and otherwise, according to age and risk factors)
5. Health education, including anticipatory guidance
6. Vision services
7. Dental services
8. Hearing services

9. Other necessary health care (diagnosis services, treatment, and other measures necessary to correct or ameliorate problems discovered by the screening services)

EPSDT also covers health care services other than periodic screenings. All mandatory and optional services covered under Medicaid—even if such services are not covered for adults—are covered by the EPSDT program. Children may be referred for an "interperiodic" screening by a parent, guardian, teacher, or other party.

The Ticket to Work and Work Incentives Improvement Act

The Ticket to Work and Work Incentives Improvement Act of 1999 (TWWIIA) expands the availability of health care services for workers with disabilities. Previously, persons with disabilities often had to choose between health care and work. TWWIIA gives states the option of allowing individuals with disabilities to purchase Medicaid coverage that is necessary to enable them to maintain employment.

New Freedom Initiative

The New Freedom Initiative was launched in 2001 as the president's comprehensive plan to reduce barriers to full community integration for people with disabilities and long-term illnesses. Under the initiative, various departments throughout the government, including the Department of Health and Human Services, were directed to partner with states to provide necessary supports to allow elders and people with disabilities to fully participate in community life. For example, through the use of Medicaid grants for community living, the initiative aims at promoting the use of at-home and community-based care as an alternative to nursing homes. Medicaid grants for aging and disability resource centers are another part of the initiative.

Spousal Impoverishment Protection

The Federal Spousal Impoverishment Legislation limits the amount of a married couples' income and assets that must be used before one of them can become eligible for Medicaid coverage in a long-term care facility. Before this legislation, a couples' income and assets were so depleted by the time one partner qualified for Medicaid that the other spouse was left with few resources.

The legislation applies to situations in which one member of the couple is in a nursing facility or medical institution and is expected to remain there for at least thirty days. When the couple applies for Medicaid coverage, their joint resources are evaluated. All resources held by both spouses are considered to be available to the spouse in the medical facility, except for certain assets, such as a home, household goods, an automobile, and burial funds.

Welfare Reform Act

Traditionally, persons considered eligible for Medicaid benefits were those who were also eligible for cash assistance through another government program, such as the Aid to Families with Dependent Children (AFDC) and Supplemental Security Income (SSI). The Personal Responsibility and Work Opportunity Reconciliation Act of 1996 (P.L. 104-193), commonly known as the **Welfare Reform Act**, replaced the AFDC program with TANF. Under this more stringent legislation, some individuals receiving TANF payments are limited to a five-year benefit period. At the end of five years, cash assistance ceases.

Eligibility for TANF assistance is determined at the county level. Answers to the following questions are taken into account:

- Is the income below set limits?
- Are the resources (including property) equal to or less than set limits?
- Is there at least one child under eighteen in the household?
- Is at least one parent unemployed, incapacitated, or absent from the home?
- Does the individual have a Social Security number and birth certificate?
- Does the individual receive adoptive or foster care assistance?

Many states use employability assessment or job search requirements for applicants, or require child immunization or school attendance, making eligibility standards more stringent. The Welfare Reform Act also affected eligibility rules for several other groups, including disabled children and immigrants. While the Welfare Reform Act made it more difficult for some groups to gain access to Medicaid benefits, individual states still have a great deal of latitude when implementing the program.

State Programs

Although the federal government sets broad standards for Medicaid coverage, there is variation among the states. The trend in recent years has been for states to offer Medicaid benefits to individuals or families who have incomes that are low, but not low enough to qualify for cash assistance programs. States set their own income limits, usually considering the applicant's income relative to the federal poverty level (FPL), taking household size into account. Most states also provide Medicaid coverage to **medically needy** individuals—people with high medical expenses and low financial resources (but not low enough to receive cash assistance). States may choose their own names for these programs. For example, California's program is called **MediCal**.

Examples of groups covered by state rules but not federal guidelines are

- Aged, blind, or disabled persons with incomes below the federal poverty level who do not qualify under federal mandatory coverage rules
- Persons who are institutionalized who do not qualify under federal rules, but who meet special state income requirements
- Persons who would be eligible if institutionalized, but who are receiving home or community care
- Children under age twenty-one who meet the TANF income and resources limits
- Infants up to one-year-old who do not qualify under federal rules, but who meet state income limit rules
- Pregnant women who do not qualify under federal rules, but who meet state income limit rules
- Optional targeted low-income children
- Recipients of state supplementary payments
- TB-infected persons who would be financially eligible for Medicaid at the SSI level (only for TB-related ambulatory services and TB drugs)
- Low-income, uninsured women identified through the Centers for Disease Control and Prevention's (CDC) National Breast and Cervical Cancer Early Detection Program (NBCCEDP) as needing breast or cervical cancer treatment

Income and Asset Guidelines

In most states, general income and asset guidelines are as follows:

- Persons who receive income from employment may qualify for Medicaid depending on their income, since a portion of their earned income is not counted toward the Medicaid income limit (income required for necessary expenditures).
- Only a portion of unearned income from Social Security benefits, Supplemental Security Income (SSI), and veterans' benefits and pensions is counted toward income limits.
- Assets are taken into account when determining eligibility. Assets include cash, bank accounts, certificates of deposit, stocks and bonds, cash surrender value of life insurance policies, and nonhome property. The applicant's residence is not counted in arriving at the total asset calculation. Assets may be owned solely by the applicant or jointly by the applicant and another party.
- Some other possessions are not counted as assets, including essential personal property such as clothing, furniture, and personal effects, and a burial plot and money put aside for burial.
- Applicants who enter a long-term care facility have their homes counted as an asset unless they are in for a short-term stay and are expected to return home shortly, or certain relatives will continue to live in the home. These relatives include a spouse, a disabled or blind child, a child who is less than twenty-one years of age, or a child or sibling under certain circumstances.
- Assets that have been transferred into another person's name are closely examined. The asset may be included in the applicant's asset total depending on when the asset was transferred, to whom it was transferred, the amount paid in return for the asset, and the state in which the applicant resides.
- Information provided on the application is checked and verified using other sources of information, including the Social Security Administration, the Internal Revenue Service, the state Motor Vehicle Agency, and the state Department of Labor, among others.

Spend-Down Programs

Some states have what are known as **spend-down** programs. In a spend-down program, individuals are required to spend a portion of their income or resources on health care until they reach or drop below the income level specified

Thinking It Through—12.1

Unlike Medicare, Medicaid eligibility coverage varies from state to state. An individual ruled ineligible in one state may qualify for coverage in another state.

1. Why do Medicaid eligibility rules and coverage vary while Medicare's do not?

2. What are the advantages and disadvantages of the current state-oriented system?

by the state. The concept is similar to an annual deductible, except that it resets at the beginning of every month. Each month, the enrollee pays a portion of incurred medical bills, up to a certain amount, before the Medicaid fee schedule takes effect and Medicaid takes over payments.

For example, a patient who has a $100 spend-down visits the physician on March 3 and is billed $75. The patient is responsible for paying the entire $75. Later in the month, she visits the physician again and is charged $60. She must pay $25, and Medicaid will pay the remaining $35. At the beginning of the next month, she is once again responsible for the first $100 of charges. The spend-down amount varies depending on the patient's financial resources.

Many states also extend benefits to other groups of individuals. For example, most states offer coverage to persons described as medically needy.

Medicaid Enrollment Verification

Medicaid cards or coupons may be issued to qualified individuals. Some states issue cards twice a month, some once a month, and others every two months or every six months. Figure 12.1 on page 426 shows sample ID cards. Figure 12.2 on page 427 displays a sample ID coupon.

Patients' eligibility should be checked each time they make an appointment and before they see the physician. Most states are moving to electronic verification of eligibility under the Electronic Medicaid Eligibility Verification System (EMEVS). Many states provide both online and telephone verification systems. In addition to eligibility dates, the system also specifies whether the patient is required to pay a copayment or coinsurance.

Some patients may require treatment before their eligibility can be checked. Figure 12.3 on page 428 is an example of an eligibility verification log for patients who have not yet been assigned ID numbers or who have misplaced their cards.

Some individuals enrolled in Medicaid are assigned **restricted status.** In restricted status, the patient is required to see a specific physician and/or use a specific pharmacy. This physician's name is listed on the patient's ID card. If the patient sees a provider other than the one listed on the card, Medicaid benefits will be denied. Likewise, a restricted status patient is limited to a certain pharmacy for filling prescriptions. Persons are assigned restricted status because of their past abuse of Medicaid benefits.

After a patient's Medicaid enrollment status has been verified, most practices also require another form of identification. A driver's license or other cards may be requested to confirm the patient's identity.

Covered and Excluded Services

Since plans are administered at a state level, each state determines coverage and coverage limits and sets payment rates, subject to federal guidelines established under Title XIX of the Social Security Act.

Covered Services

To receive federal matching funds, states must cover certain services, including

- Inpatient hospital services
- Outpatient hospital services

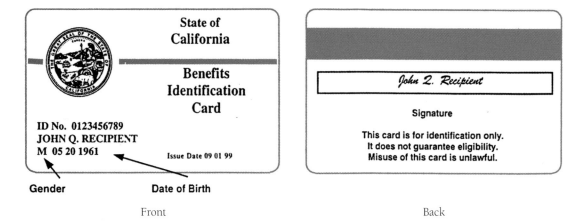

Figure 12.1 Sample Medicaid Identification Cards

- Physician services
- Emergency services
- Laboratory and X-ray services
- Prenatal care
- Early and Periodic Screening, Diagnosis, and Treatment services for persons under age twenty-one, including physical examinations, immunizations, and certain age-relevant services
- Skilled nursing facility services for persons age twenty-one or older
- Home health care services for persons eligible for skilled nursing services
- Vaccines for children

Medicaid Identification (Form 3087) Sample

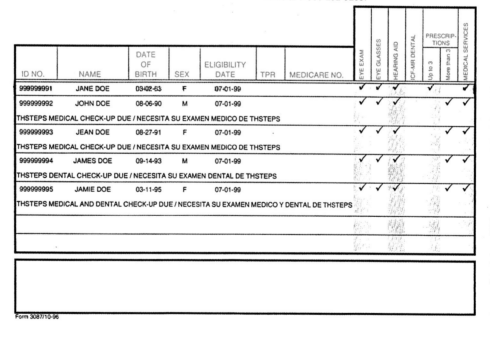

P.O. BOX 179030
AUSTIN, TEXAS

952-X
78714-9030

EROX 01-00001

TEXAS DEPARTMENT OF HUMAN SERVICES
MEDICAID IDENTIFICATION
IDENTIFICATION PARA MEDICAID

Date Run	BIN	BP	TP	Cat	Case No.	
10/25/99	610098		01	02	123456789	**GOOD THROUGH:** VALIDA HASTA: NOVEMBER 30, 1999

952-X   123456789   01   02   990930
JANE DOE
338 WEST BOONE STREET
BELVIDERE   TX   78069

ANYONE LISTED BELOW
CAN GET MEDICAID SERVICES

Under 21 years old? Please call your doctor, nurse, or dentist to schedule a checkup if you see a reminder under your name. If there is no reminder, you can still use Medicaid to get health care that you need.

A ✓ on the line to the right of your name means that you can get that service too.

Questions about Medicaid? Please call **1-800-252-8263** for help.

CADA PERSONA NOMBRADA ABAJO
PUEDE RECIBIR SERVICIOS DE MEDICAID

¿Tiene menos de 21 años? Por favor, llame a su doctor, enfermera, o dentista para hacer una cita si hay una nota debajo de su nombre. Aunque no haya ninguna nota, puede usar Medicaid para recibir la atención médica que necesite.

Las marcas ✓ a la derecha en el mismo renglón donde está su nombre significan que usted puede recibir esos servicios también.

¿Tiene preguntas sobre Medicaid? Por favor, llame al **1-800-252-8263**.

ID NO.	NAME	DATE OF BIRTH	SEX	ELIGIBILITY DATE	TPR	MEDICARE NO.	EYE EXAM	EYE GLASSES	HEARING AID	ICF-MR DENTAL	PRESCRIPTIONS Up to 3	More than 3	MEDICAL SERVICES
999999991	JANE DOE	03-02-63	F	07-01-99			✓	✓	✓		✓		✓
999999992	JOHN DOE	08-06-90	M	07-01-99			✓	✓	✓			✓	✓
THSTEPS MEDICAL CHECK-UP DUE / NECESITA SU EXAMEN MEDICO DE THSTEPS													
999999993	JEAN DOE	08-27-91	F	07-01-99			✓	✓	✓			✓	✓
THSTEPS MEDICAL CHECK-UP DUE / NECESITA SU EXAMEN MEDICO DE THSTEPS													
999999994	JAMES DOE	09-14-93	M	07-01-99			✓	✓	✓			✓	✓
THSTEPS DENTAL CHECK-UP DUE / NECESITA SU EXAMEN DENTAL DE THSTEPS													
999999995	JAMIE DOE	03-11-95	F	07-01-99			✓	✓	✓			✓	✓
THSTEPS MEDICAL AND DENTAL CHECK-UP DUE / NECESITA SU EXAMEN MEDICO Y DENTAL DE THSTEPS													

Form 3087/10-96

Figure 12.2 Sample Medicaid Identification Coupon

- Family planning services and supplies
- Nurse midwife services
- Pediatric and family nurse-practitioner services
- Rural health clinic services
- Federally qualified health-center (FQHC) services.

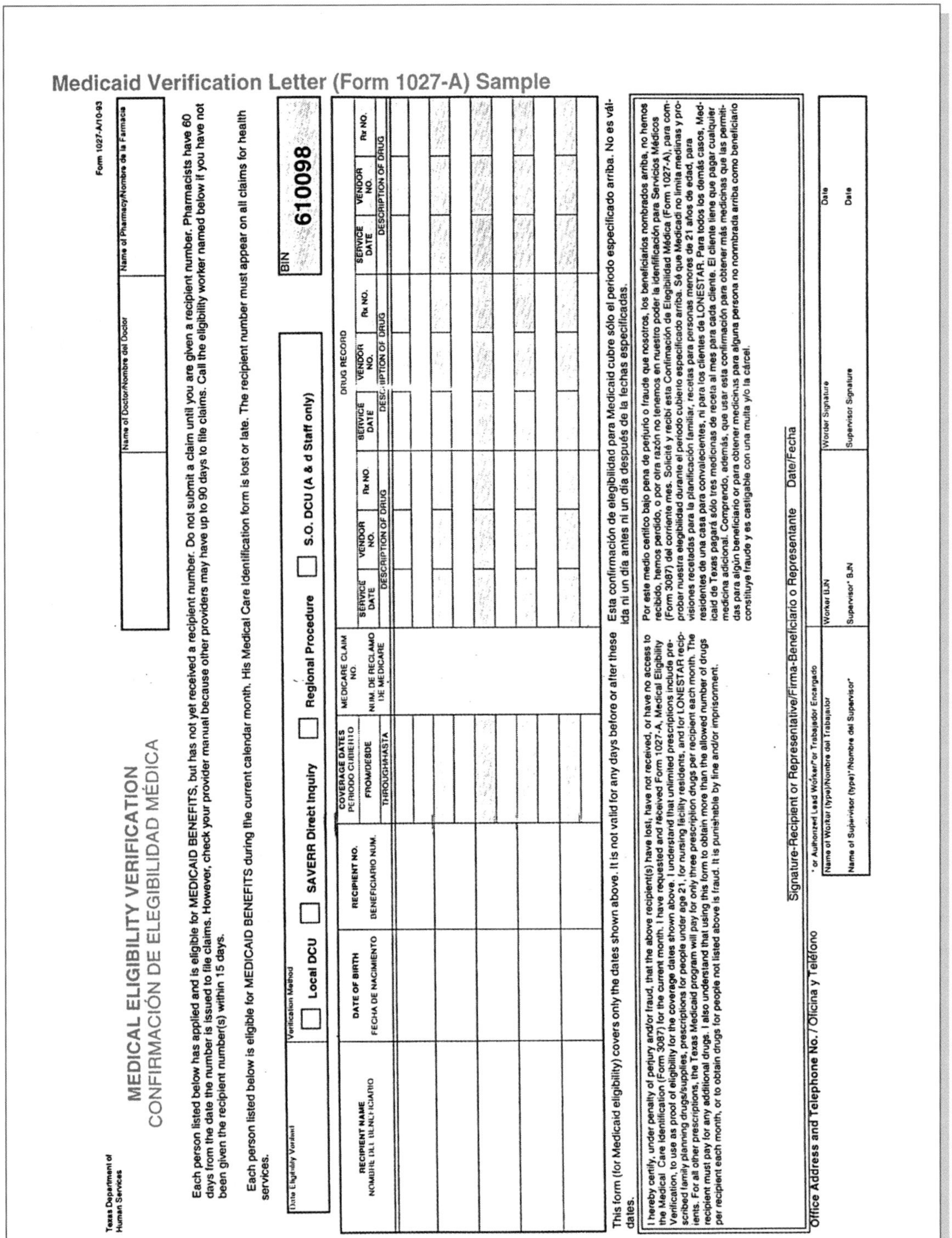

Medicaid Verification Letter (Form 1027-A) Sample

Texas Department of Human Services

Form 1027-A/10-93

MEDICAL ELIGIBILITY VERIFICATION
CONFIRMACIÓN DE ELEGIBILIDAD MÉDICA

Name of Doctor/Nombre del Doctor	Name of Pharmacy/Nombre de la Farmacia

Each person listed below has applied and is eligible for MEDICAID BENEFITS, but has not yet received a recipient number. Do not submit a claim until you are given a recipient number. Pharmacists have 60 days from the date the number is issued to file claims. However, check your provider manual because other providers may have up to 90 days to file claims. Call the eligibility worker named below if you have not been given the recipient number(s) within 15 days.

Each person listed below is eligible for MEDICAID BENEFITS during the current calendar month. His Medical Care Identification form is lost or late. The recipient number must appear on all claims for health services.

Date Eligibility Verified

Verification Method: ☐ Local DCU ☐ SAVERR Direct Inquiry ☐ Regional Procedure ☐ S.O. DCU (A & d Staff only)

BIN 610098

RECIPIENT NAME / NOMBRE DEL BENEFICIARIO	DATE OF BIRTH / FECHA DE NACIMIENTO	RECIPIENT NO. / BENEFICIARIO NUM.	COVERAGE DATES / PERIODO CUBIERTO: FROM/DESDE, THROUGH/HASTA	MEDICARE CLAIM NO. / NUM. DE RECLAMO DE MEDICARE	DRUG RECORD: SERVICE DATE, VENDOR NO., Rx NO., DESCRIPTION OF DRUG	SERVICE DATE, VENDOR NO., Rx NO., DESCRIPTION OF DRUG	SERVICE DATE, VENDOR NO., Rx NO., DESCRIPTION OF DRUG

This form (for Medicaid eligibility) covers only the dates shown above. It is not valid for any days before or after these dates.

Esta confirmación de elegibilidad para Medicaid cubre sólo el periodo especificado arriba. No es válida ni un día antes ni un día después de la fechas especificadas.

I hereby certify, under penalty of perjury and/or fraud, that the above recipient(s) have lost, have not received, or have no access to the Medical Care Identification (Form 3087) for the current month. I have requested and received Form 1027-A, Medical Eligibility Verification, to use as proof of eligibility for the coverage dates shown above. I understand that unlimited prescriptions include prescribed family planning drugs/supplies, prescriptions for people under age 21, for nursing facility residents, and for LONESTAR recipients. For all other prescriptions, the Texas Medicaid program will pay for only three prescription drugs per recipient each month. The recipient must pay for any additional drugs. I also understand that using this form to obtain more than the allowed number of drugs per recipient each month, or to obtain drugs for people not listed above is fraud. It is punishable by fine and/or imprisonment.

Por este medio certifco bajo pena de perjurio o fraude que nosotros, los beneficiarios nombrados arriba, no hemos recibido, hemos perdido, o por otra razón no tenemos en nuestro poder la identificación para Servicios Médicos (Form 3087) del corriente mes. Solicité y recibí esta Confirmación de Elegibilidad Médica (Form 1027-A), para comprobar nuestra elegibilidad durante el periodo cubierto especificado arriba. Só que Medicaid no limita medinas y provisiones recetadas para la planificación familiar, recetas para personas menores de 21 años de edad, para residentes de una casa para convalecientes, ni para los clientes de LONESTAR. Para todos los demás casos, Medicaid de Texas pagará sólo tres medicinas de receta al mes para cada cliente. El cliente tiene que pagar cualquier medicina adicional. Comprendo, además, que usar esta confirmación para obtener más medicinas que las permitidas para algún beneficiario o para obtener medicinas para alguna persona no nombrada arriba como beneficiario constituye fraude y es castigable con una multa y/o la cárcel.

Signature-Recipient or Representative/Firma-Beneficiario o Representante Date/Fecha

Office Address and Telephone No. / Oficina y Teléfono

* or Authorized Lead Worker/*or Trabajador Encargado

Name of Worker (type)/Nombre del Trabajador	Worker BJN	Worker Signature	Date
Name of Supervisor (type)*/Nombre del Supervisor*	Supervisor* BJN	Supervisor Signature	Date

Figure 12.3 Sample Medicaid Eligibility Verification Log

Some states also provide coverage for prescription drugs, dental or vision care, and other miscellaneous services such as chiropractic care, psychiatric care, and physical therapy. The federal government provides matching funds for some of these optional services, the most common of which include

- Diagnostic services
- Clinic services

- Prescription drugs
- Vision care
- Prosthetic devices
- Transportation services
- Rehabilitation and physical therapy services
- Home and community-based care to certain persons with chronic impairments

In recent years, however, because of large state budget deficits, state laws have cut back on some of these benefits, for example, prescription drug benefits and hearing, vision, and dental benefits for adults. Many states have also had to restrict eligibility for Medicaid and to reduce Medicaid payments to doctors, hospitals, nursing homes, or other providers.

Preauthorization

Some services covered under Medicaid require prior authorization before they are performed. If the provider does not obtain preauthorization, the plan may refuse to pay the claim.

Excluded Services

Rules regarding services not covered under Medicaid vary from state to state. For example, the following services may not be covered:

- Services that are not medically necessary
- Experimental or investigational procedures
- Cosmetic procedures

Types of Plans

In most states, Medicaid offers both fee-for-service and managed care plans.

Fee-for-Service

Medicaid clients enrolled in a fee-for-service plan may be treated by the provider of their choice, as long as that provider accepts Medicaid. The provider submits the claim to Medicaid and is paid directly by Medicaid.

Managed Care

Many states have shifted the Medicaid population from fee-for-service programs to managed care plans. Client enrollment in a managed care plan is either mandatory or voluntary, depending on state regulations. In 2003, thirty-eight states required some form of Medicaid managed care, and 23 million Medicaid recipients were members of HMOs (*New York Times,* February 19, 2003, C1–2). Some states, such as New York and California, regularly assign Medicaid beneficiaries to a managed care program.

Medicaid managed care plans include HMOs, prepaid health plans (PHPs), and other types of plans. The plans restrict patients to a network of physicians, hospitals, and clinics. Individuals enrolled in managed care plans must obtain all services and referrals through their primary care provider (PCP). The PCP is responsible for coordinating and monitoring the patient's care. If the patient needs to see a specialist, the PCP must provide a referral, or Medicaid will not pay for the service. In many states, a PCP may be an internist, a general practitioner, a family physician, a pediatrician, a nurse-practitioner, or a physician's assistant.

When Medicaid conducts a
post-payment review, the
following information about
a referral is expected to be
recorded in the patient
record:

PCP's name
PCP's NPI
Date the PCP contacted
    the referring provider
Reason for the referral
    (clinical data)
Patient's name
Patient's Medicaid ID
    number
Patient's date of birth

Managed care plans offer Medicaid recipients several advantages. Some Medicaid patients experience difficulty finding a physician who will treat them, in part due to the lower fee structure. Under a managed care plan, individuals choose a primary care physician who provides treatment and manages their medical care. The patient also has access to specialists should the need arise. In addition, managed care programs offer greater access to preventive care such as immunizations and health screenings.

Medicaid managed care claims are filed differently than other Medicaid claims. Claims are sent to the managed care organization instead of to the state Medicaid department. Participating providers agree to the guidelines of the managed care organization, provided that they are in compliance with federal requirements.

Payment for Services

A physician who wishes to provide services to Medicaid recipients must sign a contract with the Department of Health and Human Services (HHS). Managed care plans may also contract with HHS to provide services under Medicaid. Medicaid participating providers agree to certain provisions. For example, a provider may not discriminate on the basis of race, age, color, sex, creed, national origin, or disability; the provider must agree to treat all eligible patients.

Providers must agree to accept payment from Medicaid as payment in full for services; they may not bill patients for additional amounts. The difference must be entered into the billing system as a write-off. The amount of payment is determined by several factors, including Title XIX of the Social Security Act, HHS regulations, and state rules.

States may require Medicaid recipients to make small payments in the form of deductibles, coinsurance, or copayments. These patient payments are referred to as cost-share payments. Federal law mandates exempting emergency services and family planning services from copayments. In addition, federal law excludes certain categories of recipients from making copayments, including children under age eighteen, pregnant women, hospital or nursing home patients who contribute the majority of their income to that institution for care, and categorically needy recipients who are enrolled in HMOs.

If Medicaid does not cover a service, the patient may be billed if the following conditions are met:

- The physician informed the patient before the service was performed that the procedure would not be covered by Medicaid.
- The physician has an established written policy for billing noncovered services that applies to all patients, not just Medicaid patients.
- The patient is informed in advance of the estimated charge for the procedure, and agrees in writing to pay the charge.

However, if the physician has reason to believe a service will not be covered, the patient should be informed in advance and given a form to sign. An example of a form is shown in Figure 12.4.

If a claim is denied for the following reasons, the physician may not bill the patient for the amount:

- Necessary preauthorization was not obtained prior to procedure.
- Service was not medically necessary.
- Claim was not filed within the time period for filing (typically one year after the date of service).

Private Pay Agreement

I understand _____(Provider name)_____ is accepting me as a private pay patient for the period of _____, and I will be responsible for paying for any services I receive. The Provider will not file a claim to Medicaid for services provided to me.

Signed: _____

Date: _____

Figure 12.4 Sample Private Pay Agreement

Providers in capitated managed care plans who are paid flat monthly fees must still file claims with the Medicaid payer, since the payer uses the claim data to assess utilization. Utilization reviews examine the necessity, appropriateness, and efficiency of services delivered.

Third-Party Liability

Before filing a claim with Medicaid, it is important to determine whether the patient has other insurance coverage.

Payer of Last Resort

If the patient has coverage through any other insurance plan, or if the claim is covered by another program, such as workers' compensation, the other plan is billed first, and the remittance advice from that primary payer is forwarded to Medicaid. For this reason, Medicaid is known as the **payer of last resort**, since it is always billed after another plan has been billed, if other coverage exists.

Medicare–Medicaid Crossover Claims

Some individuals, called **Medi-Medi beneficiaries**, are eligible for both Medicaid and Medicare benefits. Claims for these patients are first submitted to Medicare and then to Medicaid with a Medicare remittance notice. Claims billed to Medicare and then submitted to Medicaid are called **crossover claims**. Some Medicare carriers automatically forward crossover claims to the state Medicaid payer.

In many instances, Medicare requires a deductible payment or coinsurance payment. When an individual has Medi-Medi coverage, these payments are sometimes paid by Medicaid. The total amount paid by Medicare and Medicaid is subject to a maximum allowed limit.

Medicaid programs in some states pay Medicare Part B premiums for Medi-Medi patients. For example, in California, MediCal pays the Medicare Part B premiums, and physicians may not bill patients for Medicare deductible and coinsurance amounts. However, MediCal does not reimburse Medicare HMO patients for any required copayments. Depending on the specific procedures and diagnoses, MediCal sometimes reimburses providers for charges denied by Medicare, including charges for services normally not covered by Medicare.

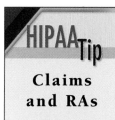

HIPAA Tip

Claims and RAs

The HIPAA 837 is used for electronic claims and for coordination of benefits. The HIPAA 835 remittance advice is the standard transaction sent by payers to Medicaid providers.

Claim Filing Guidelines

Because Medicaid is a state-based program, coordination of the requirements for completion of the HIPAA 837 are handled by a national committee called the National Medicaid EDI HIPAA workgroup (NMEH). This organization advises CMS about HIPAA compliance issues related to Medicaid.

Where to File

Claims are submitted to different agencies, depending on the particular state. Some states use fiscal intermediaries. These are private insurance companies that contract with Medicaid to process and pay claims. In other states, the state's Department of Health and Human Services may handle claims, or the county welfare agency. Medical offices obtain specific claim filing and completion requirements from the agency responsible for processing Medicaid claims in their state.

Coding

Medicaid claims are reported using the HCPCS coding system that is also used by Medicare. The ICD-9-CM is used to code diagnoses.

Unacceptable Billing Practices

Physicians who contract with Medicaid to provide services may not engage in any of the following unacceptable billing practices:

- Billing for services that are not medically necessary
- Billing for services not provided, or billing more than once for the same procedure
- Submitting claims for individual procedures that are part of a global procedure
- Submitting claims using an individual provider PIN when a physician working for or on behalf of a group practice or clinic performs services

After Filing

Once a claim has been filed and approved for payment, the provider receives payment and an 835 remittance advice. Claims that are denied may be appealed within a certain time period, usually thirty to sixty days. Appeals should include relevant supporting documentation and a note explaining why the claim should be reconsidered. The first level of appeal is the regional agent for Medicaid. If the appeal is denied, it goes to the state's welfare department for consideration. The highest level for a Medicaid appeal is the appellate court.

Fraud and Abuse

The Medicaid Alliance for Program Safeguards is an initiative to combat fraud and abuse in the Medicaid program. The alliance is composed of a central office alliance team and a network of alliance coordinators who represent all ten CMS regional offices. The central office team and coordinators are supported by a technical advisory group formed by CMS, called the Medicaid Fraud and Abuse Control Technical Advisory Group, or TAG. TAG provides a national forum for states to exchange experiences, resources, and solutions. The alliance is designed to prevent as well as detect Medicaid fraud and abuse.

Physician practice managers are responsible for supervising all nonmedical matters in the practice. They manage the billing, coding, and collection process; ensure that patients are satisfied with the care process; and are responsible for personnel policies and procedures. They are also involved in quality management (QM) and quality assurance (QA) programs that are designed to protect and ensure the quality of patient care. This part of the position entails establishing and checking the credentialing criteria for physicians and other providers, developing practice guidelines, and setting up computer systems that are used to collect and report health data.

Because their duties encompass so many areas, physician practice managers must be knowledgeable about a number of regulations. For example, access to facilities is regulated by the Americans with Disabilities (ADA) Act; hiring is regulated by the Equal Employment Opportunity Commission (EEOC); overtime compensation must be handled according to the rules of the Code of Federal Regulations; and working conditions are prescribed by the Occupational Safety and Health Administration (OSHA). Most managers use attorneys and accountants as consultants to assist in many operations of the medical practice.

Physician practice managers have at least a bachelor's degree, and many also have a Master's of Business Administration (MBA) or a Master's of Public Health (MPH).

Medicaid Claim Completion

Because Medicaid is a health plan that is categorized as a covered entity under HIPAA, Medicaid claims are usually submitted using the HIPAA 837 claim. In some situations, however, a paper claim using the CMS-1500 format may be used, or a state-specific form may be requested.

HIPAA Claims

A number of special data elements may be required for completion of HIPAA-compliant Medicaid claims. The requirements are controlled by state guidelines. These are:

Data Element	Meaning
Family Planning Indicator	Y = Family planning services involvement
	N = No family planning services involvement
EPSDT Indicator	Y = The services are the result of a screening referral
	N = The services are not the result of a screening referral
Special Program Code	Codes reported for Medicaid beneficiaries such as 03 for Special Federal Funding program and 09 for Second Opinion or Surgery
Service Authorization Exception Code	Required when providers are required by state law to obtain authorization for specific services which was not obtained for reasons such as emergency care

The physician's Medicaid number is reported as a secondary identifier.

CMS-1500 Paper Claims

If a CMS-1500 paper claim is required, follow the guidelines on page 434.

Medicaid CMS-1500 Claim Completion	
Form Locator	**Data**
1	Choose Medicaid
1a	Medicaid ID number
2	Patient's name
3	Patient's eight-digit date of birth and gender
4	Blank
5	Patient's address
6	Blank
7	Blank
8	Blank
9	Blank
9a	Blank
9b	Blank
9c	Blank
9d	Blank
10a–c	Choose No
10d	Blank
11	Blank
11a	Blank
11b	Blank
11c	Blank
11d	Choose Yes or No
12	Signature not required
13	Blank
14	Eight-digit date, if appropriate
15	Blank
16	Blank
17	*Optional:* Name/credentials of referring/ordering physician
17a	Provider's NPI
18	Blank
19	Blank
20	Choose Yes or No, or leave blank
21	Appropriate ICD codes
22	Blank
23	Preauthorization/precertification number
24A	Dates of service (eight-digit format); no consecutive dates permitted
24B	Appropriate POS code
24C	If required, appropriate TOS code
24D	Appropriate CPT/HCPCS codes with up to three modifiers
24E	Diagnosis key number for CPT/HCPCS codes
24F	Amount charged
24G	Appropriate days/units reported
24H	Enter appropriate codes if services provided under EPSDT (varies by state)
24I	Enter X if services for a medical emergency provided in emergency room
24J	Blank
24K	Blank
25	Blank
26	Blank
27	Choose Yes
28	Total of charges in form locator 24F
29	Blank or $0.00
30	Enter amount from form locator 28
31	Signature on file
32	Appropriate name/address of facility if other than provider's office or patient's home
33	Provider's name, address, and NPI

Review

Chapter Summary

1. The federal government requires the states to provide individuals in certain low-income or low-resource categories with Medicaid coverage. Coverage is available to persons receiving TANF assistance; persons eligible for TANF but not receiving assistance; persons receiving foster care or adoption assistance under the Social Security Act; children under six years of age from low-income families; some persons who lose cash assistance when their work income or Social Security benefits exceed allowable limits; pregnant women with low incomes; infants born to Medicaid-eligible pregnant women; persons age sixty-five and over or legally blind or totally disabled persons who receive Supplemental Security Income (SSI); and certain low-income Medicare recipients.

2. At times, federal programs and initiatives are enacted that give states the opportunity to expand Medicaid coverage in particular ways to targeted groups. Recent examples include the State Children's Health Insurance Program (SCHIP), Early and Periodic Screening, Diagnosis, and Treatment (EPSDT) services for children under age twenty-one who are enrolled in Medicaid, the Ticket to Work and Work Incentives Improvement Act (TWWIIA) of 1999 for persons with disabilities who want to work, and the New Freedom Initiative aimed at reducing barriers to full community integration for people with disabilities and long-term illnesses.

3. The Welfare Reform Act made it more difficult for certain groups to obtain coverage, including disabled children and immigrants.

4. Categorically needy individuals qualify for Medicaid based on their low income and resources; medically needy persons receive assistance from some states because they encounter high medical bills and have limited income and resources. Medically needy individuals may have incomes that exceed Medicaid limits.

5. States examine a person's income, current assets (some assets are not counted), and assets that have recently been transferred into another person's name when determining eligibility.

6. Medicaid usually does not pay for services that are not medically necessary, procedures that are experimental or investigational, and cosmetic procedures.

7. States offer a variety of plans, including fee-for-service and managed care plans. The trend is to shift recipients from fee-for-service plans to managed care plans. Medicaid managed care plans include HMOs, prepaid health plans (PHPs), and others.

8. When a Medicaid recipient has coverage under another insurance plan, that plan is billed first. Once the remittance advice from the primary carrier has been received, Medicaid may be billed.

Key Terms

categorically needy *page 420*

crossover claim *page 431*

Early and Periodic Screening, Diagnosis, and Treatment (EPSDT) *page 421*

Federal Medicaid Assistance Percentage (FMAP) *page 420*

MediCal *page 423*

medically needy *page 423*

Medi-Medi beneficiary *page 431*

payer of last resort *page 431*

restricted status *page 425*

spend-down *page 424*

State Children's Health Insurance Program (SCHIP) *page 421*

Temporary Assistance for Needy Families (TANF) *page 420*

Welfare Reform Act *page 422*

Review Questions

Match the key terms in the left column with the definitions in the right column.

A. medically needy

B. Temporary Assistance for Needy Families (TANF)

C. payer of last resort

D. Welfare Reform Act

E. restricted status

F. categorically needy

G. State Children's Health Insurance Program (SCHIP)

H. Federal Medicaid Assistance Percentage (FMAP) program

I. Medi-Medi beneficiaries

J. spend-down

_____ 1. The program through which the federal government makes Medicaid payments to states

_____ 2. A program that requires a patient to see a specific physician and/or use a specific pharmacy

_____ 3. Claims for patients who receive benefits from both Medicare and Medicaid

_____ 4. A description that applies to Medicaid, since it is always billed after another plan has been billed, if other coverage exists

_____ 5. Applicants who qualify based on low income and resources

_____ 6. The Personal Responsibility and Work Opportunity Reconciliation Act of 1996

_____ 7. A program that requires states to develop and implement plans for health insurance coverage for uninsured children

_____ 8. The government financial program that provides financial assistance for people with low incomes and few resources

_____ 9. A program that requires individuals to use their own financial resources to pay a portion of incurred medical bills before Medicaid makes payments.

_____ 10. Individuals with high medical expenses and low financial resources

Decide whether each statement is true or false, and write T for true or F for false.

_____ 1. Persons who see a provider for family planning services may not be charged a copayment.

_____ 2. Medicaid is known as the payer of last resort because an individual must exhaust all other resources before Medicaid pays for health care.

_____ 3. Individuals who are employed are ineligible for Medicaid.

_____ 4. After receiving payment from Medicaid, participating physicians may bill patients for the remaining amount of the charges.

_____ 5. Providers in capitated managed care plans must still submit claims to Medicaid.

_____ 6. Crossover claims are submitted to Medicare first, and then to Medicaid.

_____ 7. Individuals must receive financial assistance from the federal government to qualify for Medicaid.

_____ 8. Medicaid benefits differ from state to state.

_____ 9. The SCHIP is fully funded by individual states, without funds from the federal government.

_____ 10. States may extend health insurance coverage to groups excluded by Welfare Reform Act legislation.

Write the letter choice that best completes the statement or answers the question.

_____ 1. Applicants who have high medical bills and whose incomes exceed state limits may be eligible for health care coverage under a state _____ program.
   A. TANF
   B. categorically needy
   C. restricted status
   D. medically needy

_____ 2. Under the Federal Medicaid Assistance Program, the government makes payment directly to
   A. states
   B. individuals eligible to receive TANF
   C. individuals who are blind or disabled
   D. categorically needy individuals

_____ 3. Most individuals receiving TANF payments are limited to a _____-year benefit period.
   A. two
   B. five
   C. seven
   D. ten

_____ 4. Medicaid identification cards must be checked for eligibility
   A. once a year
   B. every six months
   C. only when there is a change in the patient's address
   D. every time the patient receives services

_____ 5. Persons classified as restricted status
   A. must select a provider within the network
   B. receive a limited set of benefits
   C. receive only emergency care
   D. must see a specific provider for treatment

_____ 6. If family planning services are provided to a patient, what data element is affected?
   A. family planning indicator
   B. the dollar amount of the charge
   C. HCPCS codes
   D. ICD-9 codes

_____ 7. If services were provided in an emergency room, what place of service code is reported?
   A. 24C
   B. 18
   C. 24i
   D. 23

_____ 8. The Medicaid Alliance for Program Safeguards
   A. specifies civil and criminal penalties for fraudulent activities
   B. audits state Medicaid payers on a regular basis
   C. is a CMS program that came about as a result of the Welfare Reform Act
   D. oversees states' fraud and abuse efforts

_____ 9. The national committee to coordinate Medicaid data elements on health care claims is called
   A. NMEH
   B. NUBC
   C. EDI
   D. HIPAA

_____ 10. Individuals apply for Medicaid benefits by contacting
   A. the Department of Health and Human Services
   B. the local Income Maintenance office
   C. the Federal Medicaid Assistance Program
   D. the insurance carrier that processes Medicaid claims in their state

Provide an answer to the following question.

What steps should be taken to verify a patient's Medicaid eligibility?

Applying your Knowledge

The objective of these two cases is to correctly complete a claim, applying what you have learned in the chapter to each case situation. Each case consists of two sections. The first section contains information about the patient, the insurance coverage, and the current medical condition. The second section is an encounter form from Valley Associates, P.C.

If you are using NDCMedisoft to complete the cases, read the Guide to NDCMedisoft before beginning. Information from the first section, the patient information form, has already been entered in the program for you. You must enter information from the second section, the encounter form, to complete the claim. If you are gaining experience by completing a paper CMS-1500 claim form, follow the instructions on page 434.

The following provider information, which is also available in the NDCMedisSoft database, should be used for the case studies in Chapter 12.

Provider Information

Name:	David Rosenberg, M.D.
Practice Name:	Valley Associates, P.C.
Address:	1400 West Center Street Toledo, OH 43601-0213
Phone:	555-321-0987
Employer ID Number	06-2345678
Medicaid PIN:	OH5678
Assignment:	Accepts
Physician Signature:	On File (1-1-2005)

Case 12.1

From the Patient Information Form:

Name	Mary Pascale
Sex	F
Birth Date	03/22/1984
SSN	246-71-0348
Address	412 Main St., apt. 2A Shaker Heights, OH 44118-2345
Telephone	555-324-6669
Employer	Unemployed
Insurance Plan	Medicaid
Member ID	246710348MC
Copayment Amount	$15
Assignment of Benefits	Y
Signature on File	Y (10-1-2008)

Condition unrelated to Employment, Auto Accident, or Other Accident

VALLEY ASSOCIATES, P.C.
David Rosenberg, M.D. - Dermatology
555-321-0987
FED I.D. #06-2345678

PATIENT NAME		APPT. DATE/TIME	
Mary Pascale		10/14/2008	10:30pm
PATIENT NO.		**DX**	
PASCAMA0		1. 693.1 contact dermatitis due to food 2. 3. 4.	

DESCRIPTION	✓	CPT	FEE	DESCRIPTION	✓	CPT	FEE
EXAMINATION				**PROCEDURES**			
New Patient				Acne Surgery		10040	
Problem Focused		99201		I&D Cyst/Abscess		10060	
Expanded Problem Focused		99202		I&D Multiple		10061	
Detailed		99203		I&D Remove Foreign Body		10120	
Comprehensive		99204		Debridement		11000	
Comprehensive/Complex		99205		Paring/Curett. (Benign)		11055	
Established Patient				Paring/Curett. (2-4)		11056	
Minimum		99211		Paring/Curett. (Over 4)		11057	
Problem Focused	✓	99212	28	Excision Skin Tags (1-15)		11200	
Expanded Problem Focused		99213		Cyrosurgery		17340	
Detailed		99214		Skin Biopsy		11000	
Comprehensive/Complex		99215		Skin Biopsy (EA additional)		+11101	

Case 12.2

From the Patient Information Form:

Name	Scott Yeager
Sex	M
Birth Date	11/17/1982
SSN	139-62-9748
Address	301 Maple Ave. Sandusky, OH 44870-4567
Telephone	555-619-7341
Employer	Unemployed
Insurance Plan	Medicaid
Member ID	139629748MC
Copayment Amount	$15
Assignment of Benefits	Y
Signature on File	Y (10-1-2008)

Condition unrelated to Employment, Auto Accident, or Other Accident

---

VALLEY ASSOCIATES, P.C.
David Rosenberg, M.D. - Dermatology
555-321-0987
FED I.D. #06-2345678

PATIENT NAME			APPT. DATE/TIME		
Scott Yeager			10/14/2008 11:00am		
PATIENT NO.			**DX**		
YEAGESC0			1. 919.7 superficial foreign body without 2. open wound, superficial 3. 4.		

DESCRIPTION	✓	CPT	FEE	DESCRIPTION	✓	CPT	FEE
EXAMINATION				**PROCEDURES**			
New Patient				Acne Surgery		10040	
Problem Focused		99201		I&D Cyst/Abscess		10060	
Expanded Problem Focused	✓	99202	50	I&D Multiple		10061	
Detailed		99203		I&D Remove Foreign Body	✓	10120	60
Comprehensive		99204		Debridement		11000	
Comprehensive/Complex		99205		Paring/Curett. (Benign)		11055	
Established Patient				Paring/Curett. (2-4)		11056	
Minimum		99211		Paring/Curett. (Over 4)		11057	
Problem Focused		99212		Excision Skin Tags (1-15)		11200	
Expanded Problem Focused		99213		Cyrosurgery		17340	
Detailed		99214		Skin Biopsy		11000	
Comprehensive/Complex		99215		Skin Biopsy (EA additional)		+11101	

Computer Exploration

1. Point your Web browser at the official Web site for California's MediCal program:

    http://www.medi-cal.ca.gov

    Look for publications that describe eligibility requirements. Also look up current information regarding HIPAA updates. What are some of the challenges unique to Medicaid HIPAA compliance?

2. Go to the Centers for Medicare and Medicaid Services Web site for Medicaid:

    http://www.cms.gov/medicaid/

    Select the *Gov't Info* link. Read the overview of the Medicaid program. Also look up information on the Medicaid program in your state. Has the SCHIP program in your state expanded in recent years?

3. Go to the Medicaid Alliance for Program Safeguards home page at the Centers for Medicare and Medicaid Services Web site:

    http://www.cms.gov/states/fraud/

    Select the underlined link at the bottom of the page for Medicaid Alliance for Program Safeguards Background. How has CMS's role evolved in overseeing states' fraud and abuse efforts? Select the underlined link for guidance and reports. Locate information about preventing Medicaid fraud and abuse in a managed care environment.

NDCMediSoft Activity

12.1 Review MediSoft Entries Specific to Medicaid

This activity explores various entries in MediSoft for a patient whose primary insurance carrier is Medicaid.

1. Alan Harcar is covered by a Medicaid managed care plan. Open the Lists menu and select Patients/Guarantors and Cases.

2. In the Search For box, key HA to display Alan Harcar's information in the Patient List dialog box.

3. Click the Edit Patient button to display the Name, Address tab.

4. Note that Alan Harcar's Social Security Number, displayed at the bottom of the box, is 321-60-5549. Click the Other Information to display Alan Harcar's employment information.

5. The bottom panel of the Other Information tab shows Alan Harcar's employment status as "Not employed." Click the Cancel button to close the Patient/Guarantor dialog box and return to the Patient List dialog box.

6. In the right side of the Patient List dialog box, click Alan Harcar's Upper Respiratory Infection case to select it, and then click the Edit Case button.

7. In the Case dialog box that is displayed, click the Policy 1 tab.

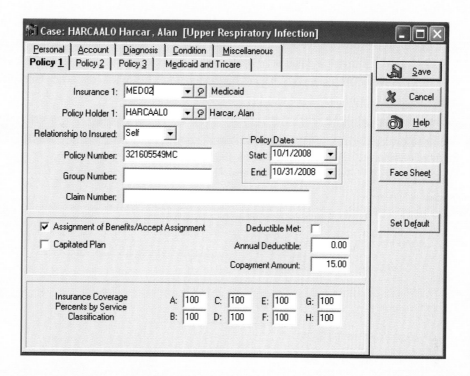

8. The Policy 1 tab shows that Medicaid is the primary carrier. Note that Alan Harcar's policy number, 321605549MC, is based on his Social Security Number. The Policy 1 tab also indicates that there is a no annual deductible and a copay of $15 per visit. The Insurance Coverage Percents by Service Classification boxes at the bottom of the tab indicate that Medicaid pays for 100 percent of covered services.

Click the Account tab.

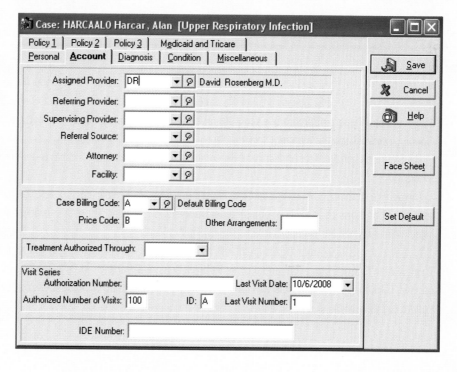

9. In the Account tab, the Price Code box reads B. In the Valley Associates, P.C. sample database, Price Code B represents the Medicare Fee Schedule. Medicare and Medicaid are the only insurance carriers that use Price Code B in this sample database. As illustrated in the NDCMediSoft activity in the previous chapter, the Price Code setting determines the amount charged for procedures in the Transaction Entry dialog box.

Click the Medicaid and Tricare tab.

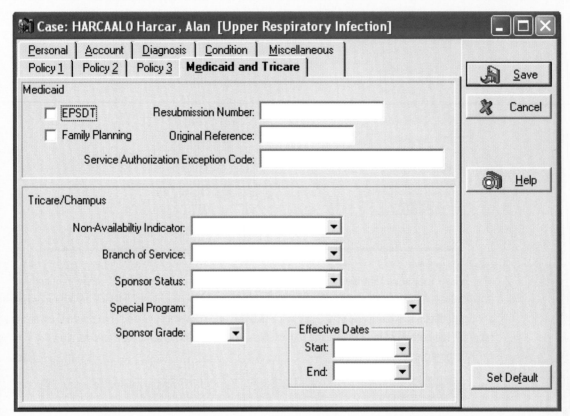

10. The top panel in the Medicaid and Tricare tab is used to record information that is specific to certain Medicaid claims. The EPST box is checked if a patient's visit is part of the Early and Periodic Screening, Diagnosis, and Treatment program, a program for patients under the age of 21. Similarly, the Family Planning box is checked if a patient's visit is part of that program.

The Resubmission Number and Original Reference boxes are used when a claim is being resubmitted to Medicaid.

The Service Authorization Exception Code is used on some Medicaid claims to describe the reason a service authorization code was not obtained before seeing the patient. There are seven exemption codes, including 1—Immediate/Urgent Care and 3—Emergency Care.

In Alan Harcar's case, these boxes are blank, as none of the circumstances apply to his claim.

11. To view Alan Harcar's procedure and payment transactions, the Transaction Entry dialog box needs to be opened. Click the Cancel button to close the Case dialog box, and then click the Close button to close the Patient List dialog box.

12. Click Enter Transactions in the Activities menu. To display Alan Harcar's transaction information, key HA in the Chart box, and press Enter.

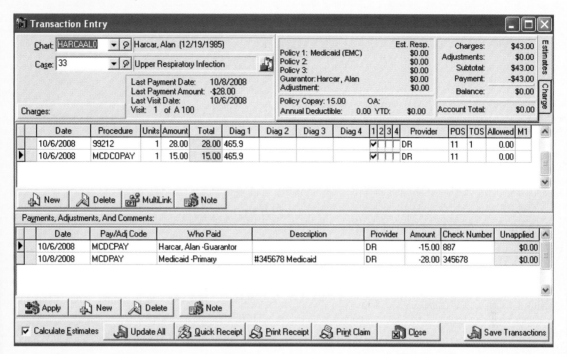

13. Study the procedures and payments in the Transaction Entry dialog box. Alan Harcar currently has a zero balance. This is because he made a copayment on the day of the visit, and because a claim was submitted for procedure 99212 (using Price Code B, this procedure is billed at $28), which Medicaid paid in full.

14. Click the Close button to exit the Transaction Entry dialog box.

TRICARE and CHAMPVA

CHAPTER OUTLINE

Objectives

After studying this chapter, you should be able to:

1. Discuss the eligibility requirements for TRICARE.
2. Compare TRICARE participating and nonparticipating providers.
3. Describe a situation in which a nonavailability statement is required.
4. Explain how the TRICARE Standard, TRICARE Prime, and TRICARE Extra programs differ.
5. Discuss the TRICARE for Life program.
6. Discuss the eligibility requirements for CHAMPVA.
7. Prepare correct TRICARE and CHAMPVA claims.

Introduction

TRICARE is the Department of Defense's health insurance plan for military personnel and their families. Implementation of this program began in 1995 and was completed in 1998. TRICARE, which includes managed care options, replaced the program known as **CHAMPUS**, the Civilian Health and Medical Program of the Uniformed Services.

The TRICARE program brings the resources of military hospitals together with a network of civilian facilities and providers to offer increased access to health care services. All military treatment facilities, including hospitals and clinics, are part of the TRICARE system. TRICARE also contracts with civilian facilities and physicians to provide more extensive services to beneficiaries.

Eligibility

Members of the following uniformed services and their families are eligible for TRICARE: the Army, Navy, Air Force, Marine Corps, Coast Guard, Public Health Service (PHS), and National Oceanic and Atmospheric Administration (NOAA). Reserve and National Guard personnel become eligible when on active duty for more than thirty consecutive days or on retirement from reserve status at age sixty. The uniformed services member is referred to as a **sponsor**, since the member's status makes other family members eligible for TRICARE coverage.

When a TRICARE patient arrives for treatment, the medical information specialist photocopies both sides of the individual's military ID card and checks the expiration date to confirm that coverage is still valid (see Figure 13.1). Decisions about eligibility are not made by TRICARE; the various branches of military service make them. Information about patient eligibility is stored in the **Defense Enrollment Eligibility Reporting System (DEERS)**. Sponsors may contact DEERS to verify eligibility; providers may not contact DEERS directly because the information is protected by the Privacy Act.

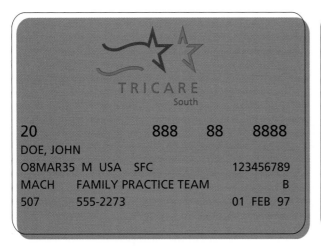
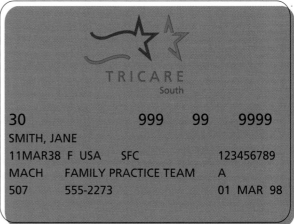

FIGURE 13.1 Sample Military Identification Cards

Provider Participation and Nonparticipation

TRICARE pays only for services rendered by authorized providers. Authorized providers are certified by TRICARE regional contractors to have met specific educational, licensing, and other requirements. Once authorized, a provider is assigned a PIN and must decide whether to participate.

Participating Providers

Providers who participate agree to accept the TRICARE allowable charge as payment in full for services. Individual providers may decide whether to participate on a case-by-case basis. Participating providers are required to file claims on behalf of patients. The regional TRICARE contractor sends payment directly to the provider, and the provider collects the patient's share of the charges. Only participating providers may appeal claims decisions.

Nonparticipating Providers

A provider who chooses not to participate may not charge more than 115 percent of the allowable charge. If a provider bills more than 115 percent, the patient may refuse to pay the excess amount. For example, if the allowed charge for a procedure is $50.00, a nonparticipating provider may not charge more than $57.50 (115 percent of $50.00). If a nonparticipating provider were to charge $75.00 for the same procedure, the patient could refuse to pay the amount that exceeds 115 percent of the allowed amount. The difference of $17.50 would have to be written off by the provider. The patient would pay the cost-share (either 20 or 25 percent) of the total charge up to the allowable charge. **Cost-share** is the TRICARE term for the amount of the charges that are the responsibility of the patient, or the coinsurance.

Once the provider submits the claim, TRICARE pays its portion of the allowable charges, but instead of going directly to the provider, the payment is mailed to the patient. The patient is responsible for paying the provider. Payment should be collected at the time of the visit.

Reimbursement

Providers who participate in the basic TRICARE plan are paid the amount specified in the Medicare Fee Schedule for most procedures. Medical supplies, durable medical equipment, and ambulance services are not subject to Medicare limits. The maximum amount TRICARE will pay for a procedure is known as the CHAMPUS Maximum Allowable Charge (CMAC). Providers are responsible for collecting the patients' deductible and their cost-share portion of the charges.

Network and Nonnetwork Providers

Providers who are authorized to treat TRICARE patients may also contract to become part of the TRICARE network. These providers serve patients in one of TRICARE's managed care plans. They agree to provide care to beneficiaries at contracted rates, and to participate on all claims in TRICARE's managed care programs.

Providers who choose not to join the network may still provide care to managed care patients, but TRICARE will not pay for the services. The patient is 100 percent responsible for the charges.

TRICARE Standard

TRICARE offers beneficiaries access to three different health care plans. **TRICARE Standard** is a fee-for-service program that replaces the CHAMPUS program, which was also fee-for-service. The program covers medical services provided by a civilian physician when the individual cannot receive treatment from a **Military Treatment Facility (MTF)**. Military families may receive services at an MTF, but the services offered vary by facility, and first priority is given to service members on active duty. When service is not available, the individual seeks treatment from a civilian provider, and TRICARE Standard benefits go into effect.

Costs

Under TRICARE Standard, medical expenses are shared between TRICARE and the beneficiary. Most enrollees pay an annual deductible. In addition, families of active-duty members pay 20 percent of outpatient charges. Retirees and their families, former spouses, and families of deceased personnel pay a 25 percent cost-share for outpatient services. If a beneficiary is treated by a provider who does not accept assignment, he or she is also responsible for the provider's additional charges, up to 115 percent of the allowable charge. See Figure 13.2 for cost-share details.

ACTIVE-DUTY FAMILY MEMBERS			
	TRICARE Prime	**TRICARE Extra**	**TRICARE Standard**
Annual Deductible	None	$150/individual or $300/family for E-5 & above; $50/$100 for E-4 & below	$150/individual or $300/family for E-5 & above; $50/$100 for E-4 & below
Annual Enrollment Fee	None	None	None
Civilian Outpatient Visit	No cost	15% of negotiated fee	20% of allowed charges for covered service
Civilian Inpatient Admission	No cost	Greater of $25 or $12.72/day	Greater of $25 or $12.72/day
Civilian Inpatient Mental Health	No cost	$20/day	$20/day
RETIREES, THEIR FAMILY MEMBERS, AND OTHERS			
	TRICARE Prime	**TRICARE Extra**	**TRICARE Standard**
Annual Deductible	None	$150/individual or $300/family	$150/individual or $300 family
Annual Enrollment Fee	$230/individual $460/family	None	None
Civilian Provider Copays:		20% of negotiated fee	25% of allowed charges for covered services
—Outpatient Visit	$12		
—Emergency Care	$30		
—Mental Health Visit	$25; $17 for group visit		
Civilian Inpatient Cost-Share	$11/day ($25 minimum)	Lesser of $250/day or 25% of negotiated charges plus 20% of negotiated professional fees	Lesser of $417/day or 25% of billed charges plus 25% of allowed professional fees
Civilian Inpatient Mental Health	$40/day	20% of institutional & negotiated professional fees	Lesser of $159/day or 25% of allowable fees

FIGURE 13.2 **Cost-Shares for TRICARE Standard Enrollees**

Patient cost-share payments are subject to an annual **catastrophic cap**, a limit on the total medical expenses that beneficiaries are required to pay in one year. For active-duty families, the annual cap is $1,000, while for all other beneficiaries the limit is $3,000. Once these caps have been met, TRICARE pays 100 percent of additional charges for covered services for that coverage year.

Covered Services

The following services are examples of services covered under TRICARE Standard:

- Ambulatory surgery
- Diagnostic testing
- Durable medical equipment
- Family planning
- Hospice care
- Inpatient care
- Laboratory and pathology services
- Maternity care
- Outpatient care
- Prescription drugs and medicines
- Surgery
- Well-child care (birth to seventeen years)
- X-ray services

TRICARE Standard also provides many preventive benefits for enrollees, including immunizations, Pap smears, mammograms, and screening examinations for colon and prostate cancer.

Noncovered Services

TRICARE Standard generally does not cover the following services:

- Cosmetic drugs and cosmetic surgery
- Custodial care
- Unproven (experimental) procedures or treatments
- Routine physical examinations
- Routine foot care

Hospital Care and Nonavailability Statements

Individuals must first seek care at a military treatment facility. If an individual lives within a certain distance of a military hospital, generally within a forty-mile radius, a nonavailability statement must be filed by the local military hospital before the patient can be treated at a civilian hospital for inpatient nonemergency care. A **nonavailability statement** (NAS) is an electronic document stating that the service the patient requires is not available at the nearby military treatment facility. The form is electronically transmitted to the DEERS database. If it is not filed, TRICARE will not pay the hospital claim. If the patient has other insurance that is primary to TRICARE, a NAS is not required. In addition, emergency services do not require a nonavailability statement.

Preauthorization Requirements

TRICARE Standard does not require outpatient nonavailability statements, except for outpatient prenatal and postpartum maternity care. A number of procedures do require preauthorization, including

- Arthroscopy
- Cardiac catheterization
- Upper gastrointestinal endoscopy
- MRI
- Tonsillectomy or adenoidectomy
- Cataract removal
- Hernia repair

TRICARE Prime

TRICARE Prime is a managed care plan similar to an HMO. After enrolling in the plan, individuals are assigned a **Primary Care Manager (PCM)** who coordinates and manages their medical care. The PCM may be a single military or civilian provider, or a group of providers. In addition to most of the benefits offered by TRICARE Standard, TRICARE Prime offers preventive care, including routine physical examinations. Active-duty service members are automatically enrolled in TRICARE Prime. TRICARE Prime enrollees receive the majority of their health care services from military treatment facilities and receive priority at these facilities.

Individuals who are not active-duty family members must pay an annual enrollment fee of $230 for an individual or $460 for a family to join the TRICARE Prime program. Under TRICARE Prime, there is no deductible, and no payment is required for outpatient treatment at a military facility. For active-duty family members, no payment is required for visits to civilian network providers, but for other beneficiaries, different copayments apply depending on the type of visit. For example, for retirees and their family members, outpatient visits with a civilian provider require a $12 copayment.

TRICARE Extra

TRICARE Extra is an alternative managed care plan for individuals who want to receive services primarily from civilian facilities and physicians rather than from military facilities. Since it is a managed care plan, individuals must receive health care services from a network of health care professionals. They may also seek treatment at a military facility, but active-duty personnel and other TRICARE Prime enrollees receive priority at those facilities, so care may not always be available.

TRICARE Extra is more expensive than TRICARE Prime, but less costly than TRICARE Standard. There is no enrollment fee, but there is an annual deductible of $150 for an individual and $300 for a family. TRICARE Extra beneficiaries pay 15 percent (5 percent less than TRICARE Standard enrollees) for civilian outpatient charges. Beneficiaries are not subject to additional charges of up to 115 percent of the allowable charge, since participating physicians agree to accept TRICARE's fee schedule.

TRICARE and Other Insurance Plans

If the individual has other health insurance coverage that is primary to TRICARE, that insurance carrier must be billed first. TRICARE is a secondary payer in almost all circumstances; among the few exceptions is Medicaid.

Many TRICARE beneficiaries purchase supplemental insurance policies to help pay deductible and cost-share or copayment fees. Most military associations offer supplementary plans, and so do private insurers. Supplemental plans are not regulated by TRICARE, so coverage varies. TRICARE is the primary payer; the purpose of a supplemental policy is simply to pick up the costs not paid by TRICARE.

TRICARE for Life

The Department of Defense offers a program for Medicare-eligible military retirees and Medicare-eligible family members called **TRICARE for Life**. Originally introduced in a trial program as TRICARE Senior Prime, TRICARE for Life offers the opportunity to receive health care at a military treatment facility to individuals age sixty-five and over who are eligible for both Medicare and TRICARE.

In the past, individuals became ineligible for TRICARE once they reached age sixty-five, and they were required to enroll in Medicare to obtain any health care coverage. Beneficiaries could still seek treatment at military treatment facilities, but only if space was available. Under TRICARE for Life, enrollees in TRICARE who are age sixty-five and over can continue to obtain medical services at military hospitals and clinics as they did before they turned sixty-five. TRICARE for Life acts as a secondary payer to Medicare; Medicare pays first and the remaining out-of-pocket expenses are paid by TRICARE. Claims are filed automatically.

Benefits are similar to those of a Medicare HMO, with an emphasis on preventive and wellness services. Prescription drug benefits are also included in TRICARE for Life. All enrollees in TRICARE for Life must be enrolled in Medicare Parts A and B and must have Part B premiums deducted from their Social Security check. (Individuals already enrolled in a Medicare HMO may not participate in TRICARE for Life.). Other than Medicare costs, TRICARE for Life beneficiaries pay no enrollment fees and no cost-share fees for inpatient or outpatient care at a military facility. Treatment at a civilian network facility requires a copay.

Filing Claims

Participating providers file claims on behalf of patients. Claims are filed with the contractor for their region. Claims are submitted to the regional contractor based on the patient's home address, not the location of the facility. Contact information for regional contractors is available on the TRICARE Web site at http://www.tricare.osd.mil. Individuals file their own claims when services are received from a nonparticipating provider, using DD Form 2642, Patient's Request for Medical Payment. A copy of the itemized bill from the provider must be attached to the form.

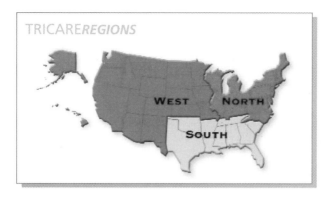

FIGURE 13.3 TRICARE Regions Map

In 2003, in an effort to simplify the administration of the TRICARE program, the Department of Defense made plans to collapse its eleven administration regions into three (see Figure 13.3). The new regions, phased in during 2004, are referred to as TRICARE North, TRICARE South, and TRICARE West. Each region is represented by one of three TRICARE contractors selected to replace the previous seven contractors. The exact perimeters of each region may change, so they should be verified through the TRICARE Web site before claims are sent.

Billing Tip

Claim Filing Deadline
TRICARE claims must be filed within one year of the date the service was provided.

HIPAA and TRICARE

The Military Health System (MHS) and the TRICARE health plan are required to comply with the HIPAA privacy policies and procedures for the use and disclosure of PHI. The MHS's Notice of Privacy Practices, which describes how a patient's medical information may be used and disclosed and how a patient can access the information, is posted at the TRICARE Web site at http://www.tricare.osd.mil.hipaa/. The HIPAA Electronic Health Care Transactions and Code Sets requirements, as well as the Security Rule, must also be followed.

Guidelines for Completing the CMS-1500

If a CMS-1500 paper claim is needed, follow the guidelines on pages 451–452.

TRICARE	
Form Locator	**Data**
1	Select CHAMPUS.
1a	Sponsor's Social Security number.
2	Patient's name.
3	Patient's eight-digit date of birth and gender.
4	Sponsor's full name, unless the sponsor is also the patient, in which case enter "Same."
5	Patient's address and phone number.
6	Patient's relationship to the sponsor.
7	If the sponsor is on active duty, enter the duty address; if retired, the home address.
8	Patient's marital and employment status.
9	Enter "None."
10a–c	If any of the boxes in 10a–c is selected, it may be necessary to file DD Form 2527, Statement of Personal Injury—Possible Third Party Liability. If the patient was treated at a hospital for an injury possibly due to a third party, or if the patient was treated in a physician's office for a possible third-party liability injury and the charges are $500 or more, the form must be filed.
11	Enter "None."
11a–c	Blank.

TRICARE (continued)

Form Locator	Data
11d	Choose Yes or No.
12	Yes, unless there is no patient contact at the time of service, for example, if laboratory tests are conducted by an outside laboratory. In these cases, enter "Patient not present."
13 – 16	Blank.
17 and 17a	Name and identification number of the referring provider or institution.
18	Hospital admission and discharge dates in eight-digit format (MMDDCCYY). If the patient has been admitted but not yet discharged, enter the admission date in From, and leave To blank.
19	Blank.
20	Yes or No.
21	Appropriate ICD codes.
22	Not required.
23	If a preauthorization other than a nonavailability indicator is required, attach a copy of the form.
24a	Date of service (eight-digit format).
24b	Place of service code.
24c	Type of service code.
24d	Appropriate CPT/HCPCS codes and any modifiers.
24e	Diagnosis key number for CPT/HCPCS codes.
24f	Amount charged.
24g	Appropriate days/units reported.
24h	Blank.
24i	Enter X if services were provided in a hospital emergency room.
24j	Blank, unless services on this claim were rendered by more than one provider. If services were rendered by more than one provider, check this box and complete form locator 24k.
24k	Enter the provider identification number of the provider who performed the procedure listed in 24a.
25	Make the appropriate selection, and enter the tax ID.
26	Optional; patient account number.
27	Choose Yes or No.
28	Total charges.
29 and 30	Blank.
31	Check with the carrier to see if an actual signature is required.
32	If the services on this claim were performed at a location other than the provider's office or the patient's home, enter the name and address of the facility where services were performed. Otherwise, enter "Same."
33	Billing provider's name, address, phone number, provider identification number, and group number.

When TRICARE is the secondary payer, six form locators on a paper claim are filled in differently than when TRICARE is the primary payer:

TRICARE (continued)

Form Locator	Data
11	Policy number of the primary insurance plan.
11a	Birth date and gender of the primary plan policyholder.
11b	Employer of the primary plan policyholder if the plan is a group plan through an employer.
11c	Name of the primary insurance plan.
11d	Select Yes or No as appropriate..
29	Enter all payments made by other insurance carriers. Do not include payments made by the patient.

Fraud and Abuse

The Program Integrity Office oversees the fraud and abuse program for TRICARE, working with the Office of the Inspector General Defense Criminal Investigative Service (DCIS) to identify and prosecute cases of TRICARE fraud and abuse. In 2001, $11.3 million was returned to the Department of Defense as a result of successful prosecution of fraudulent TRICARE payments to providers. The Fraud and Abuse link on the TRICARE Web site (http://www.tricare.osd.mil/fraud/) displays a list of frequently asked questions, news releases on fraud and abuse cases, and the names of providers who were prosecuted or sanctioned for committing health care fraud.

TRICARE providers are also subject to a quality and utilization review similar to the process used by Medicare. A qualified independent contractor (QIC) reviews claims, documentation, and records to ensure that services were medically necessary and appropriate, that procedures were coded appropriately, and that care was up to professional medical standards.

Some examples of activities considered fraudulent include

- Billing for services, supplies, or equipment not furnished or used by the beneficiary
- Billing for costs of noncovered services, supplies, or equipment disguised as covered items
- Billing more than once for the same service
- Billing TRICARE and the enrollee for the same services
- Submitting claims to TRICARE and other third-party payers without reporting payments already made
- Changing dates of service, frequency of service, or names of recipients
- Altering CPT codes to increase the amount of payment to the provider

Some examples of abusive activities include

- Failure to maintain adequate clinical documentation or financial records
- Recurrent instances of waiving beneficiary cost-share payments
- Charging TRICARE beneficiaries fees that exceed those commonly charged the general public
- Recurrent instances of submitting claims for services that are not medically necessary, or not necessary to the extent provided
- Care that is of inferior quality

Fraudulent and abusive activities can result in sanctions, exclusion from the TRICARE program, or civil or criminal penalties.

CHAMPVA

The **Civilian Health and Medical Program of the Department of Veterans Affairs (CHAMPVA)** is the government's health insurance program for veterans with a 100 percent service-related disability and their families. Under the program, health care expenses are shared between the Department of Veterans Affairs (VA) and the beneficiary.

The Veterans Health Care Eligibility Reform Act of 1996 requires veterans with a 100 percent disability to be enrolled in the program to receive benefits. Prior to this legislation, enrollment was not required.

Eligibility

The VA is responsible for determining eligibility for the CHAMPVA program. Eligible beneficiaries include

- Dependents of a veteran who is totally and permanently disabled due to a service-connected injury
- Dependents of a veteran who was totally and permanently disabled due to a service-connected condition at the time of death
- Survivors of a veteran who died as a result of a service-related disability
- Survivors of a veteran who died in the line of duty

CHAMPVA Authorization Card

Each eligible beneficiary possesses a CHAMPVA Authorization Card, known as an A-Card. The provider's office checks this card to determine eligibility and photocopies the front and back for inclusion in the patient record.

Covered Services

CHAMPVA provides coverage for most medically necessary services. The following is a partial list of services that are covered:

- **Inpatient services**
  Room and board
  Hospital services
  Surgical procedures
  Physician services
  Anesthesia
  Blood and blood products
  Diagnostic tests and procedures
  Cardiac rehabilitation programs
  Chemotherapy
  Occupational therapy
  Physical therapy
  Prescription medications
  Speech therapy
  Mental health care

- **Outpatient services**
  Maternity care
  Family planning
  Cancer screenings
  Cholesterol screenings
  HIV testing
  Immunizations
  Well-child care up to age six
  Prescription medications
  Durable medical equipment
  Mental health care
  Ambulance services
  Diagnostic tests
  Hospice services

Excluded Services

The following services are generally not covered by CHAMPVA:

- Medically unnecessary services and supplies
- Experimental or investigational procedures
- Custodial care
- Dental care (with some exceptions)

Preauthorization

Some procedures must be approved in advance, or CHAMPVA will not pay for them. It is the patient's responsibility, not the provider's, to obtain preauthorization.

A partial list of procedures that require preauthorization includes:

- Mental health and substance abuse services
- Organ and bone marrow transplants
- Dental care
- Hospice services
- Durable medical equipment in excess of $300

CHAMPVA enrollees do not need to obtain nonavailability statements, since they are not eligible to receive service in a military treatment facility (a VA hospital is not considered a military treatment facility).

Participating Providers

For most services, CHAMPVA does not contract with providers. Beneficiaries may receive care from the provider of their choice, as long as that provider is properly licensed to perform the services being delivered and is not on the Medicare exclusion list. For mental health treatment, CHAMPVA maintains a list of approved providers.

Providers who treat CHAMPVA patients are prohibited from charging more than the CHAMPVA allowable amounts. Providers agree to accept CHAMPVA payment and the patient's cost-share payment as payment in full for services. Figure 13.4 (on page 456) illustrates an online CHAMPVA provider newsletter, a resource for updating CHAMPVA information in the medical practice.

Costs

Most persons enrolled in CHAMPVA pay an annual deductible and a portion of their health care charges. Some services are exempt from the deductible and cost-share requirement. Patients' out-of-pocket costs are subject to a catastrophic cap of $3,000 per calendar year. Once the beneficiary has paid $3,000 in medical bills for the year, CHAMPVA pays claims for covered services at 100 percent for the rest of that year.

For 2002, the annual deductible was $50 per person up to $100 per family. The cost-share percentages were 75 percent for CHAMPVA, and 25 percent for the beneficiary. Beneficiaries are also responsible for the costs of health care services not covered by CHAMPVA.

CHAMPVA and Other Health Insurance Plans

When the individual has other health insurance benefits in addition to CHAMPVA, CHAMPVA is almost always the secondary payer. Two exceptions are

Health Administration Center

Department of Veterans Affairs

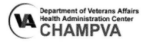
Department of Veterans Affairs
Health Administration Center
CHAMPVA

Provider News - Winter 2000

This site is designed specifically for CHAMPVA healthcare providers. In addition to important program announcements, this site offers time-saving claim tips. At a minimum, it will be updated semiannually during the months of December and June.

GENERAL ANNOUNCEMENTS

Glucose Monitor Recall

A manufacturer of blood glucose monitors is recalling and replacing some of its home blood glucose meters because of possible malfunctions. The malfunctions could cause users to fail to recognize seriously high blood glucose levels. Lifescan, Inc., announced the recall and free replacement of its SureStep meters that were manufactured before August 1997-serial numbers L6000 through L7205 and L7206-GA-00001 through 01128. Call 1-800-951-7226 immediately for more information and/or replacement.

Services

Please note that we do not automatically pay for Evaluation and Management services appended by modifier -25...appropriate documentation based on CPT guidelines must be present. If denied, you can resubmit the claim by attaching a progress note or other appropriate documentation for the date of the service.

Valid Codes

Consistent with the industry practice, claims must include codes and those codes must be valid for the date of the service-or they will be denied. New CPT and HCPCS codes are generally effective in January, while updated ICD codes are usually available in October.

New EOB

The new Explanation of Benefits (EOB) form includes modifications specifically designed to help you reconcile our Explanation of Benefits with your accounts receivables. Please take some time to review the sample, noting in particular the narrative descriptions.

Sample EOB: jpg format
Sample EOB: pdf format

Still having trouble identifying our payments?

Although we believe our new EOB makes it easier than ever before to match a CHAMPVA payment check with a particular claim, we do recognize that there may be times when identification is still difficult. While returning an unidentifiable check or one that appears to be a duplicate may occasionally be necessary, in most cases, careful review of the EOB should clarify the payment. In any case, please don't return a check without contacting us first at 303-331-7599-or FAX us a copy of the check with a brief note at 303-331-7804. In most cases, we should be able to clarify the payment and, thus, avoid the timely process of returning the check not to mention the cost of reissuing it.

FIGURE 13.4 CHAMPVA Provider News

Medicaid and supplemental policies purchased to cover deductibles, cost-shares, and other services.

Insurance claims are filed first with the primary payer. When the remittance advice from the primary plan arrives, a copy of it is attached to the claim that is then filed with CHAMPVA.

Medical billing managers, also called billing supervisors, supervise a staff of medical billers and collections specialists. Billing managers may be employed by medical group practices, hospitals, managed care organizations, and other facilities.

Medical billing managers are responsible for the quality and the quantity of the billing work that is done. They must have excellent supervisory skills for interviewing, hiring, and evaluating staff as well as planning the staff members' workload, assigning tasks, following up, and reviewing progress. Billing managers need strong computer applications skills and analytical ability in order to monitor accounts receivable. They are also required to know collection procedures, diagnostic and procedural coding,

and reimbursement under both fee-for-service and capitation contracts. Excellent communication and human relations skills are needed to resolve payer-related issues. Managers also educate physicians and other staff members about reimbursement issues and compliance requirements. They may be assigned to monitor fee schedules and to check the reimbursement sections of managed care contracts.

Success as a medical biller and additional college education in accounting, management, and supervision are often required for the position of billing manager. Employers hiring billing managers in specialized areas such as ophthalmology or radiology billing prefer candidates with a billing background in the medical specialty.

Persons under age sixty-five who are eligible for Medicare benefits and who are enrolled in Parts A and B may also enroll in CHAMPVA.

CHAMPVA for Life

CHAMPVA for Life extends CHAMPVA benefits to spouses or dependents who are age sixty-five and over. Similar to TRICARE for Life, CHAMPVA for Life benefits are payable after payment by Medicare or other third-party payers. Eligible beneficiaries must be sixty-five or older and enrolled in Medicare Parts A and B. For services not covered by Medicare, such as outpatient prescription medications, CHAMPVA acts as the primary payer.

Filing Claims

The CHAMPVA program is covered by HIPAA regulations. Most CHAMPVA claims are filed by the provider and submitted to the centralized CHAMPVA claims processing center in Denver, Colorado. The information required on a claim is the same as the information required for TRICARE.

In instances in which beneficiaries are filing their own claims, CHAMPVA Claim Form (VA Form 10-7959A) must be used. The claim must always be accompanied by an itemized bill from the provider. Claims must be filed within one year of the date of service or discharge.

Review

Chapter Summary

1. Members of the Army, Navy, Air Force, Marine Corps, Coast Guard, Public Health Service, and National Oceanic and Atmospheric Administration and their families are eligible for TRICARE. Reserve and National Guard personnel become eligible when on active duty for more than thirty consecutive days or on retirement from reserve status at age sixty.

2. Providers who participate accept the TRICARE allowable charge as payment in full for services. Participating providers are required to file claims on behalf of patients. Participating providers may appeal a decision. Nonparticipating providers may not charge more than 115 percent of the allowable charge and may not appeal a claims decision. The patient pays the provider, and TRICARE pays its portion of the allowable charges directly to the patient.

3. When an individual lives within a certain distance of a military hospital, a nonavailability statement (NAS) must be filed by the local military hospital before the patient enters the civilian hospital for inpatient nonemergency care.

4. TRICARE Standard is a fee-for-service plan in which medical expenses are shared between TRICARE and the beneficiary. Most enrollees pay an annual deductible and a cost-share percentage. TRICARE Prime is a managed care plan. After enrolling in the plan, each individual is assigned a Primary Care Manager (PCM) who coordinates and manages that patient's medical care. In addition to most of the benefits offered by TRICARE Standard, the program offers additional preventive care, including routine physical examinations. TRICARE Extra is also a managed care plan, but instead of services being provided primarily from military facilities, civilian facilities and physicians provide the majority of care. Individuals must receive health care services from a network of health care professionals.

5. Under the TRICARE for Life program, individuals age sixty-five and over who are eligible for both Medicare and TRICARE may continue to receive health care at a military treatment facility.

6. Individuals eligible for the CHAMPVA program include veterans who are totally and permanently disabled due to a service-connected injury, veterans who were totally and permanently disabled due to a service-connected condition at the time of death, and spouses or unmarried children of a veteran who is 100 percent disabled or who died as a result of a service-related disability in the line of duty.

7. Under the CHAMPVA for Life program, CHAMPVA benefits are extended to individuals age sixty-five and over who are eligible for both Medicare and CHAMPVA.

Key Terms

catastrophic cap *page 448*
CHAMPUS *page 445*
Civilian Health and Medical Program of the Department of Veterans Affairs (CHAMPVA) *page 453*
cost-share *page 446*

Defense Enrollment Eligibility Reporting System (DEERS) *page 445*
Military Treatment Facility (MTF) *page 447*
nonavailability statement (NAS) *page 448*
Primary Care Manager (PCM) *page 449*

sponsor *page 445*
TRICARE *page 445*
TRICARE Extra *page 449*
TRICARE for Life *page 450*
TRICARE Prime *page 449*
TRICARE Standard *page 447*

Review Questions

Match the key terms in the left column with the definitions in the right column.

A. Military Treatment Facility (MTF)

B. cost-share

C. TRICARE

D. TRICARE Extra

E. TRICARE Standard

F. Defense Enrollment Eligibility Reporting System (DEERS)

G. TRICARE Prime

H. catastrophic cap

I. CHAMPUS

J. Primary Care Manager (PCM)

K. nonavailability statement

L. TRICARE for Life

M. Civilian Health and Medical Program of the Department of Veterans Affairs (CHAMPVA)

N. sponsor

_____ 1. The amount of provider charges that are the responsibility of the patient

_____ 2. A program for individuals age sixty-five and over who are eligible for both Medicare and TRICARE that allows patients to receive health care at a military treatment facility

_____ 3. A place where medical care is provided to members of the military service and their families

_____ 4. The Department of Defense's new health insurance plan for military personnel and their families

_____ 5. A government database that contains information about patient eligibility for TRICARE

_____ 6. The government's health insurance program for veterans with 100 percent service-related disabilities and their families

_____ 7. The uniformed services member whose status makes it possible for other family members to be eligible for TRICARE coverage

_____ 8. An electronic document stating that the service the patient requires is not available at the local military treatment facility

_____ 9. A fee-for-service program that covers medical services provided by a civilian physician when the individual cannot receive treatment from a Military Treatment Facility (MTF)

_____ 10. A managed care plan in which most services are provided at civilian facilities

_____ 11. A provider who coordinates and manages a patient's medical care under a managed care plan

_____ 12. A managed care plan in which most services are provided at military treatment facilities

_____ 13. The Department of Defense's health insurance plan for military personnel and their families that was replaced in 1998

_____ 14. An annual limit on the total medical expenses that may be paid by an individual or family in one year

Decide whether each statement is true or false, and write T for true or F for false.

_____ 1. National Guard personnel are eligible for TRICARE whether on active duty or not.

_____ 2. Providers may elect to participate in TRICARE on a claim-by-claim basis.

_____ 3. Providers confirm an individual's eligibility for TRICARE by accessing the Defense Enrollment Eligibility Reporting System (DEERS).

_____ 4. TRICARE Standard pays a portion of charges provided by a civilian provider when treatment is not available at a military treatment facility.

_____ 5. *Cost-share* is the term TRICARE uses to describe a patient's coinsurance responsibility.

_____ 6. Under TRICARE Standard, preauthorization for treatment is not required.

_____ 7. TRICARE Prime is more expensive than TRICARE Extra.

_____ 8. Individuals enrolled in TRICARE become eligible for TRICARE for Life once they reach age sixty-five, provided they have Medicare Part A or Part B coverage.

_____ 9. In most cases, CHAMPVA does not contract with providers to offer services.

_____ 10. CHAMPVA beneficiaries must select a physician from a network of participating physicians.

Write the letter choice that best completes the statement or answers the question.

_____ 1. The TRICARE plan that is an HMO and requires a PCM is
    A. TRICARE Prime   C. TRICARE Extra
    B. TRICARE for Life   D. TRICARE Standard

_____ 2. _____ receive priority at military treatment facilities.
    A. Active duty service members   C. TRICARE Extra enrollees
    B. TRICARE Prime enrollees   D. TRICARE Standard enrollees

_____ 3. TRICARE for Life beneficiary must be at least _____ years old.
    A. seventy   C. sixty-five
    B. twenty-one   D. thirty

_____ 4. If a TRICARE Prime enrollee visits a provider outside the network, TRICARE pays _____ percent of the covered charges.
    A. 80   C. 20
    B. 100   D. 50

_____ 5. The TRICARE health care program is a covered entity and subject to privacy rules under
    A. NAS   C. TCS
    B. HIPAA   D. CHAMPVA

_____ 6. A person enrolled in CHAMPVA is responsible for _____ percent of covered charges.
    A. 20   C. 50
    B. 25   D. 60

_____ 7. Nonparticipating providers cannot bill for more than _____ percent of allowable charges.
    A. 80   C. 100
    B. 50   D. 115

_____ 8. Active-duty service members are automatically enrolled in
    A. TRICARE Prime   C. CHAMPUS
    B. TRICARE Extra   D. TRICARE Standard

_____ 9. For individuals enrolled in TRICARE for Life, the primary payer is
    A. TRICARE   C. a supplementary plan
    B. CHAMPVA   D. Medicare

_____ 10. Decisions about an individual's eligibility for TRICARE are made by the
    A. military treatment facility
    B. provider
    C. Defense Enrollment Eligibility Reporting System
    D. branch of military service

Provide answers to the following questions.

1. What is the purpose of the TRICARE program?

2. What is the priority of treatment in a military treatment facility?

Applying Your Knowledge

The objective of these three cases is to correctly complete a TRICARE claim, applying what you have learned in the chapter to each case situation. Each case consists of two sections. The first section contains information about the patient, the insurance coverage, and the current medical condition. The second section is an encounter form from Valley Associates, P.C.

If you are using NDCMedisoft to complete the cases, read the Guide to NDCMedisoft before beginning. Information from the first section, the patient information form, has already been entered in the program for you. You must enter information from the second section, the encounter form, to complete the claim. If you are gaining experience by completing a paper CMS-1500 claim form, follow the instructions on pages 451–452.

The following provider information, which is also available in the NDCMediSoft database, should be used for the case studies in Chapter 13.

Provider Information

Name	Nancy Ronkowski, M.D.
Practice Name	Valley Associates, P.C.
Address	1400 West Center Street
	Toledo, OH 43601-0213
Telephone	555-321-0987
Employer ID Number	06-7890123
Tricare PIN	TC4567
Assignment	Accepts
Physician Signature	On File (1-1-2005)

Case 13.1

From the Patient Information Form

Name	Robyn Janssen
Sex	F
Birth Date	02/12/1983
Marital Status	M
Employment	Not employed
Address	310 Wilson Ave.
	Brooklyn, OH
	44144-3456
Telephone	555-312-6649
SSN	334-62-5079
Health Plan	TRICARE
Signature	On File (1-1-2008)

Information about the Insured

Insured	Lee Janssen
Patient Relationship	
to Insured	Spouse
Date of Birth	01/05/1983
Sex	M
Address	Box 404
	Fort Dix, NJ
	08442-3456
Telephone	555-442-3600
SSN	602-37-0442
Insurance Plan	TRICARE Standard
Insurance ID Number	602370442
Copayment Amount	$10

VALLEY ASSOCIATES, P.C.

Nancy Ronkowski, M.D. - Obstetrics & Gynecology
555-321-0987
FED I.D. #06-7890123

PATIENT NAME		APPT. DATE/TIME	
Robyn Janssen		10/13/2008	10:00am

PATIENT NO.	DX
JANSSRO0	**1.** 626.0 absence of menstruation **2.** **3.** **4.**

DESCRIPTION	✓	CPT	FEE	DESCRIPTION	✓	CPT	FEE
EXAMINATION				**PROCEDURES**			
New Patient				Artificial Insemination		58322	
Problem Focused		99201		Biopsy, Cervix		57500	
Expanded Problem Focused		99202		Biopsy, Endometrium		58100	
Detailed		99203		Biopsy, Needle Asp., Breast		19100	
Comprehensive		99204		Colposcopy		57452	
Comprehensive/Complex		99205		Cyro of Cervix		57511	
Established Patient				Diaphragm Fitting		57170	
Minimum		99211		Endocervical Currettage		57505	
Problem Focused		99212		Hysteroscopy		56350	
Expanded Problem Focused	✓	99213	62	IUD Insertion		58300	
Detailed		99214		IUD Removal		58301	
Comprehensive/Complex		99215		Mammography (Bilateral)		76092	
				Marsup. of Bartholin Cyst		56440	
CONSULTATION				Norplant Insertion		11975	
Office				Norplant Removal		11976	
Problem Focused		99241		Pap Smear		88150	
Expanded Problem Focused		99242		Paracervical Block		64435	
Detailed		99243		Pessary Insertion		57160	
Comprehensive		99244		Pessary Washing		57150	
Comprehensive/Complex		99245		Polypectomy		57500	
Confirmatory							
Problem Focused		99271		**ULTRASOUND**			
Expanded Problem Focused		99272		USG, Preg Uterus, Comp.		76805	
Detailed		99273		USG, Preg Uterus, Rept.		76815	
Comprehensive		99274		USG, Gyn Complete		76856	
Comprehensive/Complex		99275		USG, Gyn Limited		76857	
				USG, Transvaginal		76830	
CULTURES							
Chlamydia		87072		**MISCELLANEOUS**			
GC Culture		87081		Wet Mount		87210	
Herpes Culture		87250		Specimen Handling		99002	
Mycoplasma/Ureoplasm		87109					
Urinalysis		8100					
Urine Culture		87088					
				TOTAL FEES			

Case 13.2

From the Patient Information Form

Name	Sylvia Evans	Telephone	555-229-3614
Sex	F	SSN	140-39-6602
Birth Date	06/10/1934	Health Plan	TRICARE
Marital Status	M	ID Number	140396602
Employment	Retired	Signature	On File (1-1-2008)
Address	13 Ascot Way Sandusky, OH 44870-1234	Copayment Amount	$10

VALLEY ASSOCIATES, P.C.
Nancy Ronkowski, M.D. - Obstetrics & Gynecology
555-321-0987
FED I.D. #06-7890123

PATIENT NAME	APPT. DATE/TIME
Sylvia Evans	10/13/2008 3:00pm

PATIENT NO.	DX
EVANSSY0	**1.** 627.1 postmenopausal bleeding **2.** **3.** **4.**

DESCRIPTION	✓	CPT	FEE	DESCRIPTION	✓	CPT	FEE
EXAMINATION				**PROCEDURES**			
New Patient				Artificial Insemination		58322	
Problem Focused		99201		Biopsy, Cervix		57500	
Expanded Problem Focused		99202		Biopsy, Endometrium		58100	
Detailed		99203		Biopsy, Needle Asp., Breast		19100	
Comprehensive		99204		Colposcopy		57452	
Comprehensive/Complex		99205		Cyro of Cervix		57511	
Established Patient				Diaphragm Fitting		57170	
Minimum		99211		Endocervical Currettage		57505	
Problem Focused	✓	99212	46	Hysteroscopy		56350	
Expanded Problem Focused		99213		IUD Insertion		58300	
Detailed		99214		IUD Removal		58301	
Comprehensive/Complex		99215		Mammography (Bilateral)		76092	
				Marsup. of Bartholin Cyst		56440	
CONSULTATION				Norplant Insertion		11975	
Office				Norplant Removal		11976	
Problem Focused		99241		Pap Smear	✓	88150	29

Case 13.3

From the Patient Information Form

Name	Eunice Walker	*Telephone*	555-772-9203
Sex	F	*SSN*	704-62-9930
Birth Date	11/03/1941	*Health Plan*	TRICARE
Marital Status	S	*ID Number*	704629930140396602
Employment	Retired	*Signature*	On File (1-1-2008)
Address	693 River Rd.	*Copayment Amount*	$10
	Toledo, OH		
	43601-1234		

VALLEY ASSOCIATES, P.C.
Nancy Ronkowski, M.D. - Obstetrics & Gynecology
555-321-0987
FED I.D. #06-7890123

PATIENT NAME	APPT. DATE/TIME	
Eunice Walker	10/13/2008	1:00pm

PATIENT NO.	DX
WALKEEU0	**1.** 611.72 lump in breast **2.** **3.** **4.**

DESCRIPTION	✓	CPT	FEE	DESCRIPTION	✓	CPT	FEE
EXAMINATION				**PROCEDURES**			
New Patient				Artificial Insemination		58322	
Problem Focused		99201		Biopsy, Cervix		57500	
Expanded Problem Focused		99202		Biopsy, Endometrium		58100	
Detailed		99203		Biopsy, Needle Asp., Breast		19100	
Comprehensive		99204		Colposcopy		57452	
Comprehensive/Complex		99205		Cyro of Cervix		57511	
Established Patient				Diaphragm Fitting		57170	
Minimum		99211		Endocervical Currettage		57505	
Problem Focused	✓	99212	46	Hysteroscopy		56350	
Expanded Problem Focused		99213		IUD Insertion		58300	
Detailed		99214		IUD Removal		58301	
Comprehensive/Complex		99215		Mammography (Bilateral)	✓	76092	134

Internet Activity

1. Point your Web browser at the official government Web site for TRICARE:

   http://www.tricare.osd.mil

   In the beneficiary section, select the link for information on claims. Read through the information displayed. Where do you file a claim if you live in Philadelphia, Pennsylvania?

2. Go to the TRICARE Web site at:

   http:// www.tricare.osd.mil

   Review the information about TRICARE Prime. In particular, study any changes in beneficiaries' cost-share requirements.

3. Visit the CHAMPVA home page at the Department of Veterans Affairs Health Administration Center Web site:

   http://www.va.gov/hac/champva/champva.html

   Select the link on how to file a claim, and read through the general claim filing instructions.

NDCMediSoft ACTIVITY

13.1 Review MediSoft Entries Specific to TRICARE

This activity explores various entries in MediSoft for a patient whose primary insurance carrier is TRICARE.

1. Mary Anne Kopelman is covered by her husband's TRICARE policy. The TRICARE policy requires a $10 copay per visit and pays for covered services in full. Open the Lists menu and select Patients/Guarantors and Cases.

2. In the Search For box, key KOPELM to display Mary Anne Kopelman's information in the Patient List dialog box.

3. In the right side of the Patient List dialog box, click Mary Anne Kopelman's Fatigue case to select it, and then click the Edit Case button.

4. The Personal tab of the Case dialog box is displayed. Notice in the Guarantor box that Arnold Kopelman is the guarantor. To determine the relationship between Arnold and Mary Anne, open the Policy 1 tab.

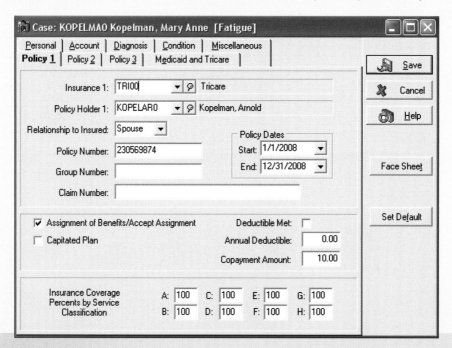

Computer Exploration

5. The Policy 1 tab shows that TRICARE is the primary carrier, that the policy holder is Arnold Kopelman, and that Arnold's relationship to Mary Anne is that of spouse.

6. Mary Anne Kopelman's policy number is 230569874. If Arnold Kopelman's patient information was accessed in the Patient/Guarantor dialog box, you would find that Mary Anne's policy number is based on her husband's Social Security Number. Because the plan is in Arnold's name, the policy number reflects his number and not hers.

7. The Policy 1 tab also indicates that the plan requires a small copay of $10 per visit and that there is no annual deductible. The Insurance Coverage Percents by Service Classification boxes at the bottom of the tab indicate that TRICARE pays for 100 percent of covered services.

   Click the Account tab.

8. Notice that the Price Code box reads A in this case. This means that Mary Anne is charged for procedures according to the default price code, rather than according to the Medicare Fee Schedule rate that corresponds to price code B in the Valley Associates, P.C., database.

   Click the Medicaid and TRICARE tab.

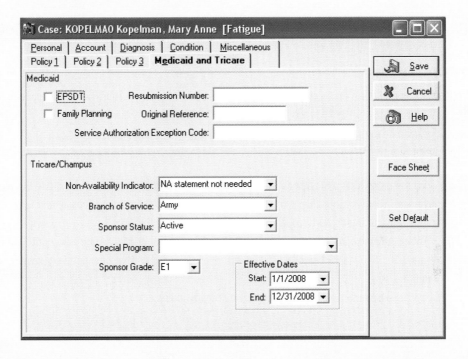

9. The bottom panel in this tab is used to record information that is specific to TRICARE/CHAMPVA claims. In Mary Anne's case, this information shows that a nonavailability statement is not needed, meaning that she is located near a military treatment facility and can obtain care there.

   The other boxes show that her husband, the sponsor, is an active-duty service member in the Army. The Sponsor Grade box indicates her husband's pay grade, E1. Code E1 corresponds to one of four codes used for enlisted members. (The MediSoft Help feature contains definitions of each of the codes displayed in the drop-down list in the Sponsor Grade box). Click the Cancel button to close the Case dialog box.

10. To view Mary Anne's procedure and payment transactions, the Transaction Entry dialog box needs to be opened. Click the Close button to close the Patient List dialog box.

Computer Exploration

11. Click Enter Transactions in the Activities menu. To display Mary Anne Kopelman's transaction information, key KOPELM in the Chart box, and press Enter.

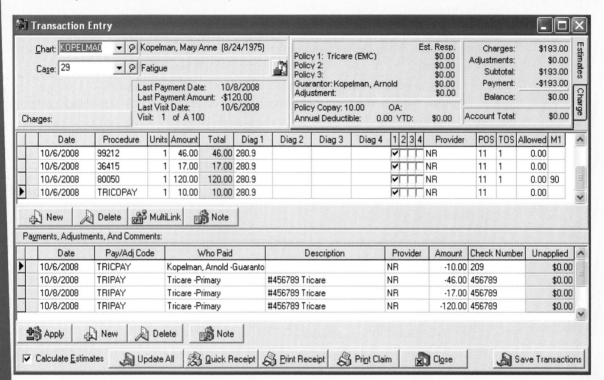

12. Study the procedures and payments displayed in the Transaction Entry dialog box. Use the scroll bars if necessary. There are four charge transactions, including a $10 copayment charge, and four payment transactions, including a $10 copayment made on the day of the visit.

  Then study the account summary information in the top panel. Mary Anne's Account Total column displays $0.00, as each charge transaction has been balanced with a corresponding payment in the full amount.

13. Click the Close button to exit the Transaction Entry dialog box.

Workers' Compensation and Disability

Objectives

After studying this chapter, you should be able to:

1. List the four federal workers' compensation plans.
2. Describe the two types of workers' compensation benefits that are offered by states.
3. List the criteria an injury must meet to be considered a covered injury or illness.
4. List the five classifications of work-related injuries.
5. List three responsibilities of the physician of record in a workers' compensation case.
6. Explain the difference between workers' compensation insurance and disability compensation programs.
7. Explain the difference between Social Security Disability Insurance (SSDI) and Supplemental Security Income (SSI).

Introduction

Workers' compensation was developed to benefit both the employer and the employee. It provides employees who are injured while on the job with a means of receiving compensation for their injuries, and it protects employers against liability for employees' injuries. Before workers' compensation was established in this country in the early 1900s, an injured workers' only recourse was to pursue legal action against the employer. To be successful, the employee had to prove that the employer was negligent. Cases were often difficult to prove and took years to settle. By 1947, all states required employers to purchase workers' compensation insurance.

Occupational Safety and Health Administration

The **Occupational Safety and Health Administration (OSHA)** was created by Congress in 1970 to protect workers from health and safety risks on the job. OSHA sets standards to guard against known dangers in the workplace, such as toxic fumes, faulty machinery, and excess noise. Businesses must meet health and safety standards set by OSHA. If they do not, they are subject to significant fines. Almost all employers are governed by OSHA legislation; the few exceptions include independent contractors, churches, domestic workers in private home settings, and federal employees.

If an employee believes the work environment is unhealthy or unsafe, a complaint may be filed directly with OSHA. The employer is prohibited from treating the employee adversely for filing a complaint with OSHA.

Federal Workers' Compensation Plans

Work-related illnesses or injuries suffered by civilian employees of federal agencies, including occupational diseases acquired by them, are covered under various programs administered by the **Office of Workers' Compensation Programs (OWCP)**. The OWCP is part of the U.S. Department of Labor. These programs are

- The Federal Employees' Compensation Program, which provides workers' compensation benefits under the **Federal Employees' Compensation Act (FECA)** to individuals employed by the federal government
- The Longshore and Harbor Workers' Compensation Program, which provides coverage under the Longshore and Harbor Workers' Compensation Act for individuals employed in the maritime field and for certain other classes of workers covered by extensions of the act
- The Federal Black Lung Program, which, under the administration of the Division of Coal Mine Workers' Compensation, provides benefits to individuals working in coal mines under the Black Lung Benefits Act
- The Energy Employees Occupational Illness Compensation Program, which went into effect on July 31, 2001, and provides benefits under the Energy Employees Occupational Illness Compensation Program Act for workers who have developed cancer and other serious diseases because they were exposed to radiation, beryllium, or silica at atomic weapons employer facilities or at certain federally owned facilities in which radioactive materials were used

Each program provides medical treatment, cash benefits for lost wages, vocational rehabilitation, or other benefits for workers of the particular employee group or industry it represents who have sustained workplace injuries or acquired occupational diseases.

State Workers' Compensation Plans

Each state administers its own workers' compensation program and has its own statutes that govern workers' compensation, so coverage varies from state to state. However, all states provide two types of workers' compensation benefits. One pays the employee's medical expenses that result from the work-related injury, and the other compensates the employee for lost wages while he or she is unable to return to work. Workers' compensation pays for all reasonable and necessary medical expenses resulting from the work-related injury.

Employers obtain workers' compensation insurance from one of the following sources: (1) a state workers' compensation fund, (2) a private insurance carrier, or (3) directly, through what is known as a self-insured fund. Under a state fund plan, companies pay premiums into a state insurance fund, and claims are paid out of that fund. Most employers contract with a private insurance carrier, which provides benefits on behalf of the company. A small number of companies that meet specific financial criteria may be allowed to self-insure. When a firm self-insures, it sets aside money in a fund that is to be used to pay workers' compensation claims. Most states require a company to obtain authorization before choosing to self-insure. Regardless of the source of workers' compensation insurance, the money that funds workers' compensation insurance is fully paid by the employer; no money is withdrawn from an employee's pay.

Employers or their insurance carriers must file proof of workers' compensation insurance with the state Workers' Compensation Board. In some states, this proof may be filed electronically through a Web-based data-entry application. In addition, the employer must post a Notice of Workers' Compensation Coverage in a place accessible to all employees. This notice must list the name, address, and telephone number of the administrator of the company's workers' compensation program.

Eligibility

Most states require public and private companies to provide workers' compensation coverage to all full-time and part-time employees, including minors. Companies that are required to carry workers' compensation insurance but fail to do so are subject to legal penalties.

The following categories of employee-employer relationships are generally not covered by workers' compensation insurance:

- Federal employees (because they are covered under a federal program)
- Railroad employees (because they are covered under a federal program)
- Self-employed individuals
- Real estate agents working on commission
- For-hire domestic, maintenance, or repair workers hired to perform a job for a homeowner on less than a full-time basis
- Drivers under a lease agreement with a carrier, such as some long-haul truck drivers

Compliance Guideline

Patient Rights
Federal workers injured on the job may select a physician from among those authorized by the OWCP. Payment is made directly to the provider, based on the Medicare Fee Schedule. The patient may not be billed for excess charges beyond the allowed charge.

Billing Tip

Workers' Compensation Fees
Some states have mandated the use of RVS (see Chapter 7) unit values as the schedule of fees for workers' compensation services. These states have often also set a conversion factor.

- Prison inmates employed by the prison
- Volunteers
- Independent contractors
- Clergy and members of religious orders
- Agricultural laborers

Benefits

Workers' compensation insurance covers injuries, illnesses, and job-related deaths. Injuries are not limited to on-the-job occurrences. They may occur while performing an off-site service for the company, such as driving to the post office on behalf of the company. Accidents such as falls in the company parking lot are also covered under workers' compensation rules.

Occupational diseases or illnesses develop as a result of workplace conditions or activities. These include lung disorders caused by poor air quality, repetitive motion illnesses such as carpal tunnel syndrome, and occupational hearing loss, among others. Illnesses may develop rapidly or over the course of many years.

Medical benefits are payable from the first day of the injury. Cash benefits vary from state to state and are generally not paid for the first seven days of disability. In most states, a worker must be disabled more than seven calendar days before benefits are payable. However, if the disability extends beyond fourteen days, a worker may become eligible for cash benefits for the first seven days retrospectively. Different states have different methods of determining wage-loss benefits. Usually, the benefits are a percentage of the worker's salary before the injury. For example, it is not uncommon for workers to be compensated at two-thirds of their average weekly wage, up to a weekly maximum. The weekly maximums differ from state to state, as do the formulas for determining a worker's average weekly wage.

When an individual is fatally injured on the job, workers' compensation pays death benefits to the employee's survivors. Funeral expenses may also be paid.

Covered Injuries and Illnesses

States determine the types of injuries that are covered under workers' compensation. Generally, an injury is covered if it meets all of the following criteria:

- It results in personal injury or death.
- It occurs by accident.
- It arises out of employment.
- It occurs during the course of employment.

An accident can be either an immediate event or the unexpected result of an occurrence over time. A worker who cuts a finger while using a box cutter is an example of an immediate accident. An employee who suffers a repetitive stress injury that developed over the course of several years is an example of an unexpected result over time.

The following are examples of covered injuries:

- Back injuries due to heavy lifting or a fall
- Repetitive stress injuries such as carpal tunnel syndrome
- Parking lot injuries such as falls
- Heat-related injuries such as heat stroke or heat exhaustion if the job requires a lot of work time in the hot sun

- Hernias if they are related to a work injury
- Personal time injuries, such as injuries that occur in the cafeteria or restroom

Some generally covered injuries may be excluded from workers' compensation, or benefits may be reduced if certain conditions were present at the time of the injury. Examples include the following:

- Employee intoxication by alcohol or illegal drugs led to the injury.
- Injury was intentionally self-inflicted.
- Employee violated the law.
- Employee failed to use safety equipment.
- Employee failed to obey safety procedures.
- Employee is also a recipient of Social Security disability benefits.
- Employee is also a recipient of unemployment insurance.
- Employee receives an employer-paid pension or disability benefit.

Classification of Injuries

Work-related injuries are grouped into five categories.

Injury without Disability

A worker is injured on the job, requires treatment, but is able to resume working within several days. All medical expenses are paid by workers' compensation insurance.

Injury with Temporary Disability

A worker is injured on the job, requires treatment, and is unable to return to work within several days. All medical expenses are paid by workers' compensation insurance, and the employee receives compensation for lost wages. Compensation varies from state to state, and is usually a percentage of the worker's salary before injury. Before an injured employee can return to work, the physician must file a doctor's **final report** indicating that the individual is fit to return to work and resume normal job activities.

Injury with Permanent Disability

A worker is injured on the job, requires treatment, is unable to return to work, and is not expected to be able to return to his or her regular job in the future. Usually this is an individual who has been on temporary disability for an extended period of time and is still unable to resume work. At that time, the physician of record files a report stating that the individual is permanently disabled. The state workers' compensation office or the insurance carrier may request an additional medical opinion before a final determination is made. An impartial physician is called in to provide an independent medical examination (IME). Once the IME report is submitted, a final determination of disability is made, and a settlement is reached. The length of coverage varies from state to state.

When an employee is rated as having a permanent disability, all medical expenses are paid by workers' compensation insurance, and the worker receives compensation for lost wages. The amount of compensation depends on a number of factors, including whether the disability is partial or total, the age of the employee, the job performed before the injury, and other factors. Partial disability is generally classified by percentage, and varies by severity. For example, a worker who has lost the use of a hand would receive less compensation than a worker paralyzed from the waist down.

Injury Requiring Vocational Rehabilitation

A worker is injured on the job, requires treatment, and is unable to return to work without vocational rehabilitation. All medical expenses are paid by workers' compensation insurance, as are the costs of the vocational rehabilitation program. **Vocational rehabilitation** is the process of retraining an employee to return to the workforce, although not necessarily in the same position as before the injury. For example, an employee who injured his or her back working in a job that required heavy lifting may be trained for work that does not involve lifting.

Injury Resulting in Death

A worker dies as a result of an injury on the job. Death benefits are paid to survivors based on the worker's earning capacity at the time of the injury.

Workers' Compensation Terminology

Physicians who examine patients under workers' compensation coverage use a set of standardized terms to describe the effects of work-related injuries and illnesses. These widely accepted terms are used by most states and insurance carriers. Different terminology is used to describe levels of pain and the effects of injuries or illnesses.

Pain Terminology

Pain is classified as minimal, slight, moderate, or severe.

- Minimal pain is annoying but does not interfere with the individual's ability to perform the job.
- Slight pain is tolerable, but the performance of some work assignments may be impaired.
- Moderate pain is tolerable, but the performance of some work assignments will show marked impairment.
- Severe pain requires avoiding activities that lead to pain.

Disability Terminology

Disabilities due to spinal injuries, heart disease, pulmonary disease, or abdominal weakness are classified as follows:

- *Limitation to light work:* Individual may work in an upright or walking position as long as no greater than minimal effort is required.
- *Precluding heavy work:* Individual has lost 50 percent or more of the ability to lift, push, pull, bend, stoop, and climb.
- *Precluding heavy lifting, repeated bending, and stooping:* Individual has lost 50 percent of the ability to perform these activities.
- *Precluding heavy lifting:* Individual has lost 50 percent of heavy lifting ability (categorization limited to lifting and does not include bending and stooping).
- *Precluding very heavy work:* Individual has lost 25 percent of the ability to lift, push, pull, bend, stoop, and climb.
- *Precluding very heavy lifting:* Individual has lost 25 percent of the ability for very heavy lifting.

Disabilities due to lower extremity injuries are described as follows:

- *Limitation to sedentary work:* Individual is able to work while in a sitting position with minimal physical effort required. Some walking and standing is possible.
- *Limitation to semisedentary work:* Individual is able to work in a job that allows 50 percent sitting and 50 percent standing or walking, with minimal physical effort demanded.

Workers' Compensation and the HIPAA Privacy Rule

Workers' compensation cases provide one of the few situations in which a health care provider may disclose a patient's protected health information to an employer without the patient's authorization. Workers' compensation claim information is not subject to the same confidentiality rules as private medical records.

Most states allow claims adjusters and employers unrestricted access to the workers' compensation files. Likewise, at the federal level, the HIPAA Privacy Rule permits disclosures of protected health information (PHI) made for workers' compensation purposes without the patient's authorization. Disclosure for any judicial or administrative proceeding in response to a court order, subpoena, or similar process is also allowed. Following the minimum necessary standard, covered entities can disclose information to the full extent authorized by state or other law. In addition, where PHI is requested by a state workers' compensation or other public official for such purposes, covered entities are permitted reasonably to rely on the official's representations that the information requested is the minimum necessary for the intended purpose.

Individuals do not have a right under the Privacy Rule to request that a physician restrict a disclosure of their PHI for workers' compensation purposes when that disclosure is required by law or authorized by, and necessary to comply with, a workers' compensation or similar law. However, for the physician to disclose information regarding an injured workers' previous condition, which is not directly related to the claim for compensation, to an employer or insurer requires the individual's written authorization.

Claims Process

When an employee is injured on the job, the injury must be reported to the employer within a certain time period. Most states require notification in writing. Once notified, the employer must notify the state workers' compensation office and the insurance carrier within a certain period of time. In some cases, the employee is given a medical service order to take to the physician who provides treatment.

In most instances, the injured employee must be treated by a provider selected by the employer or insurance carrier. Some employers contract with a managed care organization for services; in these cases, the patient must be examined and treated by a physician in the managed care plan's network. If the employee refuses to comply with the request, benefits may not be granted.

Responsibilities of the Physician of Record

The physician who first treats the injured or ill employee is known as the **physician of record**. This physician is responsible for treating the patient's condition and for determining the percentage of disability and the return-to-work date. A sample workers' compensation physician's report form is displayed in Figure 14.1.

The physician of record also files **progress reports** with the insurance carrier whenever there is a substantial change in the patient's condition that affects disability status or when required by state rules and regulations (see Figure 14.2 on page 476 for a sample physician's progress report).

Providers submit their charges to the workers' compensation insurance carrier and are paid directly by the carrier. Charges are limited to an established fee schedule. Patients may not be billed for any medical expenses. In addition, the employer may not be billed for any amount that exceeds the established fee for the service provided.

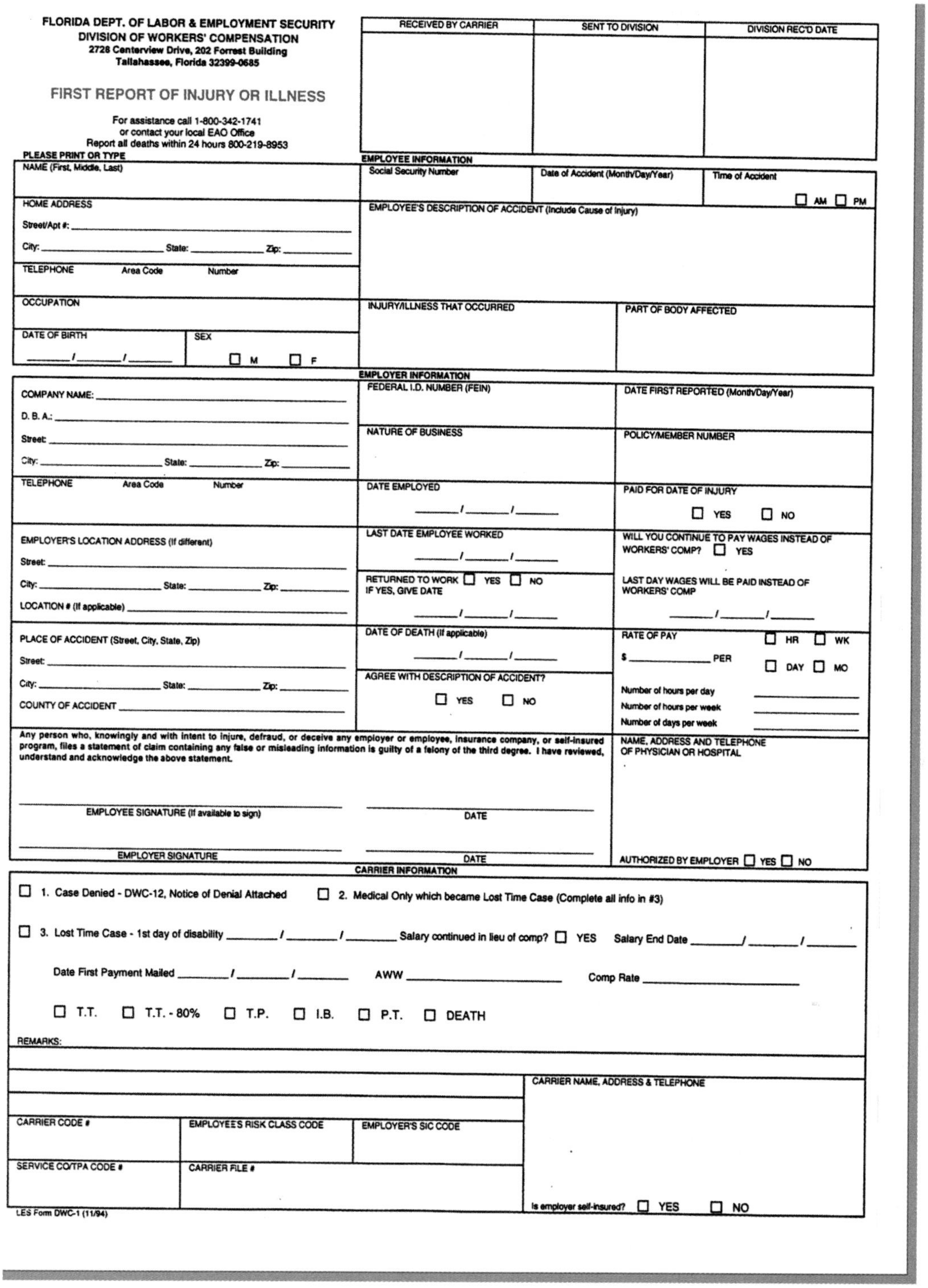

FLORIDA DEPT. OF LABOR & EMPLOYMENT SECURITY
DIVISION OF WORKERS' COMPENSATION
2728 Centerview Drive, 202 Forrest Building
Tallahassee, Florida 32399-0685

FIRST REPORT OF INJURY OR ILLNESS

For assistance call 1-800-342-1741
or contact your local EAO Office
Report all deaths within 24 hours 800-219-8953

RECEIVED BY CARRIER	SENT TO DIVISION	DIVISION REC'D DATE

PLEASE PRINT OR TYPE

EMPLOYEE INFORMATION

NAME (First, Middle, Last)

Social Security Number | Date of Accident (Month/Day/Year) | Time of Accident ☐ AM ☐ PM

HOME ADDRESS
Street/Apt #: ______
City: ______ State: ______ Zip: ______

EMPLOYEE'S DESCRIPTION OF ACCIDENT (Include Cause of Injury)

TELEPHONE Area Code Number

OCCUPATION

INJURY/ILLNESS THAT OCCURRED | PART OF BODY AFFECTED

DATE OF BIRTH ____/____/____ | SEX ☐ M ☐ F

EMPLOYER INFORMATION

COMPANY NAME: ______
D. B. A.: ______
Street: ______
City: ______ State: ______ Zip: ______

FEDERAL I.D. NUMBER (FEIN) | DATE FIRST REPORTED (Month/Day/Year)

NATURE OF BUSINESS | POLICY/MEMBER NUMBER

TELEPHONE Area Code Number

DATE EMPLOYED ____/____/____ | PAID FOR DATE OF INJURY ☐ YES ☐ NO

EMPLOYER'S LOCATION ADDRESS (If different)
Street: ______
City: ______ State: ______ Zip: ______
LOCATION # (If applicable) ______

LAST DATE EMPLOYEE WORKED ____/____/____ | WILL YOU CONTINUE TO PAY WAGES INSTEAD OF WORKERS' COMP? ☐ YES

RETURNED TO WORK ☐ YES ☐ NO
IF YES, GIVE DATE ____/____/____ | LAST DAY WAGES WILL BE PAID INSTEAD OF WORKERS' COMP ____/____/____

PLACE OF ACCIDENT (Street, City, State, Zip)
Street: ______
City: ______ State: ______ Zip: ______
COUNTY OF ACCIDENT ______

DATE OF DEATH (If applicable) ____/____/____

RATE OF PAY $ ______ PER ☐ HR ☐ WK ☐ DAY ☐ MO

AGREE WITH DESCRIPTION OF ACCIDENT? ☐ YES ☐ NO

Number of hours per day ______
Number of hours per week ______
Number of days per week ______

Any person who, knowingly and with intent to injure, defraud, or deceive any employer or employee, insurance company, or self-insured program, files a statement of claim containing any false or misleading information is guilty of a felony of the third degree. I have reviewed, understand and acknowledge the above statement.

NAME, ADDRESS AND TELEPHONE OF PHYSICIAN OR HOSPITAL

EMPLOYEE SIGNATURE (If available to sign) | DATE

EMPLOYER SIGNATURE | DATE

AUTHORIZED BY EMPLOYER ☐ YES ☐ NO

CARRIER INFORMATION

☐ 1. Case Denied - DWC-12, Notice of Denial Attached ☐ 2. Medical Only which became Lost Time Case (Complete all info in #3)

☐ 3. Lost Time Case - 1st day of disability ____/____/____ Salary continued in lieu of comp? ☐ YES Salary End Date ____/____/____

Date First Payment Mailed ____/____/____ AWW ______ Comp Rate ______

☐ T.T. ☐ T.T. - 80% ☐ T.P. ☐ I.B. ☐ P.T. ☐ DEATH

REMARKS:

CARRIER NAME, ADDRESS & TELEPHONE

CARRIER CODE #	EMPLOYEE'S RISK CLASS CODE	EMPLOYER'S SIC CODE
SERVICE CO/TPA CODE #	CARRIER FILE #	

Is employer self-insured? ☐ YES ☐ NO

LES Form DWC-1 (11/94)

Figure 14.1 Sample Workers' Compensation Physician Report Form

Responsibilities of the Employer and Insurance Carrier

The **first report of injury** form must be filed by the employer within a certain time period that varies by state. The range is normally from twenty-four hours to ten days. The form contains information about the patient, the employer, and the injury or illness. Depending on the insurance carrier, the report may be

Division of Workers' Compensation

PRIMARY TREATING PHYSICIANS PROGRESS REPORT (PR-2)

Check the box(es) which indicate why you are submitting a report at this time. If the patient is "Permanent and Stationary" (i.e., has reached maximum medical improvement), do not use this form. You may use DWC Form PR-3 or IMC Form 81556.

❑ Periodic Report (required 45 days after last report)	❑ Change in treatment plan	❑ Discharged
☒ Change in work status	❑ Need for referral or consultation	❑ Info. requested by: _____
❑ Change in patient's condition	❑ Need for surgery or hospitalization	❑ Other:

Patient:
Last _McDonald_   First _James_   M.I.___ Sex _M_ D.O.B _11/29/1964_
Address _3209 Ridge Rd_   City _Cleveland_   State _OH_ Zip _44101-2345_
Occupation _Truck driver_   SS # _602_ - _39_ - _4408_   Phone (_555_) _432-6049_

Claims Administrator:
Name _Janice Brown_   Claim Number _WC_
Address _312 East King St_   City _Toledo_   State _OH_ Zip _43601-1234_
Phone (_555_) _999-1000_   FAX (_555_) _999-1001_

Employer name: _JV Trucking_   Employer Phone (_555_) _555-5000_

The information below must be provided. You may use this form or you may substitute or append a narrative report.

Subjective complaints:

Lower back pain

Objective findings: (Include significant physical examination, laboratory, imaging, or other diagnostic findings.)

Lower back pain when bending or lifting >10 lbs.

Diagnoses:
1. _overexertion from lifting_   ICD-9 _E927_
2. _____ ICD-9 _____
3. _____ ICD-9 _____

Treatment Plan: (Include treatment rendered to date. List methods, frequency and duration of planned treatment(s). Specify consultation/referral, surgery, and hospitalization. **Identify each physician and non-physician provider.** Specify type, frequency and duration of physical medicine services (e.g., physical therapy, manipulation,acupuncture). Use of CPT codes is encouraged. Have there been any **changes** in treatment plan? If so, why?

Exam, x-rays, physical therapy, advised restricted activity.

Work Status: this patient has been instructed to:

❑ Remain off-work until _____.

☒ Return to modified work on ___10/27/2008___ with the following limitations or restrictions
(List all specific restrictions re: standing, sitting, bending, use of hands, etc.):
No bending
No lifting >10 lbs.

❑ Return to full duty on _____ with no limitations or restrictions.

Primary Treating Physician: (original signature, do not stamp)   Date of exam: _10/24/2008_

I declare under penalty of perjury that this report is true and correct to the best of my knowledge and that I have not violated Labor Code § 139.3.

Signature: _Sarah Jamison, M.D._   Cal. Lic. # _16-1234567_
Executed at: _Valley Medical Associates_   Date: _10/24/2008_
Name: _Sarah Jamison, M.D._   Specialty: _orthopedics_
Address: _1400 West Center St., Toledo, OH 43601-0123_   Phone: _555-321-0987_
Next report due no later than _11/17/2008_

DWC Form PR-2 (Rev.1/1/99)   **(Use additional pages, if necessary)**

Figure 14.2 Sample Physician's Progress Report Form

NEW HAMPSHIRE WORKERS' COMPENSATION MEDICAL FORM

This form must be completed at each health professional visit (MD, DO, DC or DDS) and must be filed with the worker's compensation insurance carrier within 10 days of the treatment (first aid excluded). Failure to comply and complete this form shall result in the provider not being reimbursed for services rendered and may result in a civil penalty of up to $2,500.

In compliance with RSA 281-A:23-b, the employer with 5 or more employees must provide temporary alternative/transitional work opportunities to all employees temporarily disabled by a work related injury or illness.

Employee _____   Employer _____

SS # _____   Work telephone # _____

Occupation _____   Employer contact _____

Date last worked _____   Employer address _____

W.C. insurer _____   _____

HEALTH PROFESSIONAL TO COMPLETE

☐ Initial visit   ☐ Follow-up visit   Date of injury _____   Time _____

Worker's statement of the incident _____

Worker's complaints _____

Diagnosis/Prognosis _____

Treatment plan _____

In your opinion is this injury and disability as a result of injury described above?   ☐ Yes   ☐ No   ☐ Unclear

EMPLOYEE WORK CAPABILITY

☐ Continue Working   Can return to work: ☐ Yes   Date _____   ☐ No
   ☐ Full Duty   ☐ With Modification. If so, for what duration? _____

Employee can	No Restrictions	Frequently	Occasionally	Unable to
bend				
kneel				
squat				
climb				
stand				
walk				
sit				
reach				
drive				
do fine motor				

No		Wrist	Elbow	Shoulder	Ankle
repetitive	Right				
motions	Left				

Employee can lift/carry maximally _____ lbs.
Employee can lift/carry frequently _____ lbs.

Employee can work a maximum of #___ hours/day, #___days /wk.
What special accommodations are required? _____
_____

Other _____
Has employee reached maximum medical improvement?
   ☐ Yes   ☐ No
Has injury caused permanent impairment?
   ☐ Yes   ☐ No   ☐ Undetermined

ALL MEDICAL NOTES MUST BE ATTACHED TO BILL

I certify that the narrative descriptions of the principal and secondary diagnosis and the major procedures performed are accurate and complete to the best of my knowledge.

_____   _____   _____
Provider's signature   Provider's Printed name   Provider's telephone#

_____   _____
Federal ID#   Date of visit

MEDICAL AUTHORIZATION: The act of the worker in applying for workers' compensation benefits constitutes authorization to any physician, hospital, chiropractor, or other medical vendor to supply all relevant medical information regarding the worker's occupational injury or illness to the insurer, the worker's employer, the worker's representative, and the department. Medical information relevant to a claim includes a past history of complaints of, or treatment of, a condition similar to that presented in the claim. [281-A:23 V(a)]

75 WCA-1 (06/94)   White - Insurer/Managed Care   Yellow - Provider   Pink - Employee/Employer

Figure 14.3 Sample First Report of Injury Form

filed electronically or mailed to the carrier. A first report of injury form is displayed in Figure 14.3.

The insurance carrier assigns a claim number to the case, determines whether the claim is eligible for workers' compensation, and notifies the employer. This determination is either an **Admission of Liability**, stating that the employer is responsible for the injury, or a **Notice of Contest**, which is a denial

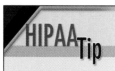
of liability. The worker must be informed of the outcome within a given number of days.

If the employee is eligible for lost wages compensation benefits, checks are sent directly to the employee, and no income taxes are withheld from the payments. If the claim is denied, the employee must pay all medical bills associated with the accident. These charges may be submitted to the individual's own health insurance carrier for payment.

Termination of Compensation and Benefits

Temporary partial and temporary total disability benefits cease when one of the following occurs:

- Employee is given a physician's release authorizing a return to his or her regular job.
- Employee is offered a different job by the employer (not the same job as before the injury) and either returns to work or refuses to accept the new assignment.
- Employee has exhausted the maximum workers' compensation benefits for the injury or illness.
- Employee cannot work due to circumstances other than the work-related injury (for example, individual is injured in an automobile accident that results in an unrelated disability).
- Employee does not cooperate with request for a medical examination (medical examinations determine the type and duration of the disability and the relationship of the injury to the patient's condition).
- Employee has returned to work.
- Employee has died (death benefits go to survivors, however).

Appeals

Individuals may appeal workers' compensation decisions. The first step in the appeals process is to request mediation. A mediator is an impartial individual who works with both parties to obtain a satisfactory resolution.

If mediation efforts on behalf of the injured employee fail, a hearing may be requested. A hearing is a formal legal proceeding. A judge listens to both sides and renders a decision, referred to as an order. If the employee is not satisfied with the judge's decision, the claim may be appealed at higher levels, for example, at a Workers' Compensation Appeals Board or, after that, at a state supreme court.

Special Billing Notes

Workers' compensation claims require special handling by the provider's billing staff. The first medical treatment report on the case must be exact; if it is not, future treatments may seem to be unrelated to the original injury and may be denied.

There are no universal rules for completing a claim form. Some plans use the HIPAA 837 or the CMS-1500, while others have their own claim forms. Although the specific procedures vary depending on the state and on the insurance carrier, the following are some general guidelines:

- Payment from the insurance carrier must be accepted as payment in full. Patients or employers may not be billed for any of the medical expenses.

- A separate file must be established when a provider treats an individual who is already a patient of the practice. Information in the patient's regular medical record (nonworkers' compensation) must not be released to the insurance carrier.
- The patient's signature is not required on any billing forms.
- The workers' compensation claim number should be included on all forms and correspondence.
- Use the eight-digit format when reporting dates such as the "date last worked."

Disability Compensation Programs

Disability compensation programs do not provide a policyholder with reimbursement for health care charges. Instead, they provide partial reimbursement for lost income that occurs due to a disability that prevents the individual from working, whether the injury is work-related or not. Benefits are paid in the form of regular cash payments. Workers' compensation coverage is a type of disability insurance; however, most disability programs do not require the injury or illness to be work-related in order to pay benefits.

To receive compensation under a disability program, an individual's medical condition must be documented in his or her medical record. The medical record often serves as substantiation for the disability benefits, and an inadequate or incomplete medical record may result in a denial of disability benefits. The more severe the disability, the greater the standard of medical documentation required. For this reason, an accurate and thorough medical record is of primary significance in disability cases.

Employers are not required to provide disability insurance. Most companies provide their employees with disability coverage and pay a substantial amount of the premiums, but others do not. Federal or state government employees are eligible for a public disability program. Individuals not covered by an employer- or government-sponsored plan may purchase disability policies from private insurance carriers.

Many individuals covered by employer-sponsored plans or private policies are also covered by a government program, such as Social Security Disability Insurance (SSDI). In these cases, the employer or private program supplements the government-sponsored coverage.

Government Programs

The federal government provides disability benefits to individuals through several different programs. The major government disability programs are

Billing Tip

Turn-around Times
It is important to track the date a workers' compensation claim is filed. Insurance carriers must pay workers' compensation claims within a certain number of days, usually thirty to forty-five days, depending on the state. If the claim is not paid within the time specified, the claimant may be eligible for interest on the payment, or a late fee may apply.

HIPAA Tip

The mandate to file claims electronically according to the HIPAA Electronic Health Care Transactions and Code Sets standards does not apply to workers' compensation plans.

- Workers' compensation (covered earlier in the chapter)
- Social Security Disability Insurance (SSDI)
- Supplemental Security Income (SSI)
- Federal Employees Retirement System (FERS) or Civil Service Retirement System (CSRS)
- Department of Veterans Affairs disability programs

Social Security Disability Insurance (SSDI)

The **Social Security Disability Insurance (SSDI)** program is funded by workers' payroll deductions and matching employer contributions. It provides compensation for lost wages due to disability. The employee payroll deductions are known as **Federal Insurance Contribution Act (FICA)** deductions.

The definition of disability used by the SSDI program and found in Section 223(d) of the Social Security Act lists the specific criteria that must be met:

> The inability to engage in any substantial gainful activity by reason of any medically determinable physical or mental impairment which can be expected to result in death, or, which has lasted or can be expected to last for a continuous period of not less than twelve months.

The SSDI program defines the categories of disability that are eligible for coverage. These are

- Presumptive legal disability, which includes cases that are specifically listed in the Social Security disability manual
- Cases that have more than one condition that together meet the disability standards
- Cases in which individuals cannot return to their former positions and also cannot obtain employment in the local area

Individuals also have to meet certain criteria to be eligible for disability benefits from the Social Security Insurance program. The following individuals are eligible:

- Disabled employed or self-employed individuals who are under age sixty-five and have paid Social Security taxes for a minimum number of quarters that varies according to age
- Individuals disabled before they reach age twenty-two who have a parent receiving Social Security benefits who retires, becomes disabled, or dies
- Disabled divorced spouses over age fifty whose former spouse paid into Social Security for a minimum of ten years and is deceased
- Disabled widows or widowers age fifty years or older whose deceased spouse paid into Social Security for at least ten years
- Employees who are blind or whose vision cannot be corrected to more than 20/200 in their better eye, or whose visual field is 20 degrees or less, even with a corrective lens

After an application for SSDI has been filed, there is a five-month waiting period before payments begin. Individuals receiving SSDI may apply for additional Medicare disability benefits twenty-four months after they become disabled.

Supplemental Security Income (SSI)

Supplemental Security Income (SSI) is a welfare program. SSI provides payments to individuals in need, including aged, blind, and disabled individuals. Eligibility is determined using nationwide standards. If the individual's income and resources are under certain limits, the individual can qualify even if he or she has never worked or paid taxes under FICA. Children under age eighteen who are disabled or blind and in need may also qualify. The basic benefit paid is the same nationwide (as of January 2003, $552 per month for an eligible individual). Many states, however, add money to the basic benefit.

Federal Worker Disability Programs

The Federal Employees Retirement System (FERS) provides disability coverage to federal workers hired after 1984. Employees hired before 1984 enrolled in the Civil Service Retirement System (CSRS). The FERS program consists of a federal disability program and the Social Security disability program. The two parts of the program have different eligibility rules, and some workers qualify for FERS benefits but not for SSDI benefits. If a worker is eligible for both, the amount of the SSDI payment is reduced based on the amount of the FERS payment.

The CSRS criteria of disability are not as strict as the SSDI criteria. CSRS determines that a worker is disabled if he or she is unable "because of disease or injury, to render useful and efficient service in the employee's current position and is not qualified for reassignment to a similar position elsewhere in the agency." Unlike the SSDI criteria, the CSRS criteria do not specifically mention the duration of the medical condition, although it may be expected to continue for at least a year. To qualify, a worker must have become disabled during the course of his or her federal career and must have completed at least five years of federal civilian service. Employees who are eligible for CSRS benefits are able to retain their health insurance coverage through the Federal Employee Health Benefit Program.

Veterans Programs

The Department of Veterans Affairs (VA) provides former armed services members with two disability programs: the Veteran's Compensation Program and the Veteran's Pension Program. Certain veterans may qualify to receive benefits from both. The Veteran's Compensation Program provides coverage for individuals with a permanent and total disability that resulted from a service-related illness or injury. In order for the veteran to be eligible for benefits, the disability must affect his or her earning capacity.

The Veteran's Pension Program provides benefits to veterans who are not and will not be able to obtain gainful employment. The disability must be service-related, and must be permanent and total.

Preparing Disability Reports

When a request is made for a medical report to support a disability claim, the physician or a member of the staff prepares the report by abstracting information from the patient's medical record. It is important to thoroughly document each examination by the physician. In many cases, an incomplete or inadequate medical report leads to denial of a disability claim.

The report for a disability claim should include the following medical information:

- Medical history
- Subjective complaints
- Objective findings

Billing Tip

Do not report 99455 or 99456 together with 99080 for completion of workers' compensation claims.

- Diagnostic test results
- Diagnosis
- Treatment
- Description of patient's ability to perform work-related activities

Supporting documents, such as X-rays, pulmonary function tests, range of motion tests, and ECGs, should also be included when appropriate.

Disability claim forms must be completed fully and accurately and must be supported by thorough and accurate medical reports. Two possible ways of billing the time spent on preparing disability claims are as follows:

1. Bill CPT code 99080 with the correct evaluation and management (E/M) office visit code. This code, which must be reported in conjunction with another service, covers the time required to complete insurance forms that convey more than a standard reporting form.

2. Bill CPT codes 99455–99456. In addition to covering medical disability examinations, these codes include the time required to complete corresponding reports and documentation.

Review

Chapter Summary

1. The workers' compensation plans that provide coverage to federal government employees are the Federal Employees' Compensation Program, the Longshore and Harbor Workers' Compensation Program, the Federal Black Lung Program, and the Energy Employees Occupational Illness Compensation Program.

2. States provide two types of workers' compensation benefits. One pays the worker's medical expenses that result from work-related illness or injury, and the other pays for lost wages while the worker is unable to return to work.

3. For an injury to be covered under a workers' compensation plan, it must (a) result in personal injury or death, (b) occur by accident, (c) arise out of employment, and (d) occur during the course of employment.

4. Work-related injuries are classified as (a) injury without disability, (b) injury with temporary disability, (c) injury with permanent disability, (d) injury requiring vocational rehabilitation, and (e) injury resulting in death.

5. The physician of record in a workers' compensation case is responsible for treating the injured worker, determining the percentage of disability, determining the return-to-work date, and filing progress notes.

6. Workers' compensation insurance pays an employee's medical bills that result from a job-related injury; disability compensation programs do not pay medical expenses. Workers' compensation insurance provides coverage for illnesses and injuries that are job-related. Most disability compensation programs provide benefits for injuries or illnesses that are not work-related.

7. Social Security Disability Insurance (SSDI) provides compensation for lost wages to individuals who have contributed to Social Security through FICA payroll taxes. Supplemental Security Income (SSI) is a welfare program that provides financial assistance to individuals in need, including aged, blind, and disabled individuals.

Key Terms

Admission of Liability *page 477*
disability compensation programs *page 479*
Federal Employees' Compensation Act (FECA) *page 468*
Federal Insurance Contribution Act (FICA) *page 480*
final report *page 471*

first report of injury *page 475*
Notice of Contest *page 477*
occupational diseases or illnesses *page 470*
Occupational Safety and Health Administration (OSHA) *page 468*
Office of Workers' Compensation Programs (OWCP) *page 468*

physician of record *page 474*
progress reports *page 474*
Social Security Disability Insurance (SSDI) *page 480*
Supplemental Security Income (SSI) *page 480*
vocational rehabilitation *page 472*

Review Questions

Match the key terms in the left column with the definitions in the right column.

A. Federal Insurance Contribution Act (FICA)

B. Notice of Contest

C. occupational diseases or illnesses

D. Office of Workers' Compensation Programs (OWCP)

E. Social Security Disability Insurance (SSDI)

F. final report

G. Federal Employees' Compensation Act (FECA)

H. Occupational Safety and Health Administration (OSHA)

I. first report of injury

J. Admission of Liability

K. Supplemental Security Income (SSI)

L. disability compensation programs

M. physician of record

N. progress reports

_____ 1. Employee payroll deductions that are used to partially fund Social Security Disability Insurance (SSDI)

_____ 2. The government agency that administers workers' compensation programs for civilian employees of federal agencies

_____ 3. Programs that provide reimbursement for lost income that occurs due to a disability that prevents the individual from working, whether the injury is work-related or not

_____ 4. Legislation that provides workers' compensation benefits to individuals employed by the federal government

_____ 5. Determination that the employer is responsible for the worker's injury or illness

_____ 6. Agency set up by Congress in 1970 to protect workers from health and safety risks on the job

_____ 7. Program funded by workers' payroll deductions and matching employer contributions that provides compensation for lost wages due to disability

_____ 8. Illnesses that develop as a result of workplace conditions or activities

_____ 9. A document indicating that an individual is fit to return to work and resume normal job activities

_____ 10. The physician who first treats an injured or ill employee

_____ 11. A welfare program that provides financial assistance to individuals in need, including aged, blind, and disabled individuals

_____ 12. Documents filed with the insurance carrier whenever there is a substantial change in the patient's condition that affects the status of an occupational illness

_____ 13. A determination that the employer is not liable for the worker's injury or illness

_____ 14. A document that contains information about the patient, the employer, and the injury or illness that must be filed by the employer, often within twenty-four hours of the incident

Decide whether each statement is true or false, and write T for true or F for false.

_____ 1. A physician who treats a patient covered by workers' compensation insurance may not charge the patient for any amount of the medical expenses.

_____ 2. Social Security Disability Insurance (SSDI) is a welfare program.

_____ 3. The Federal Employees' Compensation Act (FECA) was created to protect workers from health and safety risks on the job.

_____ 4. A disability classified as a limitation to semisedentary work allows an individual to work at a position that requires 50 percent standing and 50 percent walking.

_____ 5. Federal Insurance Contribution Act (FICA) payroll deductions provide partial funding for Social Security Disability Insurance (SSDI).

_____ 6. Most states require corporations that meet established financial standards to obtain authorization to become self-insured against workers' compensation claims.

_____ 7. Workers' compensation insurance does not cover injuries that occur in the company parking lot or cafeteria.

_____ 8. Individuals classified as permanently disabled receive compensation for lost wages as well as paid medical expenses for treatment resulting from the work-related illness or injury.

_____ 9. The physician of record is the provider who initially treats the injured or ill worker.

_____ 10. Occupational illnesses that develop over time are generally not covered by workers' compensation insurance.

Write the letter choice that best completes the statement or answers the question.

_____ 1. Once an application for Social Security Disability Insurance (SSDI) is filed, there is a _____ waiting period before benefits begin.
   A. thirty day
   B. five month
   C. fourteen day
   D. one month

_____ 2. A _____ is a denial of employer liability issued by the workers' compensation insurance carrier.
   A. First Report of Liability
   B. Notice of Contest
   C. No-Fault Notice
   D. Denial of Finding

_____ 3. An individual with a disability described as precluding heavy work has lost _____ of the capacity to push, pull, bend, stoop, and climb.
   A. 20 percent
   B. 25 percent
   C. 90 percent
   D. 50 percent

_____ 4. Before an injured employee can return to work, a physician must write a(n)
   A. progress report
   B. doctor's final report
   C. admission of liability report
   D. final report of injury

_____ 5. _____ provides workers' compensation insurance coverage to employees of the federal government.
   A. Office of Workers' Compensation Programs (OWCP)
   B. Federal Insurance Contribution Act (FICA)
   C. Supplemental Security Income (SSI)
   D. Federal Employees' Compensation Act (FECA)

_____ 6. The classifications of pain used in workers' compensation claims are
   A. minimal, moderate, severe
   B. slight, moderate, major, severe
   C. minimal, slight, moderate, severe
   D. minimal, slight, major, severe

_____ 7. A disability that limits a worker to jobs that are performed in an upright or standing position and that require no greater than minimal effort are classified as
   A. precluding very heavy work
   B. limitation to light work
   C. limitation to semisedentary work
   D. precluding heavy lifting, repeated bending, and stooping

_____ 8. Vocational rehabilitation programs provide _____ for individuals with job-related disabilities.
   A. physical therapy
   B. compensation for lost wages
   C. training in a different job
   D. payment for medical expenses

_____ 9. For a disabled widow or widower age fifty years or older to qualify for Social Security Disability Insurance (SSDI), his or her spouse must have paid into Social Security for at least

    A. six months   C. five years

    B. one year   D. ten years

_____ 10. An employee who believes the work environment to be dangerous may file a complaint with the

    A. Office of Workers' Compensation Programs

    B. local Social Security office

    C. Occupational Safety and Health Administration

    D. Workers' Compensation Board in the state in which the company is headquartered

Provide answers to the following questions.

1. How do the criteria for disability differ in the Social Security Disability Insurance (SSDI) program and the Civil Service Retirement System (CSRS) program?

2. What criteria does an injury or illness have to meet to be eligible for workers' compensation coverage?

Applying Your Knowledge

The objective of these three cases is to correctly complete workers' compensation claims, applying what you have learned in the chapter to each case situation. Each case consists of two sections. The first section contains information about the patient, the insurance coverage, and the current medical condition. The second section is an encounter form from Valley Associates, P.C.

If you are using NDCMedisoft to complete the cases, read the Guide to NDCMedisoft before beginning. Information from the first section, the patient information form, has already been entered in the program for you. You must enter information from the second section, the encounter form, to complete the claim. If you are gaining experience by completing a paper CMS-1500 claim form, follow the instructions on pages 478–479.

The following provider information, which is also available in the NDCMediSoft database, should be used for the case studies in Chapter 14.

Provider Information

Name	Sarah Jamison, M.D.	Employer ID Number	07-2345678
Practice Name	Valley Associates, P.C.	Commercial PIN	CP1234
Address	1400 West Center Street	Assignment	Accepts
	Toledo, OH 43601-0213	Physician Signature	On File (1-1-2005)
Telephone	555-321-0987		

Case 14.1

Name	Frank Puopolo	Health Plan	CarePlus Workers' Compensation
Sex	M	Insurance ID Number	2090462-37
Birth Date	05/17/1968	Group Number	OH1111
Marital Status	M	Copayment Amount	None
Employment Status	Full-time	Condition Related to:	
Employer	JV Trucking	Employment?	Yes
Address	404 Belmont Place	Auto or other Accident?	No
	Sandusky, OH	Date of Current Illness,	6/2/2008
	44870-8901	Injury, LMP	
Telephone	555-330-6467	Dates Patient Unable to Work	6/2/2008
SSN	239-04-9372	Date of Hospitalization	6/2/2008–6/4/2008
		Physician Signature on File	1/1/2005

VALLEY ASSOCIATES, P.C.
Sarah Jamison, M.D. - Orthopedic Medicine
555-321-0987
FED I.D. #07-2345678

PATIENT NAME	APPT. DATE/TIME	
Frank Puopolo	06/02/2008	12:00pm

PATIENT NO.	DX
PUOPOFR0	1. 823.22 fracture, shaft, closed, tibia & fibula 2. 3. 4.

DESCRIPTION	✓	CPT	FEE	DESCRIPTION	✓	CPT	FEE
EXAMINATION				**FRACTURES**			
New Patient				Clavicle		23500	
Problem Focused		99201		Scapula		23570	
Expanded Problem Focused		99202		Humerus, proximal		23600	
Detailed		99203		Humerus, shaft		24500	
Comprehensive		99204		Radial, colles w/manip		25605	
Comprehensive/Complex		99205		Radial, h or n w/out manip		24650	
Established Patient				Ulna, proximal		24670	
Minimum		99211		Radius & Ulna		25560	
Problem Focused		99212		Radius, colles, distal		25600	
Expanded Problem Focused		99213		Ulna, styloid		25650	
Detailed		99214		Hand MC		26600	
Comprehensive/Complex		99215		Finger/Thumb		26720	
				Coccyx		27200	
CONSULTATION				Femur, distal		27508	
Office				Tibia, prox/plateua		27530	
Problem Focused		99241		Tibia & Fibula, shaft	✓	27750	681
Expanded Problem Focused		99242		Fibula, prox/shaft		27780	
Detailed		99243		Foot, MT		28470	
Comprehensive		99244		Toe, great		28490	
Comprehensive/Complex		99245		Toe, others		28510	
Confirmatory							
Problem Focused		99271		**X-RAY**			
Expanded Problem Focused		99272		Clavicle		73000	
Detailed		99273		Humerus		73060	
Comprehensive		99274		Forearm		73090	
Comprehensive/Complex		99275		Hand, 2 views		73120	
				Hand, 3 views		73130	
EMG STUDIES				Fingers		73140	
EMG -1 extremity		95860		Femur		73550	
EMG - 2 extremities		98561		Tibia & Fibula	✓	73590	89
EMG - 3 extremities		98562		Foot, 2 views		73620	
Nerve Conduct, M w/out F		95900		Foot, 3 views		73630	
Nerve Conduct, M w/F		95903		Toes		73660	
Nerve Conduct, sensory		95904		**TOTAL FEES**			

From the Patient Information Form

Name	Marilyn Grogan
Sex	F
Birth Date	03/21/1964
Marital Status	M
Employment Status	Full-time
Employer	Microtech, Inc.
Address	23 Brookside Drive Alliance, OH 44601-1234
Telephone	555-729-4416
SSN	139-46-0589

Health Plan	CarePlus Workers' Compensation
Insurance ID Number	627422-19
Group Number	OH6319
Copayment Amount	None
Condition Related to:	
Employment?	Yes
Auto or Other Accident?	No
Date of Current Illness, Injury, LMP	3/6/2008
Dates Patient Unable to Work	3/6/2008–3/10/2008
Physician Signature on File	1/1/2005

VALLEY ASSOCIATES, P.C.
Sarah Jamison, M.D. - Orthopedic Medicine
555-321-0987
FED I.D. #07-2345678

PATIENT NAME	APPT. DATE/TIME	
Marilyn Grogan	03/06/2008	10:30am

PATIENT NO.	DX
GROGAMA0	1. 810.0 fracture, closed, clavicle 2. 3. 4.

DESCRIPTION	✓	CPT	FEE	DESCRIPTION	✓	CPT	FEE
EXAMINATION				**FRACTURES**			
New Patient				Clavicle	✓	23500	1349
Problem Focused		99201		Scapula		23570	
Expanded Problem Focused		99202		Humerus, proximal		23600	
Detailed		99203		Humerus, shaft		24500	
Comprehensive		99204		Radial, colles w/manip		25605	
Comprehensive/Complex		99205		Radial, h or n w/out manip		24650	
Established Patient				Ulna, proximal		24670	
Minimum		99211		Radius & Ulna		25560	
Problem Focused		99212		Radius, colles, distal		25600	
Expanded Problem Focused		99213		Ulna, styloid		25650	
Detailed		99214		Hand MC		26600	
Comprehensive/Complex		99215		Finger/Thumb		26720	
				Coccyx		27200	
CONSULTATION				Femur, distal		27508	
Office				Tibia, prox/plateua		27530	
Problem Focused		99241		Tibia & Fibula, shaft		27750	
Expanded Problem Focused		99242		Fibula, prox/shaft		27780	
Detailed		99243		Foot, MT		28470	
Comprehensive		99244		Toe, great		28490	
Comprehensive/Complex		99245		Toe, others		28510	
Confirmatory							
Problem Focused		99271		**X-RAY**			
Expanded Problem Focused		99272		Clavicle	✓	73000	82

Case 14.3

Name	Shih-Chi Yang
Sex	M
Birth Date	12/03/1969
Marital Status	M
Employment Status	Full-time
Employer	J&M Manufacturing
Address	6 Sparrow Road
	Brooklyn, OH
	44144-2345
Telephone	555-602-7779
SSN	334-72-9081

Health Plan	CarePlus Workers' Compensation
ID Number	1045891-22
Group Number	OH3967
Copayment Amount	None
Condition Related to:	
Employment?	Yes
Date of Current Illness,	
Injury, LMP	11/12/2008
Dates Patient Unable to Work	11/12/2008–
Physician Signature on File	1/1/2005

VALLEY ASSOCIATES, P.C.
Sarah Jamison, M.D. - Orthopedic Medicine
555-321-0987
FED I.D. #07-2345678

PATIENT NAME	APPT. DATE/TIME	
Shih-Chi Yang	11/12/2008	9:30am

PATIENT NO.	DX
YANGSHI0	**1.** 817.1 mutliple open fractures of hand bones
	2.
	3.
	4.

DESCRIPTION	✓	CPT	FEE	DESCRIPTION	✓	CPT	FEE
EXAMINATION				**FRACTURES**			
New Patient				Clavicle		23500	
Problem Focused		99201		Scapula		23570	
Expanded Problem Focused		99202		Humerus, proximal		23600	
Detailed		99203		Humerus, shaft		24500	
Comprehensive		99204		Radial, colles w/manip		25605	
Comprehensive/Complex		99205		Radial, h or n w/out manip		24650	
Established Patient				Ulna, proximal		24670	
Minimum		99211		Radius & Ulna		25560	
Problem Focused		99212		Radius, colles, distal		25600	
Expanded Problem Focused		99213		Ulna, styloid		25650	
Detailed		99214		Hand MC		26600	315
Comprehensive/Complex		99215		Finger/Thumb		26720	
				Coccyx		27200	
CONSULTATION				Femur, distal		27508	
Office				Tibia, prox/plateua		27530	
Problem Focused		99241		Tibia & Fibula, shaft		27750	
Expanded Problem Focused		99242		Fibula, prox/shaft		27780	
Detailed		99243		Foot, MT		28470	
Comprehensive		99244		Toe, great		28490	
Comprehensive/Complex		99245		Toe, others		28510	
Confirmatory							
Problem Focused		99271		**X-RAY**			
Expanded Problem Focused		99272		Clavicle		73000	
Detailed		99273		Humerus		73060	
Comprehensive		99274		Forearm		73090	
Comprehensive/Complex		99275		Hand, 2 views		73120	
				Hand, 3 views	✓	73130	91

Internet Activity

1. Point your Web browser at the federal Office of Workers' Compensation Programs home page:
   http://www.dol.gov/esa/owcp_org.htm
   Click the link for OWCP Press Releases and read some of the latest information. Click the link for Information About OWCP to read more about the Office of Workers' Compensation Programs.

2. Search for the workers' compensation Web site for your state. If you prefer, you may try entering the URL for your state: http://www.state.oh.us
   where "oh" is the two-letter abbreviation for your state (in this example, Ohio), and then locate workers' compensation information from there. What are your state's requirements for workers' compensation coverage? Try to locate a sample claim form for your state.

3. The Social Security Administration's online publications include an electronic booklet entitled "If You Are Blind or Have Low Vision—How We Can Help." It is available at the following address:
   http://www.ssa.gov/pubs/10052.html
   Read through the material in Part 1—General Information to learn about the differences between SSDI and SSI.

NDCMediSoft Activity

14.1 Review MediSoft Entries Specific to a Workers' Compensation Case

This activity explores various entries in MediSoft for a patient involved in a work-related injury. The patient, William Nisonson, is covered by CarePlus Workers' Compensation insurance.

1. Open the Lists menu and select Patients/Guarantors and Cases.
2. In the Search For box, key NI to display William Nisonson's information in the Patient List dialog box.
3. Click the Edit Patient button to display the Name, Address tab of the Patient/Guarantor dialog box.
4. As William Nisonson was injured at work, his work information should be reviewed. Click the Other Information tab.

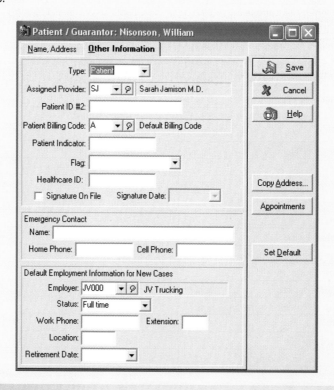

Computer Exploration

5. The bottom panel of the Other Information tab shows that William Nisonson is employed full time by JV Trucking. Click the Cancel button to close this dialog box and return to the Patient List dialog box.

6. In the right side of the Patient List dialog box, click William Nisonson's case description (Fracture, Tibia & Fibula) to select it, and then click the Edit Case button.

7. The Personal tab of the Case dialog box is displayed. Nisonson's employment information is also displayed in the Personal tab. Click the Policy 1 tab to view the details of his insurance policy for this case.

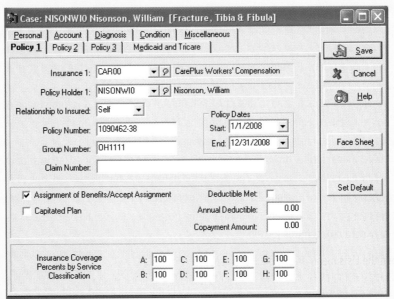

8. The Policy 1 tab shows that Nisonson is covered for the injury by CarePlus Workers' Compensation. The group plan number indicates that the plan is most likely offered through his work. The plan has no copay and pays for 100 percent of covered services.

   Click the Account tab.

9. Notice that the Price Code box reads A in this case. Click the Condition tab.

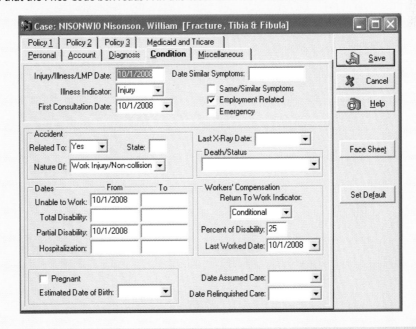

10. The Condition tab is used to report information about a patient's general status or condition, including information about a workers' compensation claim. The top panel in the Condition tab contains the Injury/Illness/LMP Date box, which is used in workers' compensation cases to indicate the date of the injury, in Nisonson's case, 10/1/2008. The other boxes in this panel are used to indicate other details about the claim, including the date of the first consultation with a health care provider (10/1/2008), and whether the injury was employment related (the check indicates Yes) and/or an emergency (the unchecked box indicates No).

11. The Accident panel in the middle of the tab contains the Related To box. If the patient's condition is related to an accident, Yes is selected in this box. Other options include No, or Auto, if the condition is related to an automobile accident. (If Auto is selected in the Related To box, then the state in which the accident occurred is entered in the State box.)

    The Nature Of box is used to describe the nature of the accident. Click the triangle button in the Nature Of box to display the drop-down list of options. In Nisonson's case, the Work Injury/Non-collision option is the correct choice. Press the Esc key to remove the drop-down list.

12. The Dates panel further down in the tab contains a series of From and To dates for recording the different stages of the patient's disability. The period the patient was unable to work due to the injury is indicated in the Unable to Work From and To boxes. In Nisonson's case, the To date is not yet known. If the patient was hospitalized during this period, the dates of the hospitalization would be provided in the Hospitalization From and To boxes in this section.

13. The last panel in the Condition tab that relates to a workers' compensation case is entitled Workers' Compensation. In this panel, the Return To Work Indicator box records the physician's estimate of the level of work the patient could participate in if he or she returned to work. Options include Limited, Normal, or Conditional. In this case, the physician has indicated Conditional.

    The physician's estimate of the patient's degree of disability is indicated in the Percent of Disability box (25 percent), and the date the patient last worked is reported in the Last Worked Date box (10/1/2008).

    Not all of this information is required for every workers' compensation case. The amount of information required depends on the insurance carrier's requirements and whether the claim is paper or electronic. Electronic claims in the HIPAA format require more details than paper claims.

14. Click the Cancel button to close the Case dialog button, and then click the Close button to close the Patient List dialog box.

Computer Exploration

15. To view William Nisonson's transaction data, click Enter Transactions on the Activities menu. Key NI in the Chart box, and press Enter.

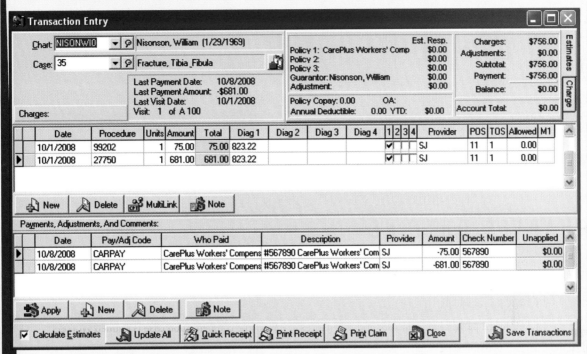

16. William Nisonson has two procedure charges, and no copayment charge. Click inside the Procedure box in the first transaction line, and then click the triangle button to display the procedure's description—NP Expanded Problem Focused. NP stands for new patient. Remember that CarePlus is a workers' compensation policy, and not Nisonson's usual plan. In a workers' compensation case, the patient is required to see the doctor connected with the workers' compensation plan. Press the Esc key to remove the drop-down list.

17. Compare the account details in the top panel with the transactions displayed in the rest of the dialog box. CarePlus has paid for both of Nisonson's procedures in full. Therefore, his account total is $0.00.

18. Click the Close button to exit the Transaction Entry dialog box.

Chapter 15

Hospital Billing and Reimbursement

Objectives

After studying this chapter, you should be able to:

1. Distinguish between inpatient and outpatient hospital services.
2. List the major steps relating to hospital billing and reimbursement.
3. Describe two differences in coding diagnoses for hospital inpatient cases and physician services.
4. Describe the classification system used for coding hospital procedures.
5. Describe the factors that affect the rate that Medicare pays for inpatient services.
6. Discuss the important items that are reported on the hospital health care claim.

Introduction

Although this text focuses on billing and reimbursement in medical practices, medical insurance specialists should be aware of the coding systems and the billing process used in hospitals. There are many financial agreements between physicians and hospitals; physicians in practices may have staff privileges at hospitals or be associated with hospitals as medical specialists. Physican practice staff also must bill for the procedures physicians perform in the hospital environment.

This chapter provides a brief overview of the types of inpatient and outpatient facilities, the various methods used by payers to pay for these services, and the coding systems that are used to report diagnoses and procedures for reimbursement.

Health Care Facilities: Inpatient Versus Outpatient

There are over 6,500 primarily nonprofit facilities that are known as acute care hospitals. Other kinds of health care facilities include psychiatric hospitals, rehabilitation facilities, clinics, nursing homes, subacute hospitals, and home health care agencies. Hospital size is measured by the number of beds.

Inpatient Care

Inpatient facilities are equipped for patients to stay overnight. In addition to hospital admission, inpatient care may be provided in

- **Skilled nursing facilities** (SNF): These facilities provide skilled nursing and/or rehabilitation services to help with recovery after a hospital stay. Skilled nursing care includes care given by licensed nurses under the direction of a physician, such as intravenous injections, tube feeding, and changing sterile dressings on a wound.
- *Long-term care facilities:* This term describes facilities such as nursing homes that provide custodial care for patients with chronic disabilities and prolonged illnesses.
- *Hospital emergency rooms or departments:* **Emergency** care involves a situation in which a delay in the treatment of the patient would lead to a significant increase in the threat to life or body part. Emergency care differs from urgently needed care, in which the condition must be treated right away but is not life-threatening.

Outpatient or Ambulatory Care

Many hospitals have expanded beyond inpatient services to offer a variety of outpatient services. Outpatient care, often called **ambulatory care**, covers all types of health services that do not require an overnight hospital stay. Most hospitals, for example, have outpatient departments that provide these services. Same-day surgery is performed in two types of facilities where patients do not stay overnight: a separate part of a hospital called an **ambulatory surgical unit** (ASU), and a free-standing facility called an **ambulatory surgical center** (ASC).

Different types of outpatient services are also provided in patients' home settings. **Home health care** services include care given at home, such as physical therapy or skilled nursing care. Home health care is provided by a **home health agency (HHA)**, an organization that provides home care services, including skilled nursing, physical therapy, occupational therapy, speech therapy, and care by home health aides. **At-home recovery care** is a different category; it includes help with the activities of daily living (ADLs), such as bathing and eating. **Hospice care** is a special approach to caring for people with terminal illnesses—that is, people who are not expected to live longer than six months—in a familiar and comfortable place, either a special hospice facility or the patient's home.

Integrated Delivery Systems

An important trend is the development of patient-centered integrated health care delivery systems, which are also called integrated networks. Health care providers from various specialties and health care facilities join together to provide patient services. At the center of the system is a single administration. Most integrated systems are locally organized, such as through the merger of local hospitals into large multifacility systems.

Integrated delivery systems change the focus of care from acute care to the continuum of care the patient needs. For example, an acute care hospital, a rehabilitation hospital, a long-term care facility, and a home care program might merge to form one system that can provide services for a stroke patient from the time of the stroke through to the resumption of normal activities. The network is set up to move the patient's record and the patient, too, from facility to facility as the patient's treatment and condition require.

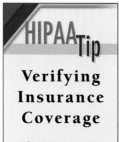

HIPAA Tip

Verifying Insurance Coverage

The HIPAA standard transaction used to verify patients' insurance is the 270/271 Eligibility for a Health Plan Inquiry/Response.

Hospital Claims Processing

Hospitals generally have large, separate departments that are responsible for major business functions. The admissions department records the patient's personal and financial information. In some hospitals, a separate insurance verification department is responsible for double-checking the patient's identity and confirming insurance coverage. The patient accounting department handles billing, and there is often a separate collections department. Organizing and maintaining patient medical records in hospitals are the duties of the **health information management (HIM)** department. Hospitals are also structured into departments for patient care. For example, there are professional services departments, such as laboratory, radiology, and surgery, as well as food service and housekeeping.

The three major steps in a patient's hospital stay from the insurance perspective are:

1. Admission, for creating or updating the patient's medical record, verifying patient insurance coverage, securing consent for release of information to payers, and collecting advance payments as appropriate
2. Treatment, during which the various departments' services are provided and charges generated
3. Discharge from the hospital or transfer to another facility, at which point the patient's record is compiled, claims and/or bills are created, and payment is followed up on

Admission

Inpatients are admitted to hospitals in a process called **registration.** Like physician practices, hospitals must keep clear, accurate records of their patients' diagnoses and treatments. The record begins at a patient's first admission to the facility or, in some facilities, during a preadmission process used to gather patient information before actual admission. Having a preadmission process gives staff members time to verify insurance coverage, calculate patients' likely financial responsibilities, and work out payment plans if necessary.

The HIM department keeps a health record system that permits storage and retrieval of clinical information by patient name or number, by physician, and by diagnosis and procedure. At almost every facility, a part or all of the records are computerized (each with a different computer system; the systems are not standardized). Each patient is listed in a patient register under a unique number. These numbers make up the **master patient index**—the main database that identifies patients. This index contains the patient's

- Last name, first name, and middle name or initial
- Birth date (eight-digit format)
- Sex
- Address
- Admission and/or treatment date
- **Attending physician**—the clinician primarily responsible for the care of the patient from the beginning of the hospital episode
- Health record number

More information is gathered for a hospital admission than is required for a visit to a physician practice. For example, in addition to hospital insurance, a patient may have long-term coverage to be recorded. Special points about the patient's care, such as language requirements, religion, or disabilities, are also entered in the record.

Outpatient department and emergency room insurance claims are often delayed because it is difficult to verify insurance coverage in these settings. The emergency department has its own registration system, because people who come for emergency and urgent treatment must receive care first by the nursing staff. Both outpatient and emergency room procedures must be set up to collect the minimum information. Many admissions departments join online insurance verification systems so that payers can be contacted during the registration process and verification received in seconds.

Consent

As in medical practices, the admission staff in hospitals must be sure patients give written consent for the work to be done and for the claim reporting that follows. Figure 15.1 (on page 498) shows an example of a consent form used in hospitals. It includes the same kinds of items patients sign in practices (the consent for medical treatment, acceptance of responsibility for payment, and assignment of benefits) and three unique items:

1. A statement covering the conditions under which the facility is responsible for the patient's personal possessions.
2. Advance directives, also called living wills, that cover how patients want to receive health care, including routine treatments and life-saving methods, if they become incapacitated. Patients may also appoint someone to make such decisions if they cannot.

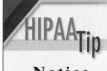

HIPAA Tip

Notice of Privacy Practices

Under the HIPAA Privacy Rule, hospitals must also present patients with a copy of their privacy practices at registration and have them sign an acknowledgment that they have received this notice.

CONSENT FOR MEDICAL TREATMENT

I, the undersigned, acknowledge and understand that, in presenting myself for voluntary registration, Inpatient, Outpatient, or Emergency Services at Memorial Hospital, authorize and consent to such diagnostic procedures, tests, or treatments as may be ordered by my physician(s) and/or emergency department physician and carried out by members of the medical staff and hospital associates. I voluntarily consent to such health care, medical and surgical, including anesthesia, X-ray, and lab procedures as may be conduced, requested, directed by delegate, or designated in the judgment of the attending physician or consulting physician. Administrative fluids, blood, and blood products/components, medications, and radiology procedures are included in this consent.

RELEASE OF MEDICAL INFORMATION

I authorize Memorial Hospital to release medical information or copies from my medical record from my date of admission through my date of discharge to insurance companies, third-party payers or authorized paying agent, or claims review organizations in order to process a claim for payment in my behalf. This information may be disseminated to any and all employers, insurance companies, or their designees present in the Hospital by the patient or the patient's representative that may provide coverage for the health care organization's charges, and to comply with the requirement of any Professional Review Organization for Joint Commission on Accreditation of Healthcare Organizations for Utilization Review and Medical Audit. I also authorize release of information to agencies that may be involved in my continuity of care. I authorize any health care provider including my physician and consulting physicians to provide to the hospital or its designee, upon request, information concerning my care, condition, and treatment for quality assurance and risk management purposes.

VALUABLES: RELEASE FROM RESPONSIBILITY

I understand that Memorial Hospital does not assume responsibility for personal possessions unless they are registered in the hospital safe. This opportunity has been offered to me.

ADVANCE DIRECTIVES

Has a living will or health care power of attorney been prepared?	Yes	No	N/A
I have provided Memorial Hospital with the most current copy.	Yes	No	N/A
I have received advance directives information.	Yes	No	N/A
The Patient's Bill of Rights has been presented to me.	Yes	No	N/A

Courtesy of Illini Hospital, Silvis, Illinois

FINANCIAL AGREEMENT AND ASSIGNMENT OF INSURANCE BENEFITS

I hereby assign, transfer, and convey all my rights, title, and interest to medical reimbursement under by insurance policy(s) to Memorial Hospital. It is understood, whether I sign as agent, patient, or as guarantor, that I am directly responsible and will pay for service rendered and not paid by insurance agency. An assignment of benefits by any insurance policy or medical reimbursement plan shall not be deemed a waiver of Memorial Hospital's right to require payment directly from the undersigned or the patient. Memorial Hospital expressly reserves the right to require such payment. Should the account be referred to any agency for collection (collection agency or attorney), the undersigned shall pay all reasonable attorney fees, collection costs, and interest. All delinquent accounts may bear a late payment penalty of not more than 10 1/2% per month thereafter charged from the date of service. I assign payment of all insurance benefits to physicians providing professional services at Memorial Hospital in conjunction with hospital services.

BILLING OF PROFESSIONAL SERVICES

I understand that I am financially responsible for professional services of the radiologist(s), pathologist(s), anesthesiologist(s), emergency department physician, and other physician charges that are not billed by the hospital. I acknowledge that the physicians providing professional services, including consultants and on-call physicians, are an independent medical staff who are not employees or agents of Memorial Hospital. I hereby authorize release of information requested by insurance/billing agencies to the aforementioned parties.

AN IMPORTANT MESSAGE FROM MEDICARE

I acknowledge that I have received a copy of *An Important Message from Medicare* and have been directed to read this brochure.

I have read this form that consists of six important areas and understand its contents. I have had an opportunity to ask questions that have been answered to my satisfaction. I voluntarily sign immediately below.

MR#_____ Date of Admission/Service _____

PA# _____ Signature: _____

Witness (name and relation) _____

Hospital Representative: _____
UCF0004   Rev: 3/97

FIGURE 15.1   Hospital Consent Form

3. Acknowledgment that the patient has received a copy of the one-page printout entitled "An Important Message from Medicare." The printout, which CMS requires hospitals to give Medicare patients on registration, explains the beneficiary's rights as a hospital patient as well as his or her appeal rights regarding hospital discharge (see Figure 15.2).

IMPORTANT MESSAGE FROM MEDICARE

YOUR RIGHTS AS A HOSPITAL PATIENT

- You have the right to receive necessary hospital services covered by Medicare, or covered by your Medicare Health Plan ("your Plan") if you are a Plan enrollee.
- You have the right to know about any decisions that the hospital, your doctor, your Plan, or anyone else makes about your hospital stay and who will pay for it.
- Your doctor, your Plan, or the hospital should arrange for services you will need after you leave the hospital. Medicare or your Plan may cover some care in your home (home health care) and other kinds of care, if ordered by your doctor or by your Plan. You have a right to know about these services, who will pay for them, and where you can get them. If you have any questions, talk to your doctor or Plan, or talk to other hospital personnel.

YOUR HOSPITAL DISCHARGE & MEDICARE APPEAL RIGHTS

Date of Discharge: When your doctor or Plan determines that you can be discharged from the hospital, you will be advised of your planned date of discharge. You may appeal if you think that you are being asked to leave the hospital too soon. If you stay in the hospital after your planned date of discharge, it is likely that your charges for additional days in the hospital will not be covered by Medicare or your Plan.

Your Right to an Immediate Appeal without Financial Risk: When you are advised of your planned date of discharge, if you think you are being asked to leave the hospital too soon, you have the right to appeal to your Quality Improvement Organization (also known as a QIO). The QIO is authorized by Medicare to provide a second opinion about your readiness to leave. You may call Medicare toll-free, 24 hours a day, at 1-800-MEDICARE (1-800-633-4227), or TTY/TTD: 1-877-486-2048, for more information on asking your QIO for a second opinion. If you appeal to the QIO by noon of the day after you receive a noncoverage notice, you are not responsible for paying for the days you stay in the hospital during the QIO review, even if the QIO disagrees with you. The QIO will decide within one day after it receives the necessary information.

Other Appeal Rights: If you miss the deadline for filing an immediate appeal, you may still request a review by the QIO (or by your Plan, if you are a Plan enrollee) before you leave the hospital. However, you will have to pay for the costs of your additional days in the hospital if the QIO (or your Plan) denies your appeal. You may file for this review at the address or telephone number of the QIO (or of your Plan).

OMB Approval No. 0938-0692. Form No. CMS-R-193 (January 2003)

FIGURE 15.2 Printout Entitled "An Important Message from Medicare"

Medicare as a Secondary Payer

Many patients are classified as MSP accounts. These patients are Medicare beneficiaries, but Medicare is the secondary payer. For example, Medicare requires automobile insurance companies to pay for patients' care after car accidents, no matter who is at fault. In these cases, the MSP information must be taken at registration to avoid delays in claim processing. The form used to determine the primary payer is shown in Figure 15.3 (on pages 500–501). If the patient does not know what insurance company covered the other person involved in the accident, the hospital may request a police accident report to obtain the information to bill the accident insurance that is primary to Medicare.

The following form lists questions to ask Medicare beneficiaries at admission. Use this chart as a guide to help identify other payers that may be primary to Medicare. Beginning with Part 1, ask the beneficiary each question in sequence. Comply with any instructions that follow an answer you have checked. If the instructions direct you to go to another part, have the beneficiary answer, in sequence, each question under the new part. If an answer you have checked is followed by the message "STOP," bill that beneficiary's services to the insurer indicated.

NOTE: There may be situations where more than one insurer is primary to Medicare (e.g., automobile insurer and EGHP). *Be sure to identify all possible insurers.*

Part I

1. Was illness/injury due to a work-related accident/condition and covered by WC plan or Federal Black Lung Program?

_____yes:

Name and address of WC plan or Federal Black Lung Program

_____

Patient's policy or identification number
STOP: WC OR FEDERAL BL PROGRAM IS PRIMARY PAYER.

_____no. GO TO PART II

Part II

1. Was illness/injury due to a non-work-related accident?

_____yes.

_____no: GO TO PART III

2. What type of accident caused illness/injury?

_____automobile

Name and address of automobile insurer

_____

Insurance claim number
STOP: AUTO INSURANCE IS PRIMARY PAYER.

_____other;

3. Was another party responsible for this accident?

_____yes;

Name and address of any liability insurer
Insurance claim number

STOP: LIABILITY INSURER IS PRIMARY PAYER.

_____no; GO TO PART III

PART III

1. Is the patient age 65 or over?

_____yes.

_____no; GO TO PART IV

2. Is the patient undergoing kidney dialysis for ESRD?

_____yes.

_____no.

FIGURE 15.3 Medicare Secondary Payer Determination Form

Pretreatment Patient Payment Collection

Most facilities attempt to collect payments that patients are responsible for—or at least a deposit—before admission and treatment. The following types of payments may be collected in advance:

3. Is the patient employed and covered by the Employer's Group Health Plan?

_____yes:

Name and address of EGHP

Patient Identification Number

    STOP: EGHP IS PRIMARY PAYER.

_____no.

4. Is the patient's spouse employed?

_____yes.

_____no; STOP; MEDICARE IS PRIMARY PAYER.

5. Is the patient covered under the group health plan of the spouse's employer?

_____yes:

Name and address of EGHP

Patient Identification Number

    STOP: EGHP IS PRIMARY PAYER.

_____no; STOP: MEDICARE IS PRIMARY PAYER.

Part IV

1. Is the patient entitled to benefits solely on the basis of ESRD?

_____yes.

_____no; GO TO PART V:

2. Is the patient covered by an EGHP?

_____yes;

Name and address of EGHP

Patient's Identification Number

_____no; STOP: MEDICARE IS PRIMARY PAYER.

3. Has the patient been undergoing kidney dialysis for more than 18 months or been entitled to Medicare for more than 18 months?

_____yes.

_____no.

4. Is the patient within an 18-month coordination period?

_____yes; STOP: EGHP IS PRIMARY PAYER.

_____no; STOP: MEDICARE IS PRIMARY PAYER.

Part V

1. Is the patient a disabled Medicare beneficiary under age 65?

_____yes.

_____no; STOP: MEDICARE IS PRIMARY PAYER.

2. Is the patient covered by a large group health plan (LGHP) based on the patient's own employment or employment of a spouse or parent?

_____yes;

Name and address of LGHP

Patient's Identification Number

    STOP: LGHP IS PRIMARY PAYER.

_____no; STOP: MEDICARE IS PRIMARY PAYER.

Source: Reprinted from CMS

FIGURE 15.3 Medicare Secondary Payer Determination Form (*continued*)

- Medicare Part A and Part B deductibles, coinsurance, and copayments.
- Medicare lifetime reserve (LTR) day amounts. Medicare pays for sixty days (over a person's lifetime) when a patient is in the hospital for more than ninety days. For each lifetime reserve day, Medicare pays all covered costs

except for a daily coinsurance ($420 in 2003). Patients without additional coverage may be required to make arrangements for paying this daily amount before admission.

- Estimated amounts for noncovered services.
- Private room differential and fees for extras, such as telephone and television services.
- Estimated amounts the patient's insurance does not cover, such as coinsurance.

Records of Treatments and Charges during the Hospital Stay

Standards for hospital patient medical records are set by the Joint Commission on Accreditation of Healthcare Organizations (JCAHO; see Chapter 1). The hospital's own bylaws and Medicare regulations for participating hospitals also influence medical record standards. The medical record contains (1) notes of the attending physician and other treating physicians, such as operative reports; (2) ancillary documents like nurses' notes and pathology, radiology, and laboratory reports; (3) patient data, including insurance information for patients who have been in the hospital before; and (4) a correspondence section that contains signed consent forms and other documents. In line with HIPAA security requirements, the confidentiality and security of patients' medical records are guarded by all hospital staff members. Both technical means, such as passwords and encryption, and legal protections, such as requiring staff to sign confidentiality pledges, are used to ensure privacy.

Patients are usually charged by hospitals for the following services:

- Room and board
- Medications
- Ancillary tests and procedures, such as laboratory workups
- Equipment used during surgery or therapy
- The amount of time spent in an operating room, recovery room, or intensive care unit

Patients are charged according to the type of accommodations and services they receive. For example, the rate for a private room is higher than the rate for a semiprivate room, and intensive care unit or recovery room charges are higher than charges for standard rooms. When patients are transferred to these services, the activity is tracked. In an outpatient or an emergency department encounter, there is no room and bed charge; instead, there is a visit charge.

Average service charges vary according to the type of care the hospital provides. For example, at a hundred-bed hospital that provides basic services, a large bill may be $15,000; but at a five-hundred-bed hospital performing complicated surgeries such as open heart procedures, a large bill may be more than $100,000.

Discharge and Billing

By the time patients are discharged from the hospital, their accounts usually have been totaled and insurance claims or bills created. The goal in most cases is to file a claim or bill within seven days after discharge. A typical bill for a patient contains many items. The items are recorded on the hospital's charge description master file, usually called the **charge master**, which is the equivalent of a medical practice encounter form. This master list contains the following information for each item:

- The hospital's code for the service and a brief description of it
- The charge for the service

- The hospital department (such as laboratory)
- The hospital's cost to provide the service
- A procedure code for the service

The hospital's computer system tracks the services in various departments. For example, if the patient is sent to the intensive care (IC) unit after surgery, the IC billing group reports the specific services received by the patient, and these charges are entered on the patient's account.

Inpatient (Hospital) Coding

The HIM department is also responsible for diagnostic and procedural coding of patients' medical records. Coding is done by inpatient medical coders as soon as a patient is discharged. Some inpatient coders are generalists; others may have special skills in a certain area, like surgical coding or Medicare. ICD-9-CM Volumes 1 and 2 are used to code inpatient diagnoses, and Volume 3 is used to code procedures performed during the hospitalization.

Hospital Diagnostic Coding

Different rules apply for assigning inpatient codes than for physician office diagnoses. These rules, found in the *Coding Clinic for ICD-9-CM,* a publication of the American Hospital Association's (AHA) Central Office on ICD-9-CM, were developed by the four groups that are responsible for the ICD-9-CM: The AHA, the American Health Information Management Association (AHIMA), the Centers for Medicare and Medicaid Services (CMS), and the National Center for Health Statistics (NCHS). The rules are based on the requirements for sequencing diagnoses and reporting procedures that are part of the **Uniform Hospital Discharge Data Set (UHDDS)**. Medicare, Medicaid, and many private payers require the UHDDS rules to be followed for reimbursement of hospital services. The rules are extensive. Three of them are briefly described below to illustrate some of the major differences between inpatient and outpatient coding.

Principal Diagnosis

For diagnostic coding in medical practices, the first code listed is the primary diagnosis, defined as the main reason for the patient's encounter with the provider. Under hospital inpatient rules, the **principal diagnosis** is listed first. The principal diagnosis is the condition established *after study* to be chiefly responsible for the admission. This principal diagnosis is listed even if the patient has other, more severe diagnoses. In some cases, the **admitting diagnosis**—the condition identified by the physician at admission to the hospital—is also reported.

Example: Inpatient admitting diagnosis: Severe abdominal pain (789.00)

Inpatient principal diagnosis after surgery: Acute appendicitis (540)

Suspected or Unconfirmed Diagnoses

When the patient is admitted for workups to uncover the cause of a problem, inpatient medical coders can also use suspected or unconfirmed conditions (rule-outs) if they are listed as the admitting diagnosis. The admitting diagnosis may not match the principal diagnosis once a final decision has been made.

Example: Inpatient admitting diagnosis: Probable acute appendicitis (540)

Inpatient principal diagnosis: Diverticulosis of the small intestine (562.00)

Comorbidities and Complications

The inpatient coder also lists all the other conditions that have an effect on the patient's hospital stay or course of treatment. A patient's other conditions at admission that affect patient care for the hospitalization being coded are called **comorbidities**, meaning coexisting conditions. Conditions that develop as complications of surgery or other treatments are coded as **complications**. Comorbidities and complications are shown in the patient medical record with the initials *CC*.

Examples: Comorbidity: The nurse's notes stated that the patient needed additional care because of chronic obstructive pulmonary disease (COPD) with emphysema.

Code: 492.8

Complication: The physician's notes indicate a diagnosis of postoperative hypertension as a postoperative complication.

Codes: Hypertension, 402.90, and 997.1, Cardiac Complications

Coding CCs is important, because their presence may increase the hospital's reimbursement level for the care. The hospital insurance claim form discussed later in this chapter allows for up to eight additional conditions to be reported.

Hospital Procedural Coding

The UHDDS requires significant procedures to be reported along with the principal diagnosis, comorbidities, and complications. Significant procedures have any of these characteristics (F. Brown, *ICD-9-CM Coding Handbook,* 2002, 47):

* They involve surgery.
* Anesthesia (other than topical) is administered.
* The procedure involves a risk to the patient.
* The procedure requires specialized training.

In inpatient coding, the ICD's Volume 3, Procedures, is used to assign procedure codes. Reporting Volume 3 codes when appropriately documented may increase the hospital's reimbursement because some procedures require more hospital time for recovery. For example, codes in range 93.31–93.39 are assigned when patients require physical therapy procedures such as whirlpool therapy.

Volume 3 Organization

Volume 3 of the ICD-9-CM has an Alphabetic Index and a Tabular List, similar to Volumes 1 and 2. The Alphabetic Index is used to locate the procedure, and the Tabular List is used to confirm the code selection. Codes are either three or four digits. The fourth digit must be assigned if available.

TABLE 15.1	ICD-9-CM Volume 3 Tabular List Organization	
Chapter		**Range**
1 Operations on the Nervous System		01–05
2 Operations on the Endocrine System		06–07
3 Operations on the Eye		08–17
4 Operations on the Ear		18–20
5 Operations on the Nose, Mouth, and Pharynx		21–29
6 Operations on the Respiratory System		30–34
7 Operations on the Cardiovascular System		35–39
8 Operations on the Hemic and Lymphatic System		40–41
9 Operations on the Digestive System		42–54
10 Operations on the Urinary System		55–59
11 Operations on the Male Genital Organs		60–64
12 Operations on the Female Genital Organs		65–71
13 Obstetrical Procedures		72–75
14 Operations on the Musculoskeletal System		76–84
15 Operations on the Integumentary System		85–86
16 Miscellaneous Diagnostic and Therapeutic Procedures		87–99

Thinking It Through—15.2

Why do the inpatient coding rules permit coding rule-outs for diagnoses, whereas the physician office coding rules do not?

Compliance Guideline

Inpatient versus Outpatient Diagnosis Coding
The UHDDS inpatient rules apply only to inpatient services. Hospital-based outpatient services and physician-office services are reported using the ICD-9-CM, Volumes 1 and 2, following the outpatient rules (see Chapter 4, Figure 4.3) and CPT.

The organization of the Tabular List and the range of codes are shown in Table 15.1.

Principal Procedure

The **principal procedure** assigned by the inpatient medical coder is the procedure that is most closely related to the treatment of the principal diagnosis. It is usually a surgical procedure. If no surgery is performed, the principal procedure may be a therapeutic procedure. Here is an example:

Inpatient principal diagnosis: Acute tonsillitis 463 (ICD-9-CM code from Volume 1, the Tabular list)

Inpatient principal procedure: Tonsillectomy 28.2 (ICD-9-CM code from Volume 3, Procedures, the Tabular List)

Payers and Payment Methods

Medicare and Medicaid both provide coverage for eligible patients' hospital services. Medicare Part A, known as hospital insurance, helps pay for inpatient hospital care, skilled nursing facilities, hospice care, and home health care. Private payers also offer hospitalization insurance. Most employees have coverage for hospital services through employers' programs.

Medicare Inpatient Payment System

Diagnosis-Related Groups

CMS's actions to control the cost of hospital services began with the implementation of **diagnosis-related groups (DRGs)** in 1983. Under the DRG classification system, the hospital stays of patients who had similar diagnoses were studied. Groupings were created based on the relative value of the resources that physicians and hospitals used nationally for patients with similar conditions. The calculations combine data about the patient's diagnosis and procedures with factors that affect the outcome of treatment, such as age, gender, comorbidities, and complications. Figure 15.4 shows the DRGs for conditions related to the circulatory system.

Prospective Payment System

At the same time the DRG system was created, CMS changed the way hospitals were paid. Payment for institutional services moved from a fee-for-service approach to the Medicare **Prospective Payment System (PPS)**. In the PPS, the payment for each type of service is set ahead of time based on the DRG. Hospitals can no longer bill Medicare their usual or customary fee. For each DRG, the PPS sets the number of hospital days and the hospital services that are reimbursed. If a patient has a principal diagnosis accompanied by comorbidities or complications, such as coma or convulsions, these additional signs are evidence of a more difficult course of treatment, and the DRG reimbursement is raised. If, however, the hospital holds the patient for longer than the DRG specifies without such circumstances, it still receives only the allowed amount and must write off the difference between the reimbursement and its actual costs. Each hospital negotiates a rate for each DRG with CMS, based on its geographic location, labor and supply costs, and teaching costs.

Quality Improvement Organizations and Utilization Review

When DRGs were established, CMS also set up Peer Review Organizations (PROs), which were later renamed Quality Improvement Organizations (QIOs). Made up of practicing physicians and other health care experts, these organizations are contracted by CMS in each state to review Medicare and Medicaid claims for the appropriateness of hospitalization and clinical care.

QIOs aim to ensure that payment is made only for medically necessary services. In many circumstances, Medicare requires precertification for inpatient or outpatient surgery, as do many private payers. While the admission or the procedure may be approved, the amount of payment is usually not determined until the QIO reviews the services. When reviewing submitted claims, QIOs may take one of the following actions:

- Review and fully approve a claim
- Review and deny portions of a claim
- Review a claim for a patient's inpatient services, and decide that no stay was medically necessary
- Decide to conduct a postpayment audit

QIOs are also resources for investigating quality of care. They review patients' complaints about the quality of care provided by inpatient hospitals, hospital outpatient departments, hospital emergency rooms, skilled nursing facilities, home health agencies, Medicare managed care plans, and ambulatory surgical centers. They also contract with private payers to perform these services.

DRG 103, Heart Transplant
DRG 104, Cardiac Valve Procedures with Cardiac Catheterization
DRG 105, Cardiac Valve Procedures without Cardiac Catheterization
DRG 106, Coronary Bypass with Cardiac Catheterization
DRG 107, Coronary Bypass without Cardiac Catheterization
DRG 108, Other Cardiothoracic Procedures
DRG 110, Major Cardiovascular Procedures with Comorbidity or Complication
DRG 111, Major Cardiovascular Procedures without Cormorbidity or Complication
DRG 112, Percutaneous Cardiovascular Procedures
DRG 113, Amputation for Circulatory System Disorders Except Upper Limb and Toe
DRG 114, Upper Limb and Toe Amputation for Circulatory System Disorders
DRG 115, Permanent Cardiac Pacemaker Implant with Acute Myocardial Infarction, Heart Failure, or Shock
DRG 116, Other Permanent Cardiac Pacemaker Implant or Generator Procedure
DRG 117, Cardiac Pacemaker Revision Except Device Replacement
DRG 118, Cardiac Pacemaker Device Replacement
DRG 119, Vein Ligation and Stripping
DRG 120, Other Circulatory System Operating Room Procedures
DRG 121, Circulatory Disorders with Acute Myocardial Infarction and Cardiovascular Complication, Discharged Alive
DRG 122, Circulatory Disorders with Acute Myocardial Infarction without Cardiovascular Complication, Discharged Alive
DRG 123, Circulatory Disorders with Acute Myocardial Infarction, Expired
DRG 124, Circulatory Disorders Except Acute Myocardial Infarction with Cardiac Catheterization and Complex Diagnosis
DRG 125, Circulatory Disorders Except Acute Myocardial Infarction with Cardiac Catheterization without Complex Diagnosis
DRG 126, Acute and Subacute Endocarditis
DRG 127, Heart Failure and Shock
DRG 128, Deep Vein Thrombophlebitis
DRG 129, Cardiac Arrest, Unexplained
DRG 130, Peripheral Vascular Disorders with Cormorbidity or Complication
DRG 131, Peripheral Vascular Disorders without Comorbidity or Complication
DRG 132, Atherosclerosis with Cormorbidity or Complication
DRG 133, Atherosclerosis without Cormorbidity or Complication
DRG 134, Hypertension
DRG 135, Cardiac Congenital and Valvular Disorders, Age Greater than 17 with Comorbidity or Complication
DRG 136, Cardiac Congenital and Valvular Disorders, Age Greater than 17 without Comorbidity or Complication
DRG 137, Cardiac Congenital and Valvular Disorders, Age 0-17
DRG 138, Cardiac Arrhythmia and Conduction Disorders with Comorbidity or Complication
DRG 139, Cardiac Arrhythmia and Conduction Disorders without Comorbidity or Complication
DRG 140, Angina Pectoris
DRG 141, Syncope and Collapse with Comorbidity or Complication
DRG 142, Syncope and Collapse without Comorbidity or Complication
DRG 143, Chest Pain
DRG 144, Other Circulatory System Diagnoses with Comorbidity or Complication
DRG 145, Other Circulatory System Diagnoses without Comorbidity or Complication
DRG 478, Other Vascular Procedures with Comorbidity or Complication
DRG 479, Other Vascular Procedures without Comorbidity or Complication

FIGURE 15.4 Diagnosis-Related Groups for Diseases and Disorders of the Circulatory System

Medicare Outpatient Payment Systems

The use of DRGs under a PPS system proved to be very effective in controlling costs. In 2000, CMS implemented a PPS approach for outpatient hospital services, which previously were paid on a fee-for-service basis. These payment programs include:

- *Hospital outpatient Prospective Payment System (PPS):* The Balanced Budget Act of 1997 authorized Medicare to begin paying for hospital outpatient services under a prospective payment system. In place of DRGs, patients are grouped under an **ambulatory patient classification (APC)** system. The APC system is based on the work of the 3M Company, which created ambulatory patient groups (APGs). Reimbursement is made according to preset amounts based on the value of each APC.
- *Ambulatory surgical centers (ASC):* CMS also sets prospective APC rates for facility services provided by Medicare-participating ASCs.
- *Skilled nursing facility (SNF) Prospective Payment System:* The Balanced Budget Act of 1997 also requires SNFs to be paid under a prospective payment system; patients are classified under the Resource Utilization Group (RUG) system.

Private Payers

Because of the expense involved with hospitalization, private payers encourage providers to minimize the number of days patients stay in the hospital. Most private payers establish the standard number of days allowed for various conditions (called the estimated length of stay, or ELOS), and compare the ELOS to the patient's actual stay as a way to control costs.

Many private payers have also adopted the UHDDS format and the DRG method of setting prospective payments for hospital services. Hospitals and the payers, which may include Blue Cross and Blue Shield or other managed care plans, negotiate the rates for each DRG.

A number of private payers use the DRG to negotiate the fees they pay hospitals. Two other payment methods are used by managed care plans. Preferred provider organizations (PPOs) often negotiate a discount from the DRG with the hospital and its affiliated physicians. The hospital may have discounted fee structures with a number of PPOs and other managed care plans—each different, depending on what was agreed to.

Health maintenance organizations (HMOs) negotiate capitated contracts with hospitals, too. The hospital agrees to provide care for a set population of prospective patients who are plan members. The HMO in turn pays the hospital a flat rate—a single set fee for each member. This rate may be a per diem (per day) rate that is paid for each day the patient is in the hospital, regardless of the specific services. Like the DRG model, when a patient is held in the hospital for longer than is stated in the agreement between the HMO and the hospital, the hospital has to write off the extra cost.

Claims and Follow-Up

Hospitals must submit claims for Medicare Part A reimbursement to Medicare fiscal intermediaries using the HIPAA health care claim called **837I**. This EDI format, similar to the 837 claim (Chapter 8), is called I for "Institutional"; physicians' claim is called 837P, for "Professional."

In some situations, a paper claim form called the **UB-92** (uniform billing 1992), also known as the **CMS-1450**, is also accepted by most other payers.

837I Health Care Claim Completion

The 837I, like the 837P, has sections requiring data elements for the billing and the pay-to provider, the subscriber and patient, and the payer, plus claim and service level details. Most of the data elements report the same information as summarized below for the paper claim.

UB-92 Claim Form Completion

The UB-92 claim form has eighty-six data fields, some of which require multiple entries (see Figure 15.5 on page 510). The information for the form locators often requires choosing from a list of codes. Table 15.2 on pages 511–514 shows required information and possible choices for a Medicare claim. (In some cases, because the list of code choices is extensive, selected entries are shown as examples.) Private-payer required fields may be slightly different, and other condition codes or options are often available. All dates should use the eight-digit format.

Remittance Advice Processing

Hospitals receive a remittance advice (RA) when payments are transmitted by payers to their accounts. The patient accounting department and HIM check that appropriate payment has been received. Unless the software used for billing automatically reports if the billed code is not the same as the paid code, procedures to find and follow up on these exceptions must be set up between the two departments.

Similar to medical practices, hospitals set up schedules when accounts receivable are due and follow up on late payments. The turnaround time for electronic claims is usually from ten to fifteen days faster than for manual paper claims, so the follow-up procedures are organized according to each payer's submission method and usual turnaround time. Payers' requests for attachments such as emergency department reports may delay payment.

Hospital Billing Compliance

Both outpatient and inpatient facilities must comply with federal and state law. In the Medicare program, compliance is as important for Part A claims as it is for Part B claims. To uncover fraud and abuse in Part A payments, the Office of the Inspector General (see Chapter 6) directs part of its annual OIG Work Plan at institutional providers. For example, CMS's annual Medical Provider Analysis and Review (MedPar) data show national averages for each DRG group in hospitals. The OIG uses these figures in preparing the part of the OIG Work Plan that is directed at hospital coding. A major target has been upcoding of DRG groups. The OIG has sought to uncover fraud when a hospital too often reports codes that result in high-relative-value DRGs.

> *Example:* A patient has a pulmonary edema (fluid in the lungs) that is due to the principal diagnosis of congestive heart failure. The correct ICD-9-CM code order leads to a DRG 127 classification. If the coder instead incorrectly reports pulmonary edema and respiratory failure, the patient is assigned DRG 87, which has a higher relative value, resulting in an improperly high payment.

The OIG has established lists of DRGs that are often the result of upcoding. Patterns of higher-than-normal reporting by a hospital of these DRGs may cause an investigation and possibly an audit of the hospital.

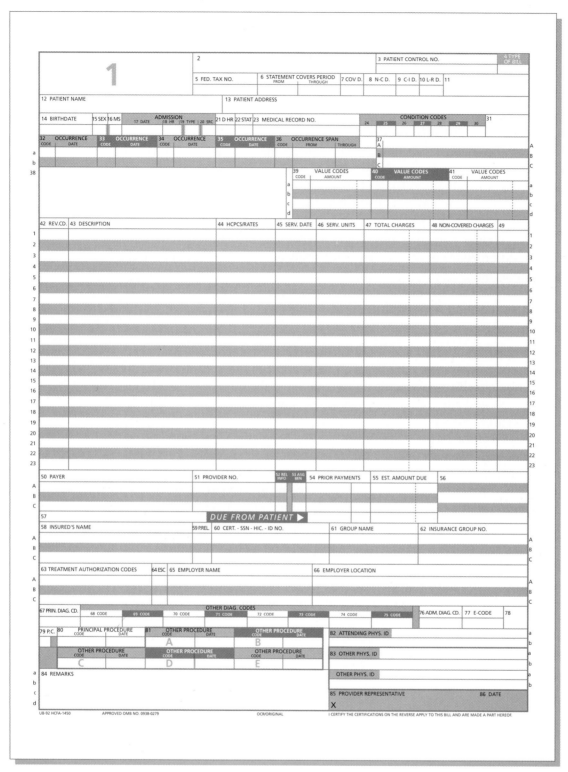

FIGURE 15.5 UB-92 Form

The OIG has also used MedPar data over the years to monitor other improper Medicare payments to hospitals. Two problem areas have been improper payments for nonphysician outpatient services and overpayments for patient transfers.

TABLE 15.2 **UB-92 Form Completion**

Form Locator	Description	Medicare Required?
1 (untitled)	Provider name, address, and telephone no.	Yes
2 (untitled)	Unassigned; for state use.	No
3 Patient Control Number	Patient's unique number assigned by the facility.	Yes
4 Type of Bill	Three-digit alphanumeric code: First digit identifies the facility type (e.g., 1 = hospital, 2 = SNF). Second digit identifies the care type (e.g., 1 = inpatient Part A, 2 = inpatient Part B, 3 = outpatient). Third digit identifies the billing sequence in this episode of care (e.g., 1 = this bill encompasses entire inpatient confinement or course of outpatient treatment for which provider expects payment from the payer).	Yes
5 Federal Tax Number	Not required.	No
6 Statement Covers Period (From—Through)	The beginning and ending dates of the period included on the bill; dates before patient's entitlement are not shown. From date is used to determine timely filing.	Yes
7 Covered Days	The total number of covered days during the billing period, including lifetime reserve days elected for which Medicare payment is requested. Should be the total of units in form locator 46.	Yes
8 Noncovered Days	The total number of noncovered days during the billing period not billable to Medicare.	Yes
9 Coinsurance Days	The number of covered inpatient hospital days after the 60th day and before the 91st day, or the number of covered inpatient SNF days after the 20th day and before the 101st day.	Yes
10 Lifetime Reserve Days	Number of lifetime reserve days applicable.	Yes
11 (untitled)	Unassigned; for state use.	No
12 Patient's Name	Patient's last name, first name, and middle initial.	Yes
13 Patient's Address	Patient's full mailing address: street number and name, PO Box or RFD; city, state, and ZIP code.	Yes
14 Patient's Birthdate	Patient's birthdate; if unavailable, use zeroes.	Yes
15 Patient Sex	M for male; F for female.	Yes
16 Patient's Marital Status	S = single; M = married; D = divorced; W = widowed; U = unknown.	No
17 Admission Date	Month, day, and year of inpatient admission.	Yes
18 Admission Hour	Time of day of admission.	No
19 Type of Admission	Required for inpatient bills: 1 = emergency, 2 = urgent, 3 = elective, 9 = information not available (rarely used).	Yes
20 Source of Admission	Source of admission: 1 = physician referral. 2 = clinic referral. 3 = HMO referral. 4 = transfer from a hospital. 5 = transfer from an SNF. 6 = transfer from another facility. 7 = emergency room. 8 = court/law enforcement. 9 = information not available. A = transfer from a rural primary care hospital.	Yes
21 Discharge Hour	Time of day of patient discharge.	No
22 Patient Status	For Part A inpatient, SNF, hospice, and outpatient hospital services: 01 = routine discharge to self or home. 02 = discharge to another short-term general hospital. 03 = discharge to SNF. 04 = discharge to ICF. 05 = discharge to another type of facility. 06 = discharge to home under care of home health organization. 07 = left against medical advice or discontinued care. 08 = discharge to home under care of home IV drug therapy provider. 09 = admitted as inpatient (after outpatient services). 20 = expired. 30 = still patient or expected to return for outpatient services. 40 = expired at home (hospice claims only).	Yes (continued)

TABLE 15.2 | UB-92 Form Completion (*continued*)

Form Locator	Description	Medicare Required?
22 Patient Status (continued)	41 = expired in a medical facility (hospice claims only). 42 = expired, place unknown (hospice claims only). 50 = hospice—home. 51 = hospice—medical facility.	
23 Medical Record Number	Assigned to patient's record by the provider.	Yes
24, 25, 26, 27, 28, 29, 30 Condition Codes*	Codes relating to bill that may affect processing; examples include: 02 = condition is employment-related. 04 = patient is HMO-enrollee. 05 = lien has been filed. 06 = ESRD patient in first eighteen months of employer group health insurance. 07 = treatment of nonterminal condition for hospice. 08 = beneficiary would not provide information about other insurance coverage. 09 = neither patient nor spouse is employed. 10 = patient and/or spouse employed, but no employer group health plan coverage exists. 31 = patient is student (full-time, day). 67 = beneficiary elects not to use lifetime reserve days.	Yes
31 (untitled)	Unassigned.	No
32, 33, 34, 35 Occurrence Codes and Dates*	Codes and date data that affect Medicare processing; examples include: 01 = auto accident. 04 = accident/employment related. 05 = other accident. 11 = onset of symptoms/illness. 17 = date occupational therapy plan established or reviewed. 18 = date of patient/beneficiary retirement. 19 = date of spouse retirement. 21 = utilization notice received. 24 = date insurance denied by primary payer. 25 = date benefits terminated by primary payer. 31 = date beneficiary notified of intent to bill for inpatient care accommodations. 32 = date beneficiary notified of intent to bill for Medicare medically unnecessary procedures or treatments. A1 = birthdate—insured A. A2 = effective date—insured A policy. A3 = benefits for insured A exhausted.	Yes
36 Occurrence Span Code and Dates	Codes and beginning/ending dates for specific events relating to the billing period, such as: 72 = first/last visit (actual dates of first and last visits in this billing period when different from form locator 6).	Yes
37 Internal Control Number or Document Control Number	For claim adjustments, providers enter the control number assigned to the original bill.	Yes
38 (untitled)	For Medicare as secondary payer, the address of the primary payer may be shown here.	No
39, 40, 41 Value Codes and Amounts*	Codes and related dollar amounts required to process the claim; examples include: 08 = Medicare lifetime reserve amount for first calendar year in billing period. 09 = Medicare coinsurance amount for first calendar year in billing period. 14 = no-fault, including auto, when primary payer payments are being applied to covered Medicare charges on this bill. 31 = patient liability amount, the amount approved by hospital or the QIO to charge the beneficiary for noncovered services. A1, B1, C1 = amounts assumed by provider to be applied to the patient's deductible amount for payer A, B, or C. A2, B2, C2 = amounts assumed by provider to be applied to the patient's coinsurance amount involving payer A, B, or C. A3, B3, C3 = amount estimated by provider to be paid by payer A, B, or C.	Yes
42 Revenue Code*	For each Medicare cost center—such as rental or purchase of durable medical equipment (DME)—for which a separate charge is billed in form locator 47, the Medicare-assigned revenue code is listed. Code 001 is placed before the total charge amount.	Yes

| TABLE 15.2 | **UB-92 Form Completion (*continued*)** |

Form Locator	Description	Medicare Required?
43 Revenue Description	Narrative description for each revenue code used in form locator 42.	No
44 HCPCS/Rates	HCPCS codes for applicable procedures.	Yes
45 Service Date	Not required.	No
46 Service Units	Number of units for each applicable service provided, such as number of months of rental for DME.	Yes
47 Total Charges	Total charges for the billing period.	Yes
48 Noncovered Charges	Total noncovered charges of those shown in form locator 42.	Yes
49 (untitled)	Unassigned.	No
50 A, B, C Payer Identification	If Medicare is primary payer, Medicare is entered on line A. If Medicare is the secondary or tertiary payer, the primary payer is entered on line A, and Medicare information on lines B or C.	Yes
51 A, B, C Provider Number	The provider's six-digit Medicare-assigned number is entered on the line corresponding to Medicare in form locator 50.	Yes
52 A, B, C Release of Information	Y = provider has on file a signed statement permitting data release to other organizations in order to adjudicate the claim. R = release is limited or restricted. N = no release is on file.	Yes
53 A, B, C Assignment of Benefits Certification Indicator	Not required; the back of the CMS-1450 contains this certification.	No
54 A, B, C Prior Payments	For other than inpatient hospital and SNF services; amount patient has paid (deductible/coinsurance).	Yes
55 A, B, C Estimated Amount Due	Not required.	No
56 (untitled)	Unassigned; for state use.	No
57 (untitled)	Unassigned.	No
58 A, B, C Insured's Name	Patient/insured's name on line corresponding to the Medicare line in form locator 50; form locators 59–66 pertain to this person.	Yes
59 A, B, C Patient's Relationship to Insured	Code for patient's relationship to insured: 01 = self. 02 = spouse. 03 = natural child/insured has financial responsibility. 04 = natural child/insured does not have financial responsibility. 05 = stepchild. 06 = foster child. 08 = employee. 09 = unknown. 11 = organ donor. 12 = cadaver donor. 15 = injured plaintiff.	Yes
60 A, B, C Certificate/Social Security Number/HI Claim/Identification Number	Patient's Medicare number; if Medicare is primary, entered in line A.	Yes
61 A, B, C Group Name	For Medicare secondary, the primary payer's insurance group or plan name.	Yes
62 A, B, C Insurance Group Number	Number for insurance named in form locator 61.	Yes
63 Treatment Authorization Code	Whenever QIO review is performed for outpatient preadmission, preprocedure, or inpatient preadmission, authorization number is shown.	Yes
64 Employment Status Code	Insured's employment status: 1 = employed full-time. 2 = employed part-time. 3 = not employed. 4 = self-employed. 5 = retired. 6 = active military duty. 7–8 = reserved. 9 = unknown.	Yes

(*continued*)

TABLE 15.2   UB-92 Form Completion (*continued*)

Form Locator	Description	Medicare Required?
65 Employer Name	Insured's employer's name.	Yes
66 Employer Location	Insured's employer's location.	Yes
67 Principal Diagnosis Code	ICD-9 diagnosis and procedure codes to highest level of specificity available.	Yes
68–75 Other Diagnoses Codes	Codes for up to eight additional conditions that coexisted at admission or developed and that had an effect on the treatment or the length of stay.	Yes
76 Admitting Diagnosis	The patient's admitting diagnosis is required if the claim is subject to QIO review.	Yes
77 E-Code	An E code is listed if applicable to the condition.	No
78 (untitled)	Unassigned.	No
79 Procedure Coding Method	Coding system used.	No
80 Principal Procedure Code and Date	ICD-9 procedure code most closely related to principal diagnosis code.	Yes—inpatient only
81 Other Procedure Codes and Dates	Up to five additional ICD-9 procedure codes as reported by the provider.	Yes—inpatient only
82 Attending/Referring Physician ID	UPIN and name of the attending or referring physician; UPIN, two spaces, last name, one space, first name, one space, middle initial.	Yes
83 Other Physician ID	UPIN and name of physician who also performed principal or surgical procedures; required on inpatient claims if a procedure is performed; required on outpatient claims if the HCPCS code is under ASC/QIO rules; use format in form locator 82.	Conditional
84 Remarks	Completed for DMEs and Medicare secondary payer.	Conditional
85 Provider Representative Signature	Not required unless a certification is required; provider representative signature required on psychiatric or TB hospital.	No
86 Date	Date of the provider representative signature.	No

*Detailed information is provided in fiscal intermediary manuals.

Focus on Careers   Medical Coder—Hospital

Medical coding specialists who work in the hospital setting are called hospital or facility coders. They may work in an inpatient setting, an outpatient clinic, or another institution such as a skilled nursing facility.

Hospital coders review patients' medical records and assign diagnosis and procedure codes. They are knowledgeable about the coding rules and procedures for hospital coding, which are regulated primarily by the American Hospital Association. Hospital coders need to become experienced in working with lengthy, complicated records of patients' stays, including operative, laboratory, pathology, and radiology reports. Accurate coding is a critical part of ensuring that claims follow the legal and ethical requirements of Medicare and other third-party payers. It is also essential for maintaining the credentials of the institution.

Certification as a professional coder or health information technician is preferred for work as a hospital coder. Two hospital-based coding certifications are available: the Certified Coding Specialist (CCS) title offered by the American Health Information Management Association's Society of Clinical Coding and the Certified Professional Coder—Hospital (CPC-H) title granted by the American Academy of Professional Coders. The American Health Information Management Association also offers the Registered Health Information Technician (RHIT) credential.

To safeguard against fraud, hospitals

- Double-check registration information. The admissions department verifies that the patient is being admitted for a medically necessary diagnosis under the payer's rules. If items will not be covered under Medicare Part A or Part B, patients must sign the Hospital-Issued Notice of Noncoverage (HINN) to acknowledge their responsibility for payment.
- Update their charge masters every year with current HCPCS, ICD-9-CM, and CPT codes.
- Compare clinical documentation with the patient's bill to make sure reported services are properly documented.
- Conduct postpayment audits to uncover patterns of denied or partially paid codes.

Thinking It Through—15.3

How are the Medicare Prospective Payment System and the use of capitated rates in managed care organizations similar? How are they different?

Review

Chapter Summary

1. Inpatient services, those involving an overnight stay, are provided by general and specialized hospitals, skilled nursing facilities, and long-term care facilities. Outpatient services are provided by ambulatory surgical centers or units, by home health agencies, and by hospice staff.

2. The first major step in the hospital claims processing sequence is admission, when the patient is registered. Personal and financial information is entered in the hospital's health record system; insurance coverage is verified; consent forms are signed by the patient; a notice of the hospital's privacy policy is presented to the patient; and some pretreatment payments are collected. In the second step, the patient's treatments and transfers among the various departments in the hospital are tracked and recorded. The third step, discharge and billing, follows the discharge of the patient from the facility and the completion of the patient's record.

3. Diagnostic coding for inpatient services follows the rules of the Uniform Hospital Discharge Data Set (UHDDS). Two ways in which inpatient coding differs from physician and outpatient diagnostic coding are that (1) the main diagnosis, called the principal rather than the primary diagnosis, is established after study in the hospital setting, and (2) coding an uncon-

firmed condition (rule-out) as the admitting diagnosis is permitted.

4. Volume 3 of the ICD-9, Procedures, is used to report the procedures for inpatient services. It is organized by surgical procedures divided into body systems, followed by diagnostic and therapeutic procedures. The three- or four-digit codes are assigned based on the principal diagnosis.

5. Medicare pays for inpatient services under its Prospective Payment System, which uses diagnosis-related groups (DRGs) to classify patients into similar treatment and length-of-hospital-stay units and sets prices for each classification group. A hospital's geographic location, labor and supply costs, and teaching costs also affect the per-DRG pay rate it negotiates with CMS.

6. The 837I—the HIPAA standard transaction for the facility claim—or, in some cases, the UB-92 form (CMS-1450) is used to report patient data, information on the insured, facility and patient type, the source of the admission, various conditions that affect payment, whether Medicare is the primary payer (for Medicare claims), the principal and other diagnosis codes, the admitting diagnosis, the principal procedure code, the attending physician, other key physicians, and charges.

Key Terms

admitting diagnosis *page 503*
ambulatory care *page 495*
ambulatory patient classification
   (APC) *page 513*
ambulatory surgical center (ASC)
   page 495
ambulatory surgical unit (ASU) *page 495*
at-home recovery care *page 496*
attending physician *page 497*
charge master *page 502*
CMS-1450 *page 508*

comorbidities *page 504*
complications *page 504*
diagnosis-related groups (DRGs)
   page 506
emergency *page 495*
health information management (HIM)
   page 496
home health agency (HHA) *page 496*
home health care *page 496*
hospice care *page 496*
inpatient *page 495*

master patient index *page 497*
principal diagnosis *page 503*
principal procedure *page 505*
Prospective Payment System (PPS)
   page 506
registration *page 497*
skilled nursing facility (SNF) *page 495*
UB-92 *page 508*
Uniform Hospital Discharge Data Set
   (UHDDS) *page 503*
837I *page 508*

Review Questions

Match the key terms in the left column with the definitions in the right column.

A. attending physician

B. principal diagnosis

C. charge master

D. inpatient

E. diagnosis-related groups (DRGs)

F. comorbidities

G. admitting diagnosis

H. principal procedure

I. ambulatory care

J. 837I Health Care Claim

_____ 1. A person admitted to a hospital for services that require an overnight stay

_____ 2. The main service performed for the condition listed as the principal diagnosis for a hospital inpatient

_____ 3. The clinician primarily responsible for the care of the patient from the beginning of the hospital episode

_____ 4. Outpatient care

_____ 5. HIPAA standard transaction for the facility claim

_____ 6. A hospital's list of the codes and charges for its services

_____ 7. The patient's condition identified by the physician at admission to the hospital

_____ 8. A system of analyzing conditions and treatments for similar groups of patients used to establish Medicare fees for hospital inpatient services

_____ 9. Conditions in addition to the principal diagnosis that the patient had at hospital admission which affect the length of the hospital stay or the course of treatment

_____ 10. The condition that after study is established as chiefly responsible for a patient's admission to a hospital

Decide whether each statement is true or false, and write T for true or F for false.

_____ 1. Skilled nursing facilities (SNF) are classified as outpatient facilities.

_____ 2. Emergency care involves a life-threatening situation.

_____ 3. An inpatient's insurance coverage is usually verified in the discharge process.

_____ 4. The master patient index contains the name of each patient's attending physician.

_____ 5. When a patient is covered by Medicare, the admissions staff must find out if Medicare is the primary payer.

_____ 6. The hospital's charge master serves the same purpose as a medical practice's encounter form.

_____ 7. The principal diagnosis is based on the admitting diagnosis.

_____ 8. Inpatient coding rules do not permit the reporting of suspected or unconfirmed diagnoses.

_____ 9. ICD-9-CM, Volume 3, is used to report inpatient procedures.

_____ 10. The UB-92 is a paper claim form that is sometimes used by hospitals.

Write the letter of the choice that best completes the statement or answers the question.

_____ 1. When the hospital staff collects data on a patient who is being admitted for services, the process is called
A. health information management
B. registration
C. MSP
D. precertification

_____ 2. Which of the following hospital departments has different procedures for collecting patients' personal and insurance information?
   A. accounting department   C. emergency department
   B. surgery department   D. collections department

_____ 3. Patient charges in hospitals vary according to
   A. their accommodations   C. their accommodations and services
   B. their services   D. their insurance coverage

_____ 4. Which of these rules governs the reporting of hospital inpatient services on insurance claims?
   A. ASC   C. APC
   B. HIM   D. UHDDS

_____ 5. Conditions that arise during the patient's hospital stay as a result of treatments are called
   A. comorbidities   C. complications
   B. admitting diagnoses   D. correlates

_____ 6. In inpatient coding, the initials CC mean
   A. chief complaint
   B. comorbidities and complications
   C. cubic centimeters
   D. convalescent center

_____ 7. The code 76.23 is an example of which type of code?
   A. CPT-4   C. ICD-9-CM Volume 2
   B. ICD-9-CM Volume 1   D. ICD-9-CM Volume 3

_____ 8. Under a Prospective Payment System, payments for services are
   A. set in advance
   B. based on the provider's fees
   C. discounts to the provider's usual fees
   D. none of the above

_____ 9. The UB-92 form locator 4 requires the
   A. type of bill   C. revenue code
   B. admission hour   D. patient status

_____ 10. Under Medicare rules for patients in car accidents, the automobile insurance is
   A. primary   C. supplemental
   B. secondary   D. tertiary

Define the following abbreviations:

1. DRG _____

2. PPS _____

3. SNF _____

4. ASC _____

5. HHA _____

Applying Your Knowledge

Follow the inpatient coding guidelines for (1) identifying the principal diagnosis, (2) coding suspected conditions, and (3) differentiating between statements of admitting, principal, comorbidity, and complication diagnoses as you analyze these cases.

Case 15.1

What is the principal diagnosis?

Discharge Date: 07/05/2007

Patient: Kellerman, Larry H.

Patient is a 59-year-old male who was recently found to have some evidence of induration of his prostate gland. He was referred for urologic evaluation and admitted to the hospital for further study and biopsy. Under general anesthesia, cystoscopy revealed early prostatic enlargement and needle biopsy was accomplished. Pathological examination of the tissue removed confirmed the presence of adenocarcinoma of the prostate.

Case 15.2

What is the admitting diagnosis?

Room: S-920

Patient: Koren, Sarah I.

Admission Date: 10/11/2007

Chief Complaint: Severe, right upper abdominal pain radiating to the back.

History of Present Illness: This 38-year-old female reports having this severe pain for two weeks. She has had some nausea and vomiting. Condition worsened by previous treatment with pain medication and Tagamet. Previous ultrasound of her gallbladder showed a very thickened gallbladder wall with a large stone, impacted at the neck of the cystic duct. Her family physician has admitted her to be taken to surgery for a cholecystectomy. She notes diarrhea a few days ago but no other change in bowel habits.

Impression: Probable acute cholecystitis.

Case 15.3

Identify the principal diagnosis, the principal procedure, the comorbidity diagnosis, and the complication in the following discharge statement.

Flora Raniculli is a 65-year-old female admitted to the hospital with a three-month history of cough, yellow-sputum production, weight loss, and shortness of breath. Chest X-ray reveals probable bronchiectasis. Patient may also have pulmonary fibrosis. She underwent a bronchoscopy that showed thick secretions in both lower lobes. Post-bronchoscopy fever finally cleared up. She is now being discharged and will call me in one week for a progress report.

Computer Exploration

1. The Centers for Medicare and Medicaid (CMS) Web site contains a designated area for hospital information. To view this information, go to the CMS hospital Web page at

    http://www.cms.hhs.gov/providers/hospital.asp

    To view the range of topics available at the site, click the Alphabetical Listings link. Scroll through the list to locate the topic Payment Systems. To learn more about the Hospital Inpatient Prospective Payment System, click this subtopic, and then read the information displayed in the Background Information and Overview links. What did you learn about the role of DRGs in this payment system?

2. As described in the activity above, go to the CMS hospital Web page at

    http://www.cms.hhs.gov/providers/hospital.asp

    Rather than use the Alphabetical Listings link, scroll to the bottom of the page and locate the highlighted topic, Medicare Secondary Payer. Click the link for Medicare Secondary Payer Questionnaire. View CMS's online version of the MSP questionnaire. In which part is information about ESRD located?

3. Go to the Medicare Quality Improvement Community's Web site at

    http://www.medqic.org/

    Look up information about the Quality Improvement Organizations program. How many QIOs make up the national network? Who do these organizations represent?

Quick Guide to MediSoft

This Quick Guide contains two parts. Part 1: *Getting Started with NDCMediSoft* provides instructions for starting the NDCMediSoft program and setting up the database files that you will use with the NDCMediSoft activities in this text. After the files are set up on your system, they will load automatically each time the program is opened. The required files for setting up the database are stored on a backup file on the Student Data Disk located inside the back cover of this text.

Part 2: *Overview and Practice* provides an introduction to the NDCMediSoft program as well as practice in creating claims in NDCMediSoft. Part 2 is contained in a PDF file on the Student Data Disk.

PART 1: *Getting Started with NDCMediSoft*

Before a medical office begins to create claims using NDCMediSoft, basic information about the practice and its patients must be entered in the program. This preliminary work has been done for you and stored in a backup file on the Student Data Disk. The medical practice with which you will work is called Valley Associates, P.C. (VAPC).

Before restoring the VAPC database file from the Student Data Disk, follow the instructions below to make a working copy of the disk so that the original copy can be kept separately in a safe place.

Note that files are supplied on both a floppy disk and a CD-ROM. If you are using the CD-ROM, alter the following instructions, accordingly, or check with your instructor.

Making a Copy of the Student Data Disk

Note: These instructions assume that Windows 98 or a later version is installed on your computer.

1. Turn on the computer and monitor.
2. After the Windows desktop is displayed, insert the Student Data Disk in the A: drive. (If you are using a different drive, please substitute that letter for "A" whenever it appears.)
3. Locate the My Computer icon, either on the desktop or in the Start menu, and click it. The My Computer window is displayed.
4. In the My Computer window, click the icon labeled 3½ Floppy (A:).
5. Open the File menu, and select Copy Disk. The Copy Disk dialog box is displayed.
6. The Copy From and Copy To windows should both list 3½ Floppy (A:). If more than one item is listed in each window, click 3½ Floppy (A:) in both windows to select them.

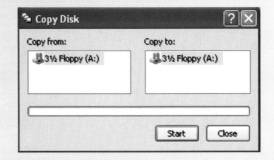

7. Click the Start button. (If a dialog box appears prompting you to insert the source disk, make sure the Student Data Disk is in the drive, and then click OK.)

8. The computer begins reading the files on the source disk. When the system prompts you to insert the disk you want to copy to (the destination disk), eject the Student Data Disk from the drive.

9. Insert a blank disk in the floppy drive, and click the OK button. The files are copied to the destination disk.

10. When the copy is completed, the message "Copy completed successfully" is displayed. Eject the disk from the drive, and label it "Working Copy VAPC."

11. Close the Copy Disk dialog box.

12. Close the My Computer dialog box.

Starting NDcMediSoft and Restoring the Backup File

The following instructions take you through the steps of restoring the backup file of the VAPC database from the working copy of the Student Data Disk. You will create a new directory and data set name for the Valley Associates, P.C., files on the hard drive, and then restore the backup file to the new directory.

1. While holding down the F7 key, click Start, Programs, NDcMediSoft, and then NDcMediSoft Advanced Patient Accounting to start NDcMediSoft. When the Find NDcMediSoft Database dialog box appears, release the F7 key. This dialog box asks you to enter the NDcMediSoft data directory.

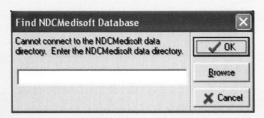

2. Click inside the data entry box to activate it. Then key C:\MediData in the space provided (where C is the letter that represents the hard drive you will be using). The dialog box should now look like this:

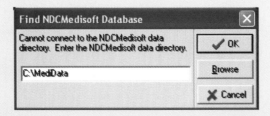

3. Click the OK button. An Information dialog box appears.

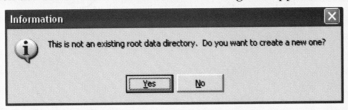

4. Click Yes. The Create Data dialog box is displayed.

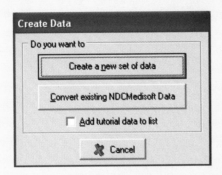

5. Click the Create a New Set of Data button. The Create a New Set of Data dialog box appears. In the upper box, key *Valley Associates PC* (this data entry box does not accept punctuation.) In the lower box, key *VAPC.* The dialog box should now look like this:

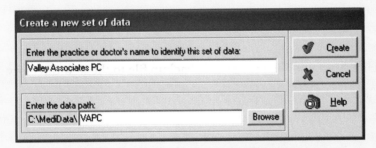

6. Click the Create button. A Confirm dialog box is displayed.

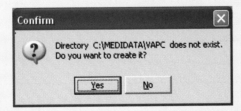

7. Click the Yes button. The Practice Information dialog box appears. In the Practice Name box, key *Valley Associates, P.C.* Leave the remaining boxes blank for now, as the backup file will fill them in later.

8. Click the Save button. The main window of the NDCMediSoft program is displayed, with the name of the new data set, Valley Associates PC, on the title bar. Your screen should look like this:

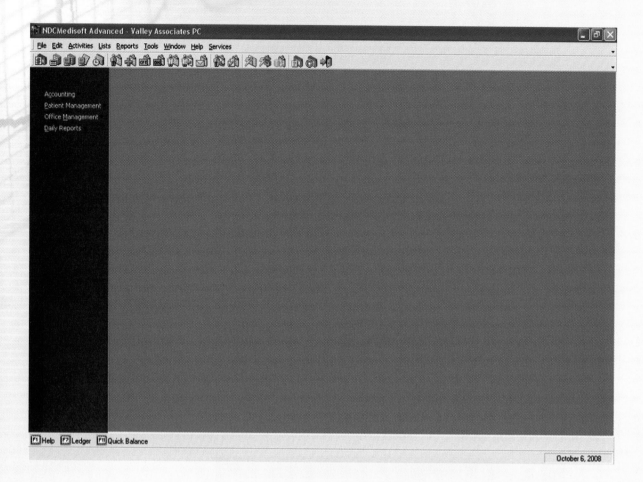

9. Insert the working copy of the Student Data Disk in the floppy drive. (This is usually the A: drive; if your computer uses a different letter to represent the floppy drive, please substitute that letter for "A:" whenever it appears in these instructions.)

10. Open the File menu at the top of the window, and locate the Restore Data option halfway down the menu.

11. Click Restore Data. A Warning dialog box is displayed.

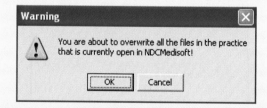

12. Click the OK button. The Restore dialog box is displayed. In the top box, key the filename *A:\VAPC.mbk* if it does not already appear. This is the name of the file on the Student Data Disk. The dialog box should now look like this:

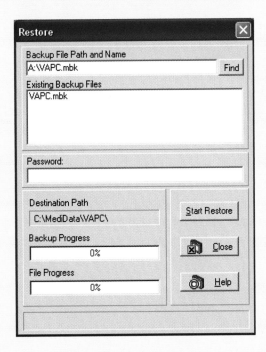

13. Click the Start Restore button. A Confirm dialog box is displayed.

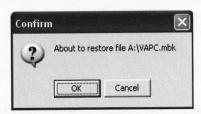

14. Click the OK button. After the program restores the database to the hard drive, an Information dialog box is displayed, indicating that the restore is complete. Click OK.
15. You are returned to the main NDCMediSoft window. (*Hint:* If the window does not fill the screen, click the Maximize button to expand it.)
16. By default, NDCMediSoft displays a sidebar with four options on the left side of the window. As the side bar is not required for this text, open the Window menu and click Show Side Bar to toggle it off.
17. The sidebar disappears. The database is now ready for use.
18. If you plan to continue with Part 2: *Overview and Practice,* click the minimize button (the first of the three small buttons displayed in the top right corner of the window) to make the NDCMediSoft program temporarily inactive.

    If you do not plan to continue with Part 2, open the File menu and click Exit (or click the X in the top right corner) to exit NDCMediSoft. When the back-up reminder dialog box appears, click the Exit Program button.

Part 2: *Overview and Practice*

Part 2 of this Guide is accessed through a PDF file contained on the Student Data Disk (a:QuickGuideP2.pdf). The PDF file contains an overview of the NDCMediSoft Advanced Patient Accounting program, including an introduction to the program's databases, an explanation of how claims are created in NDCMediSoft, and illustrations of the major dialog boxes that are used for data entry. The PDF file also contains a hands-on practice session in which you create an actual claim in NDCMediSoft.

The information and practice obtained in Part 2 will help you to carry out the NDCMediSoft activities at the end of each chapter. Therefore, it is recommended that you work with the PDF file before you begin the NDCMediSoft activities in the text.

To access the PDF file:

1. Turn on the computer and monitor.
2. After the Windows desktop is displayed, insert the Student Data Disk in the 3½″ floppy drive (drive A:).
3. Click the Start button on the Windows taskbar to display the Start menu.
4. Click the Run . . . option.
5. In the Run dialog box, key:
   a:QuickGuideP2.pdf
6. Click the OK button. The file opens in Acrobat Reader.

Note: If you do not have the Acrobat Reader program on your system, ask your instructor or lab facilitator for help in obtaining a copy.

APPENDIX A

Taxonomy Codes

This table lists the taxonomy codes for allopathic and osteopathic physicians. The *Health Care Provider Taxonomy* (Washington Publishing Company) contains codes for many other categories of providers, such as behavioral, chiropractic providers, and facilities. The Provider Taxonomy Code List is published (released) twice a year on July 1st and January 1st. The July publication is effective for use on October 1st and the January publication is effective for use on April 1st.

Code	*Definition*
193200000X	Multi-Specialty: A business group of one or more individual practitioners, who practice with different areas of specialization.
193400000X	Single Specialty: A business group of one or more individual practitioners, all of whom practice with the same area of specialization.
207K00000X	Allergy & Immunology
207KA0200X	Allergy
207K10005X	Clinical and Laboratory Immunology
207L00000X	Anesthesiology
207LA0401X	Addiction Medicine
207LC0200X	Critical Care Medicine
207LP2900X	Pain Medicine
208U00000X	Clinical Pharmacology
208C00000X	Colon & Rectal Surgery
207N00000X	Dermatology
207NI0002X	Clinical & Laboratory Dermatological Immunology
207NS0135X	Dermatological Surgery
207ND0900X	Dermatopathology
207ND0101X	MOHS-Micrographic Surgery
207NP0225X	Pediatric Dermatology
207P00000X	Emergency Medicine
207PE0004X	Emergency Medical Services
207PT0002X	Medical Toxicology
207PP0204X	Pediatric Emergency Medicine
207PS0010X	Sports Medicine
207PE0005X	Undersea and Hyperbaric Medicine
207Q00000X	Family Practice
207QA0401X	Addiction Medicine
207QA0000X	Adolescent Medicine
207QA0505X	Adult Medicine
207QG0300X	Geriatric Medicine
207QS0010X	Sports Medicine

Code	Definition
208D00000X	General Practice
208M00000X	Hospitalist
207R00000X	Internal Medicine
207RA0401X	Addiction Medicine
207RA0000X	Adolescent Medicine
207RA0201X	Allergy and Immunology
207RC0000X	Cardiovascular Disease
207RI0001X	Clinical & Laboratory Immunology
207RC0001X	Clinical Cardiac Electrophysiology
207RC0200X	Critical Care Medicine
207RE0101X	Endocrinology, Diabetes, & Metabolism
207RG0100X	Gastroenterology
207RG0300X	Geriatric Medicine
207RH0000X	Hematology
207RH0003X	Hematology & Oncology
207RI0008X	Hepatology
207RI0200X	Infectious Disease
207RI0011X	Interventional Cardiology
207RM1200X	Magnetic Resonance Imaging (MRI)
207RX0202X	Medical Oncology
207RN0300X	Nephrology
207RP1001X	Pulmonary Disease
207RR0500X	Rheumatology
207RS0010X	Sports Medicine
20980000X	Legal Medicine
	Medical Genetics
207SG0202X	Clinical Biochemical Genetics
207SC0300X	Clinical Cytogenetics
207SG0201X	Clinical Genetics
207SG0203X	Clinical Molecular Genetics
207SM0001X	Molecular Genetic Pathology
207SG0205X	Ph.D. Medical Genetics
207T00000X	Neurological Surgery
204D00000X	Neuromusculoskeletal Medicine & OMM
204C00000X	Neuromusculoskeletal Medicine, Sports Medicine
207U00000X	Nuclear Medicine
207UN0903X	In Vivo & In Vitro Nuclear Medicine
207UN0901X	Nuclear Cardiology
207UN0902X	Nuclear Imaging & Therapy
207V00000X	Obstetrics & Gynecology
207CV0200X	Critical Care Medicine
207VX0201X	Gynecological Oncology
207CG0400X	Gynecology
207VM0101X	Maternal & Fetal Medicine
207VX0000X	Obstetrics
207VE0102X	Reproductive Endocrinology
207W00000X	Opthalmology
204E00000X	Oral & Maxillofacial Surgery

Code	Definition
207X00000X	Orthopaedic Surgery
207XS0114X	Adult Reconstructive Orthopaedic Surgery
207XX0004X	Foot and Ankle Orthopaedics
207XS0106X	Hand Surgery
207XS0117X	Orthopaedic Surgery of the Spine
207XX0801X	Orthopaedic Trauma
207XX0005X	Sports Medicine
207Y00000X	Otolaryngology
207YS0123X	Facial Plastic Surgery
207YX0602X	Otolaryngic Allergy
207YX0905X	Otolaryngology/Facial Plastic Surgery
207YX0901X	Otology & Neurotology
207YP0228X	Pediatric Otolaryngology
207YX0007X	Plastic Surgery within the Head & Neck
	Pain Medicine
208VP0014X	Interventional Pain Medicine
208VP0000X	Pain Management
	Pathology
207ZP0101X	Anatomic Pathology
207ZP0102X	Anatomic Pathology & Clinical Pathology
207ZB0001X	Blood Banking & Transfusion Medicine
207ZP0104X	Chemical Pathology
207ZP0105X	Clinical Pathology/Laboratory Medicine
207ZC0500X	Cytopathology
207ZD0900X	Dermatopathology
207ZF0201X	Forensic Pathology
207ZH0000X	Hematology
207ZI0100X	Immunopathology
207ZM0300X	Medical Microbiology
207ZP0007X	Molecular Genetic Pathology
207ZN0500X	Neuropathology
207ZP0213X	Pediatric Pathology
208000000X	Pediatrics
2080A0000X	Adolescent Medicine
2080I0007X	Clinical & Laboratory Immunology
2080P0006X	Developmental–Behavioral Pediatrics
2080T0002X	Medical Toxicology
2080N0001X	Neonatal–Perinatal Medicine
2080P0008X	Neurodevelopmental Disabilities
2080P0201X	Pediatric Allergy & Immunology
2080P0202X	Pediatric Cardiology
2080P0203X	Pediatric Critical Care Medicine
2080P0204X	Pediatric Emergency Medicine
2080P0205X	Pediatric Endocrinology
2080P0206X	Pediatric Gastroenterology
2080P0207X	Pediatric Hematology–Oncology
2080P0208X	Pediatric Infectious Diseases
2080P0210X	Pediatric Nephrology
2080P0214X	Pediatric Pulmonology
2080P0216X	Pediatric Rheumatology
2080S0010X	Sports Medicine

Code	Definition
208100000X	Physical Medicine & Rehabilitation
2081P2900X	Pain Medicine
2081P0010X	Pediatric Rehabilitation Medicine
2081P0004X	Spinal Cord Injury Medicine
2081S0010X	Sports Medicine
208200000X	Plastic Surgery
2082S0099X	Plastic Surgery Within the Head and Neck
2082S0105X	Surgery of the Hand
	Preventive Medicine
203A0100X	Aerospace Medicine
2083T0002X	Medical Toxicology
2083X0100X	Occupational Medicine
2083P0500X	Preventive Medicine/Occupational Environmental Medicine
2083P0901X	Public Health & General Preventive Medicine
2083S0010X	Sports Medicine
2083P0011X	Undersea and Hyperbaric Medicine
	Psychiatry & Neurology
2084A0401X	Addiction Medicine
2084P0802X	Addiction Psychiatry
2084P0804X	Child & Adolescent Psychiatry
2084N0600X	Clinical Neurophysiology
2084F0202X	Forensic Psychiatry
2084P0805X	Geriatric Psychiatry
2084P0005X	Neurodevelopmental Disabilities
2084N0400X	Neurology
2084N0402X	Neurology with Special Qualifications in Child Neurology
2084P2900X	Pain Medicine
2084P0800X	Psychiatry
2084S0010X	Sports Medicine
2084V0102X	Vascular Neurology
	Radiology
2085B0100X	Body Imaging
2085R0202X	Diagnostic Radiology
2085U0001X	Diagnostic Ultrasound
2085N0700X	Neuroradiology
2085N0904X	Nuclear Radiology
2085P0229X	Pediatric Radiology
2085R0001X	Radiation Oncology
2085R0205X	Radiological Physics
2085R0203X	Therapeutic Radiology
2085R0204X	Vascular & Interventional Radiology

Code	Definition
208600000X	Surgery
2086S0120X	Pediatric Surgery
2086S0122X	Plastic & Reconstructive Surgery
2086S0105X	Surgery of the Hand
2086S0102X	Surgical Critical Care
2086X0206X	Surgical Oncology
2086S0127X	Trauma Surgery
2086S0129X	Vascular Surgery
208G00000X	Thoracic Surgery (Cardiothoracic Vascular Surgery)
204F00000X	Transplant Surgery
208800000X	Urology

APPENDIX B

Place of Service Codes

Codes designated as F are facility codes; those with NF are nonfacility physician practice codes. The rate calculations for nonfacility locations take into account the higher overhead expenses such as the cost of clinical staff, supplies, and equipment, collectively called practice expense, generally borne by providers in these settings. The facility rates paid to providers usually are lower because the hospital/facility is reimbursed separately for overhead costs associated with patient care.

03	school NF
04	homeless shelter NF
05	Indian Health Service freestanding facility
06	Indian Health Service provider-based facility
07	Tribal 638 freestanding facility
08	Tribal 638 provider-based facility
11	office NF
12	home NF
13	assisted living facility NF
14	group home NF
15	mobile unit NF
20	urgent care facility NF
21	inpatient hospital F
22	outpatient hospital F
23	emergency room, hospital F
24	ambulatory surgical center F, or NF for payable procedures not on ASC list
25	birthing center NF
26	military treatment facility F
31	skilled nursing facility F
32	nursing facility NF
33	custodial care facility NF
34	hospice F
41	ambulance, land F
42	ambulance, air or water F
49	independent clinic NF
50	federally qualified health center NF
51	inpatient psychiatric facility F
52	psychiatric facility, partial hospitalization F
53	community mental health center F
54	intermediate care facility/mentally retarded NF
55	residential substance abuse treatment facility NF
56	psychiatric residential treatment center F
57	nonresidential substance abuse treatment facility NF
60	mass immunization center NF
61	comprehensive inpatient rehabilitation facility F

62	comprehensive outpatient rehabilitation facility NF
65	end-stage renal disease treatment facility NF
71	state or local public health clinic NF
72	rural health clinic NF
81	independent laboratory NF
99	other place of service NF

Abbreviations

AACP	American Academy of Professional Coders
AAMA	American Association of Medical Assistants
AAMT	American Association for Medical Transcription
ABN	advance beneficiary notice
AHIMA	American Health Information Management Association
AMA	American Medical Association
AMT	American Medical Technologists
ANSI	American National Standards Institute
APC	ambulatory patient classification
A/R	accounts receivable
ASU	ambulatory surgical unit
ASC	ambulatory surgical center
BCBS	Blue Cross and Blue Shield
CC	(1) physicians' records: chief complaint, (2) hospital documentation: comorbidities and complications
CCA	certified coding associate
CCI	Correct Coding Initiative (National; Medicare)
CCS	certified coding specialist
CCS-P	certified coding specialist: physician-based
CE	covered entity
CHAMPVA	Civilian Health and Medical Program of Veterans Affairs
CLIA	Clinical Laboratory Improvement Amendment
CMA	certified medical assistant
CMS	Centers for Medicare and Medicaid Services
COB	coordination of benefits
COBRA	Consolidated Omnibus Budget Reconciliation Act of 1985
COP	conditions of participation
CPC	Certified Professional Coder
CPC-H	Certified Professional Coder: Hospital Outpatient Facility
CPT	Current Procedural Terminology
CRCS	Civil Service Retirement System
DEERS	Defense Enrollment Eligibility Reporting System
DME	durable medical equipment
DOS	date of service
DRG	Diagnosis-Related Groups
DRS	designated record set
Dx	diagnosis
E/M code	Evaluation and Management code
EDI	electronic data interchange
EFT	electronic funds transfer
EMC	electronic media claim
EMR	electronic medical record
EOB	explanation of benefits
EOC	episode of care
EP	established patient
EPSDT	Early and Periodic Screening, Diagnosis, and Treatment
ERISA	Employee Retirement Income Security Act of 1974
FECA	Federal Employee Compensation Act.
FEHBP	Federal Employees Health Benefits Program
FERS	Federal Employees Retirement System
FI	fiscal intermediary
FICA	Federal Insurance Contribution Act
FMAP	Federal Medicaid Assistance Percentage
GPCI	geographic practice cost index
HBA	health benefits advisor
HCPCS	Healthcare Common Procedure Coding System
HEDIS	Health Employer Data and Information Set
HHA	home health agency
HHS	Department of Health and Human Services
HIM	health information management
HIPAA	Health Insurance Portability and Accountability Act
HMO	health maintenance organization
ICD-9-CM	International Classification of Diseases, 9th Revision, Clinical Modification
IPA	individual practice association
JCAHO	Joint Commission on Accreditation of Healthcare Organizations
LCD	local coverage determination
MCM	Medicare Carriers Manual
MCO	managed care organization
MFS	Medicare fee schedule
MMA	Medicare Modernization Act
MSA	Medicare savings account
MRN	Medicare remittance notice; Medicare redetermination notice
MSN	Medicare summary notice
MTF	military treatment facility
MTS	Medicare Transaction System
NCCI	National Correct Coding Initiative
NCQA	National Committee for Quality Assurance
NEC	not elsewhere classified
NEMB	notice of exclusion from Medicare benefits
nonPAR	nonparticipating
NOS	not otherwise specified
NP	new patient
NPI	national provider identifier
NPP	Notice of Privacy Practices
NUCC	National Uniform Claim Committee
OCR	The Office of Civil Rights
OIG	Office of the Inspector General
OSHA	Occupational Safety and Health Administration
OWCP	Office of Workers' Compensation Programs
PCM	primary care manager (TRICARE)
PCP	primary care physician
PECOS	Provider Enrollment Chain and Ownership System
PHI	protected health information
PIN	provider identifier number
PMPM	per member per month
POS	place of service
PPO	preferred provider organization
PPS	prospective payment system
PSO	provider-sponsored organization
QIO	quality improvement organization
RA	remittance advice
RBRVS	Resource-Based Relative Value Scale (Medicare)
RHIA	registered health information manager

RHIT	registered health information technologist	SSDI	Social Security Disability Insurance
RMA	registered medical assistant	SSI	Supplemental Security Income
RUG	Resource Utilization Group	TANF	Temporary Assistance for Needy Families
RVS	relative value scale	TCS	(HIPAA Electronic) Transaction and Code Sets
RVU	relative value unit.	TPA	third-party claims administrator
SCHIP	State Children's Health Insurance Program	TPO	treatment, payment, and operations
SDI	state disability insurance	UCR	usual, customary, reasonable
SNF	skilled nursing facility	UHDDS	Uniform Hospital Discharge Data Set
SOAP	Subjective/Objective/Assessment/Plan		

Glossary

270 and 271 The HIPAA (ASC X12N) eligibility for a health plan's benefits inquiry and response transactions.

276 and 277 The HIPAA (ASC X12N) claim status inquiry and response transactions.

278 The HIPAA (ASC X12N) request for services inquiry and response that is used for precertification and referral authorization.

835 The HIPAA (ASC X12N) payment and remittance advice (explanation of benefits) transaction.

837I The HIPAA (ASC X12N) institutional claim transaction.

837P (HIPAA 837 claim) The HIPAA (ASC X12N) professional claim transaction.

ASC X12N Refers to the Accredited Standards Committee X12, Insurance Subcommittee.

A

abuse Actions that improperly use another's resources.

acceptance of assignment (V. accept assignment) A participating physician's agreement to accept the allowed charge as payment in full.

access The ability or means necessary to read, write, modify, or communicate data/information or otherwise use any system resource.

accounts receivable (A/R) Monies owed to a medical practice by its patients and third-party payers.

Acknowledgment of Receipt of Notice of Privacy Practices Form accompanying a covered entity's Notice of Privacy Practices; covered entities must make a good-faith effort to have patients sign the acknowledgment.

acute Describes an illness or condition having severe symptoms and a short duration; can also refer to a sudden exacerbation of a chronic condition.

addenda Updates to the ICD-9-CM diagnostic coding system.

add-on code Procedures that are performed and reported only in addition to a primary procedure; indicated in CPT by a plus sign (+) next to the code.

adjudication The process followed by health plans to examine claims and determine benefits.

adjustment An amount (positive or negative) entered in a patient billing program to change a patient's account balance.

administrative code set Under HIPAA, required codes for various data elements, such as taxonomy codes and place of service (POS) codes.

Admission of Liability Carrier's determination that an employer is responsible for an employee's claim under workers' compensation.

admitting diagnosis The patient's condition determined by a physician at admission to an inpatient facility.

advance beneficiary notice (ABN) Medicare form used to inform a patient that a service to be provided is not likely to be reimbursed by the program.

adverse effect Condition due to the correct usage of a drug.

advisory opinion An opinion issued by CMS or the OIG which becomes legal advice for the requesting party, who, if they act according to the advice, are immune from investigation on that matter; provides guidance for others in similar matters.

allowed charge The maximum charge that a health plan pays for a specific service or procedure; also called allowable charge, maximum fee, and other terms.

Alphabetic Index The section of the ICD-9-CM in which diseases and injuries with corresponding diagnosis codes are presented in alphabetical order.

ambulatory care Outpatient care.

ambulatory patient classification (APC) A Medicare payment classification for outpatient services.

ambulatory surgical center (ASC) A clinic that provides outpatient surgery.

ambulatory surgical unit (ASU) A hospital department that provides outpatient surgery.

American Academy of Professional Coders (AAPC) National association that fosters the establishment and maintenance of professional, ethical, education, and certification standards for medical coding.

American Association of Medical Assistants National association that fosters the profession of medical assisting.

American Association for Medical Transcription National association fostering the profession of medical transcription.

American Health Information Management Association (AHIMA) National association of health information management professionals; promotes valid, accessible, yet confidential health information and advocates quality health care.

American Medical Association (AMA) Member organization for physicians; goals are to promote the art and science of medicine, improve public health, and promote ethical, educational, and clinical standards for the medical profession.

American National Standards Institute (ANSI) Organization that sets standards for electronic data interchange on a national level.

Accredited Standards Committee X12, Insurance Subcommittee (ASC X12N) The ANSI-accredited standards development organization that maintains the administrative and financial electronic transactions standards adopted under HIPAA.

appeal A request sent to a payer for reconsideration of a claim adjudication.

assignment of benefits Authorization by policyholder that allows a health plan to pay benefits directly to a provider.

assumption coding Reporting undocumented services that the coder assumes have been provided because of the nature of the case or condition.

at-home recovery care Assistance with the activities of daily living provided for a patient in the home.

attending physician The clinician primarily responsible for the care of the patient from the beginning of a hospitalization.

audit Methodical review; in medical insurance, a formal examination of a physician's accounting or patient medical records.

audit-edit claim response Report from a receiver of an electronic claim transmitted to its sender regarding the status and completeness of the claim.

authentication Corroboration that a person is the one claimed.

authorization Document signed by a patient that permits release of particular medical information under the specific stated conditions.

auto-posting Software feature that enables automatic entry of payments on a remittance advice to credit an individual's account.

B

balance billing Collecting the difference between a provider's usual fee and a payer's lower allowed charge from the insured.

benefits The amount of money a health plan pays for services covered in an insurance policy.

billing provider The person or organization (often a clearinghouse or billing service) sending a HIPAA claim, as distinct from the pay-to provider that receives payment.

billing service Company that provides billing and claims processing services.

birthday rule The guideline that determines which of two parents with medical coverage has the primary insurance for a child; the parent whose day of birth is earlier in the calendar year is considered primary.

BlueCard A Blue Cross and Blue Shield program that provides benefits for plan subscribers who are away from their local areas.

Blue Cross A primarily nonprofit corporation that offers prepaid medical benefits for hospital services, and some outpatient, home care, and other institutional services.

Blue Cross and Blue Shield Association (BCBS) The national licensing agency of Blue Cross and Blue Shield Plans.

Blue Shield A primarily nonprofit corporation which offers prepaid medical benefits for physician, dental, and vision services, and other outpatient care.

bundled code Single procedure code used to report a group of related procedures.

business associate A person or organization that performs a function or activity for a covered entity but is not part of its workforce.

C

CHAMPUS Now the TRICARE program; formerly the Civilian Health and Medical Program of the Uniformed Services (Army, Navy, Air Force, Marine Corps, Coast Guard, Public Health Service, and the National Oceanic and Atmospheric Administration) that serves spouses and children of active-duty service members, military retirees and their families, some former spouses, and survivors of deceased military members.

CHAMPVA The Civilian Health and Medical Program of the Department of Veterans Affairs which shares health care costs for families of veterans with 100 percent service-connected disability and the surviving spouses and children of veterans who die from service-connected disabilities.

CMS See Centers for Medicare and Medicaid Services.

CMS-1450 Paper claim for hospital services; also known as the UB-92.

CMS-1500 Paper claim for physician services.

CPT The abbreviation that refers to the American Medical Association's publication *Current Procedural Terminology*.

capitation Payment method in which a prepayment covers the provider's services to a plan member for a specified period of time.

capitation rate (cap rate) The contractually set periodic prepayment to a provider for specified services to each enrolled plan member.

carrier Health plan; also known as insurance company, payer, or third-party payer.

carve out A part of a standard health plan that is changed under a negotiated employer-sponsored plan; also refers to subcontracting of coverage by a health plan.

cash flow The inflow of payments from patients and payers to a medical practice and the outflow from the practice of payments to suppliers and staff; based on the actual movement of money rather than amounts that are receivable or payable.

catastrophic cap The maximum annual amount a TRICARE beneficiary must pay for deductible and cost share.

category In the ICD-9-CM, a three-digit code used to classify a particular disease or injury.

Category II codes Optional CPT codes that track performance measures for a medical goal such as reducing tobacco use.

Category III codes Temporary codes for emerging technology, services, and procedures; to be used, rather than an unlisted code, when available.

categorically needy A person who receives assistance from government programs such as Temporary Assistance for Needy Families (TANF).

Centers for Medicare and Medicaid Services (CMS) Federal agency within the Department of Health and Human Services (HHS) that runs Medicare, Medicaid, Clinical Laboratories (under the CLIA program), and other governmental health programs.

certificate Term for Blue Cross and Blue Shield medical insurance policy.

certification number Number returned electronically by a health plan when approving a referral authorization request.

charge-based fee structure Fees based on the amounts typically charged for similar services.

charge master A hospital's list of the codes and charges for its services.

chief complaint (CC) A patient's description of the symptoms or other reasons for seeking medical care from a provider.

chronic An illness or condition with a long duration.

Civilian Health and Medical Program of the Veterans Administration See CHAMPVA.

claimant Person or entity exercising the right to receive benefits.

claim adjustment reason code Code used by a health plan on a remittance advice to describe payment information.

claim attachment Documentation that a provider sends to a payer in support of a health care claim.

claim control number Unique number assigned by the sender to a health care claim.

claim frequency code (claim reason submission code) A code reported on a HIPAA 837 claim that identifies the claim as original, replacement, or void/cancel action.

claim scrubber Software that checks claims to permit error correction for "clean" claims.

claim turnaround time The time period in which a health plan is obligated to process a claim.

clean claim A claim that is accepted by a health plan for adjudication.

clearinghouse A company that converts, for a fee, nonstandard data formats into HIPAA standard transactions and transmits the data to health plans; or also handles the reverse process, changing HIPAA formatted transactions from health plans into nonstandard formats for providers.

Clinical Laboratory Improvement Amendments (CLIA) 1988 federal law establishing standards for laboratory testing performed in hospital-based facilities, physician's office laboratories, and other locations; administered by CMS.

code edits A computerized screening system used to identify improperly or incorrectly reported codes.

code linkage The connection between a service and a patient's condition or illness; establishes the medical necessity of the procedure.

code set Alphabetic and/or numeric representations for data. Medical code sets are systems of medical terms that are required for HIPAA transactions. Administrative (nonmedical) code sets, such as taxonomy codes and Zip codes, are also used in HIPAA transactions.

coding The process of assigning numerical codes to diagnoses and procedures/services.

coexisting condition Additional illness that either has an effect on the patient's primary illness or is also treated during the encounter.

coinsurance The portion of charges that an insured person must pay for health care services after payment of the deductible amount; usually stated as a percentage.

combination code A single code that classifies both the etiology and the manifestation of an illness or injury.

comorbidity Admitted patient's coexisting condition which affects the length of the hospital stay or the course of treatment.

compliance plan A medical practice's written plan for (a) the appointment of a compliance officer and committee, (b) a code of conduct for physicians' business arrangements and employees' compliance, (c) training plans, (d) properly prepared and updated coding tools such as job reference aids, encounter forms, and documentation templates, (e) rules for prompt identification and refunding of overpayments, and (f) ongoing monitoring and auditing of claim preparation.

complication Condition an admitted patient develops after surgery or treatment that affects the length of hospital stay or the course of further treatment.

concurrent care Medical situation in which a patient receives extensive, independent care from two or more attending physicians on the same date of service.

conditions of participation (Medicare) (COP) Regulations concerning provider participation in the Medicare program.

Consolidated Omnibus Budget Reconciliation Act of 1985 (COBRA) Federal law requiring employers with more than 20 employees to allow terminated employees (except for cases of gross misconduct) to remain covered under the employer's group health plan for 18 months, at the employee's expense.

consultation Service performed by a physician to advise a requesting physician about a patient's condition and care; the consultant does not assume responsibility for the patient's care and must send a written report back to the requestor.

consumer-driven health plan Type of employment-sponsored medical insurance that combines a high-deductible plan with a medical savings plan that covers some out-of-pocket expenses.

contract An enforceable, voluntary agreement in which specific promises are made by one party in exchange for some consideration by the other party.

convention Typographic techniques or standard practices that provide visual guidelines for understanding printed material.

conversion factor Dollar amount used to multiply a relative value unit to arrive at a charge.

coordination of benefits (COB) A clause in an insurance policy that explains how the policy will pay if more than one insurance policy applies to the claim.

copayment An amount that a health plan requires a beneficiary to pay at the time of service for each health care encounter.

corporate integrity agreement A compliance action under which a provider's Medicare billing is monitored by the Office of the Inspector General.

Correct Coding Initiative See **National Correct Coding Initiative.**

cost share The term meaning coinsurance for a TRICARE or CHAMPVA beneficiary.

covered entity (CE) Under HIPAA, a health plan, clearinghouse, or provider that transmits any health information in electronic form in connection with a HIPAA transaction. In the law, "health plan" does not specifically include workers' compensation programs, property and casualty programs, or disability insurance programs.

counseling Physician's discussion with a patient and/or family concerning diagnostic results, prognosis, treatment options, and/or instructions.

credentialing The process of periodic verification that a provider or facility meets the professional standards of a certifying organization. Physician credentialing involves screening and evaluating qualifications and other credentials, including licensure, required education, relevant training and experience, and current competence.

crossover claim Claim for services to a Medicare/Medicaid beneficiary; Medicare is the primary payer and automatically transmits claim information to Medicaid as the secondary payer.

cross-reference Directions in printed material that tell a reader where to look for additional information.

crosswalk A comparison or map of the codes for the same or similar classifications under two coding systems that provides a guide for selecting the closest match.

Current Procedural Terminology (CPT) Publication of the American Medical Association containing the HIPAA-mandated standardized classification system for reporting medical procedures and services performed by physicians.

D

database An organized collection of related data items having a specific structure.

data element The smallest unit of information in a HIPAA transaction.

data format An arrangement of electronic data for transmission.

date of service The date of a patient encounter for medical services.

day sheet In a medical office, a report that summarizes the business day's charges and payments, drawn from all the patient ledgers for the day.

deductible An amount that an insured person must pay, usually on an annual basis, for health care services before a health plan's payment begins.

Defense Enrollment Eligibility Reporting System (DEERS) The worldwide database of TRICARE and CHAMPVA beneficiaries.

de-identified health information Medical data from which individual identifiers have been removed; also known as a redacted or blinded record.

dependent A person other than the insured, such as a spouse or child, who is covered under a health plan.

descriptor The narrative part of a CPT code that identifies the procedure or service.

designated record set (DRS) A covered entity's records that contain protected health information (PHI). For providers, the designated record set is the medical/financial patient record.

destination payer In HIPAA claims, the health plan receiving the claim.

determination A payer's decision regarding the benefits due for a claim.

diagnosis A physician's opinion of the nature of a patient's illness or injury.

diagnosis code The number assigned to a diagnosis in the *International Classification of Diseases.*

diagnosis-related groups (DRG) A system of analyzing conditions and treatments for similar groups of patients used to establish Medicare fees for hospital inpatient services.

diagnostic statement A physician's description of the main reason for a patient's encounter; may also describe related conditions or symptoms.

direct provider Provider of medical services who treats the patient face-to-face, as opposed to an indirect provider such as a laboratory.

disability compensation program A plan that reimburses the insured for lost income when the insured cannot work because of an illness or injury, whether or not it is work-related.

disallowed charge An item on a remittance advice that identifies the difference between the allowable charge and the amount the physician charged for a service.

disclosure The release, transfer, provision of, access to, or divulging in any other manner of information outside the entity that holds it.

discounted fee-for-service A negotiated payment schedule for health care services based on a reduced percentage of a provider's usual charges.

documentation The systematic, logical, and consistent recording of a patient's health status—history, examinations, tests, results of treatments, and observations—in chronological order in a patient medical record.

documentation template Physician practice form used to prompt the physician to document a complete review of systems (ROS) when done and the medical necessity for the planned treatment.

domiciliary care Care provided in the home; or providing care and living space, such as a home for disabled veterans.

downcode A payer's review and reduction of a procedure code (often an E/M code) to a lower level than reported by the provider.

durable medical equipment (DME) Medicare term for reusable physical supplies such as wheelchairs and hospital beds that are ordered by the provider for use in the home; reported with HPCPS Level II codes.

E

E code An alphanumeric ICD code for an external cause of injury or poisoning.

E/M See evaluation and management code.

Early and Periodic Screening, Diagnosis, and Treatment (EPSDT) Medicaid's prevention, early detection, and treatment program for eligible children under the age of 21.

elective surgery Nonemergency surgical procedure that can be scheduled in advance.

electronic data interchange (EDI) The exchange (system to system) of data in a standardized format.

electronic funds transfer (EFT) Electronic routing of funds between banks.

electronic claim A health care claim that is transmitted electronically; also known as an electronic media claim (EMC).

electronic media Electronic storage media, such as hard drives and removable media, and transmission media used to exchange information already in electronic storage media, such as the Internet. Paper transmission via fax and voice transmission via telephone are not electronic transmissions.

electronic medical record (EMR) Creation and/or maintenance of patient medical records in electronic form, such as computer files.

electronic remittance Payment made through electronic funds transfer.

electronic remittance advice See remittance advice.

emancipated minor A person who has reached the legal age for an emancipated minor under state law.

emergency A situation in which a delay in the treatment of the patient would lead to a significant increase in the threat to life or body part.

Employee Retirement Income Security Act of 1974 (ERISA) A federal law that provides incentives and protection against litigation for companies that set up employee health and pension plans.

encounter An office visit between a patient and a medical professional.

encounter form A listing of the diagnoses, procedures, and charges for a patient's visit; also called the superbill.

encryption A method of scrambling transmitted data so it cannot be deciphered without the use of a confidential process or key.

episode-of-care (EOC) option A flat payment by a health plan to a provider for a defined set of services, such as care provided for a normal pregnancy, or for services for a certain period of time, such as a hospital stay.

eponym A name or phrase that is formed from or based on a person's name; usually describes a condition or procedure associated with that person.

established patient A patient who has received professional services from a provider (or another provider with the same specialty in the same practice) within the past three years.

ethics Standards of conduct based on moral principles.

etiology The cause or origin of a disease.

etiquette Standards of professional behavior.

evaluation and management (E/M) codes Procedure codes that cover physicians' services performed to determine the optimum course for patient care; listed in the Evaluation and Management section of CPT.

excluded parties Individuals/companies who, because of reasons bearing on professional competence, professional performance, or financial integrity, are not permitted by the OIG to participate in any federal health care programs.

excluded service A service specified in a medical insurance contract as not covered.

explanation of benefits (EOB) A document from a payer sent to a patient that shows how the amount of a benefit was determined.

explanation of Medicare benefits (EOMB) See Medicare Summary Notice.

external audit Audit conducted by an organization outside of the practice, such as a federal agency.

F

family deductible A fixed, periodic amount that must be met by the combination of payments for covered services to each individual of an insured/dependent group before benefits from a payer begin.

Federal Employee Compensation Act (FECA) A federal law that provides workers' compensation insurance for civilian employees of the federal government.

Federal Employees Health Benefits Program (FEHBP) The health insurance program that covers employees of the federal program.

Federal Employees Retirement System (FERS) Disability program for employees of the federal government.

Federal Insurance Contribution Act (FICA) The federal law that authorizes payroll deductions for the Social Security Disability Program.

Federal Medicaid Assistance Percentage (FMAP) Basis for federal government Medicaid allocations to individual states.

fee-for-service Method of charging under which a provider's payment is based on each service performed.

fee schedule List of charges for services performed.

final report A report filed by the physician in a state workers' compensation case when the patient is discharged.

firewall A software system designed to block unauthorized entry to a computer's data.

first report of injury or illness A report filed in state workers' compensation cases that contains the employer's name and address, employee's supervisor, date and time of accident, geographic location of injury, and the patient's description of what happened.

fiscal intermediary A government contractor that processes claims for government programs; for Medicare, the fiscal intermediary (FI) processes Part A claims.

formulary A list of a health plan's selected drugs and their proper dosages; often a plan pays only for the drugs it lists.

fragmented billing Incorrect billing practice in which procedures covered under a single bundled code are "unbundled" and separately reported.

fraud Intentional deceptive act to obtain a benefit.

G

gatekeeper See primary care physician.

gender rule A coordination of benefits rule for a child insured under both parents' plans under which the father's insurance is primary

geographic practice cost index (GPCI) A Medicare factor used to adjust providers' fees to reflect the cost of providing services in a particular geographic area relative to national averages.

global period The number of days surrounding a surgical procedure during which all services relating to the procedure—preoperative, during the surgery, and post-operative—are considered part of the surgical package and are not additionally reimbursed.

global surgical concept See surgical package.

group health plan Under HIPAA, an employee health plan that either has 50 or more participants or is administered by another business entity.

guardian An adult legally responsible for care and custody of a minor.

H

HCFA See Centers for Medicare and Medicaid Services.

HCFA-1450 See CMS-1450.

HCFA-1500 See CMS-1500.

Health and Human Services (HHS) The U.S. Department of Health and Human Services, whose agencies have authority for creating and enforcing HIPAA regulations.

health care claim An electronic transaction or a paper document filed with a health plan to receive benefits.

Health Care Financing Administration See Centers for Medicare and Medicaid Services.

Healthcare Common Procedure Coding System (HCPCS) Procedure codes for Medicare claims, made up of CPT codes (Level I) and national codes (Level II).

Health Care Fraud and Abuse Control Program Government program to uncover misuse of funds in federal health care programs; run by the Office of the Inspector General (OIG).

Health Employer Data and Information Set (HEDIS) Set of standard performance measures on the quality of a health care plan collected and disseminated by the National Committee for Quality Assurance (NCQA).

health information management (HIM) Hospital department that organizes and maintains patient medical records; also profession devoted to managing, analyzing, and utilizing data vital for patient care, making it accessible to healthcare providers.

Health Insurance Portability and Accountability Act (HIPAA) of 1996 Federal act that set forth guidelines for standardizing the electronic data interchange of administrative and financial transactions, exposing fraud and abuse in government programs, and protecting the security and privacy of health information.

health maintenance organization (HMO) A managed health care system in which providers agree to offer health care to the organization's members for fixed periodic payments from the plan; usually members must receive medical services only from the plan's providers.

health plan Under HIPAA, an individual or group plan that either provides or pays for the cost of medical care, including group health plan, health insurance issuer, health maintenance organization, Medicare Part A or B, Medicaid, TRICARE, and other governmental and nongovernmental plans.

health savings account An insurance plan under which an employer sets aside an annual amount an employee can use to pay for certain types of health care costs; also known as a medical savings account.

HIPAA claim Generic term for the HIPAA ASC X12N 837 professional health care claim transaction.

HIPAA Claim Status–Inquiry The HIPAA ASC X12N 276 transaction in which a provider asks a health plan for information on a claim's status.

HIPAA Claim Status–Response The HIPAA ASC X12N 277 transaction in which a health plan answers a provider's request for information on a claim's status.

HIPAA Coordination of Benefits The HIPAA ASC X12N 837 transaction that is sent to a secondary or tertiary payer on a claim with the primary payer's remittance advice.

HIPAA Electronic Health Care Transactions and Code Sets (TCS) The HIPAA rule governing the electronic exchange of health information.

HIPAA Eligibility for a Health Plan–Inquiry The HIPAA ASC X12N 270 transaction in which a provider asks a health plan for information on a patient's eligibility for benefits.

HIPAA Eligibility for a Health Plan–Response The HIPAA ASC X12N 271 transaction in which a health plan answers a provider's request for information on a patient's eligibility for benefits.

HIPAA Health Care Claims or Equivalent Encounter Information The HIPAA ASC X12N 837 transaction used by a provider to report professional, institutional, or dental claims.

HIPAA Health Care Payment and Remittance Advice The HIPAA ASC X12N 835 transaction used by a health plan to describe a payment in response to a health care claim.

HIPAA National Identifier HIPPA-mandated identification systems for employers, health care providers, health plans, and patients; the NPI, National Provider System, and employer system are in place, health plan and patient systems are to be created.

HIPAA Privacy Rule Law that regulates the use and disclosure of patients' protected health information (PHI).

HIPAA Referral Certification and Authorization The HIPAA ASC X12N 278 transaction in which a provider asks a health plan for approval of a service and the health plan responds; an approved request has a certification number.

HIPAA Security Rule Law that requires covered entities to establish administrative, physical, and technical safeguards to protect the confidentiality, integrity and availability of health information.

HIPPA transaction General term for the electronic transactions, such as claim status inquiries, health care claim transmittal, and coordination of benefits regulated under the HIPAA Health Care Transactions and Code Sets standards.

home health agency (HHA) Organization that provides home care services to patients.

home health care Care given to patients in their homes, such as skilled nursing care.

home plan A Blue Cross and Blue Shield plan in the community where the subscriber has contracted for coverage.

hospice A public or private organization that provides services for terminally ill people and their families.

hospice care Palliative care for people with terminal illnesses.

host plan A participating provider's local Blue Cross and Blue Shield plan.

I

ICD-9-CM Abbreviated title of International Classification of Diseases, 9th Revision, Clinical Modification.

ICD code A system of diagnostic codes based on the International Classification of Diseases.

incident-to Term for services of allied health professionals, such as nurses, technicians, and therapists, provided under the physician's direct supervision that may be billed under Medicare.

indemnity A health plan's agreement to reimburse a policyholder for covered losses.

indirect provider Provider that does not interact face-to-face with the patient, such as a laboratory.

individual practice association (IPA) A type of health maintenance organization in which physicians are self-employed and provide services to both HMO members and nonmembers.

individual deductible   A fixed, periodic amount that must be met by each individual of an insured/dependent group before benefits from a payer begin.

information technology   (IT) The development, management, and support of computer-based hardware/software systems.

informed consent   The process by which a patient authorizes medical treatment after discussion regarding the nature, indications, benefits, and risks of a treatment a physician recommends.

inpatient   A person admitted to a medical facility for services that require an overnight stay.

insurance aging report   A report grouping unpaid claims transmitted to payers by the length of time that they remain due, such as 30, 60, 90, or 120 days.

insurance commission   A state's regulatory agency for the insurance industry that serves as liaison between the patient and payer, and the provider and payer.

insured   The policyholder or subscriber to a health plan or medical insurance policy; also known as guarantor.

intermediary   See fiscal intermediary.

internal audit   A self-audit conducted by a staff member or consultant as a routine check of compliance with reporting regulations.

International Classification of Diseases, 9th Revision, Clinical Modification   (ICD-9-CM) A publication containing the HIPAA-mandated standardized classification system for diseases and injuries; developed by the World Health Organization and modified for use in the United States.

J

job reference aid   A list of a medical practice's frequently reported procedures and diagnoses.

Joint Commission on Accreditation of Healthcare Organizations   (JCAHO) Organization that reviews accreditation of hospitals and other organizations/programs.

L

LCD   Local Coverage Determination.

late effect   Condition that remains after an acute illness or injury has completed its course.

liable   Legally responsible.

limiting charge   In Medicare, the highest fee (115 percent of the Medicare Fee Schedule) that nonparticipating physicians can charge for a particular service.

line item control number   On a HIPAA claim, the unique number assigned by the sender to each service line item reported.

Local Coverage Determination (LCD)   Notices sent to physicians that contain detailed and updated information about the coding and medical necessity of a specific Medicare service.

Local Medicare Review Policy   (LMRP) See Local Coverage Determination.

M

M code   A classification number that identifies the morphology of neoplasms.

main number   The five-digit procedure code listed in the CPT.

main term   The word in bold-faced type that identifies a disease or condition in the Alphabetic index in ICD-9-CM.

managed care   A system that combines the financing and the delivery of appropriate, cost-effective health care services to its members.

managed care organization   (MCO) Organization offering some type of managed health care plan.

manifestation   A characteristic sign or symptom of a disease.

master patient index   A hospital's main patient database.

maximum benefit limit   The amount an insurer agrees to pay for an insured's covered expenses over the course of the insured person's lifetime.

Medicaid   A federal and state assistance program that pays for health care services for people who cannot afford them.

MediCal   California's state Medicaid program name.

medical error   Failure of a planned action to be completed as intended or the use of a wrong plan to achieve an aim. Errors that result in patient harm are "adverse effects," those that did not are "near misses." The most common form of errors is drug errors.

medical insurance   A financial plan that covers the cost of hospital and medical care due to illness or injury.

medical insurance specialist   The person in a medical office who handles patients' health care claims.

medical malpractice   Failure to use an acceptable level of professional skill when giving medical services that results in injury or harm to a patient.

medical necessity   Payment criterion of payers that requires medical treatments to be appropriate and provided in accordance with generally accepted standards of medical practice. The reported procedure or service (1) matches the diagnosis, (2) is not elective, (3) is not experimental, (4) has not been performed for the convenience of the patient or the patient's family, and (5) has been provided at the appropriate level.

medical necessity denial   Refusal by a health plan to pay for a reported procedure that does not meet its medical necessity criteria.

medical record   A file that contains the documentation of a patient's medical history, record of care, progress notes, correspondence, and related billing/financial information.

medical review program   A payer's procedures for ensuring that providers give patients the most appropriate care in the most cost-effective manner.

medical terminology   The terms used to describe diagnoses and procedures; based on anatomy.

medically indigent   Medically needy.

medically needy   Medicaid classification for people with high medical expenses and low financial resources, although not sufficiently low to receive cash assistance.

Medicare   The federal health insurance program for people 65 or older and some people with disabilities.

Medicare Advantage   Medicare plans other than the Original Medicare Plan.

Medicare beneficiary   A person covered by Medicare.

Medicare carrier   A private organization under contract with CMS to administer Medicare Part B claims in an assigned region.

Medicare Fee Schedule   (MFS) The RBRVS-based allowed fees that are reimbursable to Medicare participating physicians.

Medicare Modernization Act   Short name for the Medicare Prescription Drug, Improvement, and Modernization Act of 2003, which includes a number of changes that will roll out over a period of years, including a prescription drug benefit.

Medicare Part A   The part of the Medicare program that pays for hospitalization, care in a skilled nursing facility, home health care, and hospice care.

Medicare Part B   The part of the Medicare program that pays for physician services, outpatient hospital services, durable medical equipment, and other services and supplies.

Medicare-participating agreement   A phrase that describes physicians and other providers of medical services who have signed agreements with Medicare to accept assignment on all Medicare claims.

Medicare Redetermination Notice   (MRN) Resolution of a first appeal for Medicare fee-for-service claims; a written decision notification letter due within 60 days of the appeal.

Medicare Remittance Notice   (MRN) Remittance advice from Medicare to providers that explains how payments for a batch of Medicare claims were determined.

Medicare Summary Notice   (MSN) Type of remittance advice from Medicare to plan beneficiaries to explain how their benefits were determined.

Medigap   Insurance plan offered by a private insurance carrier to supplement Medicare Original Plan coverage.

Medi-Medi beneficiary   Person who is eligible for both Medicare and Medicaid benefits.

Military Treatment Facility   (MTF) Government facility providing medical services for members and dependents of the Uniformed Services.

minimum necessary standard   Principle that individually identifiable health information should be disclosed only to the extent needed to support the purpose of the disclosure.

modifier   A number that is appended to a code to report particular facts. CPT modifiers report special circumstances involved with a procedure or service. HCPCS modifiers are often used to designate a body part, such as left side or right side.

monthly enrollment list   Document of eligible members of a capitated plan registered with a particular PCP for a monthly period.

moribund   Approaching death.

multiple modifiers   Two or more modifiers used to augment a procedure code.

N

National Committee for Quality Assurance (NCQA) Organization that collects and disseminates the HEDIS information rating the quality of health maintenance organizations.

National Correct Coding Initiative   (NCCI) Computerized Medicare system to prevent overpayment for procedures.

National Correct Coding Initiative edits   Pairs of CPT or HCPCS Level II codes that are not separately payable by Medicare except under certain circumstances. The edits apply to services by the same provider for the same beneficiary on the same date of service.

National Patient ID (Individual Identifier)   Unique individual identification system to be created under HIPAA National Identifiers.

National Payer ID (Health Plan ID)   Unique health plan identification system to be created under HIPAA National Identifiers.

National Provider Identifier   (NPI) Under HIPAA, unique 10-digit identifier assigned to each provider by the National Provider System; replaces both the UPIN and Medicare PIN.

National Uniform Claim Committee   (NUCC) Organization responsible for the content of health care claims.

negligence   In the medical profession, failure to perform duties properly according to the state-required standard of care.

network model HMO   A type of health maintenance organization where physicians remain self-employed and provide services to both HMO members and nonmembers.

new patient A patient who has not received professional services from a provider (or another provider with the same specialty in the same practice) within the past three years.

nonavailability statement A form required for pre-authorization when a TRICARE member seeks medical services in other than military treatment facilities.

nonparticipating (nonPAR) physician A physician or other health care provider who chooses not to join a particular government or other program or plan.

nontraumatic injury A condition caused by the work environment over a period longer than one work day or shift. Also known as occupational disease or illness.

not elsewhere classified (NEC) An ICD-9-CM abbreviation indicating the code to be used when an illness or condition cannot be placed in any other category.

not otherwise specified (NOS) An ICD-9-CM abbreviation indicating the code to be used when no information is available for assigning the illness or condition a more specific code.

Notice of Contest Carrier's determination to deny liability for an employee's workers' compensation claim.

Notice of Exclusions from Medicare Benefits (NEMB) CMS form that can be used by participating providers to give Medicare patients, before providing an uncovered service such as a screening test, written notification that Medicare will not pay and the estimated charge for which the patient will be responsible.

Notice of Privacy Practices (NPP) A HIPAA-mandated description of a covered entity's principles and procedures related to the protection of patients' health information.

O

occupational disease/illness A condition caused by the work environment over a period longer than one work day or shift; also known as nontraumatic injury.

Occupational Safety and Health Administration (OSHA) Federal agency that regulates workers' health and safety risks in the workplace.

Office of Civil Rights (OCR) Government agency that enforces the HIPAA Privacy Act.

Office of the Inspector General (OIG) Government agency that investigates and prosecutes fraud against government health care programs such as Medicare.

Office of Workers' Compensation Programs The office of the U.S. Department of Labor that administers the Federal Employees' Compensation Act.

OIG Compliance Program Guidance for Individual and Small Group Physician Practices OIG publication that explains the recommended features of compliance plans for small providers.

OIG Fraud Alert Notices issued by the OIG to advise providers about potentially fraudulent or non-compliant actions regarding billing and reporting practices.

OIG Work Plan The OIG's annual list of planned projects under the Medicare Fraud and Abuse Initiative.

open-access plans Type of health maintenance organization in which members can visit any specialists in the HMO's network without a referral.

open enrollment period Period of time during which a policyholder can choose to switch a health plan or options without penalty; often used to describe the fourth quarter of the year for employees in employer-sponsored health plans, or the designated period for enrollment in a Medicare or Medigap plan.

operations (health care) Activities such as conducting quality assessment and improvement, protocol development, reviewing the competence or qualifications of health care professionals, and actions to implementation of compliance with regulations.

Original Medicare Plan The Medicare fee-for-service plan.

out-of-pocket Expenses the insured must pay before benefits begin.

outpatient A patient who receives health care in a hospital setting without admission; the length of stay is generally less than 23 hours.

overpayment An improper or excessive payment to a provider as a result of billing or claims processing errors for which a refund is owed by the provider.

P

PECOS Provider Enrollment Chain and Ownership System.

panel In CPT, a single code grouping laboratory tests that are frequently done together.

participating (PAR) physician/provider A physician/provider who agrees to provide medical services to a payer's policyholders according to the terms of the plan or program's contract.

password Confidential authentication information composed of a string of characters.

patient aging report A report grouping unpaid patients' bills by the length of time that they remain due, such as 30, 60, 90, or 120 days.

patient information form A form that includes a patient's personal, employment, and insurance company data needed to complete a health care claim; also known as a registration form.

patient ledger A record of all charges and payments made on a particular patient's account.

patient statement A report that shows the services provided to a patient, the total payments made, total charges, adjustments, and the balance due.

payer of last resort Regulation that Medicaid pays last on a claim when a patient has other insurance coverage.

pay-to provider The person or organization that is to receive payment for services reported on a HIPAA claim; may be the same as or different from the billing provider.

per member per month (PMPM) A periodic capitated prospective payment to a provider that covers only services listed on the schedule of benefits.

permanent disability A condition that prevents a person with a disability compensation program from doing any job.

pharmacy benefit manager A company that operates an employer's pharmacy benefits program, buying drugs, setting up the formulary, and pricing the prescriptions for the insured.

physical status modifier A code used in the Anesthesia Section of CPT with procedure codes to indicate the patient's health status.

physician of record Provider under a workers' compensation claim who first treats the patient and assesses the level of disability.

place of service (POS) code A HIPAA administrative code that indicates where medical services have been provided, such as an office or hospital.

point-of-service (POS) option In HMOs, a plan that permits patients to receive medical services from non-network providers; this choice requires a larger patient payment than visits with network providers.

policyholder A person who buys an insurance plan; the insured, subscriber, or guarantor.

preauthorization Prior authorization from a payer for services to be provided; if not received, the charge is not usually covered.

precertification Prior authorization from a payer that must be received before elective hospital-based or outpatient surgeries are covered.

preexisting condition An illness or disorder of a beneficiary that existed before the effective date of insurance coverage.

preferred provider organization (PPO) A managed care organization structured as a network of health care providers who agree to perform services for plan members at discounted fees; usually, plan members can receive services from non-network providers for a higher charge.

premium The periodic amount of money the insured pays to a health plan for a health care policy.

preventive medical services Care that is provided to keep patients healthy or to prevent illness, such as routine checkups and screening tests.

primary care manager (PCM) Provider who coordinates and manages the care of TRICARE beneficiaries.

primary care physician (PCP) A physician in a health maintenance organization who directs all aspects of a patient's care, including routine services, referrals to specialists within the system, and supervision of hospital admissions; also known as a gatekeeper.

primary diagnosis A diagnosis that represents the patient's major illness or condition for an encounter.

primary insurance (payer) The health plan that pays benefits first when a patient is covered by more than one plan.

primary procedure The most resource-intensive (highest paid) CPT procedure done during a patient's encounter.

principal diagnosis The condition that after study is established as chiefly responsible for a patient's admission to a hospital.

principal procedure The main service performed for the condition listed as the principal diagnosis for a hospital inpatient.

prior authorization number An identifying code assigned by a government program or health insurance plan when preauthorization is required; also called the certification number.

private disability insurance An insurance plan that can be purchased to provide the insured benefits when illness or injury prevents employment.

privileging The process of determining a health care professional's skills and competence to perform specific procedures as a participant in, or an affiliate of, a health care facility or system. Once a facility privileges a practitioner, the practitioner may perform those specific procedures.

procedure code A code that identifies medical treatment or diagnostic services.

professional component The part of the relative value associated with a procedure code that represents a physician's skill, time, and expertise used in performing it, as opposed to the technical component.

prognosis The physician's prediction of outcome of disease and likelihood of recovery.

progress report A report filed by the physician in state workers' compensation cases when a patient's medical condition or disability changes; also known as a supplemental report.

prospective audit An internal audit of particular claims conducted before they are transmitted to payers.

prospective payment Payment for health care made before the services are provided.

Prospective Payment System (PPS) Medicare system for payment for institutional services.

protected health information (PHI) Individually identifiable health information that is transmitted or maintained by electronic media.

provider A person or entity that supplies medical or health services and bills for or is paid for the services in the normal course of business. A provider may be a professional member of the health care team, such as a physician, or a facility, such as a hospital or skilled nursing home.

Provider Enrollment Chain and Ownership System (PECOS) CMS national database of participating providers.

provider-sponsored organization (PSO) Capitated Medicare managed care plan in which the physicians and hospitals that provide treatment also own and operate the plan.

provider withhold An amount withheld from a provider's payment by a MCO under contractual terms; may be paid if stated financial requirements are met.

Q

quality improvement organization (QIO) State-based group of physicians who are paid by the government to review aspects of the Medicare program, including the quality and appropriateness of services provided and fees charged.

qui tam "Whistle-blower" cases in which a relator accuses another party of fraud or abuse against the federal government.

R

reasonable fee The lower of either the fee the physician bills or the usual fee, unless special circumstances apply.

real-time Information technology term for computer systems that update information at the same time as they receive it; the sender and receiver "converse" by inquiring and responding to data while remaining connected.

referral Transfer of patient care from one physician to another.

referral number Authorization number given by a referring physician to the referred physician.

referring provider The physician who refers the patient to another physician for treatment.

registration The process of gathering personal and insurance information about a patient during admission to a hospital.

relative value scale (RVS) System of assigning unit values to medical services based on an analysis of the skill and time required of the physician to perform them.

relative value unit (RVU) A factor assigned to a medical service based on the relative skill and time required to perform it.

relator Person who makes an accusation of fraud or abuse in a *qui tam* case.

remittance The statement of the results of the health plan's adjudication of a claim.

remittance advice (RA) Health plan document describing a payment resulting from a claim adjudication; also called an explanation of benefits (EOB).

rendering provider Term used to identify the physician or other medical professional who provides the procedure reported on a health care claim if other than the pay-to provider.

reprice Contractual reduction of a physician's fee schedule.

resource-based fee structure Setting fees based on the relative skill and time required to provide similar services.

resource-based relative value scale (RBRVS) Federally mandated relative value scale for establishing Medicare charges.

respondeat superior Doctrine making the employer responsible for employees' actions.

responsible party Person or entity other than the insured or the patient who will pay a patient's charges.

restricted status A category of Medicaid beneficiary.

retention schedule A practice policy that governs which information from patients' medical records is to be stored, for how long it is to be retained, and the storage medium to be used.

retroactive payment Payment for health care after the services are provided

retrospective audit An internal audit conducted after claims are processed by payers and after RAs have been received for comparison with submitted charges.

rider Document that modifies an insurance contract.

roster billing Under Medicare, simplified billing for pneumococcal, influenza virus, and hepatitis B vaccines.

S

SOAP *Subjective/Objective/Assessment/Plan* Documentation format in which encounter information is grouped into four sections containing the patient's subjective descriptions of signs and symptoms; the physician's notes on the objective information regarding the condition and examination/test results; the physician's assessment, or diagnosis, of the condition; and the plan of treatment.

schedule of benefits A list of the medical expenses that a health plan covers.

secondary insurance (payer) The health plan that pays benefits after the primary plan when a patient is covered by more than one plan.

secondary condition Additional diagnosis(ses) that occurs at the same time as a primary diagnosis and that affects its treatment.

secondary procedure A procedure performed in addition to the primary procedure.

secondary provider identifier On HIPAA claims, identifiers that may be required by various plans in addition to the NPI, such as a plan identification number.

section guidelines Usage notes provided at the beginnings of CPT sections.

self-insured employer A company that creates its own insurance plan for its employees, rather than using a carrier; the employer assumes all payment risk, contracts with physicians, and pays for claims from a company fund.

self-pay patient A patient who does not have insurance coverage.

separate procedure Descriptor used in the Surgery Section of CPT for a procedure that is usually part of a surgical package but may also be performed separately or for a different purpose, in which case it may be reported separately.

service line information On a HIPAA claim, information about the services being reported.

skilled nursing facility (SNF) Health care facility in which licensed nurses under a physician's direction provide nursing and/or rehabilitation services.

small health plan Under HIPAA, a health plan with under $5 million in annual receivables.

SNODENT Systemized nomenclature of dentistry.

SNOMED Systemized nomenclature of medicine.

Social Security Disability Insurance (SSDI) The federal disability compensation program for salaried and hourly wage earners, self-employed people who pay a special tax, and widows, widowers, and minor children with disabilities whose deceased spouse/parent would qualify for Social Security benefits if alive.

special report A note prepared to detail the reasons for a new, variable, or unlisted procedure or service; explains the patient's condition and justifies the procedure's medical necessity.

spend-down State-based Medicaid program requiring beneficiaries to pay part of their monthly medical expenses.

sponsor The uniformed service member in a family qualified for TRICARE or CHAMPVA.

staff model HMO A type of HMO in which member providers are employees of the organization and provide services for only HMO-member patients.

standards of care (medical) State-specified performance measures for the delivery of health care by medical professionals.

State Children's Health Insurance Program (SCHIP) Program to offer health insurance coverage for uninsured children under Medicaid.

stop-loss provision Contractual guarantee against participating provider's financial loss due to an unusually large demand for high-cost services.

subcapitation Arrangement under which a capitated provider prepays an ancillary provider for specified medical services for plan members.

subcategory In ICD-9-CM, a four-digit code number.

subclassification In ICD-9-CM, a five-digit code number.

subpoena A order of a court for a party to appear and testify in a court of law.

subpoena *duces tecum* An order of a court directing a party to appear, to testify, and to bring specified documents or items.

subscriber The insured.

subterm A word or phrase that describes a main term in the Alphabetic Index of the ICD-9-CM.

superbill A listing of the diagnoses, procedures, and charges for a patient's visit; also called the encounter form.

supplemental insurance An insurance plan, such as Medigap, that provides benefits for services which are not normally covered by a primary plan.

supplemental report A report filed by the physician in state workers' compensation cases when a patient's medical condition or disability changes; also known as progress report.

Supplemental Security Income (SSI) A government program that helps pay living expenses for low-income older people and those who are blind or have disabilities.

supplementary term A nonessential word or phrase that helps to define a code in the ICD-9-CM; usually enclosed in parentheses or brackets.

surgical package A combination of services included in a single procedure code for some surgical procedures in CPT.

T

TPO Health care treatment, payment, and operations; under HIPAA, patients' protected health information may be shared for TPO.

Tabular List The section of the ICD-9-CM in which diagnosis codes are presented in numerical order.

taxonomy code Administrative code set under HIPAA that is used to report a physician's specialty when it affects payment.

technical component The part of the relative value associated with a procedure code that reflects the technician's work and the equipment and supplies used in performing it, as opposed to professional component.

Temporary Assistance for Needy Families (TANF) A government program that provides cash assistance for low-income families.

temporary disability A condition that keeps a person with a private disability compensation program from working at the usual job for a short time, but from which the worker is expected to recover completely and return to work.

third-party administrator (TPA) Company that provides administrative services for health plans but is not a contractual party.

third-party payer A private or governmental organization that insures or pays for health care on the behalf of beneficiaries: The insured person is the first party, the provider the second party, and the payer the third party.

trace number A number assigned to a HIPAA 270 electronic transaction sent to a health plan to inquire about patient eligibility for benefits.

transaction Under HIPAA, a structured set of data transmitted between two parties to carry out financial or administrative activities related to health care; in a medical billing program, a financial exchange that is recorded, such as a patient's copayment or deposit of funds into the provider's bank account.

traumatic injury An injury caused by a specific event or series of events within a single work day or shift.

TRICARE A government health program that serves dependents of active-duty service members, military retirees and their families, some former spouses, and survivors of deceased military members; formerly called CHAMPUS.

TRICARE Extra TRICARE'S managed care health plan that offers a network of civilian providers.

TRICARE for Life Program for beneficiaries who are both Medicare and TRICARE eligible.

TRICARE Prime The basic managed care health plan offered by TRICARE.

TRICARE Standard The fee-for-service health plan offered by TRICARE.

truncated coding Diagnoses that are not coded at the highest level of specificity available.

U

UB-92 Paper hospital claim, formerly a Medicare-required Part A (hospital) form; also known as the CMS-1450.

unbundling The incorrect billing practice of breaking a panel or package of services/procedures into component parts and reporting them separately.

uncollectible accounts Monies that cannot be collected from the practice's payers or patients and must be written off.

Uniform Hospital Discharge Data Set (UHDDS) Classification system for inpatient health data.

unlisted procedure A service that is not listed in CPT; reported with an unlisted procedure code and requires a special report when used.

unspecified An incompletely described condition which must be coded with an unspecified ICD code.

upcode Use of a procedure code that provides a higher payment than the code for the service actually provided.

urgently needed care In Medicare, a beneficiary's unexpected illness or injury requiring immediate treatment; Medicare plans pay for this service even if it is provided out of a plan's service area.

usual, customary, and reasonable (UCR) Setting fees by comparing the usual fee the provider charges for the service, the customary fee charged by most providers in the community, and what is reasonable considering the circumstances.

usual fee Fee for a service or procedure that is charged by a provider for most patients under typical circumstances.

utilization A pattern of usage for a medical service or procedure.

utilization review A payer's process to determine the appropriateness of hospital-based health care services delivered to a member of a plan.

utilization review organization (URO) An organization hired by a payer to evaluate the medical necessity of procedures before they are provided to a member of a plan.

V

V code An alphanumeric code in the ICD-9-CM that identifies factors that influence health status and encounters that are not due to illness or injury.

verification report A report created by a medical billing program to permit double-checking of basic claim content before transmission.

vocational rehabilitation Retraining program covered by workers' compensation to prepare a patient for reentry into the workforce.

W

waiting period The time period between an insured's date of enrollment and the date insurance coverage is effective.

walkout receipt A medical billing program report given to a patient that lists the diagnoses, services provided, fees, and payments received and due after an encounter.

Welfare Reform Act 1996 law that established the Temporary Assistance for Needy Families program in place of the Aid to Families with Dependent Children program and tightened Medicaid eligibility requirements.

workers' compensation insurance A state or federal plan that covers medical care and other benefits for employees who suffer accidental injury or become ill as a result of employment.

write off (N. write-off) To deduct an amount from a patient's account because of a contractual agreement to accept a payer's allowed charge or other reason.

Index

Longshoremen's and Harbor Workers'
Compensation Act
(LHWCA), 468
Lozenge (ICD-9-CM), 118

M

M (morphology) codes, 131–132
Main term
  CPT, 146
  ICD-9-CM, 112
Managed care, 11
Managed care organizations (MCOs),
    11–17, 331, 333
  Blue Cross/Blue Shield plans, 335–336
  comparison of, 17, 333
  consumer-driven health plans, 15–17,
    333–334
  growth of, 11, 13
  Medicaid coverage, 429–430
  medical billing programs, 73–74
  Medicare coverage, 377–378
  origins of, 11
  participation contracts, 337–347
    billing and reimbursement
      information, 341–347
    contract provisions, 337–347
    notice of participation, 337
  plan types, 11–17
    health maintenance organization
      (HMO), 11, 12–15, 17
    independent practice associations
      (IPAs), 14, 17, 333
    point-of-service option, 17
    preferred provider organization
      (PPO), 11, 15, 17, 333, 508
  TRICARE Extra, 447, 449
  TRICARE Prime, 447, 449
Manifestation, 114
Manual review, 298–299
Marginally uniform conversion
    factor, 227
Master patient index, 497
Maximum benefit limit
  defined, 233
  over-limit services, 233
Medi-Medi beneficiaries, 431
Mediation, 478
Medicaid, 419–435
  administration of, 19, 420
  appeals, 432
  claims processing, 433–434
    coding, 432, 433–434
    electronic transmission, 433
    fee-for-service plan, 429
    managed care, 430
    payment for services, 430–431
    submission of claims, 432
    unacceptable billing practices, 432
  coordination of benefits, 84
  covered services, 425–429
  defined, 18
  eligibility requirements
    enrollment verification,
      425–428
    federal, 420–423
    state, 423–425
  enrollment verification, 425, 426,
    427, 428
  establishment of, 420
  excluded services, 429
  fraud detection and investigation, 190,
    193–194, 318, 432
  payment for services, 430–431
  preauthorization, 429
  spend-down programs, 422, 424–425
  state programs for, 421, 423–425

third-party liability, 431
  crossover claims, 431
  payer of last resort, 431
types of plans
  fee-for-service, 429
  managed care, 429–430
write-offs, 318, 351
Medicaid Alliance for Program
    Safeguards, 432
Medicaid Fraud and Abuse Control
    Technical Advisory Group
    (TAG), 432
MediCal, 423, 431
Medical assistants, 5, 23
Medical assisting certification, 23
Medical billers. See Medical insurance
    specialists
Medical coders
  certification, 23, 122
  hospital, 514
  physician office, 122
  physician practice, 122
  strategies to avoid fraud and abuse,
    200–206
Medical coding manager, 171
Medical insurance. See also specific
    programs
  accrediting organizations, 20
  career opportunities. See Career
    opportunities
  contract, 6
  extent of coverage, 17
  payers, 17–18
    communications with, 79–80,
      84–85, 350
    government-sponsored, 18
    insurance companies, 17
    private-sector, 17
    self-insured health plans, 17, 334
  plan types, 10–18
    indemnity, 10–11
    managed care, 11–17
  policy types, 7–8
  regulation, 18–20
    federal, 19
    state, 19–20
  reimbursement, 8–10
    capitation, 8–10
    fee-for-service, 8, 9
Medical insurance specialists, 4–6, 20–27
  certification, 22–23
    Certified Coding Specialist
      (CCS), 23
    Certified Coding Specialist—
      Physician-based (CCS-P), 122
    Certified Medical Assistant
      (CMA), 23
    Certified Professional Coder (CPC;
      CPC-H), 23, 122
    Registered Health Information
      Technician (RHIT), 23
    Registered Medical Assistant
      (RMA), 23
  characteristics for success, 21
  communications skills of. See
    Communications skills
  continuing education opportunities, 23
  described, 7, 22
  diagnosis codes and, 109–110
  education, 22–23
  information technology and. See
    Information technology (IT)
  medical ethics and etiquette, 25–27
  obtaining a position, 23–25
  procedure codes and, 144
  professional organizations, 23

requests for information, 48–49
roles and responsibilities, 22
strategies to avoid fraud and abuse,
    200–206
Medical necessity denial, 206, 299, 389
Medical necessity reduction, 299
Medical necessity review, 92–93, 196, 299
  coding errors relating to, 199–200
  Medicare, 368–369
  postpayment audit, 309–310
Medical professional liability, 41–42
Medical Provider Analysis and Review
    (MedPar), 509–510
Medical records, 40–47. See also Patient
    information; Protected health
    information (PHI)
  confidentiality of, 50–57
  contents of, 43
  defined, 40
  disability compensation and, 478,
    481–482
  documentation standards, 41–47
    discharge summaries, 46–47
    medical record formats, 40–41
    medical standards of care, 41
    patient encounters, 43–47
    patient examinations, 44–45, 160
    progress reports, 45–46
    termination of provider-patient
      relationship, 47
  electronic, 40–41, 319
  formats
    problem-oriented medical record
      (POMR) format, 44
    SOAP format, 44
  during hospitalization, 498–499
  paper-based, 40–41
Medical review program, 297, 391, 393
Medical Review Unit (MRU), 393
Medical secretaries, 5
Medical standards of care, 41
Medically needy persons, 423
Medicare, 364–394
  administration of, 19, 365
  appeals, 305, 308–309, 389–390
  audits, 193–195, 197, 391–392,
    509–515
  comprehensive medical review,
    391, 393
  types, 391
  CHAMPVA for Life, 457
  claim preparation and processing,
    252–270, 382–389
  claims process, 365
  clearinghouses, 385
  CMS-1500, 91, 267–270
  CMS-1500 form locators, 268–269,
    387–388
  electronic billing, 383–386, 389
  electronic transmission,
    383–386, 389
  exclusions, 368–369, 370, 371
  fiscal intermediaries, 365
  global surgical package, 384–385
  HCPCS codes required for,
    144–145, 174–177, 383
  hospitalization, 498–500, 502
  ICD-9 codes required for, 109–110
  incident-to billing, 385
  Local Coverage Determinations
    (LCDs), 383, 389
  Medicare as secondary payer,
    382–383, 389, 499–500
  Medicare Remittance Notice
    (MRN), 389
  MSP claims, 389, 499–500